Essentials of
HEMATOLOGY

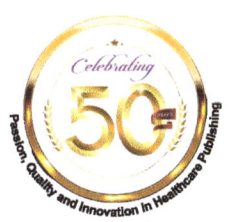

Essentials of
HEMATOLOGY

Third Edition

Shirish M Kawthalkar MD (Pathology)
Associate Professor
Department of Pathology
Government Medical College
Nagpur, Maharashtra, India

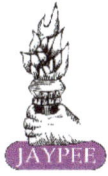

JAYPEE BROTHERS MEDICAL PUBLISHERS
The Health Sciences Publisher
New Delhi | London

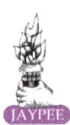 **Jaypee Brothers Medical Publishers (P) Ltd**

Headquarters
Jaypee Brothers Medical Publishers (P) Ltd
4838/24, Ansari Road, Daryaganj
New Delhi 110 002, India
Phone: +91-11-43574357
Fax: +91-11-43574314
Email: jaypee@jaypeebrothers.com

Overseas Offices
J.P. Medical Ltd
83 Victoria Street, London
SW1H 0HW (UK)
Phone: +44 20 3170 8910
Fax: +44 (0)20 3008 6180
Email: info@jpmedpub.com

Website: www.jaypeebrothers.com
Website: www.jaypeedigital.com

© 2020, Jaypee Brothers Medical Publishers

The views and opinions expressed in this book are solely those of the original contributor(s)/author(s) and do not necessarily represent those of editor(s) of the book.

All rights reserved. No part of this publication may be reproduced, stored or transmitted in any form or by any means, electronic, mechanical, photocopying, recording or otherwise, without the prior permission in writing of the publishers.

All brand names and product names used in this book are trade names, service marks, trademarks or registered trademarks of their respective owners. The publisher is not associated with any product or vendor mentioned in this book.

Medical knowledge and practice change constantly. This book is designed to provide accurate, authoritative information about the subject matter in question. However, readers are advised to check the most current information available on procedures included and check information from the manufacturer of each product to be administered, to verify the recommended dose, formula, method and duration of administration, adverse effects and contraindications. It is the responsibility of the practitioner to take all appropriate safety precautions. Neither the publisher nor the author(s)/editor(s) assume any liability for any injury and/or damage to persons or property arising from or related to use of material in this book.

This book is sold on the understanding that the publisher is not engaged in providing professional medical services. If such advice or services are required, the services of a competent medical professional should be sought.

Every effort has been made where necessary to contact holders of copyright to obtain permission to reproduce copyright material. If any have been inadvertently overlooked, the publisher will be pleased to make the necessary arrangements at the first opportunity. The **CD/DVD-ROM** (if any) provided in the sealed envelope with this book is complimentary and free of cost. **Not meant for sale.**

Inquiries for bulk sales may be solicited at: jaypee@jaypeebrothers.com

Essentials of Hematology

First Edition: 2006

Second Edition: 2013

Third Edition: **2020**

ISBN 978-93-89188-02-8

Preface to the Third Edition

Modern hematology is a complex, diverse, and constantly changing field in medical science. Due to rapid technological advances especially in molecular genetic testing, blood disorders are now being more precisely defined, rapid sophisticated diagnostic tools are becoming available and newer effective modes of therapy are being introduced.

The third edition remains connected to the previous two editions in being concise, well-illustrated, and conceptual. In the third edition, additionally, recent advances have been incorporated where required. This edition uses the classification, nomenclature, and diagnostic approach to malignant hematologic diseases as per the recently updated revised *World Health Organization Classification of Tumors of Hematopoietic and Lymphoid Tissues* published in 2017.

The scope of the book encompasses students of MBBS, postgraduates in pathology and medicine, and students of medical laboratory technology.

I am grateful to my parents who encouraged my individuality and desire for learning and writing. I am thankful to my wife Dr Anjali, for her perpetual belief and unstinted support of my academic and professional goals, and to my sons Dr Ameya and Dr Ashish, who energized my life and provided their valuable feedback from student's perspective.

I thank Dr Sajal Mitra, Dean, Government Medical College, Nagpur, Maharashtra, India and Dr WK Raut, Professor and Head, Department of Pathology, for their encouragement and support.

I thank Shri Jitendar P Vij (Group Chairman), Mr Ankit Vij (Managing Director) and Mr MS Mani (Group President) of M/s Jaypee Brothers Medical Publishers (P) Ltd, New Delhi, India, and their team, for invaluable assistance during all phases of the development of this book.

Shirish M Kawthalkar

Preface to the First Edition

This book is an attempt to present hematology and blood transfusion in a concise and simplified manner and is primarily intended for undergraduate students (second and final year MBBS and BDS). At the same time, it will also be useful for postgraduate students of pathology, medicine, pediatrics, and obstetrics and gynecology. One comes across a hematological problem frequently in all branches of medicine. Hematology and blood transfusion are closely related, and blood bank forms an integral and life-saving support system of a multidisciplinary hospital. A concise textbook of hematology and blood transfusion is needed for undergraduates who have to take on major subjects during their MBBS years. The coverage of hematology in available books is either too extensive or too short for their requirements. I have tried to strike a balance based on my experience in teaching and in diagnostic hematology.

This book was published in 1998 as *Essentials of Hematology and Blood Transfusion.* Changes are constantly occurring in hematology especially in molecular diagnostics, classification, and treatment of malignant disorders. I have tried to update each chapter to ensure that current knowledge and practices are reflected. Laboratory investigations play a major role in proper diagnosis and management of blood diseases. Therefore, laboratory aspects have been given relatively more coverage. As the scope of this book is limited, it has not been possible to give treatment of blood disorders in detail, especially dosages and drug schedules.

During preparation of this book help has been taken from various well-known textbooks and numerous journals that have been duly acknowledged at the end of each chapter. Figures of blood and bone marrow cells have been presented in a manner that highlights the important morphological details and helps in better understanding. Undoubtedly, there will be errors of omission and commission for which I take the full responsibility. Suggestions and constructive criticism are most welcome.

I am indebted to my parents for their constant support, value-based guidance, and blessings that I have received throughout my life. The friendship, love, care, and support of my wife Anjali, herself a gynecologist, can never be adequately acknowledged and my children Ameya and Ashish, have made everything in life meaningful, worthwhile, and enjoyable.

I am thankful to Dr (Mrs) VS Dani, Dean, Government Medical College, Nagpur, Maharashtra, India and Dr SK Bobhate, Professor and Head, Department of Pathology, Government Medical College, Nagpur, for their valuable guidance. I express my appreciation and gratitude to M/s Jaypee Brothers Medical Publishers (P) Ltd, New Delhi, India for their sensible and valuable advice during publication of this book and also for bringing out the book in an excellent, easy-to-read format.

Shirish M Kawthalkar

Contents

SECTION 1: PHYSIOLOGY OF BLOOD

1. **Overview of Physiology of Blood**   3
   - Normal Hematopoiesis   3
   - Red Blood Cells   9
   - White Blood Cells   18
   - Immune System   33
   - Megakaryopoiesis   38
   - Normal Hemostasis   39

SECTION 2: DISORDERS OF RED BLOOD CELLS (ANEMIAS)

2. **Approach to Diagnosis of Anemias**   61
   - Approach to Diagnosis   62
   - Classification of Anemia   73
3. **Anemias due to Impaired Red Cell Production**   81

   Iron Deficiency Anemia   81
   - Normal Iron Metabolism   81
   - Causes of Iron Deficiency Anemia   85
   - Clinical Features   86
   - Laboratory Features   87
   - Differential Diagnosis   91
   - Treatment of Iron Deficiency Anemia   92

   Megaloblastic Anemias   93
   - Normal Vitamin B_{12} Metabolism   93
   - Normal Folate Metabolism   96
   - General Morphological Features of Megaloblastic Anemia   97
   - Causes of Megaloblastic Anemia   100

   Aplastic Anemia and Related Disorders   109
   - Acquired Aplastic Anemia   109
   - Constitutional Aplastic Anemia   118
   - Pure Red Cell Aplasia   119

Anemia of Chronic Disorders 119
- Pathogenesis 120
- Clinical Features 121
- Laboratory Features 121
- Differential Diagnosis 122
- Treatment 122

Sideroblastic Anemia 122
- Sideroblasts 122
- Types and Causes 123
- Pathogenesis 124

Anemia of Chronic Renal Failure 125
- Pathogenesis 125
- Clinical and Laboratory Features 126
- Treatment 126

Anemia of Liver Disease 127

Myelophthisic Anemia 127

Congenital Dyserythropoietic Anemias 128
- CDA Type I 129
- CDA Type II 130
- CDA Type III 130

4. Anemias due to Excessive Red Cell Destruction 133

Disorders of Red Cell Membrane 133

Hereditary Spherocytosis 134
- Etiopathogenesis 134
- Inheritance 135
- Clinical Features 135
- Laboratory Features 136
- Diagnosis of Hereditary Spherocytosis 140
- Differential Diagnosis 140
- Treatment 140

Hereditary Disorders of Hemoglobin 140
- General Features and Approach to Diagnosis 140
- The Thalassemias 152
- Sickle-Cell Disorders 181

Disorders of Red Cell Enzymes 194
- Glucose-6-Phosphate Dehydrogenase Deficiency 194

Immune Hemolytic Anemias 200
- Classification 200
- Autoimmune Hemolytic Anemias due to Warm-reacting Autoantibodies 201
- Autoimmune Hemolytic Anemias due to Cold-reacting Autoantibodies 205
- Drug-induced Immune Hemolytic Anemias 208

Hemolytic Disease of the Fetus and Newborn 210
- Rh Hemolytic Disease of the Fetus and Newborn 211
- ABO Hemolytic Disease of Newborn 218

Paroxysmal Nocturnal Hemoglobinuria 219
- Pathogenesis 220
- Clinical Features 222
- Laboratory Features 223
- Treatment 226
- Prognosis 226

Mechanical Hemolytic Anemias 226
- Microangiopathic Hemolytic Anemia 227
- March Hemoglobinuria 228
- Cardiac Hemolytic Anemia 228

Hemolytic Anemia due to Direct Action of Physical, Chemical, or Infectious Agents 228
- Physical Agents 228
- Chemical Agents 228
- Infectious Agents 228

Hypersplenism 229
- Normal Structure and Function of Spleen 229
- Causes of Splenomegaly 230
- Diagnostic Criteria 230

SECTION 3: DISORDERS OF WHITE BLOOD CELLS

5. **Acute Leukemias** 235
   - Diagnosis and Classification 235
   - Predisposing Factors 235
   - Mechanisms of Oncogenesis in Acute Leukemias 236
   - Classification of Acute Leukemias 240
   - Clinical Features of Acute Leukemias 244
   - Diagnosis of Acute Leukemias 244
   - Acute Lymphoblastic Leukemia 258
   - Acute Myeloid Leukemia 271

6. **Myelodysplastic Syndromes** 287
   - Pathogenesis 287
   - Classification of Myelodysplastic Syndromes 289
   - Clinical Features 291
   - Laboratory Features 291
   - Differential Diagnosis 295
   - Prognosis 295
   - Treatment 297

7. **Myeloproliferative Neoplasms** 299
   - Clonal Origin 299
   - Chronic Myeloid Leukemia, BCR-ABL1 Positive 301
   - Polycythemia Vera 313
   - Primary Myelofibrosis 319
   - Essential Thrombocythemia 322

8. **Chronic Lymphoid Leukemias** 325
   - Chronic Lymphocytic Leukemia   325
   - Prolymphocytic Leukemia   333
   - Hairy Cell Leukemia   335

9. **Plasma Cell Dyscrasias** 341
   - Investigations in Plasma Cell Dyscrasias   341
   - Plasma Cell Myeloma (Multiple Myeloma)   350
   - Waldenström's Macroglobulinemia   363
   - Monoclonal Gammopathy of Undetermined Significance   366

10. **Malignant Lymphomas** 369
    - Hodgkin's Lymphoma   370
    - Non-Hodgkin's Lymphoma   377

11. **Quantitative and Qualitative Disorders of Leukocytes** 389
    Disorders of Granulocytes   389
    - Neutrophilia   389
    - Leukoerythroblastic Reaction   392
    - Leukemoid Reaction   392
    - Neutropenia   393
    - Eosinophilia   394
    - Basophilia   396
    - Disorders of Phagocytic Leukocytes Characterized by Morphologic Changes   396

    Disorders of Monocyte–Macrophage System   399
    - Monocytosis   399
    - Storage Disorders   400

    Lymphocytosis   403

    Plasma Cells in Peripheral Blood   404
    - Infectious Mononucleosis   404

    Immunodeficiency Diseases   407
    - Classification of Immunodeficiency Diseases   408

12. **Hematopoietic Stem Cell Transplantation** 414
    - Types of Hematopoietic Stem Cell Transplantation   414
    - Sources of Hematopoietic Stem Cells   418
    - Recent Advances in Hematopoietic Stem Cells Transplantation   419

SECTION 4: DISORDERS OF HEMOSTASIS

13. **Approach to the Diagnosis of Bleeding Disorders** 423
    - Clinical Evaluation   423
    - Laboratory Evaluation   425
    - Screening Tests   426
    - Specific Tests   433

14. **Bleeding Disorders Caused by Abnormalities of Blood Vessels (The Vascular Purpuras)** 442
    - Anaphylactoid Purpura (Henoch-Schönlein Purpura, Allergic Purpura)   442

- ❑ Infections 443
- ❑ Scurvy 443
- ❑ Senile Purpura 443
- ❑ Purpura Simplex 443
- ❑ Mechanical Purpura 443
- ❑ Hereditary Hemorrhagic Telangiectasia (Osler-Weber-Rendu Disease) 444

15. Bleeding Disorders Caused by Abnormalities of Platelets 445
- ❑ Thrombocytopenia 445
- ❑ Evaluation of a Thrombocytopenic Patient 456
- ❑ Thrombocytosis 457
- ❑ Disorders of Platelet Function 457

16. Disorders of Coagulation 462

Inherited Disorders of Coagulation 462
- ❑ Hemophilia A 462
- ❑ Von Willebrand Disease 472
- ❑ Hemophilia B 478
- ❑ Inherited Disorders of Fibrinogen 478

Acquired Disorders of Coagulation 479
- ❑ Vitamin K Deficiency 480
- ❑ Liver Disease (Cirrhosis of Liver) 481
- ❑ Disseminated Intravascular Coagulation 482
- ❑ Acquired Inhibitors of Coagulation (Circulating Anticoagulants) 486
- ❑ Heparin Therapy 489
- ❑ Oral Anticoagulants 490
- ❑ Other Acquired Coagulation Disorders 492

SECTION 5: BLOOD TRANSFUSION

17. Blood Group Systems 497
- ❑ ABO System 498
- ❑ The Rh System 500

18. Serologic and Microbiological Techniques 504
- ❑ Serologic Techniques 504
- ❑ Microbiologic Techniques 513

19. Collection of Donor Blood, Processing, and Storage 517
- ❑ Types of Blood Donors 517
- ❑ Criteria for Selection of Blood Donors 518
- ❑ Collection of Donor Blood 521
- ❑ Processing of Donor Blood 524
- ❑ Storage of Donor Blood Unit 524

20. Whole Blood, Blood Components, and Blood Derivatives 526
- ❑ Whole Blood 528
- ❑ Blood Components 529
- ❑ Blood Derivatives 534

21. Transfusion of Blood to the Recipient — 536
- Selection of Donor Blood for Whole Blood or Packed Red Cell Transfusion   536
- Selection of Donor Plasma   537
- Antibody Screening and Identification   538
- Compatibility Test   538
- Issue of Donor Blood Unit   538
- Transfusion of Blood Unit   539

22. Adverse Effects of Transfusion — 541
- Immediate Complications   542
- Delayed Complications   545
- Complications Associated with Massive Blood Transfusion   550

23. Autologous Transfusion — 551
- Predeposit Autologous Blood Transfusion   551
- Acute Normovolemic Hemodilution   552
- Blood Salvage   552

24. Alternatives to Blood Transfusion — 554
- Hematopoietic Growth Factors   554
- Red Cell Substitutes   555

APPENDICES

Appendix A: Reference Ranges   557
Appendix B: Selected Cluster of Differentiation Antigens   560
Appendix C: Critical Values in Hematology   566
Appendix D: Association of Morphology, Special Stains, and Laboratory Tests with Disease   567

Index   579

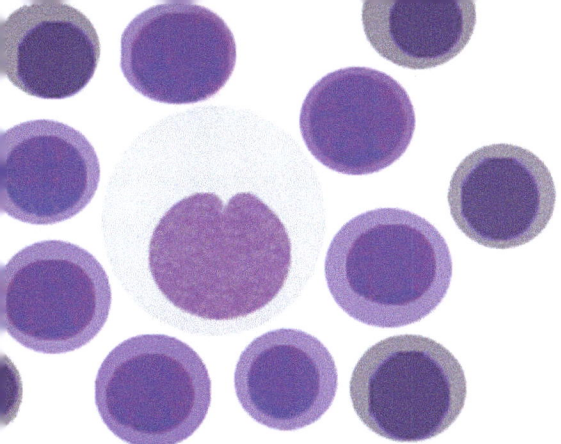

Physiology of Blood

Section Outline

1. Overview of Physiology of Blood 3

SECTION 1

CHAPTER 1

Overview of Physiology of Blood

NORMAL HEMATOPOIESIS

The physiologic process of formation of blood cells is known as hematopoiesis. It proceeds through different stages starting from early embryonic life—mesoblastic stage (yolk sac), hepatic stage, and myeloid (bone marrow) stage. *Primitive hematopoiesis* begins in the extraembryonic yolk sac during the 3rd week of embryonic life; it is transient, and mostly, nucleated erythroid cells (megaloblastic) are produced that contain embryonic hemoglobins (Gower I, Gower II, and Portland). *Definitive hematopoietic stem cells* arise subsequently intraembryonically at the site of the dorsal aorta called the aorta-gonads-mesonephros (AGM) region. These hematopoietic stem cells (HSCs) migrate to the liver, spleen, and bone marrow; and liver and spleen become the main sites of hematopoiesis from 2 to 7 months. Recent evidence indicates that hematopoietic cells and endothelium originate from common precursors called hemangioblasts. The bone marrow starts producing blood cells around 3rd to 4th month and by birth becomes an exclusive site of blood cell formation (Fig. 1.1). In younger age, whole of the skeletal marrow participates in blood cell production. By late childhood, hematopoiesis

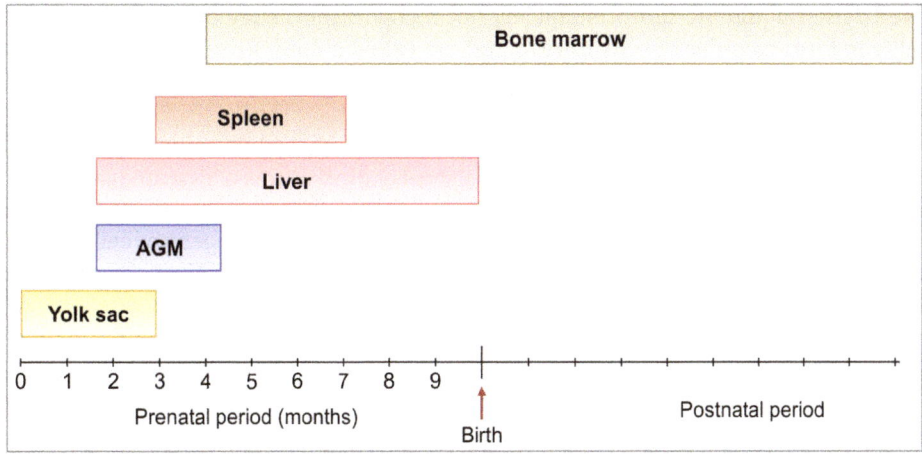

Fig. 1.1: Stages of hematopoiesis.
(AGM: aorta-gonad-mesonephros region)

becomes restricted to the flat bones, such as sternum, ribs, iliac bones, and vertebrae, and the proximal ends of long bones. At other skeletal sites, hematopoietic areas are replaced by fat cells. However, when there is increased demand for blood cell production, conversion of yellow fatty inactive marrow to red active marrow can occur. In extremely severe cases (e.g. severe chronic anemia), resumption of hematopoietic activity in organs other than bone marrow, such as liver and spleen (extramedullary hematopoiesis) can occur.

Hierarchy of Hematopoiesis (Figs. 1.2 and 1.3)

Hematopoietic precursor cells (all the cells prior to mature cells) are divided into three compartments:
- Hematopoietic stem cells
- Hematopoietic progenitor cells
- Hematopoietic maturing cells

1. **Hematopoietic stem cells (HSCs):** Hematopoietic stem cells comprise about 0.5% of total hematopoietic precursor cells. They have the ability of proliferation, differentiation along all the lineages of blood cells, and self-renewal (nondifferentiating cell division to ensure lifelong maintenance of stem cell population). Most of the HSCs at a given time are quiescent and nondividing. HSCs are morphologically nonrecognizable and resemble small lymphocytes. The currently recognized immunophenotypes of HSCs is CD34+, CD38-, Lin-, Thy-1 (CD90)+, CD49f+, c-Kit+, and HLADR-.

    HSCs can be long-term repopulating cells (LT-HSCs) and short-term repopulating cells (ST-HSCs). LT-HSCs are HSCs that are usually quiescent in a steady state and have a permanent reconstitutional ability in lethally irradiated animals.

    ST-HSCs can sustain hematopoiesis only for 8–12 weeks after HSC transplantation. Estimated number of HSCs in humans is about 2×10^4.

2. **Hematopoietic progenitor cells:** HSCs when committed to differentiation, enter into progenitor cell compartment which comprises 3% of total precursor cell population. Initially, the cells retain the capacity to generate all hematopoietic lineages (multipotential progenitor cells or MPP). With additional divisions, cells lose multilineage potential and ultimately cells with restricted unilineage potential develop. They do not have the ability of self-renewal and are morphologically not recognizable. They can be assayed by their ability to form colonies of cells in vitro and are called colony-forming units (CFUs). They are mitotically more active than HSCs and can expand the size of progenitor compartment when required.

3. **Hematopoietic maturing cells:** They comprise >95% of total precursor cells. They have morphologically recognizable nuclear and cytoplasmic features which are used to identify their lineage and stage of development.

    The factors which influence the commitment of stem cells and progenitor cells to different lineages, are unknown; the bone marrow microenvironment and responsiveness of progenitors to hematopoietic growth factors appear to play a role. There is also enhanced expression of lineage-specific genes and silencing of other alternate lineage genes by epigenetic modification of chromatin structure.

    Distinction between various hematopoietic precursor cells is based on cell marker analysis (Table 1.1).

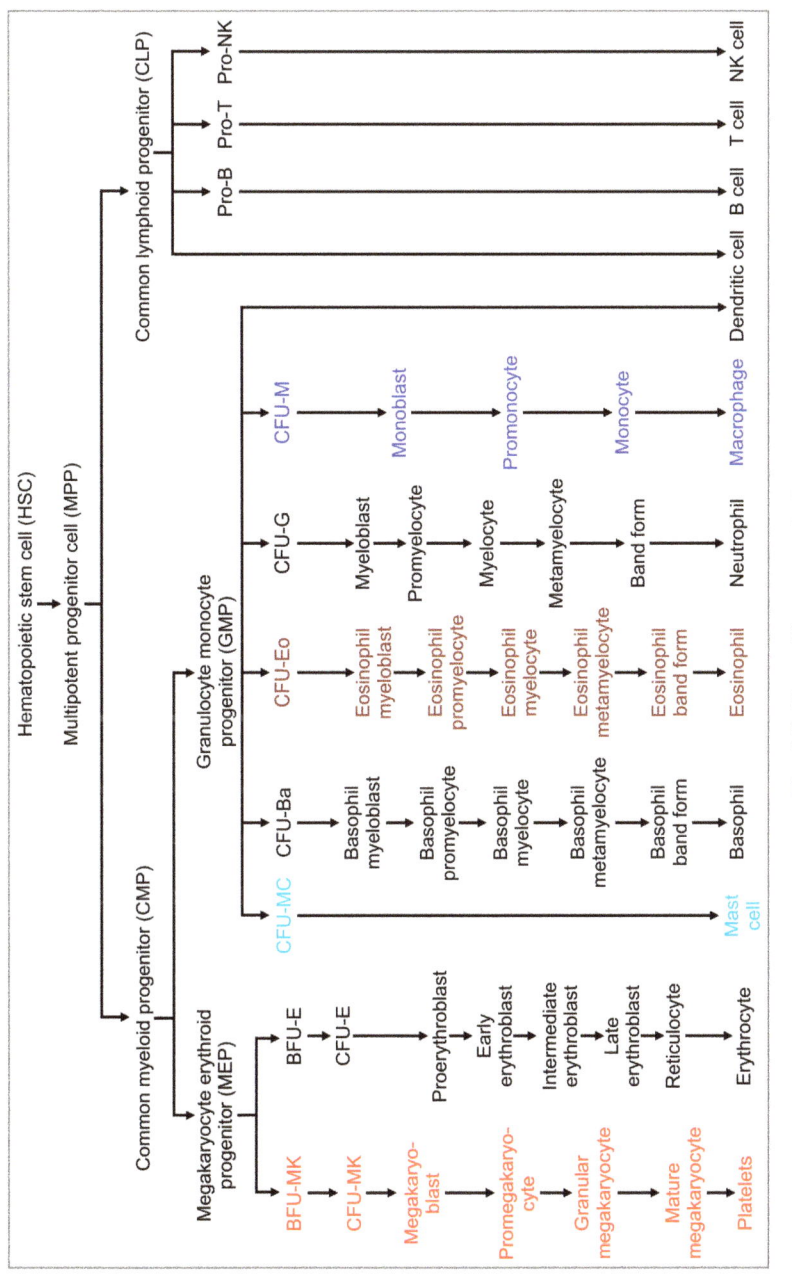

Fig. 1.2: Normal hematopoiesis.

(BFU-MK: burst-forming unit megakaryocyte; CFU-MK: colony-forming unit megakaryocyte; BFU-E: burst-forming unit erythroid; CFU-E: colony-forming unit erythroid; CFU-MC: colony-forming unit mast cell; CFU-G: colony-forming unit granulocyte; CFU-M: colony-forming unit macrophage; CFU-Eo: colony-forming unit eosinophil; CFU-Ba: colony-forming unit basophil; NK: natural killer).

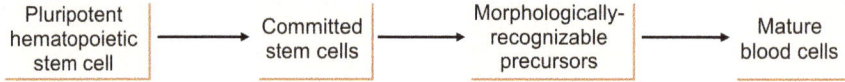

Fig. 1.3: Principal steps in hematopoiesis.

Hematopoietic Growth Factors

Hematopoietic growth factors (HGFs) are a group of proteins that (i) regulate proliferation, differentiation, and maturation of hematopoietic progenitor cells; (ii) influence the commitment of progenitors to specific lineages; and (iii) affect the function and survival of mature blood cells. HGFs are produced by different types of cells, which include T lymphocytes, macrophages, fibroblasts, endothelial cells and renal interstitial cells (Fig. 1.4 and Table 1.2).

Table 1.1: CD markers of hematopoietic precursor cells.

Cell	CD markers
Hematopoietic stem cell (HSC)	CD34+, c-Kit (CD117 or SCF-R)+, CD38-, Lin-, CD45RA-, Thy1 (CD90)+, CD49f+, CD150+, Sca-1+, CD244-, CD48-
Multipotent progenitor cell (MPP)	CD34+, c-Kit (CD117 or SCF-R)+, CD38-, Lin-, CD45RA-, Thy1 (CD90)-, CD49f-, CD150-, Sca-1+, CD244+, CD48-
Common myeloid progenitor (CMP)	CD34+, c-Kit (CD117 or SCF-R)+, Lin-, CD45RA-, Sca-1 Low, IL7R (CD127)-, FCγR Low
Common lymphoid progenitor (CLP)	CD34+, c-Kit (CD117 or SCF-R) Low, Lin-, Sca-1 low, Thy1 (CD90) Low, IL-7R (CD127)+, CD10+, CD19-, CD45RA+
Granulocyte macrophage progenitor (GMP)	CD34+, c-Kit (CD117 or SCFR)+, FCγR High+, CD33+, CD13+, Sca-1-, CD45RA+
Megakaryocyte erythroid progenitor (MEP)	CD34-, c-Kit (SCFR)+, FCγR-, CD33-, CD13-, Sca-1-

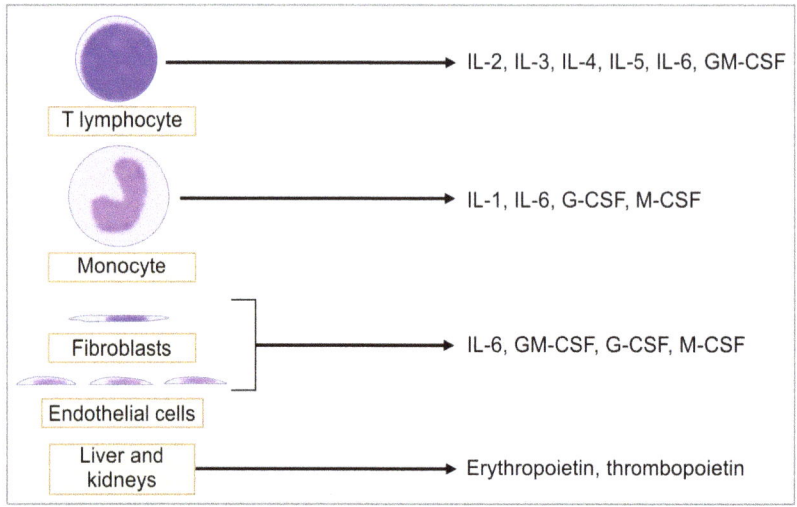

Fig. 1.4: Selected HGFs and their sources.

Chapter 1: Overview of Physiology of Blood

Table 1.2: Selected growth factors, their sources, and actions.

Growth factor	Source	Action
1. Interleukin-1 (IL-1)	Activated macrophages	Mediates synthesis and release of acute phase proteins by liver cells; synthesis of other cytokines
2. Interleukin-2 (IL-2)	T lymphocyte	Growth factor for activated T cells
3. Interleukin-3 (IL-3)	T lymphocyte	Growth factor for myeloid progenitor cells
4. Interleukin-6 (IL-6)	T lymphocytes, monocytes/macrophages, fibroblasts	Growth factor for hematopoietic progenitor cells and for B and T lymphocytes; mediates acute phase response
5. C-kit ligand (stem cell factor)	Fibroblasts, endothelial cells, stromal cells	Early hematopoietic stem cells
6. GM-CSF	T cells, stromal cells, macrophages	Multilineage growth factor for neutrophils, monocyte/macrophage, eosinophils, red cells, platelets
7. G-CSF	Monocytes/macrophages, fibroblasts	Lineage-restricted growth factor for neutrophils
8. M-CSF	Monocytes/macrophages, fibroblasts, endothelial cells	Lineage-restricted growth factor for monocytes and macrophages
9. Erythropoietin	Kidneys and liver	Lineage-restricted growth factor for erythrocytes
10. Thrombopoietin	Kidneys and liver	Lineage-restricted growth factor for platelets

HGFs may bind to specific cell receptors on the surface of the cells to directly induce their proliferation and differentiation or may stimulate the production of other cytokines that then act on the target cells.

Two types of HGFs may be distinguished—multilineage HGFs that have action on more than one cell line and lineage-restricted HGFs that act on one specific cell line. Examples of multilineage HGFs are GM-CSF (granulocyte macrophage-colony stimulating factor) and interleukin-3 (IL-3) while lineage-restricted HGFs are erythropoietin, G-CSF (granulocyte-colony stimulating factor), and M-CSF (macrophage-colony stimulating factor). For proliferation and differentiation of myeloid progenitors, either GM-GSF or IL-3 and a lineage-specific cytokine (erythropoietin, G-CSF, or M-CSF) are required.

Many of the HGFs have been produced by the recombinant DNA technology and are undergoing clinical trials in various disorders. Recently, recombinant GM-CSF, G-CSF, and erythropoietin have been approved for clinical use in certain conditions in USA.

GM-CSF (Sargramostim)

- GM-CSF stimulates proliferation, differentiation, and maturation of lineages committed to neutrophil and monocyte/macrophage cell lines (CFU-GEMM and CFU-GM) and also enhances the functional activity of mature neutrophils and monocytes.

- Recombinant GM-CSF is used to enhance the myeloid recovery following autologous bone marrow transplantation in nonmyeloid malignancies. It is also being used to increase stem cell harvest from peripheral blood in peripheral blood stem cell transplantation. It is being tried in chemotherapy-induced myelosuppression and in myelodysplastic syndrome with neutropenia.

G-CSF (Filgrastim)

- G-CSF stimulates myeloid progenitor cells (CFU-G) to form mature neutrophils.
- Recombinant G-CSF is used to reduce duration and severity of neutropenia in nonmyeloid malignancies that are being treated with myelosuppressive chemotherapy and in autologous bone marrow transplantation.

Erythropoietin (Epoetin Alfa)

- Erythropoietin is a glycoprotein produced in kidneys (90%) and in liver (10%). It stimulates progenitor cells committed to erythroid lineage (CFU-E and BFU-E) to proliferate and differentiate.
- It is indicated in patients with anemia of chronic renal failure who are on dialysis. It is also being tried in zidovudine—treated human immunodeficiency virus positive patients having anemia, and in anemia of cancer.

Thrombopoietin Receptor Agonists (Eltrombopag, Romiplostin)

- Thrombopoietin is produced constitutively in liver and binds to its receptor C-Mpl on stem cells and megakaryocytes/platelets. It is a major regulator of megakaryocyte and platelet development.
- It is indicated in patients with idiopathic (autoimmune) thrombocytopenic purpura as second- or third-line therapy after steroids and intravenous immunoglobulin, and is being tried in myelodysplastic syndrome.

The Hematopoietic Microenvironment

The existence of hematopoietic microenvironment is suggested by the fact that formation of blood cells is restricted specifically to bone marrow. The hematopoietic microenvironment is essential for development and maintenance of hematopoietic cells throughout life. The exact nature of the microenvironment is poorly understood; however, it appears to be composed of (1) cellular components: Endothelial cells, fibroblasts, osteoblasts, adipocytes, macrophages, monocytes, and T lymphocytes and (2) extracellular matrix (composed of collagen, glycoproteins, glycosaminoglycans, and adhesion molecules). Bone marrow microenvironment provides supporting stroma, growth and differentiation factors for hematopoiesis. Stem cells and progenitors are bound to the stromal cells or to adhesion molecules within the matrix. Release of mature blood cells from the marrow is regulated by the microenvironment.

Organization of bone marrow: Organization of normal bone marrow is shown in Figure 1.5.

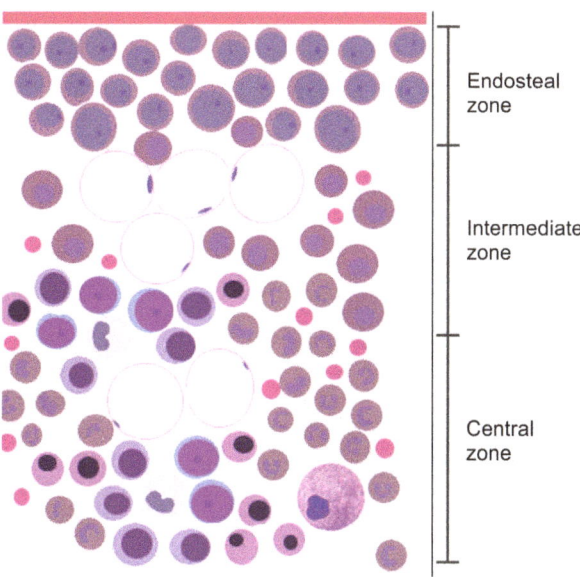

Fig. 1.5: Bone marrow organization. Bone marrow is located in the intertrabecular space beneath the cortex. Organization of various cells in the normal bone marrow is characteristic. (1) Endosteal zone: Myeloid precursors (myeloblasts, promyelocytes); (2) Intermediate zone: Myelocytes, erythroid islands; and (3) Central zone: Metamyelocytes, bands, segmented neutrophils, erythroid islands, and megakaryocytes. Megakaryocytes abut against a sinusoid.

RED BLOOD CELLS

Stages of Erythropoiesis

Within the bone marrow, erythroid cells are arranged in the form of islands (Fig. 1.6). The earliest morphologically identifiable erythroid cell in the bone marrow is the **proerythroblast** (pronormoblast), a large (15–20 µm) cell with a fine, uniform chromatin pattern, one or more nucleoli, and dark blue cytoplasm.

The next cell in the maturation process is the **basophilic (early) normoblast**. This cell is smaller in size (12–16 µm) and has a coarser nuclear chromatin with barely visible nucleoli. The cytoplasm is deeply basophilic.

The more differentiated erythroid cell is the **polychromatic (intermediate) normoblast** (size 12–15 µm). The nuclear size is smaller and the chromatin becomes clumped. Polychromasia of cytoplasm results from admixture of blue ribonucleic acid and pink hemoglobin. This is the last erythroid precursor capable of mitotic division. The orthochromatic (late) normoblast is 8–12 µm in size. The nucleus is small, dense, pyknotic and commonly eccentrically located. The cytoplasm stains mostly pink due to hemoglobinization. It is called orthochromatic because cytoplasmic staining is largely similar to that of erythrocytes. The nucleus is ultimately expelled from the orthochromatic normoblast with the formation of a reticulocyte. The reticulocyte still has remnants of ribosomal RNA in the form of a cytoplasmic reticulum. After 1–2 days in the bone marrow and 1–2 days in peripheral blood reticulocytes lose RNA and become mature pink-staining erythrocytes (Figs. 1.7 and 1.8).

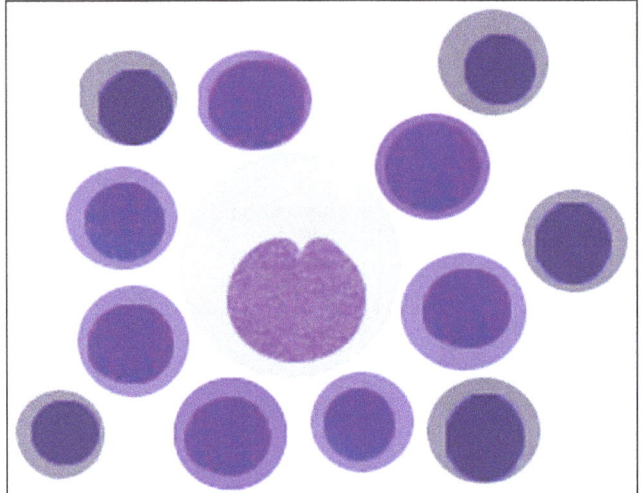

Fig. 1.6: Erythroid island: Within the bone marrow, erythroid progenitors are found in the form of 'islands' (erythroid colonies). An erythroid island is composed of erythroblasts surrounding a central macrophage. The more immature precursors are present close to the macrophage and maturing forms are towards the periphery. The macrophage has dendritic processes which extend between erythroid progenitors, support them, and supply iron for hemoglobin synthesis.

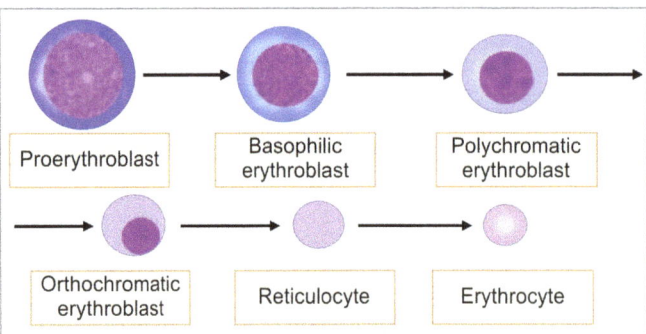

Fig. 1.7: Stages in the formation of a mature red cell. With each stage, cell size and nuclear size become smaller, chromatin clumping increases, and ultimately nucleus is extruded. Color of cytoplasm gradually changes from basophilic to orange-red.

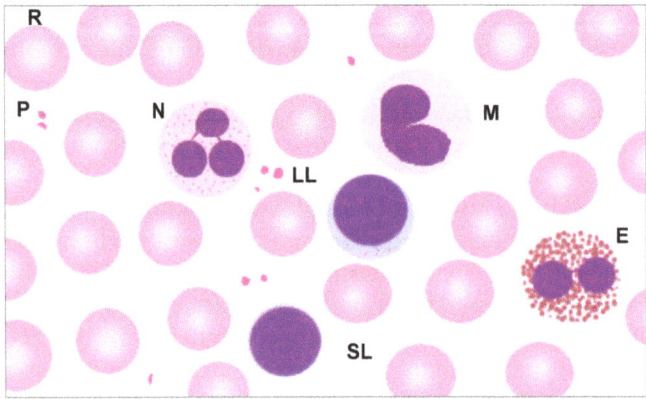

Fig. 1.8: Normal peripheral blood smear showing normocytic normochromic—red cells (R), neutrophil (N), eosinophil (E), monocyte (M), small lymphocyte (SL), large lymphocyte (LL), and platelets (P).

About four mitotic divisions and continued differentiation lead to the production of 16 mature erythrocytes from each pronormoblast.

Structure and Function of Erythrocytes

Mature erythrocyte is a round biconcave disc about 7 to 8 µm in diameter. Basic structural properties of various red cell components (hemoglobin, enzymes, and membrane) are outlined below.

Hemoglobin

Hemoglobin is responsible for transport of oxygen from lungs to the tissues and of carbon dioxide from tissues to the lungs. Hemoglobin (MW 64,500 daltons) is composed of heme (consisting of iron and protoporphyrin) and globin. The globin portion of the molecule consists of four (or two pairs of) polypeptide chains. One heme group is bound to each polypeptide chain.

Variants of hemoglobin: Hemoglobin is not homogeneous and normally different variants exist, such as A, A2, F, Gower I, Gower II, and Portland (Box 1.1). The last three are present only during embryonic life. Others are present in varying proportions during fetal and adult life. The relative proportions of different hemoglobins are: Adults— HbA 97%, HbA2 2.5%, and HbF 0.5%; Newborns— HbF 80% and HbA 20%.

> **Box 1.1:** Normal hemoglobin variants.
> - Hb Gower I: $\zeta_2\epsilon_2$
> - Hb Gower II: $\alpha_2\epsilon_2$
> - Hb Portland: $\zeta_2\gamma_2$
>   The above three hemoglobins are embryonic hemoglobins.
> - HbF: $\alpha_2\gamma_2$: Predominates in fetal life
> - HbA: $\alpha_2\beta_2$: Predominates in adult life
> - HbA2: $\alpha_2\delta_2$

Hemoglobin A (HbA), the principle hemoglobin of adults, consists of a pair each of alpha (α) and of beta (β) polypeptide chains and its structure is designated as $\alpha_2\beta_2$. Fetal hemoglobin (HbF), the predominant hemoglobin in fetal life contains a pair of alpha (α) and a pair of gamma (γ) chains. Two types of γ chains are distinguished, Gγ and Aγ, which have different amino acids (either glycine or alanine) at position 136. Thus, HbF is heterogeneous and contains $\alpha_2\gamma_2$ 136Gly and $\alpha_2\gamma_2$ 136Ala. During embryonic life, there are three hemoglobins: Gower I ($\zeta_2\epsilon_2$), Gower II ($\alpha_2\epsilon_2$), and Portland ($\zeta_2\gamma_2$). With fetal development, synthesis of zeta (ζ) and epsilon (ϵ) chains is replaced by that of α and γ chains, respectively. After birth, production of γ chains switches to that of β and delta (δ) chains.

Structure of globin genes: Normal hemoglobin is a tetramer composed of a pair of α-like and a pair of β-like polypeptide chains. Each chain is linked to one molecule of heme. The α-like polypeptide chains (ζ and α) and β-like polypeptide chains (ϵ, γ, β, and δ) are encoded by α- *and* β-*globin* gene clusters on chromosomes 16 and 11, respectively. The order of genes in α-*globin* gene cluster from 5' to 3' end is ζ-$\psi\zeta$-$\psi\alpha2$-$\psi\alpha1$-$\alpha2$-$\alpha1$. The order of genes in β-globin gene cluster from 5' to 3'end is $\psi\beta2$-ϵ-Gγ-Aγ-$\psi\beta1$-δ-β (Fig. 1.9).

The $\psi\zeta$, $\psi\alpha2$, $\psi\alpha1$, and $\psi\beta$ are pseudogenes. A pseudogene (ψ) contains sequences similar to a functional gene but is rendered inactive due to mutation during evolutionary process. In humans, autosomal chromosomes occur in pairs. As each member of chromosome 16 has two α gene loci (a locus refers to specific physical position of a gene on chromosome), there are total four α genes. However, there is only one β-globin gene locus on chromosome 11, and therefore *β genes* are two in number.

Genes are the base sequences which are present along the DNA strands and are necessary for the formation of a protein. The different functional areas of a globin gene are:
1. Exons and introns: The regions of DNA strand which encode amino acids in the protein product are known as exons, while noncoding regions which interrupt the coding sequences

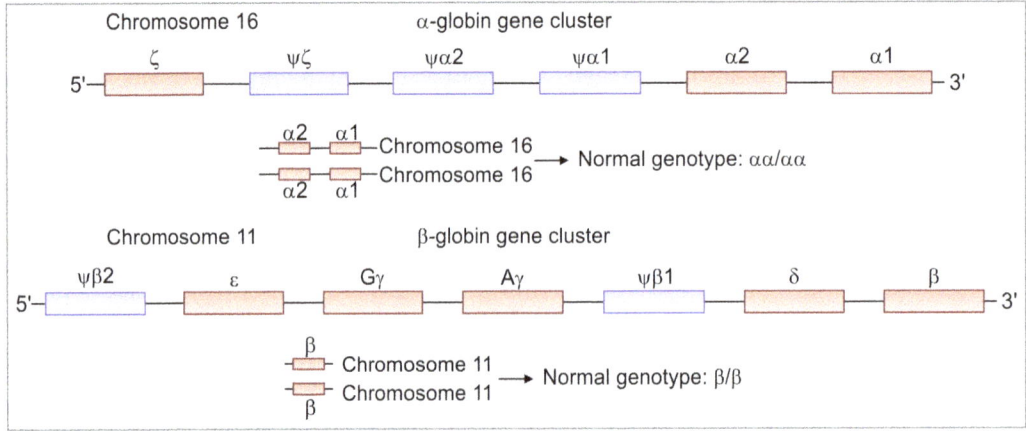

Fig. 1.9: α- and β-globin gene clusters. Purple boxes represent pseudogenes while light red boxes represent active genes. Normal genotype is shown below each gene cluster.

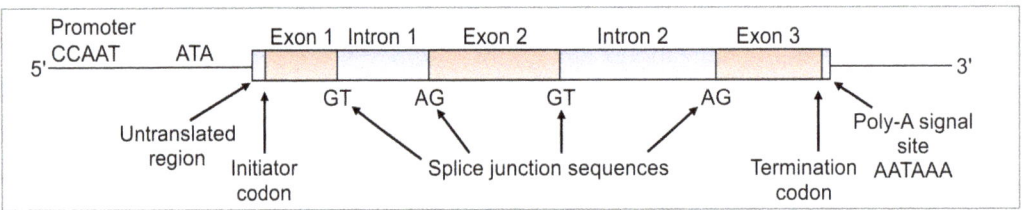

Fig. 1.10: A schematic diagram of β-globin gene.

are known as introns or intervening sequences. Each globin gene contains three exons and two introns.
2. *Splice junction sequences*: These are sequences at the junction of exons and introns and are required for precise splicing (or removal) of introns during the formation of mRNA.
3. *Promoter*: The promoter region is present toward 5' end of the gene and contains sequences to which the RNA polymerase binds; it is necessary for correct initiation of transcription. Two promoter sequences are TATA and CCAAT.
4. *Polyadenylation signal*: The 3' end of the globin gene contains the sequence AATAAA that serves as a signal for the addition of a poly-A track to the mRNA transcript (Fig. 1.10).

Steps in the synthesis of globin: Globin synthesis involves three steps—transcription, processing of mRNA, and translation (Fig. 1.11).
1. *Transcription*: Transcription involves synthesis of a single strand of RNA from DNA template by the enzyme RNA polymerase. The base sequence of RNA which is produced is complementary to the base sequence of DNA. Binding of RNA polymerase to the promoter is essential for accurate initiation of transcription. RNA polymerase slides along the DNA strand in a 5' to 3' direction and builds the RNA molecule. Transcription continues through exons and introns and when a chain terminating sequence is encountered, RNA polymerase gets separated from the DNA strand. The RNA strand thus formed is called messenger RNA (mRNA).

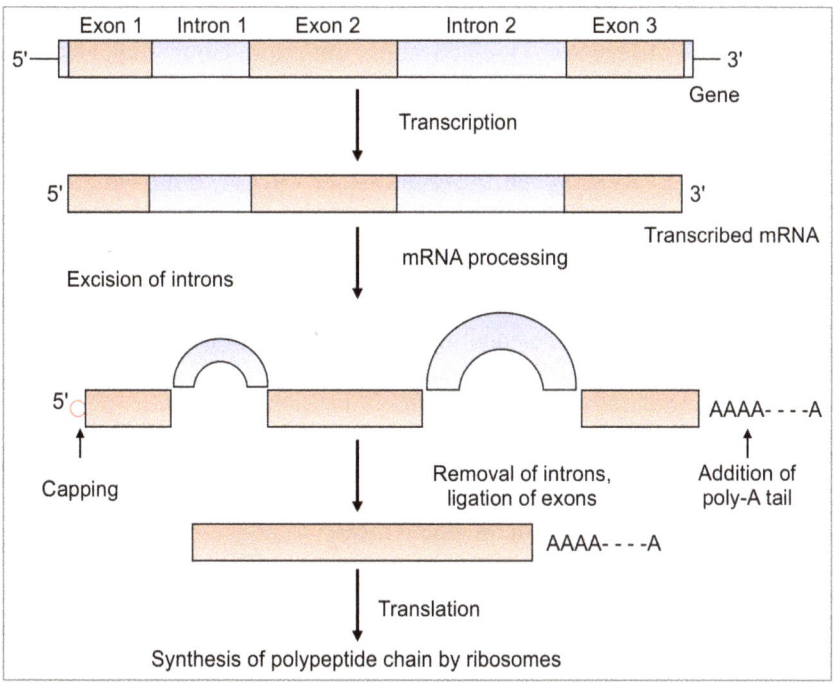

Fig. 1.11: Globin chain synthesis.

2. *Processing of mRNA*: In the next stage, mRNA molecule is processed by addition of a cap structure and a poly-A tail and by removal of introns. A cap structure (modified nucleotides) is added at the 5'end of mRNA; though the exact role is unknown, capping appears to be necessary for initiation of translation. At the 3' end a poly-A tail consisting of about 150 adenylic acid residues is added. AAUAAA sequence at the 3' end signals the addition of poly-A tail about 20 bases downstream from the polyadenylation site. Polyadenylation is required for stability of the transcript and its transport to the cytoplasm.

   Excision of introns and joining together of exons in the mRNA transcript are essential before mRNA is transported from the nucleus to the cytoplasm. Accurate splicing is guided by the presence of GT dinucleotide at the exon-intron boundary (5' end of intron) and AG dinucleotide at the intron-exon boundary (3' end of intron). Intron 1 is excised before intron 2. During splicing, excision at 5'exon-intron boundary occurs initially with the formation of 'lariat' structures; subsequently excision at the 3' intron-exon boundary occurs followed by joining of exons.

3. *Translation*: This process which occurs on ribosomes consists of synthesis of a polypeptide chain according to the directions provided by the mRNA template. There are three kinds of RNA which take part in the synthesis of polypeptides—messenger RNA (mRNA), transfer RNA (tRNA), and ribosomal RNA (rRNA). The mRNA, transcribed from the DNA template, carries the genetic code from the nucleus to the cytoplasm and determines the sequence of amino acids in the formation of a polypeptide. The tRNA transports specific amino acids from the cytoplasm to the specific locations (codons) along the mRNA strand; each tRNA binds and transports a specific amino acid. The rRNA along with certain structural proteins

constitutes the ribosome which serves as a site for protein synthesis. The different steps of protein synthesis (translation) are activation, initiation, elongation, and termination. In activation, an amino acid combines with its specific tRNA molecule in the cytoplasm; such tRNA is called activated or charged tRNA. Translation always begins at a codon that specifies methionine (AUG, the initiator codon). The process of translation is initiated when a methionine-bearing specific tRNA binds with initiator codon in mRNA. Elongation of polypeptide chain occurs when successive amino acids are added after methionine according to the pattern provided by the genetic code. During this process, movement of ribosomes occurs along the mRNA strand and ribosome slides to the next codon when an amino acid specified by preceding codon is added to the growing polypeptide chain. Amino acids are attached to each other by peptide bonds. Termination of translation occurs when a chain-terminating (or a stop) codon is encountered (UAA, UAG, or UGA). This is followed by release of the completed polypeptide chain from the ribosomes.

The primary polypeptide chain is then organized into a secondary and a tertiary structure from interactions in its amino acids. One molecule of heme is attached to each polypeptide chain. Two different pairs of polypeptide chains with their attached heme moieties associate with each other to form a tetrameric hemoglobin molecule.

Changes in globin gene expression during development (Globin "switching"): Hb Gower I, Hb Gower II, and Hb Portland are the predominant hemoglobins during embryonic life (up to 12 weeks). HbF ($\alpha 2 \gamma 2$) is the major hemoglobin of fetal life; it starts gradually declining after 36 weeks of gestation and constitutes less than 1% of hemoglobin in adults. Beta (β) chain synthesis starts around 10th week of gestation and is significantly augmented around the time of birth. HbA ($\alpha 2 \beta 2$) gradually becomes the predominant hemoglobin by 3-4 months of age. Delta (δ) globin gene is expressed late in the third trimester but HbA2 ($\alpha 2 \delta 2$) remains at a low level (about 2.5%) in adults.

The developmental changes in the expression of the globin genes can be correlated with the time of appearance of clinical features in hemoglobinopathies. Thus, α-thalassemia manifests at birth while clinical features of β-thalassemia appear a few months after birth.

Biosynthesis of heme: Heme is a complex of protoporphyrin and iron. Biosynthesis of heme requires mitochondrial (as well as cytosolic) enzymes and therefore only erythroid precursors but not mature red cells can synthesize heme.

Structure and function of hemoglobin: Hemoglobin is a tetramer composed of four polypeptide chains ($\alpha 1$, $\alpha 2$, $\beta 1$, and $\beta 2$) and four heme groups. α chain consists of 141 amino acids, while β chain has 146 amino acids. Each polypeptide chain is arranged in a helical conformation. There are eight helical segments designated A to H. Iron of heme is covalently bound to histidine at the eighth position of the F helical segment. Charged or polar residues are arranged on the outer surface, while the uncharged or nonpolar residues are arranged towards the inner part of the molecule. Heme is suspended in a "pocket" formed by the folding of the polypeptide chain and residues in contact with heme are nonpolar. The four polypeptide chains make contact at $\alpha 1 \beta 1$ and $\alpha 1 \beta 2$ interfaces. The former is a stabilizing contact, while the latter is the functional contact across which movement of chains occurs during oxygenation and deoxygenation.

The function of hemoglobin is transport of oxygen from the lungs to the tissues. As partial pressure of oxygen increases, hemoglobin shows progressively increasing affinity for oxygen. When first oxygen binds to the heme group, it successively increases the oxygen affinity of the remaining three heme groups. When the percent saturation of hemoglobin with oxygen is plotted against the partial pressure of oxygen, a sigmoid-shaped oxygen dissociation curve is obtained. Small changes in oxygen tension allow significant amount of oxygen to be released or bound.

Factors affecting oxygen affinity of hemoglobin are pH, temperature, intraerythrocyte level of 2,3-diphosphoglycerate or 2,3-DPG (also known as 2,3-bisphosphoglycerate or 2,3-BPG) and presence of hemoglobin variants. The Bohr effect refers to the alteration in oxygen affinity due to alteration in pH. Low pH (e.g. in tissues) reduces the oxygen affinity while higher pH (e.g. in lungs) increases the oxygen affinity of hemoglobin. High temperature reduces the oxygen affinity while low temperature increases the oxygen affinity. 2,3-DPG binds to deoxyhemoglobin with considerably more affinity than to oxyhemoglobin and stabilizes the deoxyhemoglobin state. Low levels of 2,3-DPG in red cells in stored blood in blood bank are associated with reduced release of oxygen after blood transfusion. Hemoglobin variants with high oxygen affinity are methemoglobin, Hb Bart's, and HbH.

Red Cell Enzymes

The mature red cell requires energy to preserve the integrity of the cell membrane, for active transport of cations, for nucleotide salvage, and for synthesis of glutathione. This is mostly provided by glycolysis (Embden–Meyerhof pathway). In this metabolic pathway, glucose is converted to pyruvate and lactate through a series of enzymatic reactions with generation of ATP (Fig. 1.12). Catabolism of 1 mole of glucose leads to net generation of 2 moles of ATP. ATP is required for active cation transport and maintaining red cell deformability. In the middle of the glycolytic pathway, a Rapoport–Luebering shunt exists in red cells for the synthesis of 2,3-DPG. When this shunt is utilized, there is no net gain of ATP since. 1,3-diphosphoglycerate is diverted to produce 2,3-DPG. 2,3-DPG is an important determinant of the oxygen affinity of hemoglobin. The activity of Rapoport–Luebering shunt is stimulated in the presence of hypoxia to improve oxygen delivery to the tissues. 2,3-DPG binds to hemoglobin and reduces its affinity for hemoglobin so that more oxygen is delivered to the tissues. Apart from ATP and 2,3-DPG, another important product of glycolysis is NADH that is required for reduction of methemoglobin to oxyhemoglobin.

The aerobic hexose monophosphate shunt (pentose phosphate shunt) is another metabolic pathway in red cells.

The two dehydrogenase enzymes, glucose-6-phosphate dehydrogenase (G6PD) and 6-phosphogluconate dehydrogenase (6-PGD), cyclically generate NADPH from NADP. These two enzymes also convert glucose-6-phosphate to pentose which is returned to the main glycolytic pathway. NADPH and the enzyme glutathione reductase are required for the regeneration of reduced glutathione (GSH) from oxidized glutathione (GSSG). GSH along with glutathione peroxidase detoxifies hydrogen peroxide and protects hemoglobin from oxidant damage.

Most of the methemoglobin produced in the normal cell is reduced to hemoglobin by NAD-linked methemoglobin reductase. Methemoglobin reductase that is linked to NADP requires methylene blue for its activation and is more effective in drug-induced methemoglobinemia (Fig. 1.12).

Various metabolic pathways in the red cell are summarized in Box 1.2.

Section 1: Physiology of Blood

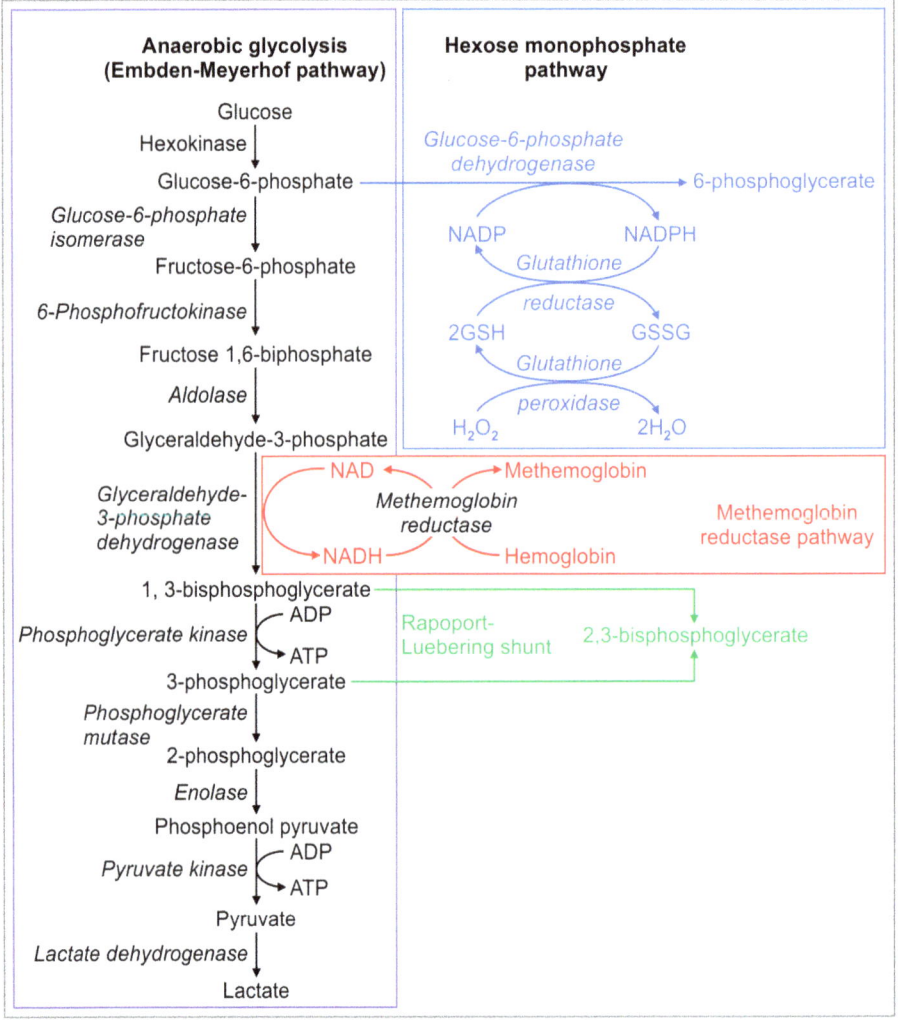

Fig. 1.12: Metabolic pathways in red cell.

Box 1.2: Metabolic pathways in the red cell.
- Embden–Meyerhof pathway (anaerobic glycolysis): Generates 90% of ATP to provide energy for reactions like maintenance of membrane integrity, regulation of the intracellular and extracellular pumps, maintenance of hemoglobin function, etc.
- Rapoport–Luebering shunt: Synthesis of 2,3-DPG, a determinant of oxygen affinity of hemoglobin
- Hexose monophosphate shunt (pentose phosphate pathway): Provides 5–10% of ATP and protects hemoglobin from oxidant damage
- Methemoglobin reductase pathway: Maintains hemoglobin iron in the ferrous state by reducing NAD to NADH and prevents accumulation of methemoglobin in red cell.

Red Cell Membrane

The red cell membrane (Fig. 1.13) is composed of lipids, a complex network of proteins, and a small amount of carbohydrates. The membrane lipids include phospholipids, cholesterol,

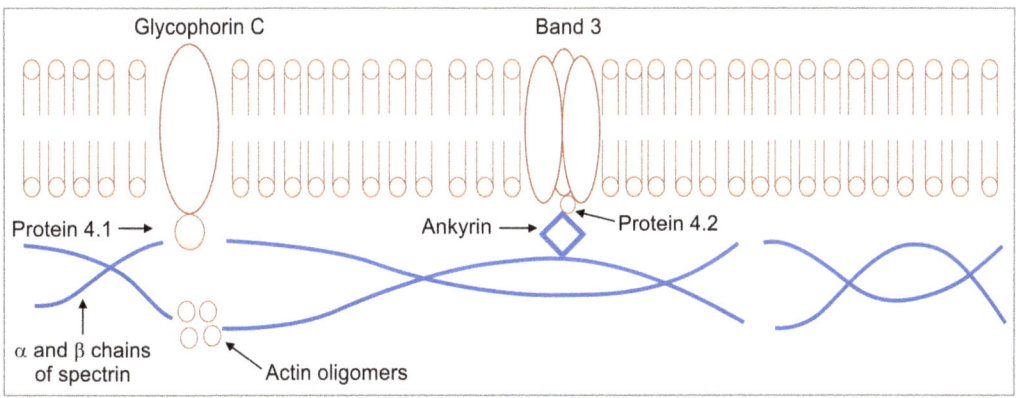

Fig. 1.13: Schematic illustration of red cell membrane.

and glycolipids. The phospholipids are arranged in the form of a bilayer. The distribution of phospholipids is asymmetrical with aminophospholipids and phosphatidyl inositols located preferentially in the inner part of the bilayer and choline phospholipids in the outer part. The polar head groups are oriented both internally and externally, while the fatty acid chains are oriented toward each other. The red cell membrane proteins are embedded within the lipid bilayer (transmembranous proteins) and also form an extensive network beneath the bilayer (submembranous proteins). The transmembranous and submembranous proteins constitute the red cell cytoskeleton. Red cell membrane proteins can be separated according to molecular size by sodium dodecyl sulfate polyacrylamide gel electrophoresis (SDS-PAGE). Different bands can be visualized when stained with a protein stain, such as Coomassie blue. The important skeletal proteins are spectrin (bands 1 and 2), ankyrin (band 2.1), anion exchange protein (band 3), protein 4.1, and actin (band 5). Spectrin is the major cytoskeletal protein; it consists of two dissimilar chains, alpha and beta which are intertwined together. The head ends of the spectrin dimers interact with those of the other spectrin dimers to form spectrin tetramers and oligomers. The tail ends of spectrin tetramers interact with actin and this association is stabilized by protein 4.1. On electron microscopy, the skeletal proteins appear to be organized in the form of a hexagonal lattice; the arms of the hexagon are formed by spectrin and corners by actin, protein 4.1, and adducin. The anchorage of the cytoskeleton to the overlying lipid bilayer is achieved by two associations: Band 3-ankyrin-spectrin association and glycophorin C-protein 4.1 association. Band 3 is the anion exchange channel through which the exchange of HCO_3^- and Cl^- occurs.

There are two types of red cell membrane protein and lipid interactions:
1. Vertical interactions: These are perpendicular to the plane of the membrane and stabilize the lipid bilayer. These interactions are between skeletal lattice proteins on the cytoplasmic side of the membrane and integral proteins and lipids of the membrane. Defects in vertical interactions result from defects in ankyrin, band 3, protein 4.2, α-spectrin, and β-spectrin. These defects lead to uncoupling of lipid bilayer from the underlying membrane proteins with selective loss of portions of lipids. Defect in vertical interactions result in hereditary spherocytosis.
2. Horizontal interactions: These are parallel to the plane of the membrane and are significant in formation of the supporting protein framework beneath the membrane and impart mechanical stability. Defects in horizontal interactions result from defects in protein

4.1, glycophorin C, α-spectrin, and β-spectrin. Defects in horizontal interactions cause disruption of protein lattice beneath the membrane, membrane destabilization, and fragmentation of red cells (hereditary elliptocytosis, hereditary pyropoikilocytosis).

Disorders that affect content of membrane lipid bilayer lead to the formation of acanthocytes or stomatocytes.

The membrane provides mechanical strength and flexibility to the red cell to withstand the shearing forces in circulation. The cell membrane also serves to maintain the red cell volume by the cation pump. The cation pump operated by the membrane enzyme ATPase, regulates the intracellular concentration of Na^+ and K^+. The membrane ATPase also drives the calcium pump which keeps the intracellular Ca^{++} at a very low level. The red cells exchange HCO_3^- (formed from tissue CO_2) in the lungs with Cl^- through the anion exchange channel (band 3) in the membrane.

Red cell destruction: The life span of normal erythrocytes is about 120 days. The senile red cells are recognized by macrophages of reticuloendothelial system and are destroyed mainly in the spleen. Globin is converted to amino acids which are stored to be recycled again. Degradation of heme liberates iron and porphyrin. Iron is stored as ferritin in macrophages or is released in circulation where it is taken up by transferrin and transported to erythroid precursors in bone marrow. The porphyrin is converted to bilirubin.

WHITE BLOOD CELLS

Neutrophils

Stages of Granulopoiesis

The maturation sequence in granulopoiesis is—myeloblast, promyelocyte, myelocyte, metamyelocyte, band cell, and segmented granulocyte (Fig. 1.14). This process occurs within the marrow.

Myeloblast: Myeloblast is the earliest recognizable cell in the granulocytic maturation process. It is about 15-20 µm in diameter, with a large round to oval nucleus, and small amount of basophilic cytoplasm. The nucleus contains 2-5 nucleoli and nuclear chromatin is fine and reticular.

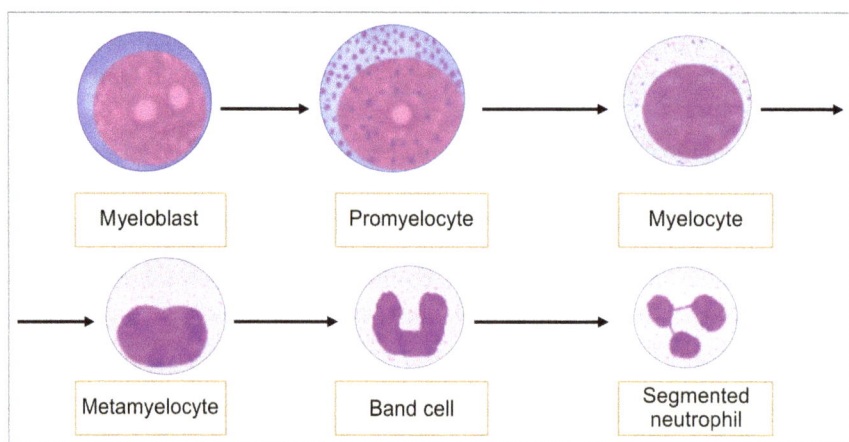

Fig. 1.14: Stages in the formation of mature neutrophils.

Promyelocyte: The next stage in the maturation is promyelocyte which is slightly larger in size than myeloblast. Primary or azurophil granules appear at the promyelocyte stage. The nucleus contains nucleoli as in myeloblast stage, but nuclear chromatin shows slight condensation.

Myelocyte: Myelocyte stage is characterized by the appearance of secondary or specific granules (neutrophilic, eosinophilic, or basophilic). Initially, specific neutrophilic granules appear only in Golgi region near the nucleus; this is sometimes called as "dawn of neutrophilia". Myelocyte is a smaller cell with round to oval eccentrically placed nucleus, more condensation of chromatin than in promyelocyte stage, and absence of nucleoli. Cytoplasm is relatively greater in amount than in promyelocyte stage and contains both primary and secondary granules as well as secretory vesicles. It is the last cell capable of cell division.

Metamyelocyte: In the metamyelocyte stage, the nucleus becomes indented and kidney shaped, and the nuclear chromatin becomes moderately coarse. Cytoplasm contains both primary and secondary granules. Tertiary granules are synthesized during this stage.

Band stage (stab form): This is characterized by band-like shape of the nucleus with constant diameter throughout and condensed nuclear chromatin.

Segmented neutrophil (polymorphonuclear neutrophil): With Leishman's stain, nucleus appears deep purple with 2-5 lobes which are joined by thin filamentous strands. Nuclear chromatin pattern is coarse. The cytoplasm stains light pink. Neutrophils with less than 3 lobes are called as hyposegmented, while those with more than 5 lobes are called as hypersegmented (Fig. 1.15).

In normal females (XX), an appendage is present attached to the neutrophil nucleus and is called as a drumstick or Barr body. It represents one inactivated X chromosome. (Random inactivation of one X chromosome in females during embryogenesis is called as lyonization). Barr bodies are observed in 2–3% of circulating neutrophils in females; they are also seen in males with Klinefelter's syndrome (XXY).

Neutrophil granules (Box 1.3): The neutrophil granules are of four types: Primary or azurophilic granules (acquired at promyelocyte stage), secondary or specific granules (acquired at

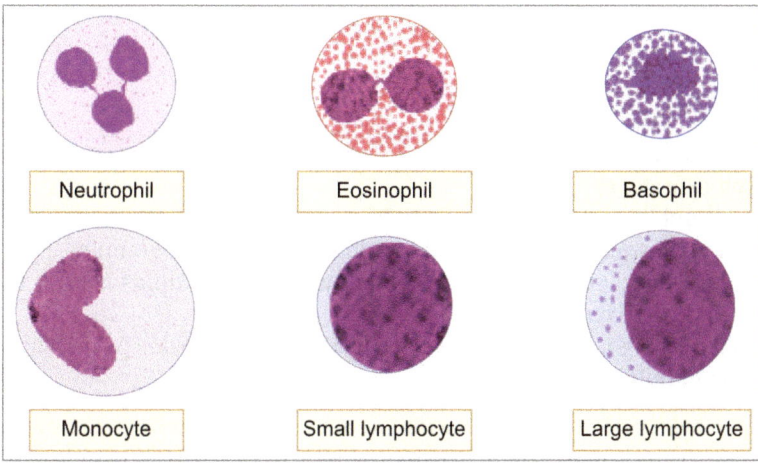

Fig. 1.15: Mature white blood cells.

Box 1.3: Neutrophil granules and their contents.

- **Primary (azurophilic) granules:**
  - Antimicrobials: Myeloperoxidase. Lysozyme, defensins, bactericidal permeability increasing protein
  - Proteases: Elastase (ELANE), cathepsin G
  - Acid hydrolases
- **Secondary (specific) granules:** Lactoferrin, collagenase, lysozyme, transcobalamin 1, plasminogen activator
- **Tertiary granules:** Gelatinase
- **Secretory vesicles:** Leukocyte alkaline phosphatase (LAP), cytochrome b_{558}, complement receptor 1 (CD35)

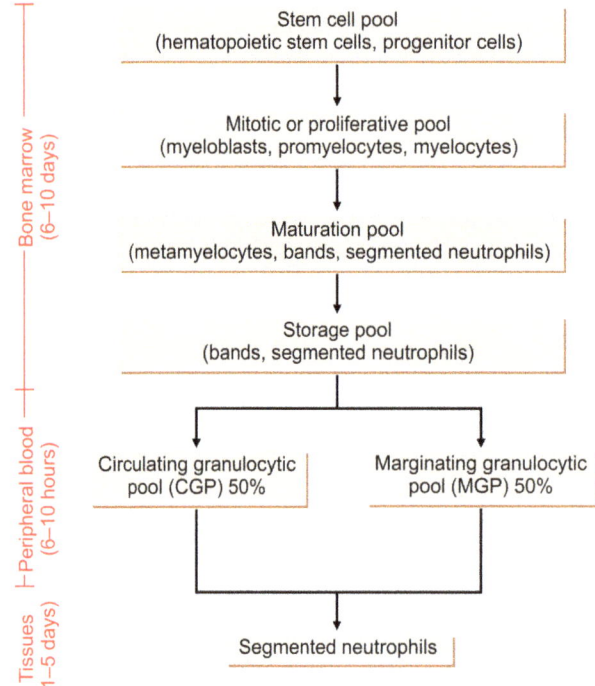

Fig. 1.16: Neutrophil kinetics. After release from the marrow, neutrophils in peripheral blood can be divided into two compartments: circulating pool (measured by leukocyte count) and marginating pool (neutrophils adhering to endothelium via adhesion molecules; this portion is not measured by leukocyte count).

myelocyte stage), tertiary granules (acquired at metamyelocyte stage), and secretory vesicles (appear at myelocyte stage).

Lipids in neutrophils and precursors include phospholipids, cholesterol, and triglycerides; they are present in plasma membrane and membranes of various granules. Lymphocytes do not contain lipids. Therefore Sudan black B stain which stains lipids is used to distinguish between myeloblasts and lymphoblasts.

Carbohydrate (glycogen) present in neutrophils precursors stains positively with periodic acid Schiff stain (granular positivity).

Function of neutrophils: After their formation, neutrophils remain in marrow for 5 more days as a reserve pool. Neutrophils have a life span of only 6-10 hours in circulation. Neutrophil compartments and kinetics are shown in Figure 1.16.

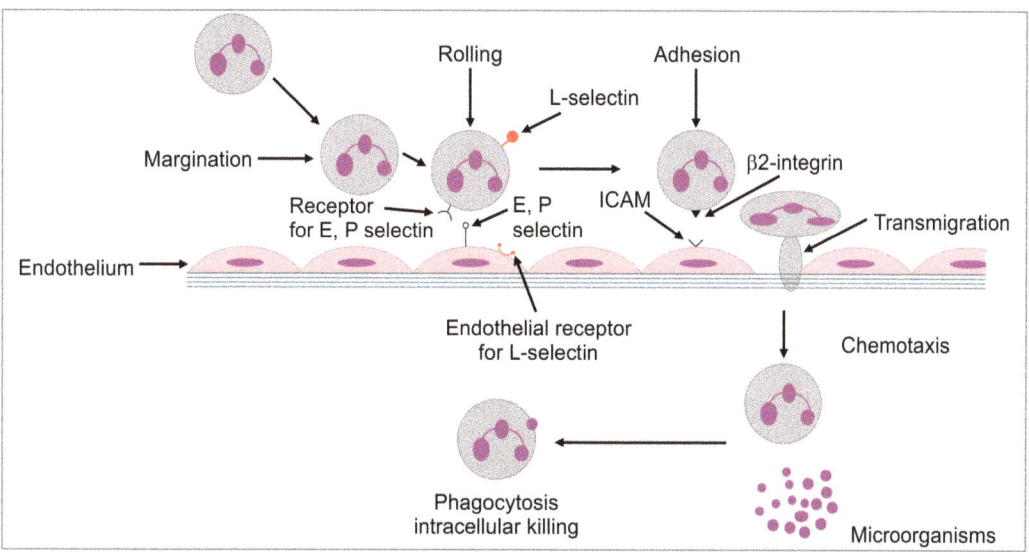

Fig. 1.17: Neutrophil adhesion and migration. The sequence of neutrophil 'events' in acute inflammation is: margination, rolling, adhesion (sticking), transmigration or emigration, chemotaxis, accumulation of neutrophils at the site of injury, and phagocytosis. The movement of leukocytes which are normally moving in the center of the blood vessel towards the periphery of the blood vessel is called as margination. During rolling, neutrophils attach weakly and transiently to endothelium of venules, then detach, and bind again. This is mediated by expression of selectin adhesion molecules on the surface of neutrophils (L-selectin) and endothelial cells (E- and P-selectins). Adhesion results from interaction of integrin adhesion molecules on neutrophils (CD11b/CD18 or β2-integrins) with their ligands (ICAM) on endothelial cells. Following adhesion, the leukocytes insert pseudopods into the junctions between the endothelial cells and squeeze through the interendothelial junction. They eventually traverse the basement membrane by dissolving it through release of type IV collagenase and escape into the interstitium. The molecules required for transmigration or diapedesis of leukocytes are platelet endothelial cell adhesion molecules (PECAM-1 or CD31) expressed by endothelial cells and leukocytes.

In response to infection and inflammation, neutrophils come to lie closer to endothelium (margination) and adhere to endothelial surface (sticking) (Fig. 1.17). This is followed by escape of neutrophils from blood vessels to extravascular tissue (emigration). The escape of neutrophils is guided by chemotactic factors present in the inflammatory zone. Chemotactic factors for neutrophils include bacterial factors, complement components, such as C3a and C5a, breakdown products of neutrophils, fibrin fragments, and leukotriene B4. Phagocytosis follows which involves three steps—antigen recognition, engulfment, and killing of organism. Neutrophils have receptors for Fc portion of immunoglobulins and for complement. Many organisms are identified by neutrophils after they are coated with opsonins (IgG1, IgG3, and C3b). Cytoplasm of the neutrophil extends in the form of pseudopods around the microorganism, and the organism is eventually completely enclosed within the membrane-bound vacuole (phagosome). Lysosomal granules fuse with phagosome and discharge their contents into the phagolysosome. The last step in phagocytosis is killing of microorganism which may be either oxygen-dependent or oxygen-independent. Oxygen-dependent mechanism involves conversion of oxygen to hydrogen peroxide by oxidase in phagolysosome; myeloperoxidase in the presence of halide ion (e.g. Cl^-) converts hydrogen peroxide to HOCl that has a strong bactericidal activity.

Another oxygen-dependent bactericidal mechanism is independent of myeloperoxidase and involves formation of superoxide radicals, hydroxyl radicals, and singlet oxygen. Oxygen-independent bactericidal mechanism occurs in lysosomal granules and is mediated by substances like lysozyme, major basic protein, bactericidal permeability increasing protein, lactoferrin, defensins, hydrolases, and acid pH of phagosomes.

Eosinophils

Eosinophil forms via the same stage as the neutrophil and the specific granules first become evident at the myelocyte stage. The major cytokine required for production and differentiation of eosinophils is interleukin-5. The size of the eosinophil is slightly larger than that of neutrophil. The nucleus is often bilobed and the cytoplasm contains numerous large, bright orange-red granules. Eosinophils contain three main types of granules: Primary, secondary (specific), and small. Primary granules contain Charcot-Leyden crystal (CLC) protein (also called galectin-10), which has lysophospholipase activity. CLC protein is released in large amounts in body fluids, secretions, and tissues in eosinophilic inflammatory conditions, resulting in formation of needle-shaped crystals. Exact role of CLC protein is unclear. Secondary or specific granules contain major basic protein (MBP), eosinophil cationic protein (ECP), eosinophil peroxidase (EPO), and eosinophil-derived neurotoxin (EDN). MBP, ECP, and EPO are highly toxic for larval parasites. ECP and EDN are toxic to viruses, bacteria, and helminths. Small granules contain acid phosphatase and arylsulfatase enzymes. Maturation time for eosinophils in bone marrow is 9 days and half-life in blood is about 18 hours. In tissues, eosinophils reside in skin, lungs, and gastrointestinal tract.

Basophils

The main cytokine involved in basophil growth and differentiation is IL-3. Basophils originate from granulocyte monocyte progenitor (GMP), which is derived from CMP. Basophils are small (5–7 μ), round to oval cells which contain very large, coarse, deep purple granules. The multilobed nucleus has condensed chromatin and is covered by granules. The granules are metachromatic and contain histamine, heparin, peroxidase, major basic protein, cathepsin G, and lysophospholipase. Basophils have surface receptors (FcεRI) for IgE. Upon reaction of IgE with receptor, granular contents are released (degranulation) which play a role in immediate hypersensitivity (or type I) reaction.

Similar to basophils, mast cells in tissues have surface receptors for IgE and have granules containing histamine. Recent evidence indicates that mast cells have a distinct pathway of origin from HSCs. Both basophils and mast cells are derived from common myeloid progenitor cell but have different committed progenitor cells (CFU-baso and CFU-MC, respectively). Mast cells in connective tissues differ from basophils in following respects. In contrast to basophils, mast cells are larger (10–15 μ) in size, have a single round to oval eccentrically placed nucleus, mature in connective tissue (not in bone marrow), have a proliferative potential, have a longer life span (weeks to months in contrast to days for basophils), and contain many large granules.

Monocytes, Macrophages, and Dendritic Cells

Monocytes, macrophages, and dendritic cells play a major role in host defense and immune regulation. Monocytes originate in bone marrow from granulocyte monocyte progenitor (GMP) under the action of GM-CSF, IL-3, and M-CSF. Morphologically identifiable initial

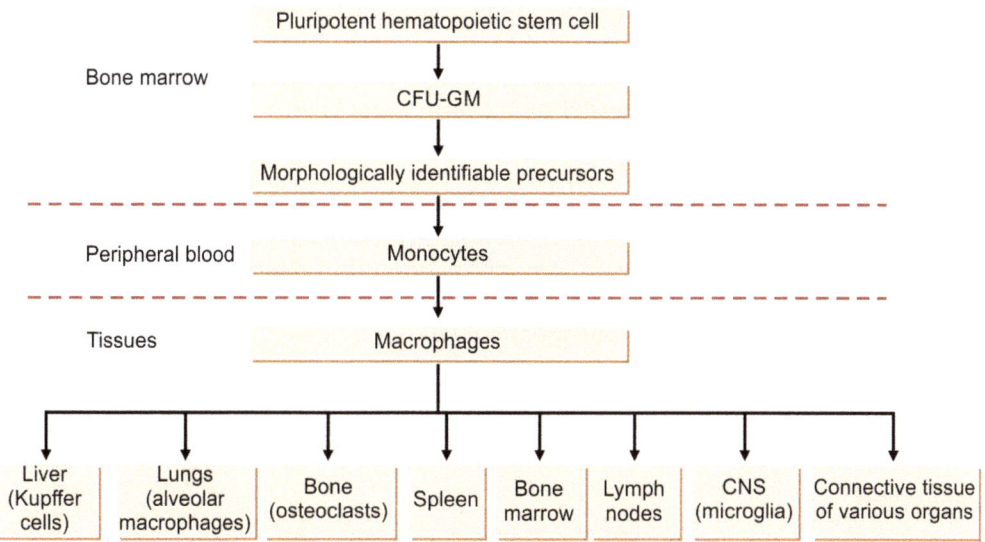

Fig. 1.18: Mononuclear phagocyte system.

cell in development is monoblast which is indistinguishable from myeloblast. The next cell is promonocyte which has an oval or clefted nucleus with fine chromatin pattern and 2 to 5 nucleoli. The monocyte is a large cell (15–20 μm), with irregular shape, oval or clefted (often kidney-shaped) nucleus and fine, delicate chromatin. Cytoplasm is abundant, blue-gray with ground glass appearance and often contains fine azurophil granules and vacuoles. Monocyte granules contain myeloperoxidase, lysozyme, nonspecific esterases, and lysosomes.

Monocytes circulate in blood for about 1-3 days and then enter and settle in tissues where they are called as macrophages or histiocytes. In some organs, macrophages have distinctive morphologic and functional characteristics (Fig 1.18).

Monocytes, macrophages, and dendritic cells have abundant receptors for Fc portion of IgG. A variety of pattern recognition receptors are found on macrophages and dendritic cells through which phagocytes directly attach to microorganisms.

In acute inflammation, monocytes play a key role in antigen presentation, phagocytosis, and repair.

On flow cytometry, CD14, CD36, and CD64 are considered as monocyte-associated markers. CD14 is the most specific monocyte marker.

Dendritic cells are classified into plasmacytoid and myeloid types based on their origin, surface receptor expression, and functions. Dendritic cells are specialized antigen presenting cells that are located mainly in skin, mucosal surfaces, and lymph nodal germinal centers. Their main action is presentation of processed antigen to T-helper cells.

Macrophage phagocytosis is slower as compared to neutrophils. Macrophages have receptors for Fc portion of IgG and C3b and cause phagocytosis of organisms that are coated with these substances. Macrophages also recognize and phagocytose some target substances by their surface characteristics.

Macrophages may be activated by certain stimuli, such as lymphokines (interferon γ secreted by T lymphocytes), direct contact with microorganism, phagocytized material, and complement components. Activated macrophages are larger and have enhanced metabolic and phagocytic activity.

Activated macrophages secrete a variety of biologically active substances:
1. Cytokines—interleukin-1, tumor necrosis factor α, interferons α and β;
2. Growth factors—fibroblast growth factors, hematopoietic growth factors (GM-CSF and G-CSF), angiogenesis factor, transforming growth factor β;
3. Complement proteins;
4. Coagulation factors, e.g. thromboplastin;
5. Oxygen-derived free radicals—hydrogen peroxide, superoxide, hydroxyl radical;
6. Prostaglandins and leukotrienes which are chemical mediators in inflammation;
7. Enzymes—elastases, collagenases, lysozyme, plasminogen activator, lipases;
8. Fibronectin;
9. Transferrin, transcobalamin II, apolipoprotein E.

The major functions of macrophages are processing and presentation of antigens to T lymphocytes during immune response, killing of intracellular pathogens, tumoricidal activity, and phagocytosis of organisms and of injured and senescent cells.

Lymphocytes

These are of two types—small and large. Most of the lymphocytes in peripheral blood are small (7–10 μm). The nucleus is round or slightly clefted with coarse chromatin and occupies most of the cell. The cytoplasm is basophilic, slight and is visible as a thin border around the nucleus.

Around 10–15% of lymphocytes in peripheral blood are large (10–15 μm). Their nucleus is similar to that of small lymphocytes but their cytoplasm is relatively more and contains few azurophilic (dark red) granules.

On immunophenotyping, there are two major types of lymphocytes in peripheral blood: B lymphocytes (10–20%) and T lymphocytes (60–70%). Differences between B and T lymphocytes are presented in Table 1.3. About 10–15% of lymphocytes are of natural killer (NK) cell type.

B Lymphocytes

B lymphocytes arise from the lymphoid stem cells in the bone marrow. Initial development occurs in primary lymphoid organ (bone marrow) from where B cells migrate to the secondary lymphoid organs (lymph nodes and spleen) where further differentiation occurs on antigenic stimulation. On activation by antigen, B cells undergo differentiation and proliferation to

Table 1.3: Comparison of B and T lymphocytes.

Parameter	B lymphocytes	T lymphocytes
1. Origin	Lymphoid stem cell in bone marrow	Lymphoid stem cell in bone marrow, maturation in thymus
2. Surface antigens	CD19, CD20, CD22	CD2, CD5, CD7, CD4/CD8
3. Surface receptor	Surface membrane immunoglobulin (SmIg)	T-cell receptor associated with CD3
4. Percentage in peripheral blood	30%	70%
5. Location in lymph node	Follicles, medullary cords	Paracortex, medullary sinuses
6. Function	Humoral immunity (maturation into plasma cell which produce immunoglobulins)	Cell-mediated immunity, graft rejection, delayed hypersensitivity, regulation of B-cell function

form plasma cells and memory cells. Plasma cells secrete immunoglobulins, while memory cells have a lifespan of many years and upon restimulation with the same antigen undergo proliferation and differentiation. Plasma cell is a round to oval cell with eccentrically placed nucleus and deeply basophilic cytoplasm. Nuclear chromatin is dense and arranged in a radiating or cartwheel pattern. The function of B lymphocytes is production of antibodies after differentiation to plasma cells. Antibodies can cause destruction of target cells/organisms either directly or by opsonization. B lymphocytes also can process antigen and serve as antigen-presenting cell via major histocompatibility complex (MHC) class II. B-cell antigen receptor (BCR) complex consists of membrane immunoglobulin associated with two proteins (CD79a and CD79b) that binds antigen and initiate B cell transformation by signal transduction.

Antigen-presenting cells in the body are monocytes/macrophages, dendritic cells, and B lymphocytes

Immunoglobulin gene rearrangement: There are five classes of immunoglobulins: IgM, IgG, IgA, IgD, and IgE. Each immunoglobulin molecule consists of two heavy chains and two light chains. Heavy chain (μ, δ, γ, ε, and α) determines the class of the immunoglobulin molecule. The two light chains are kappa (κ) and lambda (λ). Both heavy and light chains have constant and variable regions. The antigen-specificity of a particular immunoglobulin molecule depends upon amino acid sequence in the variable region (antigen-binding site). To react with a vast array of antigens, the immune system must have the capability to produce a large number of antigen-specific variable regions. The amino acid sequences in constant regions of heavy and light chains remain same for particular class and do not determine antigen specificity.

The heavy chain genes are located on chromosome 14. Light chain genes are located on chromosomes 2 (κ chain) and 22 (λ chain).

An immunoglobulin gene consists of V (Variable) and J (Joining) exons which code for amino acid sequences in variable region, and C (Constant) exon which codes for amino acid sequences in constant region. In heavy chain genes, another exon called D (Diversity) is present which codes for amino acids in variable region (in addition to V and J) (Fig. 1.19). There are several gene segments in V, D, and J regions, and therefore numerous antigen specificities can arise by various combinatorial rearrangements.

The un rearranged heavy and light chain genes are present in all the cells of the body (germ-line configuration); complete rearrangement occurs only in B cells. During development of B cells, rearrangement of heavy chain genes precedes the rearrangement of light chain genes.

Heavy chain gene rearrangement (Fig. 1.19): First, a *D* gene segment combines with a J segment (to form DJ), followed by combination of DJ with a *V* gene segment. The VDJ thus formed codes for amino acid sequence in variable region. From the C region, initially Cμ segment (which is located immediately 3' to the VDJ exon) is transcribed so as to form VDJCμ mRNA. This causes expression of μ heavy chains in the cytoplasm of pre-B cells, and after rearrangement of light chain genes expression of IgM on the surface of early B cells. Usually Cδ locus which lies very close to Cμ locus is also transcribed so that the cell expresses both IgM and IgD (with identical variable region sequences) on the surface.

Light chain gene rearrangement: During light chain gene rearrangement, initially a VJ exon is formed by fusion of one V and one J segment. The VJ exon is transcribed along with C exon and after splicing forms VJC mRNA.

Second immunoglobulin gene rearrangement can occur in activated B cells in which switching to new C segment of heavy chain gene occurs, i.e. Cμ to Cγ1 or Cα1 or Cε, etc.

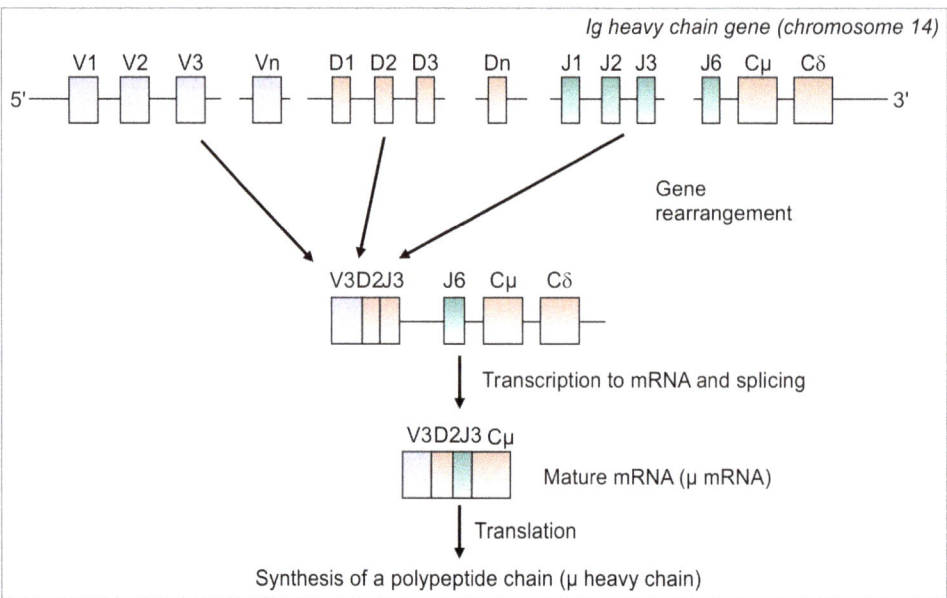

Fig. 1.19: Immunoglobulin heavy chain gene rearrangement. DJ rearrangement occurs first followed by VDJ joining (V3D2J3 in this example). V and D regions other than V3 and D2 are deleted. The rearranged gene is transcribed into mRNA and intervening sequences between J3 and Cμ are spliced. The mRNA formed is translated into a μ heavy chain in cytoplasm.

This causes change in the class of the immunoglobulin molecule, i.e. IgM to IgG1 or IgA or IgE, etc. Switching does not affect VDJ exon so that antigen specificity is not altered.

B-cell ontogeny (Fig. 1.20): During B-cell development, sequential genotypic and phenotypic changes occur which can be detected by immunological markers and gene rearrangement studies. Important features in B-cell ontogeny are outlined below:

i. There are two stages of B-cell development: Antigen-independent and antigen-dependent. Antigen-independent development occurs in bone marrow, while antigen-dependent development occurs in peripheral lymphoid tissues.

ii. Rearrangement of immunoglobulin genes and immunoglobulin expression: Initially, there is rearrangement of heavy chain genes which is followed by rearrangement of light chain genes. In pre-B cell, rearrangement of heavy chain gene causes appearance of μ heavy chain in cytoplasm (Cμ). This is followed by rearrangement of light chain genes. Light chains associate with μ heavy chain in cytoplasm and IgM is expressed on the cell surface. Mature B cells express both IgM and IgD. In activated B cells, class switching of heavy chains occurs such as IgM to IgG or IgA or IgE. Plasma cells do not have surface expression of immunoglobulin but synthesize and secrete large amounts of immunoglobulins of one class.

iii. Cell surface antigens: The earliest antigens expressed during B-cell development are TdT (within the nucleus) and HLA-DR (on cell surface); these are, however, not specific for B-cells. There is a sequential appearance of antigens on developing B-cells: CD10, CD19, and CD20. With development and maturation new antigens are expressed, while some of the previous ones are lost. Plasma cells express specific antigens, such as CD38 (Fig. 1.20).

iv. According to the fundamental theory of lymphoid neoplasms, the neoplastic cells represent cells arrested at various stages of normal lymphocyte development.

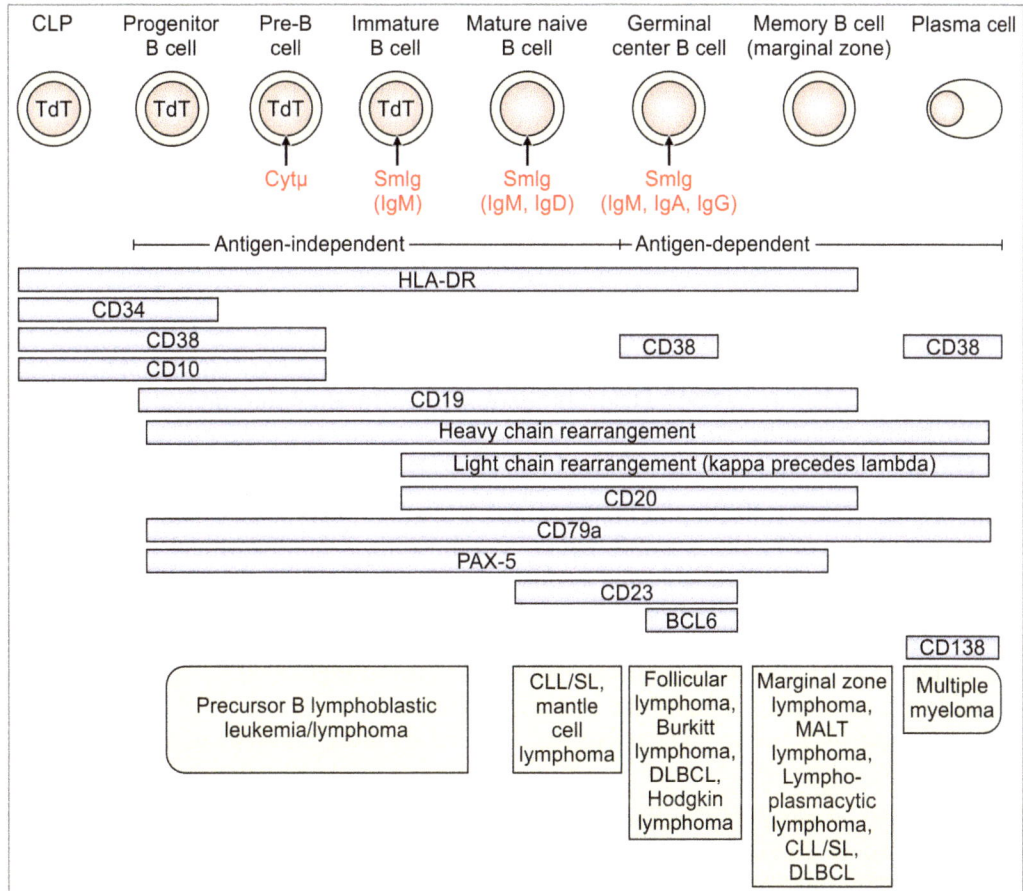

Fig. 1.20: Normal stages of B-cell development showing sequential expression of various antigens and heavy and light chain gene rearrangement. As shown at the bottom, lymphoid neoplasms represent cells arrested at various stages of normal development.
CLL/SL: chronic lymphocytic leukemia/small lymphocytic lymphoma; DLBCL: diffuse large B-cell lymphoma; MALT: mucosa-associated lymphoid tissue; HLA-DR: Human leukocyte antigen-DR isotype)

Functions of B lymphocytes include (1) production of immunoglobulins after differentiating into plasma cells, and (2) antigen presentation via MHC class II.

T Lymphocytes

T lymphocytes originate from the progenitor cells in the bone marrow and undergo maturation in thymus. After their release from thymus, T cells circulate in peripheral blood and are transported to secondary lymphoid organs (i.e. paracortex of lymph nodes and periarteriolar lymphoid sheaths in spleen).

T lymphocytes comprise 80–90% of circulating lymphocytes. T cells differentiate into helper T cells (CD4+), cytotoxic T cells (CD8+), and regulatory T cells.

CD4+ T cells predominate in peripheral blood over CD8+ cells. They are subclassified into T_H1, T_H2, and T_H17 CD4+ T cells. T_H1 cells are produced from naïve CD4+ T cells after release of IL-12 from activated macrophages in delayed type of hypersensitivity. T_H1 cells secrete IFN-γ that activates macrophages and cytotoxic T cells. T_H2 cells are produced from naïve CD4+ T

Section 1: Physiology of Blood

Box 1.4: Functions of T lymphocytes.
- **CD4+ T helper cells:** (1) recognition of antigen presented by antigen-presenting cells in association with MHC class II molecules, (2) assisting macrophages to kill intracellular pathogens via release of IFN-γ, (3) stimulation of B cells to produce antibodies; (4) activation of CD8+ cytotoxic T cells via secretion of IL-2, (5) Recruitment of eosinophils in allergic reactions as well as for defense against helminths by T_H2 cells.
- **CD8+ cytotoxic cells:** Recognize antigen in association with MHC class I molecules and kill target cells (virus-infected cells, tumor cells, and donor graft cells) via release of granzymes and perforins.
- **Regulatory T cells:** Restrict immune responses and prevent reactions against self-antigens.

cells after release of IL-4 from antigen presenting cells. T_H2 cells secrete IL-4, IL-5, and IL-13, which recruit eosinophils for defense against helminth parasites and are important in allergic reactions. TH17 cells secrete IL-17 which is important for recruiting neutrophils and monocytes in inflammatory reaction.

Functions of T lymphocytes are shown in Box 1.4.

T-cell receptor: The T-cell receptor (TCR) complex consists of seven polypeptide chains. In the majority (95%) of T cells, α and β chains form the antigen-binding site of TCR (αβTCR); each of these chains has a variable and a constant region similar to immunoglobulins. α-and β chains are linked together by a disulfide bond to form α-β heterodimer. The α-β heterodimer is noncovalently associated with CD3 molecular complex which is composed of six polypeptide chains (Fig. 1.21). The variable regions of α and β chains bind antigen, while CD3 converts this antigenic recognition into intracellular activating signals.

In a minority of T cells, γ and δ polypeptide chains are present instead of α- and β chains (γδTCR).

TCR gene rearrangement: The genetic structure of TCR bears resemblance to that of immunoglobulins. The TCR β chain gene is located on chromosome 7 and TCR α chain gene is located on chromosome 14.

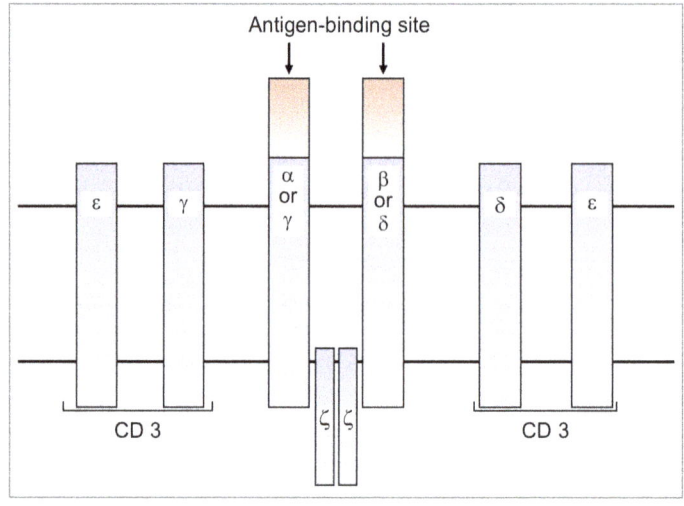

Fig. 1.21: T-cell receptor complex.

Although all somatic cells contain T-cell receptor gene in germ-line configuration, rearrangement occurs only in T cells. The TCR β gene consists of variable (V), diversity (D), joining (J), and constant (C) regions. One segment each from V, D, and J regions join together with deletion of intervening sequences. The rearranged gene is transcribed into mRNA. Splicing in transcribed mRNA causes fusion of VDJ to C region to generate TCR βmRNA. Rearrangement of other polypeptide chain occurs similarly. As there are a number of V, D, and J segments which code for amino acid sequences in variable region, it is possible to generate T-cell receptors with different antigen specificities by various combinations during rearrangement. Rearrangement of TCR β gene precedes the rearrangement of TCR α gene.

T-cell ontogeny (Fig. 1.22): Progenitor T cells from the bone marrow are transported to thymus where they undergo maturation. During maturation, there is rearrangement of *TCR* genes, expression of some cell surface proteins, and acquisition of ability to distinguish self-antigen from foreign antigens.

Initially, immature cortical thymocytes express CD7, TdT, and cytoplasmic CD3 (cCD3). Those T cells which subsequently are going to form α and β polypeptides (αβ TCR) first rearrange TCR β gene followed by TCR α gene. Expression of αβ TCR occurs in association with expression of CD3 on surface of cells. Initially, both CD4 and CD8 antigens are acquired; with further maturation cell retains either CD4 or CD8 antigen. CD4+ cells are called helper-inducer T cells whereas CD8+ cells are called cytotoxic T cells. The mature T cells are released from thymus, circulate in peripheral blood, and are transported to peripheral lymphoid organs.

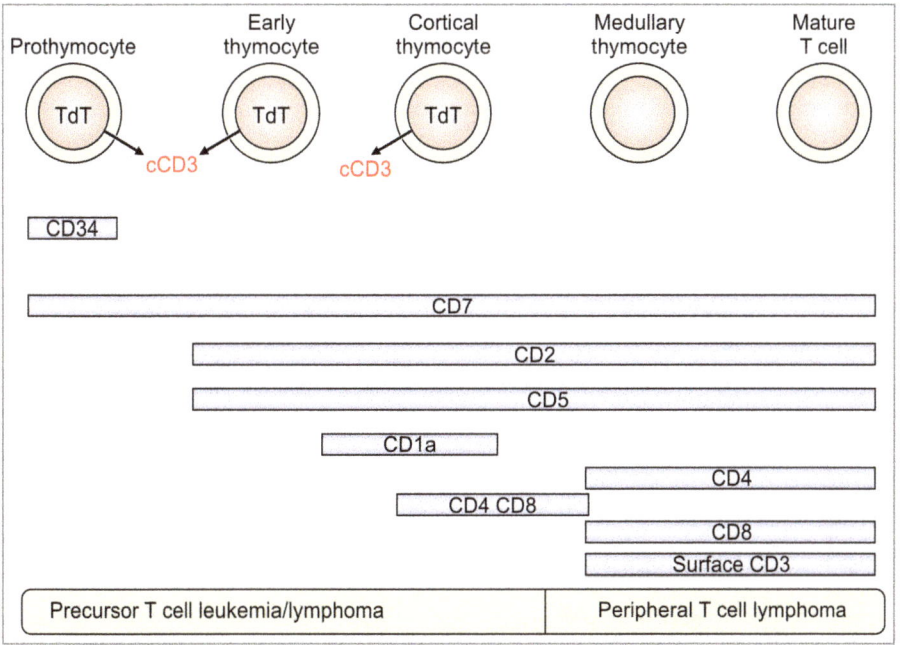

Fig. 1.22: Stages of T-cell development. Correlation of stages with T-cell neoplasms is shown at the bottom.

Natural Killer Cells

About 10–15% of peripheral blood lymphocytes are natural killer cells. These cells do not require previous exposure or sensitization for their cytotoxic action. They play a significant role in host defense against tumor cells and virally infected cells. Morphologically, these cells are large granular lymphocytes.

Both natural killer cells and cytotoxic T cells kill virus-infected cells, and tumor cells. However, NK cells are MHC-unrestricted while cytotoxic T cells are MHC class I-restricted.

White Cell Antigens

Human Leukocyte Antigens System

Human leukocyte antigens (HLA) are encoded by a cluster of genes on short arm of chromosome 6 called major histocompatibility complex (MHC). There are numerous allelic genes at each locus which makes the HLA system extremely polymorphic. The antigens are called HLA because they were first detected on white blood cells, although they are present on several other cells also.

Types of HLA antigens: There are three types of HLA antigens: Class I, class II, and class III.

Class I antigens: Genes at HLA-A, HLA-B, and HLA-C positions specify class I antigens. Class I antigens are glycoproteins which are associated noncovalently with β2 microglobulin. Almost all nucleated cells possess class I antigens (Fig. 1.23).

Class II antigens: HLA-D region (HLA-DR, HLA-DQ, and HLA-DP) encodes class II antigens. These consist of two glycoprotein chains α and β which are bound noncovalently. Class II antigens are present on monocytes, macrophages, B-lymphocytes, and stimulated T lymphocytes (Fig. 1.23).

Comparison of class I and class II HLA antigens is presented in Table 1.4.

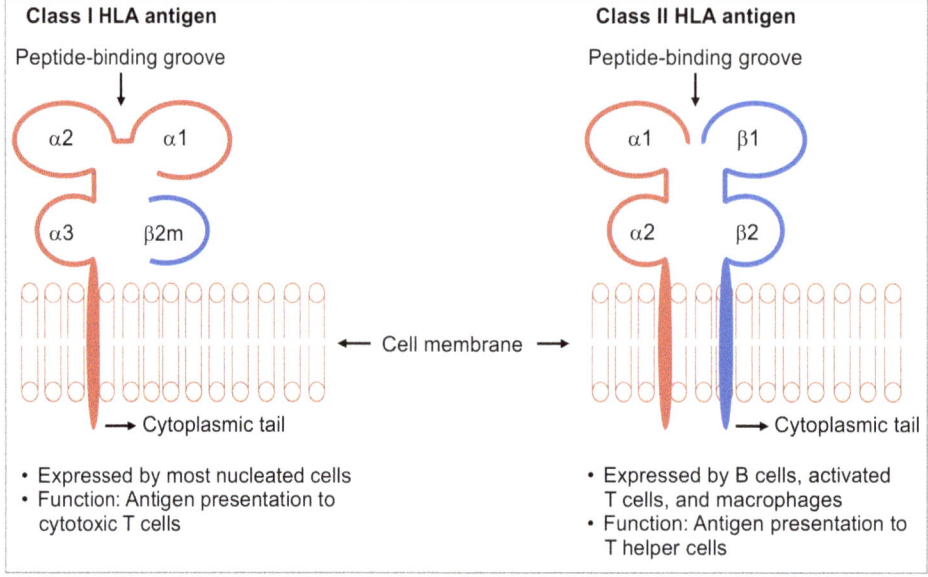

Fig. 1.23: Structure of class I and class II HLA antigens.

Table 1.4: Comparison of MHC class I and MHC class II molecules.

Parameter	MHC class I	MHC class II
Location of genes	Polymorphic α-chain genes on chromosome 6; invariant or constant β-chain gene on chromosome 15	Polymorphic α- and β- chain genes on chromosome 6
Genes	HLA-A, HLA-B, HLA-C	HLA-D (HLA-DP, HLA-DQ, HLA-DR)
Cell distribution	All nucleated cells and platelets, except red cells	Antigen presenting cells (B cells, macrophages, dendritic cells)
Recognized by	CD8 T lymphocytes	CD4 T lymphocytes
Function	Presentation of endogenous antigens from intracellular pathogens (e.g. viruses) to CD8+ T cells	Presentation of exogenous antigens from extracellular pathogens (e.g. bacteria) to CD4+ T cells
Structure	α chain (α1, α2, α3 domains) linked noncovalently to β2 microglobulin	Noncovalently associated α (α1, α2 domains) and β (β1, β2 domains) chains
Multiple alleles	Yes	Yes

Class III antigens: Genes specifying class III antigens are situated between genes which specify class I and class II antigens. Class III genes encode certain complement components and cytokines (tumor necrosis factor).

The HLA genes are closely linked and are inherited by an individual as a haplotype from each parent. In a given population, certain HLA haplotypes occur much more frequently than expected by chance alone (linkage disequilibrium).

Significance of HLA antigens: (1) They are important as histocompatibility antigens in organ transplantation; (2) HLA antigens play a major role in recognition of foreign antigens and in immunity; (3) in transfusion medicine, HLA antigens are responsible for alloimmunization against platelet antigens and refractoriness to platelet transfusions, febrile transfusion reactions, and graft-versus-host disease; (4) a relationship exists between presence of some HLA antigens and susceptibility to certain diseases (Table 1.5); and (5) HLA antigen typing can be used for paternity testing.

Applications for HLA typing include:
- Hematopoietic stem cell transplantation (HSCT) and solid organ transplantation
- Selection of platelets for patients refractory to platelet transfusion
- Disease association with certain HLA phenotypes (diagnosis and prognosis)
- Paternity testing

Tests for HLA typing are of following types:
A. Serologic typing of class I and class II molecules: Lymphocytotoxicity test (complement-dependent microlymphocytotoxicity typing)
B. Cellular typing of class II molecules: Mixed lymphocyte culture (MLC) or mixed lymphocyte reaction (MLR), primed lymphocyte typing (PLT)
C. Molecular or DNA-based typing of class I and class II alleles:
    - Sequence-specific primer (SSP) typing
    - Sequence-specific oligonucleotide probe (SSOP) hybridization
    - Sequence-based typing (SBT)
    - Next generation sequencing

Table 1.5: Association of HLA with disease.

Disease	HLA type
Seronegative* arthropathies (ankylosing spondylitis, Reiter syndrome, psoriatic arthritis, IBD-associated arthritis)	HLA-B27
Narcolepsy	HLA-DQB1
Type 1 diabetes mellitus	HLA-DR3, HLA-DR4
Systemic lupus erythematosus	HLA-DR2, HLA-DR3
Multiple sclerosis	HLA-DR2
Rheumatoid arthritis	HLA-DR4
Primary hemochromatosis	HLA-A3
Hashimoto thyroiditis	HLA-DR3, HLA-DR5
Graves disease	HLA-B8, HLA-DR3
Addison disease	HLA-B8, HLA-DR3, HLA-DR4
21-hydroxylase deficiency	HLA-BW47
Celiac disease	HLA-DQ2, HLA-DQ8

*Negative for rheumatoid factor in serum; IBD: Inflammatory bowel disease

Based on specificity, HLA typing is also classified as low resolution, intermediate resolution, and high resolution typing. Low resolution typing specifies HLA locus and the antigen family only; it produces a result similar to serologic lymphocytotoxicity testing. Intermediate resolution typing identifies specific allele within the HLA family. High resolution typing involves complete nucleotide sequencing of the HLA gene cluster. Low resolution typing is adequate for solid organ transplantation (kidney), while high resolution typing is necessary for HSCT.

Tests for detection of HLA antigens:
1. *Lymphocytotoxicity test:* Class I HLA antigens are detected by lymphocytotoxicity test. In this test, lymphocytes are first isolated from peripheral blood by density-gradient separation. These lymphocytes are then added to known specific antisera in microwell plates and incubated to allow the antibodies to bind to target antigens. Complement is added to the lymphocyte-antiserum mixture followed by further incubation. If particular antigen is present on lymphocytes, then antigen-antibody reaction occurs which activates and fixes the complement leading to cell membrane injury and cell death. A vital dye (eosin Y or trypan blue) is then added to differentiate living from dead cells. Damaged cells take up the dye due to the increased permeability of injured cell membrane, while living cells remain unstained.

    For detection of class II antigens (HLA-DR and HLA-DQ), lymphocytotoxicity test is carried out on B lymphocytes. This is because class II antigens are present on B lymphocytes and not on unstimulated T cells. Separation of B lymphocytes is usually achieved by magnetic beads which are coated with monoclonal antibodies against B cells.
2. *Mixed lymphocyte culture (MLC) or mixed lymphocyte reaction (MLR):* This test is used for detection of class II antigens. Lymphocytes from two different individuals are cultured together. Lymphocytes from one individual are inactivated by irradiation or by mitomycin C before the test to suppress their division; these lymphocytes are called stimulator cells. During incubation in culture, lymphocytes from the other individual recognize the foreign class II HLA antigens on stimulator cells and respond by enlarging in size, synthesizing

DNA, and proliferating (blastogenic response); these cells are called responder cells. If HLA class II antigens on responder and stimulator cells are identical, there is no blastogenic response. After 5–7 days 3H-thymidine is added to the culture and radioactive material incorporated into the dividing (responder) cells is quantitated. The amount of radioactive thymidine incorporated into the dividing cells is proportional to DNA synthesis.
3. *Primed lymphocyte typing (PLT) test:* This test is used for detection of HLA-DP antigens. It is based on mixed lymphocyte culture. In this method, the culture of lymphocytosis extended for 2 weeks during which death of stimulator cells occurs and proliferation of responder cells halts. As these responder cells have been primed (i.e. sensitized), their re-encounter with the cells which carry the same HLA-DP antigen as the initial stimulator cells causes their rapid proliferation.
4. Molecular or DNA-based typing of class I and class II alleles: DNA-based typing has replaced serological lymphocytotoxicity test and is now the most common method for HLA typing. Various molecular methods are outlined below.
   - *Sequence-specific primer (SSP):* Primers that are specific for a unique DNA sequence are used for HLA typing. A primer is specific for an allele or a group of alleles. If the sample being tested exactly matches both the primers, DNA is amplified. Presence of absence of amplification is detected by agarose gel electrophoresis.
   - *Sequence-specific oligonucleotide probe (SSOP) hybridization:* In this technique, a set of oligonucleotide probes (conjugated with a fluorescent marker) which can identify each allele is hybridized to the denatured PCR-amplified DNA. The oligonucleotide probe will anneal to the denatured DNA if complementary sequence is present.
   - *Sequence-based typing (SBT):* The nucleotide sequence of the entire HLA gene is determined and compared with known HLA sequences to determine the genotype.

Neutrophil-specific Antigens

Apart from HLA antigens, granulocytes also possess neutrophil-specific antigens. According to the new human neutrophil antigen (HNA) nomenclature system introduced by the International Society of Blood transfusion Working Party, the antigens include HNA-1 (HNA-1a, HNA-1b, HNA-1c, HNA-1d), HNA-2, HNA-3, HNA-4, and HNA-5. Neutrophil-specific antigens play an important role in alloimmune neonatal neutropenia, febrile nonhemolytic transfusion reaction, and transfusion-related acute lung injury (TRALI).

IMMUNE SYSTEM

As white cells play a major role in immunity, it is appropriate to consider antibodies and complement here.

Antibodies

Antibodies are immunoglobulins that react with antigens. They are produced by plasma cells, which in turn are derived from B lymphocytes.

Structure of Immunoglobulins

The immunoglobulin molecule consists of two identical heavy (H) chains and two identical light (L) chains. The H and L chains are linked together by disulfide (s-s) bonds. Five classes of immunoglobulins are recognized based on the type of H chain: IgA (α or alpha H chain), IgD (δ or delta), IgE (ε or epsilon), IgG (γ or gamma), and IgM (μ or mu). Light chains are of two varieties—κ (kappa) and λ (lambda).

A molecule of immunoglobulin consists of light chains of the same type (either κ or λ); both types of light chains are never present together. Kappa and lambda chains are present in 2:1 proportion in immunoglobulins.

Each chain has a constant and a variable region (Fig. 1.24). Amino acid composition in the carboxy terminal region of heavy chain and light chain is the constant region; in the heavy chain it determines the class of the immunoglobulin molecule. The CH2 domain in IgG binds complement, while CH3 domain binds to Fc receptor of monocytes. The variable region of the molecule (VL and VH) is the specific antigen-binding site and is in the aminoterminal part of the molecule. The area J of the heavy chains in the constant regions between CH1 and CH2 domains is flexible and is called hinge region; due to this the two antigen-binding sites can move in relation to each other spanning variable distances.

Each immunoglobulin molecule can be digested by a proteolytic enzyme papain just above the disulfide bond joining the two heavy chains into three parts: One Fc and two Fab fragments. The fragment which contains the carboxy terminal and constant parts of both heavy chains, is called the Fc (Fragment crystallizable) fragment. Each Fab (Fragment antigen binding) fragment contains amino-terminal portion of H chain and complete light chain and has the antigen-combining site (Fig. 1.24).

Classes of Immunoglobulins

IgG: This is the major immunoglobulin in plasma comprising about 75% of all circulating immunoglobulins. IgG is the monomer of the basic immunoglobulin structure. There are four subclasses of IgG: IgG1, IgG2, IgG3, and IgG4. Relative concentration in serum can be represented as IgG1 > IgG2 > IgG3 > IgG4. IgG is usually produced during secondary immune response. It is the only immunoglobulin which is transferred transplacentally to the fetus from the mother. The fetus cannot synthesize IgG and therefore IgG antibodies in the newborn represent those passively gained from the mother. IgG is capable of fixing complement with

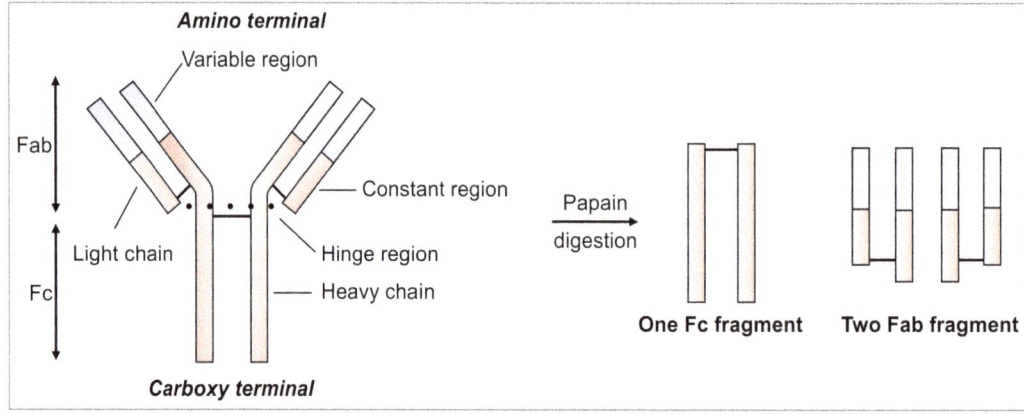

Fig. 1.24: Structure of immunoglobulin molecule. Broken line indicates site of papain digestion.

order of efficacy being IgG3, IgG1, and IgG2. IgG4 cannot bind complement in the classical pathway. Only IgG3 and IgG1 can bind to Fc receptors on macrophages.

IgM: This has high molecular weight and is also called macroglobulin due to its large size. IgM molecules have a pentameric structure (i.e. five immunoglobulin units joined together) and also have an additional short polypeptide chain (J or joining chain). It comprises 5–10% of circulating immunoglobulins. IgM is the first antibody produced in response to the antigen (primary response). In contrast to IgG, IgM cannot cross the placenta. The fetus is able to produce IgM after maturation of its immune system. IgM is highly efficient in binding complement. A single molecule of IgM can bind complement, while two molecules of IgG (IgG doublets) are necessary for complement binding. The order of efficiency of complement binding of immunoglobulins is IgM, IgG3, IgG1, and IgG2. There are no receptors on macrophages for IgM.

IgA: There are two subclasses of IgA: IgA1 and IgA2. IgA is present mostly in body secretions such as gastrointestinal and respiratory mucosal secretions, saliva, tears, etc. Secretory IgA is mostly IgA2 and exists as a dimer. Serum IgA which is mostly IgA1 is a monomer.

IgD and IgE: Both are present in trace amounts in serum and are monomeric.

Most IgD is expressed on the surface of resting B lymphocytes where it serves as an antigen receptor.

Most IgE is bound to basophils or mast cells through heavy chain. When a specific antigen combines with IgE, vasoactive substances are released from these cells and lead to anaphylaxis.

Alloantibodies versus autoantibodies: Alloantibodies are those which are produced by an individual against antigens present in another individual of the same species. Autoantibodies are those which are produced by an individual against one's own antigens.

Warm-versus cold antibodies: Warm antibodies react maximally at 37°C, while cold antibodies show maximum activity at 0–4°C. Most IgG antibodies are of warm type, while most IgM antibodies are of cold type. Characteristic features of different immunoglobulins are presented in Table 1.6.

Table 1.6: Characteristics of immunoglobulins.

Parameter	IgM	IgG	IgA	IgE	IgD
1. Approx. % of total Ig	5%	80%	15%	Trace	Trace
2. Molecular weight	900,000	150,000	150,000 or 300,000	190,000	180,000
3. Heavy chain	μ	γ	α	ε	δ
4. Structure	Pentamer	Monomer	Dimer (secretions), monomer (serum)	Monomer	Monomer
5. Half-life (days)	5	21	6	2	3
6. Complement activation	Yes	Yes	No	No	No
7. Placental transfer	No	Yes	No	No	No
8. Main function	Primary immune response	Secondary immune response	Mucosal immunity	Anaphylactic reaction	Unknown

Complement

Complement are serum proteins which when activated react in an orderly manner with each other to cause immunologic destruction of target cells. They play an important role in innate immunity and in pathological inflammation. Most of the complement components are synthesized in liver, except C1 components which are synthesized in intestinal epithelial cells. Normally, complement components are present in an inactive form in plasma.

The most important step in complement activation is proteolysis of C3 component.

There are three pathways of complement activation: Classical, alternate, and lectin-binding pathways (Fig 1.25).
1. Classical pathway: Activated by antigen-antibody (IgG or IgM) combination; complement is best fixed by IgM.
2. Alternate pathway: Activated by microbial surface molecules (e.g. endotoxin), complex polysaccharides, cobra venom, etc.
3. Lectin pathway: Activated by binding of mannose-binding lectin in plasma to mannose or other sugars on microbial surface (Lectins are proteins that bind to carbohydrates).

Classical Pathway

Classical pathway is usually initiated by reaction of antibody (IgG or IgM) with antigen (e.g. red cells). Binding of only a single IgM pentameric molecule or of IgG doublet to an antigen is necessary for complement activation.

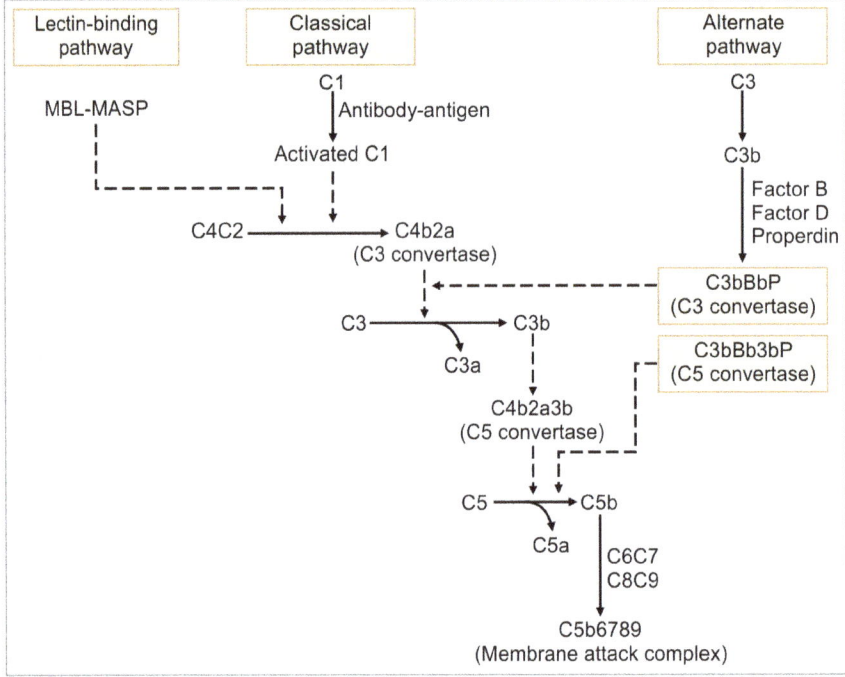

Fig. 1.25: The complement pathway. Solid arrow indicates transformation of a complement component. Dashed arrow indicates enzymatic action of complement component that causes cleavage of that component.
(MBL: mannose-binding lectin; MASP: mannose-associated serine protease)

The complements are activated in the following order: Ag–Ab complex—C1, C4, C2, C3, C5, C6, C7, C8, C9. This process occurs on the surface of target cells (e.g. red cells). Binding of antibody to antigen causes exposure of complement-binding site on immunoglobulin. The activated C1 cleaves C4 to form C4a and C4b; C4a is released into the body fluid, while C4b attaches to the red cell membrane. Activated C1 also cleaves C2 to form C2a. The C4b2a complex (C3 convertase) is formed. The C4b2a complex attached to cell membrane has enzymatic activity and can cleave several hundred C3 molecules. The C3a is released into plasma, while C3b attaches to the cell membrane. C3b however is rapidly degraded into C3dg. C3b is not enzymatically active by itself, but presence of C3b on the cell surface is recognized by specific receptors on the surface of macrophages and this causes phagocytosis of C3b-bearing cells. C3dg cannot adhere to macrophages because macrophages do not have receptors for C3dg. Once C3b is converted to C3dg, then complement cascade is terminated; C3dg-coated red cells in circulation are resistant to further complement-mediated cell destruction.

Some C3b joins C4b2a to form C4b2a3b (C5 convertase). C5 convertase cleaves C5 into C5a and C5b. C5a is released in circulation. C5b joins with C6, C7, C8, C9 to form membrane attack complex (MAC) which fixes on cell membranes and causes cell lysis. The MAC creates pores in red cell membrane through which water enters into red cells, cells swell and are lysed.

Alternate Pathway

In alternate pathway, C3 is activated directly with no role of earlier complement components. It does not require antigen-antibody reaction.

C3 can be activated by endotoxins, complex carbohydrates, such as are present on some microorganisms, and aggregates of IgA. A serum protein called properdin, factors B and D, and magnesium ions are needed for activation of alternate pathway.

Normally, C3 is being continuously cleaved at low level probably by factor B resulting C3b is rapidly cleared from the plasma. However, when C3b comes in contact with certain substances (e.g. complex carbohydrates on the surface of microorganisms) then association of C3bB occurs on the surface of micro-organisms in the presence of Mg^{++} ions. Factor B is cleaved by factor D to form C3bBb. Properdin may stabilize C3bBb. C3bBb splits C3 to generate more C3b thus forming an amplification loop.

Alternate pathway plays an important role in initial defense against infection in nonimmune persons.

Mannose-binding lectin pathway: Mannose-binding lectin directly binds to target cell surface; this resembles binding of C1 to immune complexes and directly activates the classical pathway (without the need for immune complex formation).

Regulation of Complement Activity

Following factors act as a control mechanism against prolonged complement action:
- Specific inhibitors of activation of some complement components (e.g. C1 esterase inhibitor) are present in plasma, Complement activation on own cells is prevented by decay-accelerating factor or DAF (CD55).
- Enzymatically active complement components have a very short life and are rapidly degraded to inactive forms.
- Active fragments are rapidly cleared from circulation.

Various Effects of Complement Activation
- Opsonization: Macrophages have specific receptors for C3b and thus target cells coated with C3b are recognized and phagocytozed by them (Opsonins are substances which when present on the surface of the antigen, such as red cells facilitate immune phagocytosis; these are C3b and Fc portion of immunoglobulin which are recognized by specific receptors on the surface of macrophages).
- Target cell lysis by membrane attack complex C5b-9.
- Acute inflammation: Certain complement components play a role in acute inflammation. C3a and C5a are anaphylatoxins and increase vascular permeability. C5a, in addition, causes neutrophil chemotaxis and activates lipoxygenase pathway of arachidonic acid metabolism with further release of chemical mediators of inflammation..

Disorders of complement include:
- C1 esterase inhibitor deficiency: Causes hereditary angioedema
- Deficiency of decay accelerating factor (CD55): Causes of paroxysmal nocturnal hemoglobinuria
- Deficiency of C3 and C5: Recurrent pyogenic infections by encapsulated bacteria
- Deficiency of C6, C7, C8, and C9: Recurrent infections by *Neisseria* species.

MEGAKARYOPOIESIS

The process of development of megakaryocytes and platelets in bone marrow is known as megakaryopoiesis. It is divided into four stages (Fig. 1.26). Megakaryoblasts (stage I) are the earliest morphologically recognizable precursors; they are 6–24 μ in diameter contain a single, large, oval, kidney-shaped, or lobed nucleus with loose chromatin and multiple nucleoli, and have deeply basophilic agranular cytoplasm. Promegakaryocytes (stage II) are larger than megakaryoblasts (15–30 μ), have lobulated or horseshoe-shaped nucleus, more abundant and less basophilic cytoplasm which may contain azurophil granules. Granular megakaryocytes (stage III) are 40–60 μ in diameter contain a large multilobed nucleus with coarsely granular chromatin, and have abundant mildly basophilic cytoplasm containing numerous azurophil granules. Mature megakaryocytes (stage IV) are of similar size, contain a tightly packed multilobed and pyknotic nucleus, and have acidophilic cytoplasm; granules are arranged as "platelet fields" (groups of 10-12 azurophil granules). Sometimes neutrophils or other marrow cells are seen traversing through the cytoplasm (emperipolesis); it has no clinical significance.

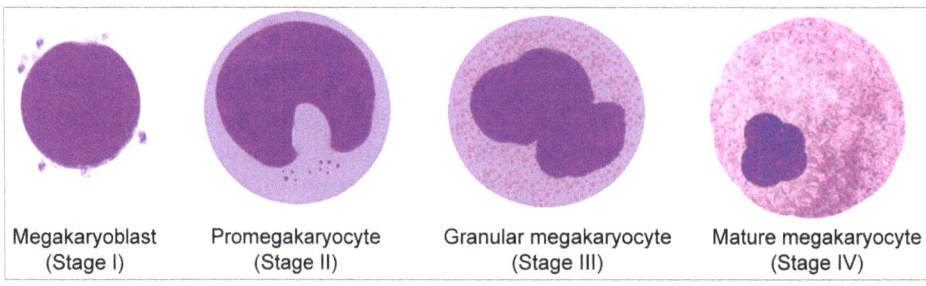

Fig. 1.26: Megakaryopoiesis.

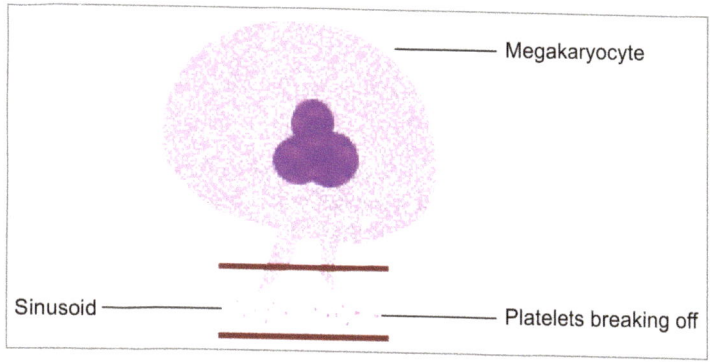

Fig. 1.27: Formation and release of platelets from a megakaryocyte.

Mature megakaryocytes extend long and slender cytoplasmic processes (proplatelets) between endothelial cells of sinusoids in bone marrow and platelets are released from fragmentation of these processes. Each megakaryocyte produces 1,000–5,000 platelets, leaving behind a "bare" nucleus which is removed by macrophages.

A unique feature of thrombocytopoiesis is endomitosis. This refers to nuclear division with cytoplasmic maturation but without cell division. As the cell matures from megakaryoblast to the megakaryocyte, there is gradual increase in cell size, number of nuclear lobes, and red-pink granules and gradual decrease in cytoplasmic basophilia. Megakaryocytes, the most abundant cells of the platelet series in the marrow are large and contain numerous nuclear lobes with dense nuclear chromatin, and small aggregates of granules in the cytoplasm. The megakaryocytes possess well-developed membrane demarcation system. Upon complete maturation, megakaryocytes extend pseudopods through the walls of the marrow sinusoids and individual platelets break-off into the peripheral circulation (Fig. 1.27). There is evidence that some of the megakaryocytes are carried to the lungs where platelets are released. A humoral factor, thrombopoietin, controls the maturation of megakaryocytes.

Thrombopoietin or TPO, a glycoprotein, binds to C-Mpl receptors (also called as TPO receptors) on cell surface and directs growth and development of megakaryocytes. Biallelic mutation of TPO receptor gene causes congenital amegakaryocytic thrombocytopenia.

Markers for megakaryocytic differentiation are FVIII, CD41 (GPIIb), CD42 (GPIb), and CD61 (GPIIIa).

NORMAL HEMOSTASIS

Hemostasis is the mechanism by which loss of blood from the vascular system is controlled by a complex interaction of vessel wall, platelets, and plasma proteins. Following vessel injury, hemostasis can be considered as occurring in two stages: Primary and secondary. Primary hemostasis is the initial stage during which vascular wall and platelets interact to limit the blood loss from damaged vessel. During secondary hemostasis, a stable fibrin clot is formed from coagulation factors by enzymatic reactions. Although formation of blood clot is necessary to arrest blood loss, ultimately blood clot needs to be dissolved to resume the normal blood flow. The process of dissolution of blood clot is called fibrinolysis.

The roles of vascular wall, platelets, and plasma proteins in normal hemostasis are briefly outlined below.

Vascular Wall

Endothelial cells synthesize certain substances which have inhibitory influence on hemostasis. These include—thrombomodulin, protein S, heparin-related substances, prostacycline (PGI2), and tissue plasminogen activator (tPA). Binding of thrombomodulin to thrombin causes activation of protein C. Protein C inactivates factors V and VIII:C and is a potent inhibitor of coagulation. Protein S is a cofactor for protein C. Deficiency of protein C or protein S is associated with tendency towards thrombosis. Heparin-like substances on the surface of endothelial cells potentiate the action of antithrombin. Prostacycline, a prostaglandin synthesized by endothelial cells, induces vasodilatation and also inhibits platelet aggregation. Endothelial cells also synthesize tissue plasminogen activator which converts plasminogen to plasmin, and activates fibrinolytic system.

Certain factors synthesized by endothelial cells promote hemostasis and include tissue factor, von Willebrand factor (vWF), and platelet activating factor. Tissue factor or thromboplastin activates extrinsic system of coagulation. vWF mediates adhesion of platelets to subendothelium. Platelet activating factor induces aggregation of platelets (Fig. 1.28).

Another vascular factor promoting hemostasis is vasoconstriction of small vessels following injury.

Subendothelial collagen promotes platelet adhesion and also activates factor XII (intrinsic pathway).

Weibel-Palade bodies are unique structures within vascular endothelial cells that store P-selectin and vWF. P-selectin causes adhesion of neutrophils and monocytes to endothelium during inflammation, while vWF mediates platelet adhesion.

Platelets

Platelets are derived from cytoplasmic fragmentation of bone marrow cells called megakaryocytes. They measure 2-3 μ in diameter. The platelet volume normally ranges from 7-11 fl (called mean platelet volume or MPV). Young platelets retain most of their RNA when they are released from the bone marrow (called reticulated platelets) and can be differentiated from older platelets based on their RNA content. Normal platelet count in peripheral blood is 1.5-4 lacs/mm³. Platelets remain viable in circulation for approximately 10 days. About one-

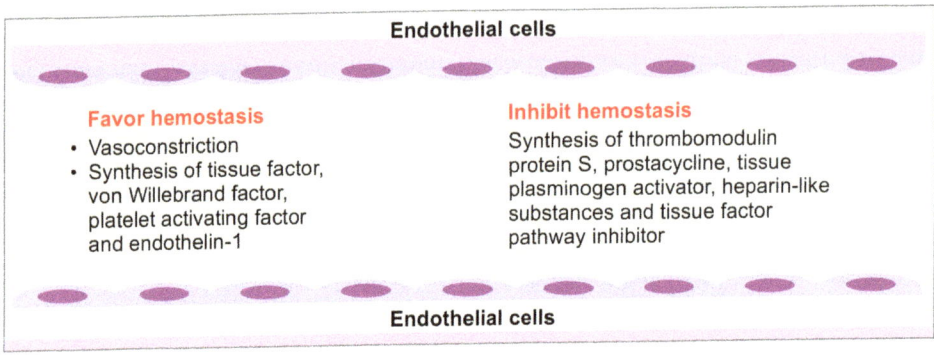

Fig. 1.28: Role of blood vessels in hemostasis.

third of the total platelets in the body are in the spleen and remainder in peripheral blood. Under light microscope, in peripheral blood smears stained with one of the Romanowsky stains, platelets appear as small, irregular with fine cytoplasmic processes. Cytoplasmic granules are often visible.

These granules may be packed in the central portion (granulomere) with peripheral cytoplasm appearing clear (hyalomere).

The number of platelets in circulation is regulated by TPO, which is synthesized constitutively in liver and kidney. TPO binds to megakaryocytes, platelets, and HSCs through TPO receptor (C-Mpl). Platelet count is maintained by TPO by a mechanism called as "sponge" model. Free TPO in circulation binds to high-affinity TPO receptors on platelets where it is internalized and degraded. TPO that is not bound to platelets stimulates megakaryopoiesis in bone marrow. Thus, low platelet count is associated with increased free TPO and stimulation of megakaryopoiesis. High platelet count is associated with less free TPO to bind to megakaryocytes in bone marrow.

Ultrastructure of Platelets

Ultrastructurally, following three zones can be distinguished: (1) Peripheral zone: Exterior coat (glycocalyx), cell membrane, and open canalicular system; (2) Sol-gel zone: Microfilaments, circumferential microtubules, and dense tubular system; and (3) Organelle zone: Alpha granules, dense granules, mitochondria, lysosomes, peroxisomes, and glycogen (Fig. 1.29).

Peripheral zone: Exterior or surface coat (glycocalyx) overlies the cell membrane. It is made of proteins, glycoproteins, and mucopolysaccharides. Some of the glycoproteins are polysaccharide side chains of the integral membrane proteins while others are adsorbed from the plasma.

The cell membrane is a trilaminar membrane composed of proteins, lipids, and carbohydrates. The chief membrane lipids are phospholipids which are arranged as a bilayer; the polar head groups are oriented both externally (towards plasma) and internally (towards cytoplasm) while the fatty acid chains are oriented towards each other. Phospholipids are distributed asymmetrically in the membrane with negatively charged phospholipids (phosphatidylserine, phosphatidylethanolamine, and phosphatidylinositol) concentrated on the inner half of the bilayer and neutral phospholipids (phosphatidylcholine and sphingomyelin) on the outer half. As the negatively charged phospholipids are located on

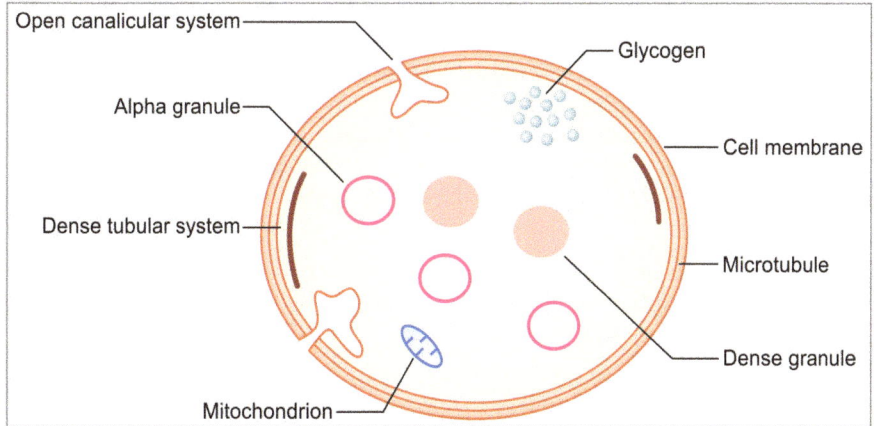

Fig. 1.29: Ultrastructure of platelet.

the inner surface, they are separated from the coagulation proteins in plasma thus preventing inappropriate activation of coagulation. The phospholipids play an important role in prostaglandin synthesis and in platelet procoagulant activity. The cell membrane also contains glycoproteins (like Ib/IX, IIb/IIIa, and Ia/IIa) that play important role in platelet adhesion and aggregation.

An extensive open canalicular system (also called as surface-connected canalicular system or SCCS) formed by invagination of the cell membrane communicates with the exterior. It functions as a route through which platelet contents are secreted outside the cell. It facilitates platelet spreading and filopedia formation after adhesion. The number of GPIIb/IIIa receptors also increase on platelet surface after activation, since SCCS acts as their storage reservoir.

Sol-gel zone: Microtubules provide structural support to the platelets and maintain its discoid shape. Microfilaments have contractile function. The dense tubular system derived from smooth endoplasmic reticulum is the site of pooling of calcium and formation of prostaglandin and thromboxane (arachidonic acid metabolism).

Organelle zone: Platelet organelles are alpha granules, dense granules, lysosomes, and peroxisomes. Contents of platelet organelles are shown in Box 1.5.

Platelet Membrane Glycoproteins

The cell membrane contains integral membrane glycoproteins (Gp) which play an important role in hemostasis. Important platelet membrane glycoproteins and their functions are as follows:

GPIb/V/IX (CD42 a-d): Interaction of GPIb/V/IX causes adhesion of platelets to subendothelium in high shear stress at the site of injury. Following adhesion, signal transduction causes platelet shape change, activation, and granule secretion. There is also activation of GPIIb/IIIa, which is necessary for platelet aggregation and firm platelet adhesion. GPIb/V/IX consists of several

---

Box 1.5: Platelet organelles and their contents.

Alpha granules
1. Platelet-specific proteins: Platelet factor 4, β-thromboglobulin, multimerin
2. Coagulant proteins: Fibrinogen, factor V, factor XI, factor XIII, von Willebrand factor
3. Anticoagulant proteins: Antithrombin, protein S, tissue factor pathway inhibitor, plasminogen activator inhibitor-1, plasminogen, α2-antiplasmin
4. Adhesion proteins: thrombospondin-1, fibronectin, vitronectin, P-selectin
5. Growth factors: Epidermal growth factor, transforming growth factor-β
6. Angiogenic factors: Vascular endothelial growth factor, platelet-derived growth factor

Dense granules
1. Cations: Calcium, magnesium
2. Nucleotides: Adenosine diphosphate, adenosine triphosphate
3. Bioactive amines: Serotonin, histamine

Lysosomes
Enzymes: Acid hydrolases, cathepsins, elastase, collagenases, galactosidase, glucuronidase

subunits like GPIbα, GPIbβ, GPIX, and GPV. Qualitative or quantitative defects in GPIbα, GPIbβ, and GPIX cause Bernard-Soulier syndrome.

GPIIb/IIIa (CD41/CD61, Integrin αIIbβ3): Activation of integrin αIIbβ3 (GPIIb/IIIa) is required for binding of fibrinogen and aggregation. It is also necessary for final firm adhesion of platelets to subendothelium. GPIIb/IIIa receptor is activated by (1) binding of vWF to GPIb/V/IX, binding of platelet agonists like thromboxane A2 and ADP to platelets, and binding of thrombin to platelet thrombin receptor. Antiplatelet drugs like abciximab, eptifibatide, and tirofiban block fibrinogen binding to GPIIb/IIIa, thus inhibiting platelet aggregation. Quantitative or qualitative defects in GPIIb/IIIa due to mutation in *ITGA2B* or *ITGB3* genes cause Glanzmanns thrombasthenia (a moderate to severe congenital bleeding disorder).

GPIa/IIa (CD49b/CD29, Integrin α2β1): This is a receptor for collagen and mediates platelet adhesion independent of vWF. GPIa/IIa deficiency is extremely rare and cause mild bleeding disorder.

GPVI: GPVI occurs on platelet surface in complex with Fc receptor (FcR) γ-chain. GPVI is required for interaction of platelets with collagen at the site of vessel injury under high shear condition. This initiates platelet activation and promotes integrin αIIbβ3 activation, which is necessary for platelet aggregation.

GP Ic/IIa (Integrin α5β1): This is a major platelet receptor for fibronectin and plays supplemental role in platelet adhesion.

Platelet Antigens

Platelets possess HLA antigens, ABO antigens, and platelet-specific antigens. HLA class I antigens induce alloimmunization and cause refractoriness to platelet transfusions when platelets are obtained from random donors. The platelet-specific antigen systems are now known as human platelet antigen (HPA) systems. Platelet-specific antigens play an important role in neonatal alloimmune thrombocytopenic purpura (NATP) and in post-transfusion purpura.

Role of Platelets in Hemostasis

Activation of platelets refers to adhesion, aggregation, and release reaction of platelets which occurs after platelet stimulation (i.e. after vascular damage).

Adhesion: This means binding of platelets to nonendothelial surfaces particularly subendothelium which is uncovered following vascular injury. vWF mediates adhesion of platelets to subendothelium via GpIb on the surface of platelets (Fig. 1.30).

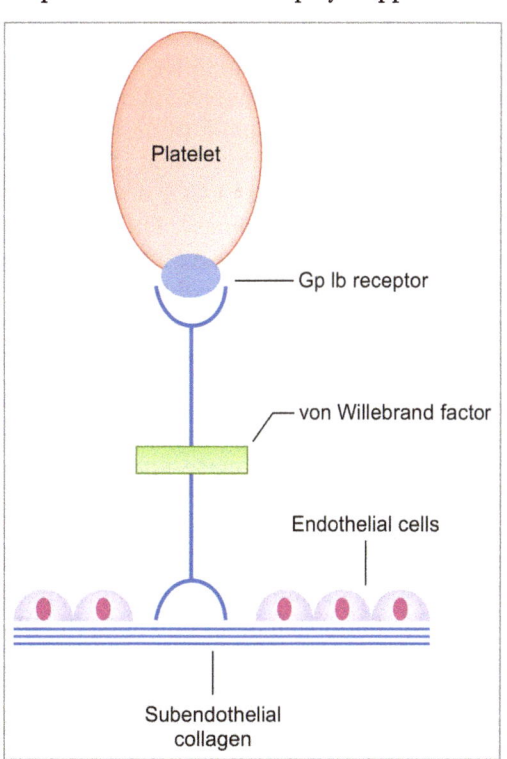

Fig. 1.30: Platelet adhesion to subendothelial collagen. Gp Ib receptor on platelets and von Willebrand factor are necessary for attachment of platelets to subendothelial collagen.

Congenital absence of glycoprotein receptor GpIb (Bernard–Soulier syndrome) or of vWF in plasma (von Willebrand's disease) causes defective platelet adhesion and bleeding disorder.

Platelets normally circulate as round to oval disc-like structures. With activation, platelets undergo shape change, i.e. they become more spherical and form pseudopodia.

This shape change is due to reorganization of microtubules and contraction of actomyosin of microfilaments.

Release reaction (secretion): Immediately after adhesion and shape change, process of release reaction or secretion begins. In this process, contents of platelet organelles are released to the exterior. ADP released from dense granules promotes platelet aggregation. Platelet factor 4 released from alpha granules neutralizes the anticoagulant activity of heparin, while platelet-derived growth factor stimulates proliferation of vascular smooth muscle cells and skin fibroblasts and plays a role in wound healing.

Activated platelets also synthesize and secrete thromboxane A2 (TxA2) (Fig. 1.31). Platelet agonists, such as ADP, epinephrine, and low-dose thrombin bind to their specific receptors on platelet surface, and activate phospholipase enzymes which release arachidonic acid from membrane phospholipids. Arachidonic acid is converted to cyclic endoperoxides PGG2 and PGH2 by the enzyme cyclo-oxygenase. These are then converted to thromboxane A2 by thromboxane synthetase. Thromboxane A2 has a very short half-life and is degraded into thromboxane B2 which is biologically inactive. TxA2 causes shape change and stimulates release reaction from alpha and dense granules. TxA2 also induces aggregation of other platelets and local vasoconstriction.

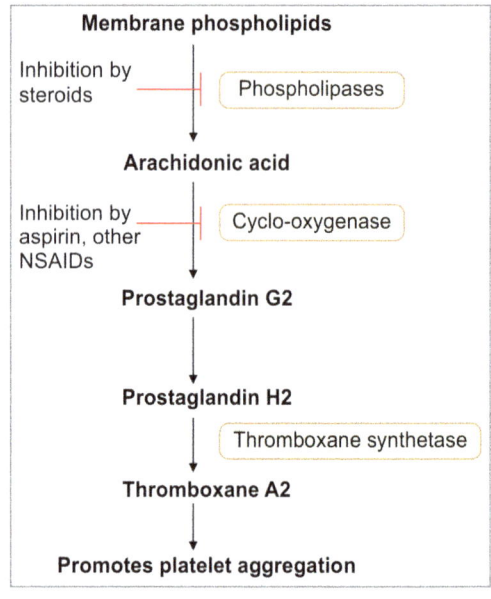

Fig. 1.31: Synthesis of thromboxane A2. Modes of action of certain antiplatelet drugs are also shown.

Aggregation: This may be defined as binding of platelets to each other. ADP released from platelets or from damaged cells binds to specific receptors on platelet surface. This causes inhibition of adenylcyclase and reduction in the level of cyclic AMP in platelets. A configurational change in the membrane occurs so that receptors for fibrinogen (Gp IIb and IIIa) become exposed on the surface. Binding of fibrinogen molecules to GPIIb/IIIa receptors on adjacent platelets causes platelet aggregation (Fig. 1.32). The activated platelets release ADP and TxA2 and so a self-sustaining reaction is generated leading to the formation of a platelet plug. Thrombin generated from activation of coagulation system is a potent

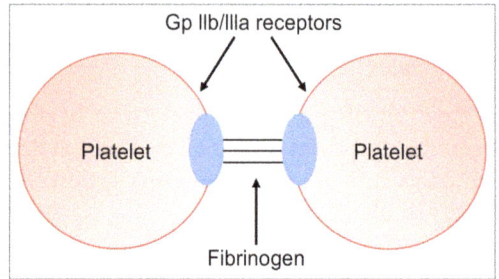

Fig. 1.32: Platelet aggregation. This requires binding of fibrinogen molecules to Gp IIb/IIIa receptors on platelets.

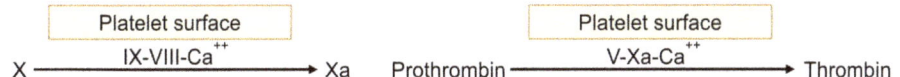

Fig. 1.33: Platelet procoagulant activity. Platelets provide surface for some important coagulation reactions.

platelet-aggregating agent and also converts fibrinogen to fibrin. Fibrin and aggregated mass of platelets at the site of injury constitute the hemostatic plug.

Platelet procoagulant activity: When platelets are activated, negatively charged phospholipids (phosphatidylserine and phosphatidylinositol) located in the inner half of the lipid bilayer become exposed on the outer surface. These phospholipids play active role in coagulation by providing surface for interaction of some coagulation factors. Critical coagulation reactions for which activated platelets provide a negatively charged phospholipid (PL) surface are shown in Figure 1.33.

Platelets may play a role in the activation of F XII in the presence of ADP and kallikrein. Platelets also can directly activate F XI independent of F XII. This may explain the absence of bleeding diathesis in persons with F XII deficiency.

In addition, platelets also secrete calcium, F V, fibrinogen, and F XII and contribute to the coagulation system.

Platelet microparticles: When platelets are activated and phosphatidylserine is exposed on surface, small blebs form over the plasma membrane. These microparticles increase the surface area for coagulation reactions (especially generation of FXa and thrombin). These small blebs also express GPIIb/IIIa and GPIb/V/IX. Circulating microparticles (0.1 to 1 μ) are derived from megakaryocytes as well as platelets; they are prothrombotic since phosphatidylserine on their surface promotes thrombin generation.

Plasma Proteins in Hemostasis

Plasma proteins in hemostasis can be divided into following groups:
1. Coagulation system: Factors I, II, III, IV, V, VII, VIII, IX, X, XI, XII, XIII, prekallikrein, high molecular weight kininogen.
2. Fibrinolytic system: Plasminogen, plasmin, tissue plasminogen activator (tPA), urokinase plasminogen activator (uPA), plasminogen activator inhibitor-1 (PAI-1), plasminogen activator inhibitor-2 (PAI-2), α2-antiplasmin, thrombin-activatable fibrinolysis inhibitor (TAFI).
3. Inhibitor system: Protein C, protein S, and antithrombin.

Coagulation System

A number of coagulation proteins (factors) participate in coagulation reactions, which ultimately lead to the formation of a fibrin clot. According to the International System of Nomenclature, coagulation factors are designated by Roman numerals (I–XIII). Table 1.7 lists the blood coagulation factors; common names and synonyms are given on the right side. Coagulation proteins can be divided into following categories: (1) Fibrinogen (F I); (2) Serine proteases: (a) Vitamin K-dependent factors—II, VII, IX, X, (b) Contact factors—XI, XII, high molecular weight kininogen, prekallikrein; (3) Cofactors—V, VIII, tissue factor (F III); and (4) Transglutaminase: F XIII.

Section 1: Physiology of Blood

Table 1.7: Blood coagulation factors.

Factor	Synonym
I	Fibrinogen
II	Prothrombin
III	Tissue factor, thromboplastin
IV	Calcium
V	Labile factor, proaccelerin
VI	F VI has been determined to be activated form of F V and the term F VI is no longer used
VII	Stable factor
VIII	Antihemophilic factor or globulin
IX	Christmas factor, plasma thromboplastin component
X	Stuart–Prower factor
XI	Plasma thromboplastin antecedent
XII	Hageman factor
XIII	Fibrin stabilizing factor, Laki–Lorand factor
Fletcher factor	Prekallikrein
Fitzgerald factor	High molecular weight kininogen

The coagulation factors have been assigned Roman numerals according to the order of their discovery. Except calcium and thromboplastin, all the coagulation factors listed in Table 1.7 are glycoproteins. When coagulation factors become activated, they are converted from an inactive zymogen form to a serine protease. However, factors V and VIII, when activated, do not develop enzymatic activity but become modified and are called cofactors; in their absence the reactions, which they modify, become markedly slow. Activation of fibrinogen denotes cleavage of fibrinopeptides A and B from the molecule with formation of fibrin. Factors II, VII, IX, and X are called vitamin K-dependent factors. Vitamin K is required for γ-carboxylation of these proteins which is necessary for calcium binding. Calcium in turn, is necessary for binding of these coagulation factors to phospholipid surface. Attachment of coagulation factors to phospholipid is essential for coagulation reactions to occur. In the absence of vitamin K, carboxylation fails to occur and functionally inactive forms of vitamin K-dependent factors are produced. Factors XII, XI, high molecular weight kininogen, and prekallikrein are called contact factors; they are involved in the activation of coagulation via intrinsic pathway.

The liver is the site of synthesis of most coagulation factors. However, F XIII is derived from megakaryocytes, while vascular endothelial cells and megakaryocytes synthesize vWF.

Individual coagulation factors are considered briefly below:

Fibrinogen [Molecular weight (MW) 340,000; 1/2 life 90 hours)]: The level of fibrinogen in plasma is the greatest among the coagulation proteins and ranges from 200 to 400 mg/dL. Fibrinogen molecule consists of three pairs of polypeptide chains Aα, Bβ, and γ which are held together by disulfide bonds. The complete molecule is represented as Aα2 Bβ2 γ2. Fibrinogen consists of three domains—two outer D domains and a central E domain. Fibrinopeptides A and B are located in the central domain at the N-terminals of Aα and Bβ chains, respectively.

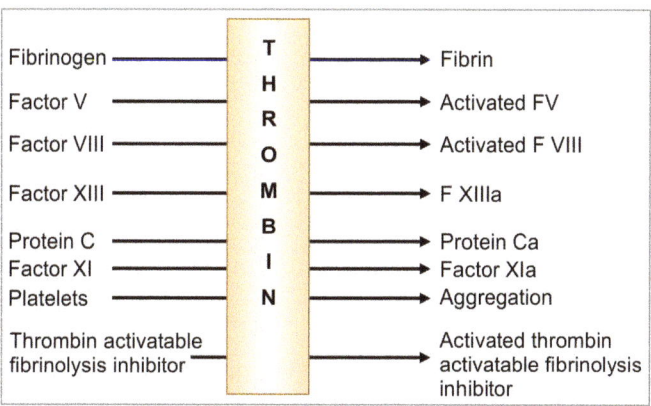

Fig. 1.34: Multiple actions of thrombin in hemostasis.

Thrombin releases fibrinopeptides A and B from these chains to form fibrin monomers (*See* Fig. 1.38). Fibrinogen is an acute phase reactant and its concentration rises in a variety of nonspecific conditions, such as inflammation, trauma, and myocardial infarction. In addition to plasma, fibrinogen is also present in α granules of platelets. In addition to formation of a fibrin clot, fibrinogen plays a crucial role in platelet aggregation by binding to GPIIb/IIIa on adjacent platelets.

Prothrombin (MW 72,000; 1/2 life 60 hours): Factor II or prothrombin is converted to thrombin by the enzyme complex Xa-V-phospholipid-calcium (called prothrombinase). Thrombin has multiple functions in hemostasis (Fig. 1.34).
1. Thrombin splits fibrinopeptides A and B from fibrinogen to form fibrin monomers;
2. Thrombin activates F XIII which is necessary for cross-linking of fibrin and stabilization of the clot;
3. Thrombin activates factors VIII and V which in turn enhance the activation of F X and prothrombin, respectively;
4. Thrombin is a powerful platelet agonist;
5. Thrombin activates protein C, a natural anticoagulant
6. Thrombin activates thrombin-activatable fibrinolysis inhibitor (TAFI) which protects clot from fibrinolysis.

Thromboplastin: Tissue factor is required for activation of F VII in extrinsic pathway. It is composed of two parts: Protein and phospholipid. Tissue factor is distributed in all tissues, but especially high concentrations are present in brain, placenta, and lungs. Tissue factor (TF) is normally constitutively expressed on most cells, except endothelial cells and circulating blood cells. TF is expressed on endothelial cells and monocytes following exposure to endotoxin, C5a, immune complexes, IL-1, and tumor necrosis factor.

Factor V (MW 330,000; 1/2 life 12–36 hours): F V is a heat-labile factor which is inactivated rapidly at room temperature in vitro. F V is activated by thrombin and functions as a cofactor in the conversion of prothrombin to thrombin by the prothrombinase complex. About one-fifth of the F V in blood is stored in platelet alpha granules which is released when platelets are activated.

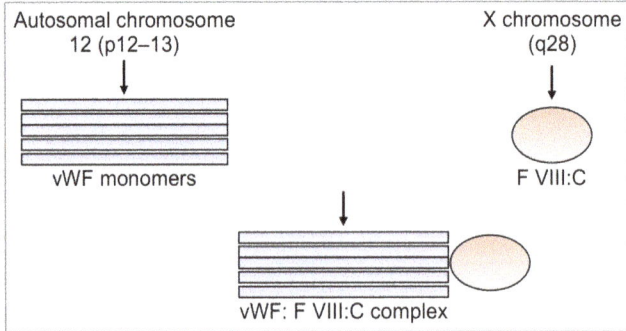

Fig. 1.35: Formation of FVIII: vWF complex.

Factor VII (MW 48,000; 1/2 life 6 hours): Tissue injury results in the formation of a complex between single chain form of F VII, tissue factor, and calcium which generates small amount of F Xa from F X. Factor Xa then in the reverse reaction cleaves F VII to yield F VIIa (two chain form); the F VIIa—tissue factor-calcium complex has greatly increased activity. This complex can also activate F IX.

Factor VIII (MW of F VIII: C-200,000; 1/2 life of F VIII:C approx. 12 hours): The F VIII circulates in plasma as a noncovalently bound complex of two components—F VIII:C and vWF. F VIII:C is the low molecular weight portion which has procoagulant activity and its synthesis is X-linked. F VIII mRNA is detected in various tissues; liver however, appears to be the primary source of F VIII. vWF is the high molecular weight component which is autosomal in inheritance and synthesized by endothelial cells and megakaryocytes (Fig. 1.35). vWF functions as a carrier protein for F VIII:C and also mediates adhesion of platelets to the subendothelium at sites of vessel damage.

The gene that codes for F VIII is located on the long arm of the X chromosome. It is 186 kilobases long and consists of 26 exons. The RNA is approximately 9 kilobases in length. The F VIII protein is composed of various domains, which are arranged as A1-A2-B-A3-C1-C2. A1 and A2 domains constitute the heavy chain of the molecule, while A3, C1, and C2 make up the light chain. B is the connecting region (Fig. 1.36).

Thrombin proteolytically cleaves F VIII molecule at three different positions to form activated F VIII. Activated F VIII functions as a cofactor in the reaction F X × F Xa and enhances the velocity of this reaction several thousand-fold. Further cleavage by thrombin and activated protein C in activates VIII.

Various terms and definitions related to F VIII and vWF are given below:
- *Vlll vWF:* Complex of F VIII procoagulant protein and vWF
- *F VIII:C:* F VIII coagulant activity which is measured by clotting assay
- *F VIII:C Ag:* Antigenic expression of F VIII measured by immunologic technique
- *VWF:* A multimeric protein necessary for platelet adhesion
- *VWF:RCo:* Ristocetin cofactor activity, the activity of vWF required for ristocetin-induced platelet aggregation
- *VWFAg:* Antigenic expression of vWF measured by immunological technique.

Factor IX (MW 57,000; 1/2 life 24 hours): F IX, a vitamin K-dependent glycoprotein, is activated by F XIa or by F VIIa-tissue factor complex to F IXa, a two-chain molecule. F IX is inherited in a sex-linked manner.

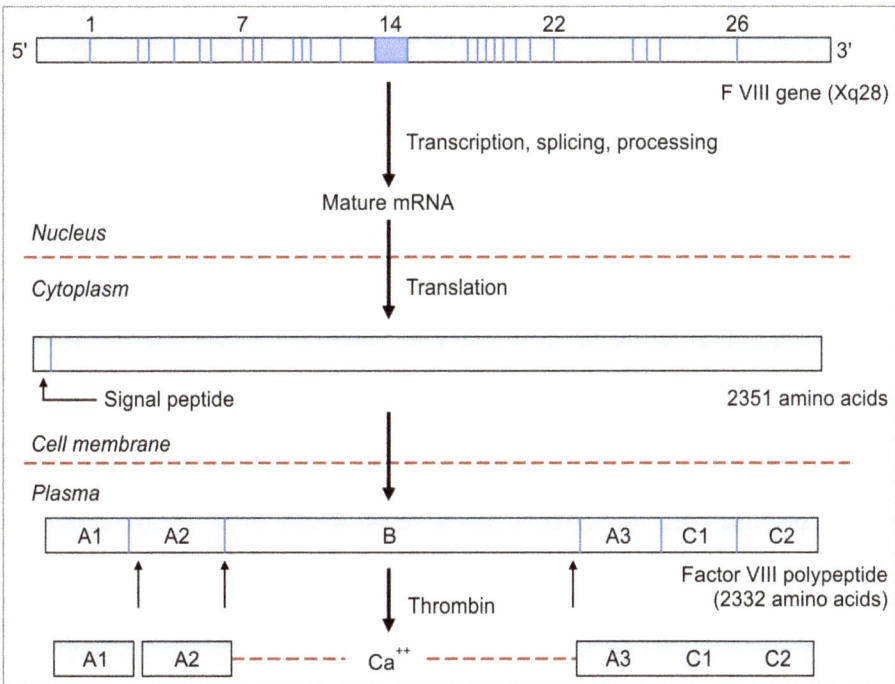

Fig. 1.36: Factor VIII gene and factor VIII molecule. F VIII gene has 26 exons and 25 introns. Polypeptide chain encoded by the gene has six regions: A1, A2, B, A3, C1, and C2. Proteolytic action by thrombin (small arrows) produces activated F VIII molecule.

Factor X (MW 58,000; 1/2 life 20–40 hours): F X, a vitamin K-dependent protein, is activated by both intrinsic (i.e. F IXa-VIII-phospholipid-calcium complex) and extrinsic (i.e. tissue factor-VII complex) pathways. It is necessary for the formation of prothrombinase (Xa-V-phospholipid-calcium) in the common pathway.

Factor XI (MW 160,000; 1/2 life 40–80 hours): F XI is activated by F XIIa in the presence of high molecular weight kininogen. Its activity increases upon storage.

Factor XII (MW 80,000; 1/2 life 40–50 hours): F XII is activated when it comes in contact with substances, such as collagen, glass, celite, ellagic acid, etc. F XIIa converts F XI to its active form and also prekallikrein to kallikrein. F XII plays a role in contact activation of coagulation system, inflammatory response, complement system, fibrinolysis, and formation of kallikrein and kinin.

Factor XIII (MW 320,000; 1/2 life 3–7 days): In contrast to all other coagulation factors, F XIII is a transglutaminase. Activated F XIII catalyzes the formation of covalent bonds between adjacent molecules of fibrin monomer (cross-linking) which provides stability to the fibrin clot.

Prekallikrein (MW 88,000; 1/2 life 35 hours): Prekallikrein is activated by F XIIa to kallikrein. Kallikrein in turn further activates F XII and thus serves to amplify the initial stimulus. Kallikrein plays a role in chemotaxis and in activation of fibrinolysis. Kallikrein also converts high molecular weight kininogen to bradykinin, a chemical mediator of inflammation.

High molecular weight kininogen (MW 110,000; 1/2 life 6.5 days): This circulates in plasma complexed to prekallikrein and F XI. It promotes contact activation.

Role of von Willebrand factor (vWF) in hemostasis: vWF is synthesized by both endothelial cells (Weibel-Palade bodies) and platelets (alpha granules). It circulates in plasma in the form of multimers. Its size is regulated by proteolysis of ultralarge multimers by ADAMTS13. The two main functions of vWF are (1) adhesion of platelets to subendothelium, and (2) binding to FVIII:C in circulation to protect it from proteolysis.

Mechanism of Blood Coagulation

Scheme of blood coagulation is divided into intrinsic, extrinsic, and common pathways (Fig. 1.37). The intrinsic pathway is initiated by contact activation and consists of interaction of contact factors (F XII, F XI, prekallikrein, and high molecular weight kininogen), F IX, F VIII, phospholipid, and calcium; these reactions generate a complex which causes activation of F X to F Xa. The extrinsic pathway is initiated by tissue injury with release of tissue thromboplastin which causes activation of F VII; the enzyme which is formed activates F X. Both intrinsic and extrinsic pathways proceed to common pathway which begins with activation of F X, involves interaction of F X, F V, prothrombin, phospholipid, calcium, and F XIII and leads to the formation of fibrin.

Intrinsic pathway: Initiation of intrinsic pathway occurs when plasma comes in contact with a negatively charged surface, such as glass, kaolin, celite, or ellagic acid in vitro. In vivo, this surface is probably provided by subendothelium of a damaged vessel. Following contact with a negatively charged surface, a conformational change in F XII with exposure of enzymatically active site probably occurs and in this way a small amount of F XIIa is formed. F XIIa converts prekallikrein to kallikrein and F XI to F XIa in the presence of high molecular weight kininogen.

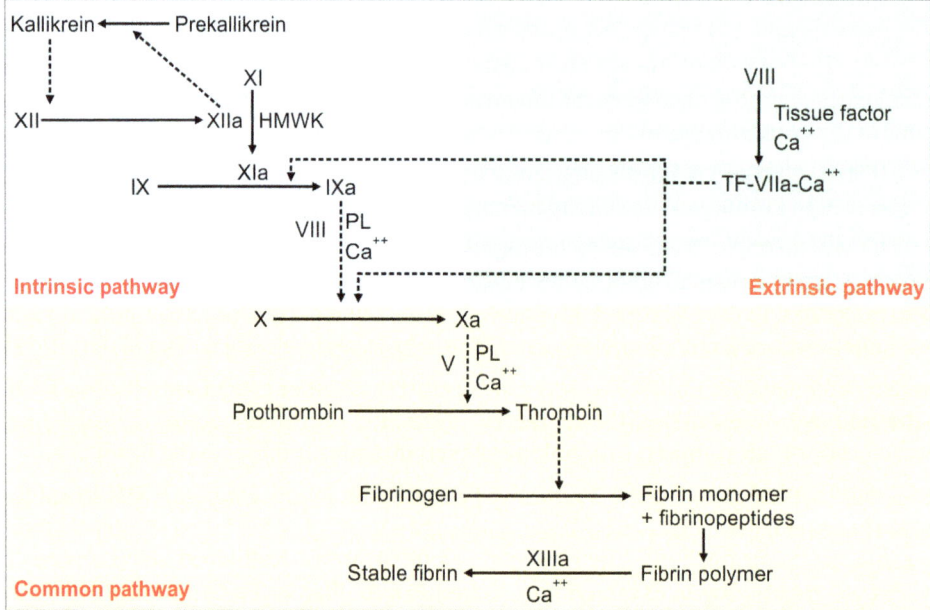

Fig. 1.37: Scheme of blood coagulation. Solid arrows indicate transformation. Broken lines indicate action.
(HMWK: high molecular weight kininogen; TF: tissue factor; PL: phospholipid; Ca^{++}: calcium).

Kallikrein in turn activates more F XII thus providing autoamplification of the reaction. F XIa cleaves F IX to yield F IXa; this reaction requires the presence of phospholipid and calcium. F IX a complexes with activated F VIII, phospholipid, and calcium and activates F X to F Xa. F VIII is activated by thrombin and also by F Xa. F VIII does not possess enzymatic activity but functions as a cofactor; in its presence the reaction rate is enhanced several thousand times.

Extrinsic pathway: F VII complexes with tissue factor released after tissue injury in the presence of calcium ions and activates F X and F IX. F Xa and thrombin convert the single-chain form of F VII to the two-chain form which has greatly increased enzymatic activity as compared to the single-chain form. This reciprocal activation of F VII leads to autoamplification of the reaction.

The concept of intrinsic and extrinsic pathways of blood coagulation is applicable to in vitro blood clotting. It is uncertain whether intrinsic pathway plays any significant role in vivo. This is because of observed absence of hemorrhagic tendencies in patients of F XII, prekallikrein, or HMWK deficiency. Also, in addition to F VII of extrinsic pathway, tissue factor has also been shown to activate F IX to F IXa in intrinsic pathway. In vivo, blood clotting seems to be initiated primarily by tissue factor.

Common pathway: Common pathway begins with the activation of F X. F Xa generated by intrinsic or extrinsic pathway complexes with F V, phospholipid, and calcium. This is called prothrombinase complex which activates prothrombin to thrombin. F V is modified by thrombin or F Xa to form activated F V which functions as a cofactor in the above reaction. Thrombin removes fibrinopeptides A and B from α and β chains of the fibrinogen molecule to form fibrin monomer. Free fibrin monomers spontaneously polymerize by forming end-to-end and side-to-side noncovalent bonds with each other. This is called fibrin polymer. F XIIIa (generated from F XIII by thrombin), in the presence of calcium, mediates the formation of covalent bonds between adjacent polypeptide chains. This cross-linking of fibrin monomers imparts structural stability to the clot (Fig. 1.38).

Cell-based model of hemostasis: According to the recent concept, coagulation process in vivo occurs in three overlapping phases: Initiation, amplification, and propagation (Fig 1.39).

Initiation: Initiation phase occurs on the surface of TF-expressing cells (usually endothelium). It begins with exposure of TF to coagulation factors upon endothelial injury or upon endothelial activation. TF is exposed on endothelial cells by endotoxins (bacterial lipopolysaccharides), IL-1, tissue necrosis factor-α, C5a, or immune complexes. TF complexes with both factor VII and the small proportion of factor VII that is circulating in the activated form. Inactive factor VII is then rapidly activated after complexing with TF. Complex of TF with FVIIa is called as TF-VIIa complex. This complex converts FIX to FIXa and FX to FXa. If FXa diffuses from the cell surface on which it was activated, it is quickly inhibited by the TF pathway inhibitor (TFPI) or antithrombin (AT). However, the FXa that remains on the TF cell surface combines with FVa ((FXa-FVa-Ca++) to generate small amounts of thrombin.

The FVIIa/TF complex formed initially is subsequently inhibited by TFPI. However, FIXa is not inhibited by TFPI and it slowly moves in the fluid phase from TF-bearing cells to adjacent platelets located at the site of injury.

Amplification or priming: Low concentration of thrombin generated in the initiation phase activates platelets adhering to the injury site which release FV from their α-granules. Thrombin activates FV and FVIII to their activated forms. These activated factors bind to platelet surfaces.

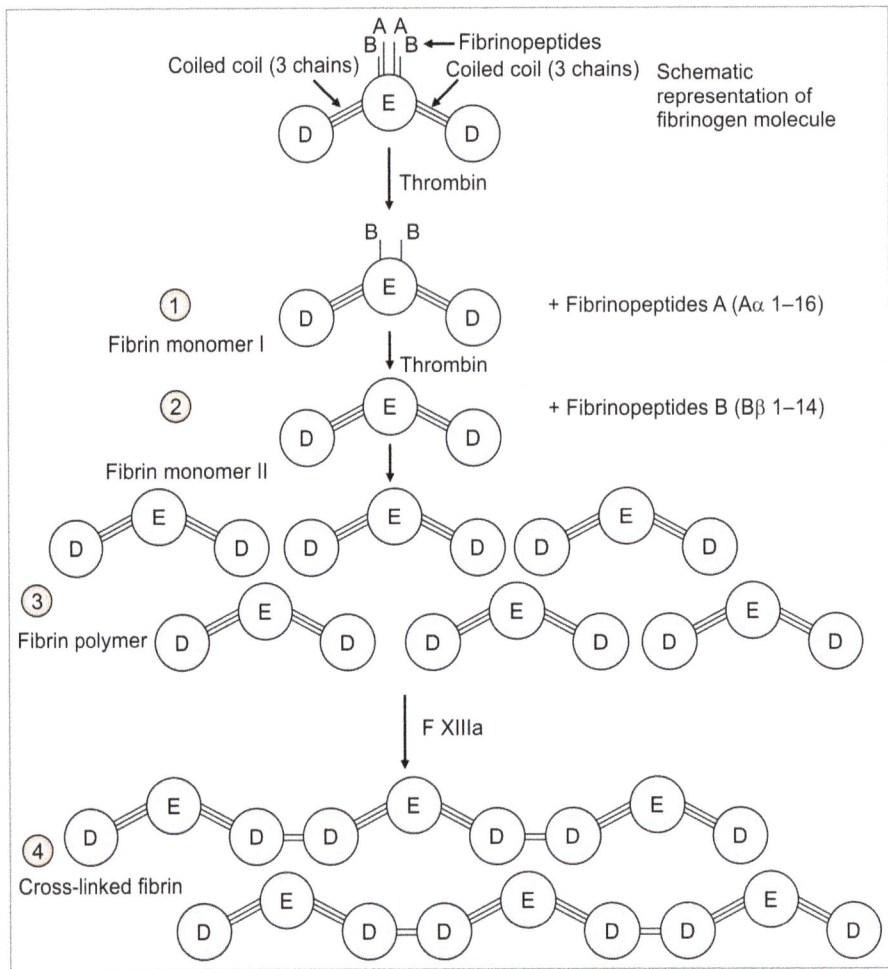

Fig. 1.38: Steps in the formation of cross-linked fibrin. 1 and 2: Cleaving of fibrinopeptides from fibrinogen by thrombin to form fibrin monomers. 3: Spontaneous polymerization of fibrin monomers. 4: Cross-linking of fibrin monomers mediated by F XIIIa. During this stage, covalent bonds form mainly between adjacent γ chains. For simplicity Aα chains are not shown.

Propagation: The FIXa-FVIIIa-Ca^{++} complex is formed on the surface of activated platelets. This complex activates FX; subsequently, FXa complexes with FVa to produce a burst of thrombin. Adequate thrombin is generated which cleaves fibrinogen to fibrin. Thrombin activates FXIII to FXIIIa which stabilizes fibrin to form a stable clot.

Fibrinolytic System

Fibrinolysis is the process of dissolution of blood clots which is necessary to maintain the free flow of blood in the vascular system. The major enzyme of the fibrinolytic system is plasmin, which is generated from proteolytic cleavage of plasminogen. Plasmin can cause cleavage of both fibrinogen as well as fibrin. Plasmin digests insoluble or cross-linked fibrin to release fibrin

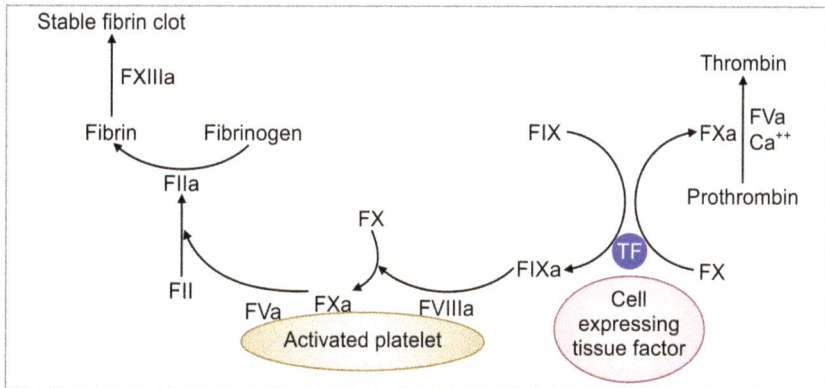

Fig. 1.39: Cell-based model of coagulation.

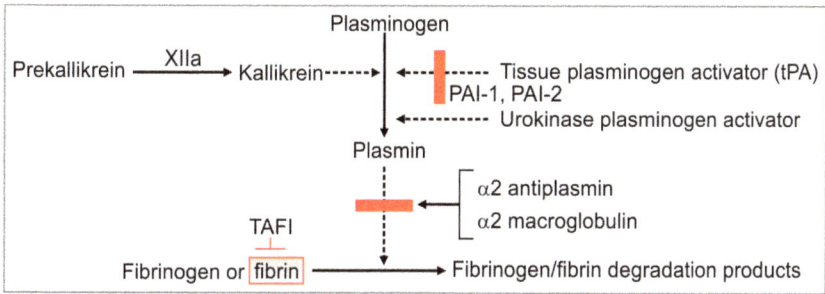

Fig. 1.40: The fibrinolytic system.

degradation products or FDPs which are then cleared from the circulation by macrophages of the mononuclear phagocytic system.

Plasminogen is converted to plasmin by plasminogen activators. This reaction occurs on the surface of fibrin. The plasminogen activators include—(1) tissue plasminogen activator (tPA): This is synthesized by endothelial cells and is the most important physiological plasminogen activator. tPA most efficiently converts plasminogen to plasmin when plasminogen is bound to the fibrin clot; (2) kallikrein (formed from prekallikrein by the action of F XIIa) converts plasminogen to plasmin (Fig. 1.40).

Inhibitors of fibrinolysis: These include (1) α2-antiplasmin which combines rapidly with plasmin in circulation to form plasmin-antiplasmin complex; (2) α2-macroglobulin which inhibits plasmin; (3) plasminogen activator inhibitors PAI-1 and PAI-2 released from endothelial cells which neutralize tPA; and (4) thrombin-activated fibrinolytic inhibitor (TAFI) which cleaves specific fibrin lysine residues, thus removing binding sites for plasminogen and tPA.

Components of fibrinolytic system are shown in Table 1.8.

Fibrinogen degradation products: Plasmin initially attacks α chains of the fibrinogen molecule and removes small fragments designated as A, B, and C from the C-terminals of the A α chains. This is followed by degradation of B β chains with removal of first 42 amino acids. This leads to the formation of a large fragment X that still retains fibrinopeptide A. The next cleavage involves

Table 1.8: Components of the fibrinolytic system.

Name	Site of synthesis	Function
Fibrinolytic agents		
Plasminogen	Liver	Zymogen; inactive precursor of plasmin
Plasmin	-	Serine protease enzyme that cleaves fibrin
Plasminogen activators		
Tissue plasminogen activator (tPA)	Endothelium	Extrinsic activator; converts plasminogen to plasmin when bound to fibrin
Urokinase type plasminogen activator (uPA)	Endothelium, kidney	Extrinsic activator; converts plasminogen to plasmin; reaction is amplified when cleaved by plasmin to tcuPA
Intrinsic or accessory activators	Liver	Kallikrein, FXIIa, FXIa; activate plasminogen directly
Fibrinolytic inhibitors		
Plasminogen activator inhibitor-1 (PAI-1)	Endothelium, monocytes/macrophages, liver cells, fat cells	**Ser**ine **p**rotease **in**hibitor (Serpin); primary physiologic inhibitor of tPA and uPA
Plasminogen activator inhibitor-2 (PAI-2)	Placenta, monocytes/macrophages, tumor cells	Serine protease inhibitor (serpin) of tPA and uPA
α2-antiplasmin (α2-plasmin inhibitor)	Liver, kidney	Inhibitor of plasmin
Thrombin-activatable fibrinolysis inhibitor (TAFI)	Liver	Carboxypeptidase; removes lysine residues from fibrin and thus interferes with the binding of plasminogen and tPA to fibrin
C1-esterase inhibitor	Liver	Protease inhibitor (Serpin); Inhibits complement proteins C1q and C1s, kallikrein, FXIIa, and plasmin
Activation receptors		
uPA Receptor (uPAR)	Located on endothelial cells, monocytes, and macrophages	Ligand for uPA
Annexin A2	Located on endothelial cell, monocytes, and macrophages	Ligand for tPA and plasminogen

Note: Prothrombin, tPA, uPA, and plasminogen have "kringle" domains (named after Danish Pastry) that helps them to bind to fibrinogen

all the three chains in an asymmetrical manner with the release of fragment Y and fragment D. Fragment Y is rapidly degraded by plasmin liberating two fragments D and E (Fig. 1.41).

Fibrin degradation products: Degradation of cross-linked fibrin is different from that of fibrinogen. Firstly, the fibrin degradation products are different because of the presence of covalent bonding. Thus, the characteristic fragments are oligomers of X and Y, D-dimer, D2E complex, and Y-D complex. Secondly, fibrin degradation is slower due to the presence of cross-linkages (Fig. 1.42).

Effects of FDPs: Normally, the FDPs are cleared from the circulation by macrophages of the reticuloendothelial system. However, when FDPs increase they have a potent anticoagulant

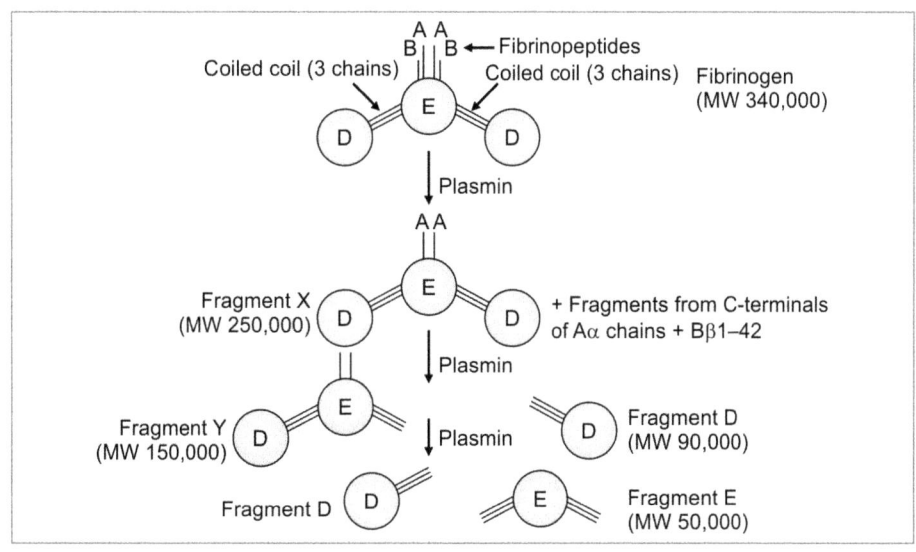

Fig. 1.41: Fibrinogen degradation products.

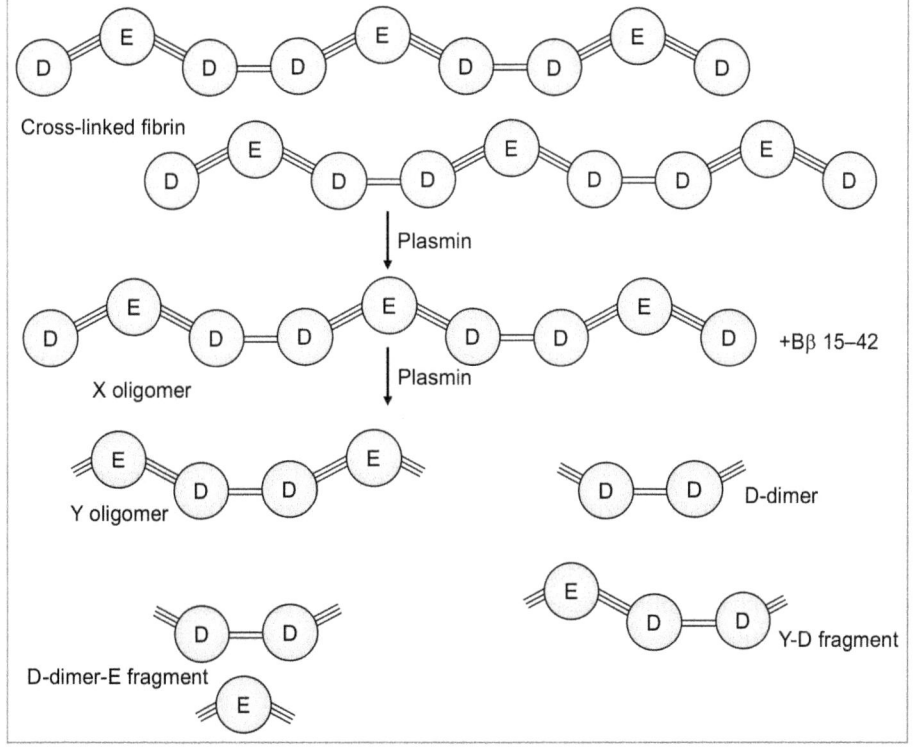

Fig. 1.42: Fibrin degradation products.

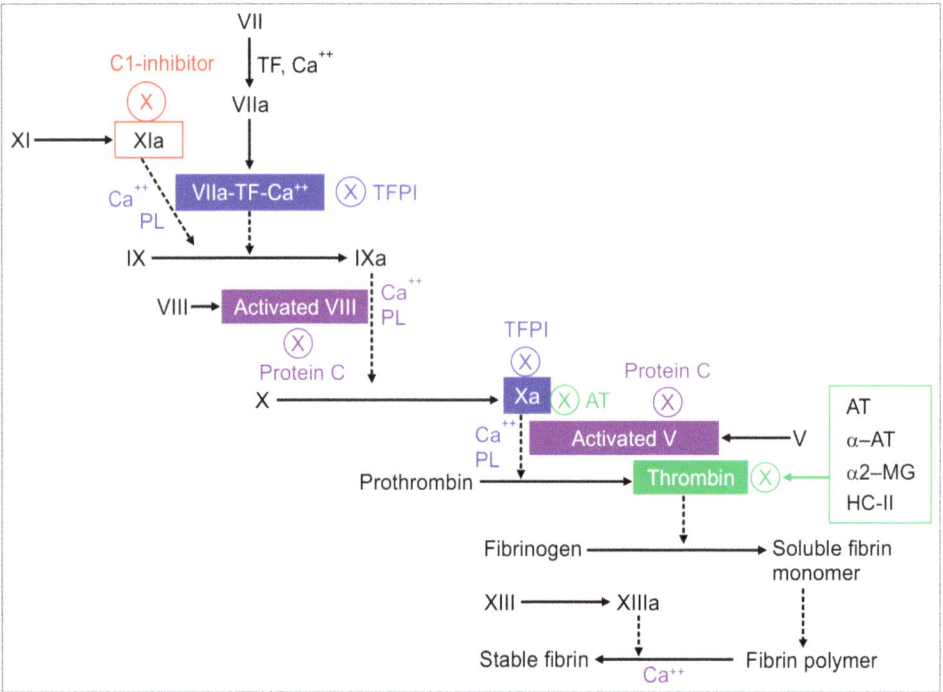

Fig. 1.43: Natural inhibitors of coagulation: These include (1) tissue factor pathway inhibitor (TFPI) (binds to F Xa and then to VIIa-TF-Ca++ complex), (2) antithrombin (AT) (inhibits mainly thrombin and F Xa), (3) protein C pathway (inactivates activated forms of F VIII and F V), (4) α1-antitrypsin (a-AT), α2-macroglobulin (α2-MG), and heparin cofactor-II (HC-II) inhibit thrombin, and (5) C1-inhibitor inhibits F XIa.

action in the form of inhibition of polymerization of fibrin, antithrombin activity, and impairment of platelet function.

Natural Inhibitors of Coagulation

There are three main physiologic inhibitors of coagulation that are present in normal plasma. These are antithrombin (previously called antithrombin III), protein C and protein S system, and tissue factor pathway inhibitor (Fig. 1.43 and Table 1.9).

Antithrombin (AT): AT is the most important physiologic inhibitor of coagulation. This is a single chain glycoprotein synthesized by the liver. AT possesses inhibitory activity principally against thrombin and to a lesser extent against factors Xa, XIa, XIIa, and IXa. AT binds with thrombin and other serine proteases to form a stable complex. Heparin-like substances present on the luminal surface of blood vessels promote activity of AT. The importance of AT as a natural anticoagulant derives from the fact that AT deficiency is associated with increased risk of thrombosis.

Heparin binds with AT and potentiates its action. This is the basis of efficacy of heparin as a therapeutic anticoagulant.

Table 1.9: Natural inhibitors of coagulation.

Name	Nature	Function
Antithrombin	Serine protease inhibitor (Serpin)	Inhibits thrombin, FXa, XIa, XIIa, and IXa
Protein C	Serine protease	Inactivates FVa and FVIIIa
Protein S	Inhibitory cofactor	Cofactor for activated protein C in inactivating FVa and FVIIIa
Protein Z-dependent protease inhibitor	Serine protease inhibitor (Serpin)	Inhibits FXa along with cofactor protein Z
Protein Z	Inhibitory cofactor	Cofactor for inhibition of FXa by protein Z-dependent protease inhibitor
Tissue factor pathway inhibitor	Protease inhibitor	Inhibitor of FVIIa and FXa
Thrombomodulin	Cofactor/Modulator	Cofactor for activation of protein C
Heparin cofactor II	Serine protease inhibitor (Serpin)	Thrombin inhibitor
α1-protease inhibitor (α1-antitrypsin)	Serine protease inhibitor (Serpin)	Inhibitor of FXIa
α2-macroglobulin	Protease inhibitor	Inhibitor of thrombin, kallikrein, and plasmin
C1-esterase inhibitor	Serine protease inhibitor (Serpin)	Inhibitor of complement (C1r and C1s), kallikrein, FXIa, FXIIa
Protein C inhibitor	Serine protease inhibitor (Serpin)	Inhibitor of activated protein C

Protein C: Protein C is a vitamin K-dependent glycoprotein synthesized in the liver. It circulates in an inert zymogen form and is activated by thrombin in the presence of thrombomodulin on the surface of vascular endothelial cells. It causes proteolytic destruction of activated factors V and VIII. Protein S, another vitamin K-dependent protein, functions as a cofactor in this reaction and enhances the action of protein C. It also appears to enhance fibrinolysis.

An inhibitor of protein C is present in plasma; it is thought that deficiency of this inhibitor accounts for cases of combined deficiency of F V and F VIII.

Deficiency of protein C or S is associated with risk of thrombosis.

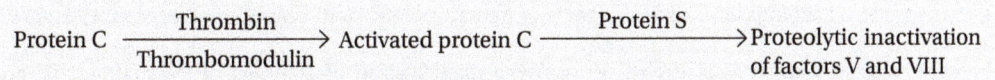

Tissue factor pathway inhibitor (TFPI): This binds to F Xa, and F Xa-TFPI complex then attaches to tissue factor-VII complex to neutralize it.

BIBLIOGRAPHY

1. Baugh RF, Hougie C. Structure and function in blood coagulation. In: Poller L (Ed). Recent Advances in Blood Coagulation. No. 3. Edinburgh, Churchill Livingstone; 1981.
2. Bottomley SS, Muller-Eberhard U. Pathophysiology of heme synthesis. Semin Hematol. 1988;25:282-302.
3. Brommer EJP, Brakman P. Developments in fibrinolysis. In: Poller L (Ed): Recent Advances in Blood Coagulation. No. 5. Edinburgh, Churchill Livingstone; 1991.
4. Cannistra SA, Griffin JD. Regulation of the production and function of granulocytes and monocytes. Semin Hematol. 1988;25:173-88.
5. Collen D, Lijnen HR. Basic and clinical aspects of fibrinolysis and thrombolysis. Blood. 1991;78: 3114-24.
6. Dacie JV, Lewis SM. Practical Haematology. 7th edition. Edinburgh, Churchill Livingstone; 1991. pp. 54-79
7. Furie B, Furie BC. Molecular and cellular biology of blood coagulation. N Engl J Med. 1992;326: 800-806.
8. Gerrard JM, Didisheim P. Platelet structure, biochemistry and physiology. In Poller L (Ed): Recent Advances in Blood Coagulation. No. 3. Edinburgh, Churchill Livingstone; 1981.
9. Greer JP, Foerster J, Rodgers GM, et al. Wintrobe's Clinical Hematology. 12 th edition. Philadelphia. Lippincott Williams & Wilkins; 2009.
10. Groopman JE. Colony-stimulating factors: Present status and future applications. Semin Hematol. 1988;25: 30-7.
11. High KA, Benz EJ. The ABC of molecular genetics. A haematologist's introduction. In: Hoffbrand, AV (Ed): Recent Advances in Haematology. Vol. 4. Edinburgh, Churchill Livingstone; 1985.
12. Holmsen H. Platelet metabolism and activation. Semin Hematol. 1985;22: 219-40.
13. Imboden JB, Jr. T lymphocytes and natural killer cells. In: Stites DP, Terr AL, Parslow TG (Eds). Basic and Clinical Immunology. 8th edition. Connecticut, Appleton and Lange; 1994.
14. Johnston RB. Monocytes and macrophages. N Engl J Med. 1988;318:747-52.
15. Kumar V, Abbas AK, Fausto N, et al. Robbins and Cotran Pathologic basis of disease. 8th edition. Philadelphia, Saunders Elsevier; 2010.
16. Lenting PJ, van Mourik JA, Mertens K. The life cycle of coagulation factor VIII in view of its structure and function. Blood. 1998;92:3983-96.
17. McPherson RA, Pincus MR (Eds). Henry's Clinical Diagnosis and Management by Laboratory Methods. 21st edition. Philadelphia, Elsevier Saunders; 2007.
18. Mohandas N, Chasis JA. Red blood cell deformability, membrane material properties and shape: Regulation by transmembrane, skeletal, and cytosolic proteins and lipids. Semin Hematol. 1993;30: 171-92.
19. Nathan CF. Secretory products of macrophages. J Clin Invest. 1987;79:319-26.
20. Ogston D, Bennett B. Blood coagulation mechanism. In: Poller L (Ed). Recent Advances in Blood Coagulation. No. 5. Edinburgh, Churchill Livingstone; 1991.
21. Parslow TG. Immunoglobulin genes, B cells, and the humoral immune response. In: Stites DP, Terr AL, Parslow TG (Eds). Basic and Clinical Immunology. 8th edition. Connecticut, Appleton and Lange; 1994.
22. Sixma JJ. The haemostatic plug. In Poller L (Ed): Recent Advances in Blood Coagulation. No. 3. Edinburgh, Churchill Livingstone; 1981.
23. Spangrude GJ. Biologic and clinical aspects of hematopoietic stem cells. Annu Rev Med. 1994;45:93-104.
24. Swerdlow SH, Campo E, Harris NL, et al. WHO Classification of Tumours of Haematopoietic and Lymphoid Tissues. 4th edition. Lyon. International Agency for Research on Cancer. 2008.
25. Van der Valk P, Herman CJ. Leucocyte functions. Lab Invest. 1987;56:127-37.
26. Williams D, Nathan DG. Introduction: the molecular biology of hematopoiesis. Semin Hematol. 1991;28:114-16.

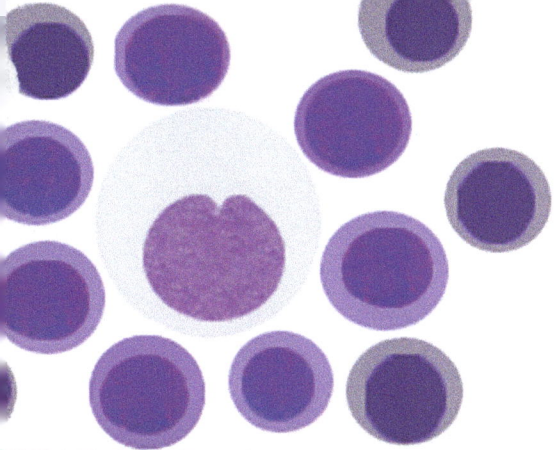

Disorders of Red Blood Cells (Anemias)

Section Outline

2. Approach to Diagnosis of Anemias *61*
3. Anemias due to Impaired Red Cell Production *81*
4. Anemias due to Excessive Red Cell Destruction *133*

SECTION 2

CHAPTER 2

Approach to Diagnosis of Anemias

INTRODUCTION

Anemia is defined as a reduction in the concentration of circulating hemoglobin or oxygen-carrying capacity of blood below the level that is expected for healthy persons of same age and sex in the same environment. Normal hemoglobin (and packed cell volume or PCV) levels are given in Table 2.1. Anemia exists if hemoglobin or PCV level is below the lower limit of normal for the particular age and sex.

The normal hemoglobin level depends upon age and sex of the individual and the environment. The difference in hemoglobin level between sexes is related to the androgens that have stimulatory effect on erythropoiesis. The lower level of hemoglobin during pregnancy as compared to the nonpregnant state is due to hemodilution caused by expansion of plasma volume. The normal hemoglobin level in newborn period is highest; subsequently hemoglobin level falls and reaches minimum level by 2 months of age. Hemoglobin level reaches adult levels by puberty. Adult levels of hemoglobin remain similar until the age of 70 years. Over the next two decades of life, hemoglobin level falls by about 0.2 g/dL in females, while in males, it falls by more than 1 g/dL due to fall in androgen level. Persons living at high altitudes who are exposed to low oxygen tensions have a higher hemoglobin concentration than persons living at sea level.

Hemoglobin level is highest at birth and gradually falls during infancy; this is called as physiological anemia of infancy and is due to physiologic adaptation in response to

Table 2.1: Normal levels of hemoglobin and packed cell volume.

Age/sex	Hemoglobin (g/dL)	PCV (%)
Adult males	13–17	40–50
Adult females (nonpregnant)	12–15	38–45
Adult females (pregnant)	11–14	36–42
Children, 6–12 years	11.5–15.5	37–46
Children, 6 months–6 years	11–14	36–42
Infants, 2–6 months	9.5–14	32–42
Newborns	13.6–19.6	44–60

transition from relative hypoxemia of intrauterine life to oxygenated environment after birth. Hemoglobin level remains low as compared to adults during childhood. This physiological anemia of childhood possibly results from lower oxygen affinity of hemoglobin secondary to hyperphosphatemia during growth period with associated elevated 2,3-diphosphoglycerate content in red cells.

APPROACH TO DIAGNOSIS

Anemia can result from a variety of causes. Investigations in a case of anemia should be directed toward answering following questions: (1) Is anemia present and if so, what is its severity? (2) What is the cause of anemia? In most cases, presence of anemia can be established and its cause determined with the help of clinical findings and a few simple investigations.

Establishing the Presence and Severity of Anemia

The tests used for this purpose are estimation of **hemoglobin concentration and packed cell volume**. The results of these tests are influenced by plasma volume. Increase in plasma volume with red cell count remaining normal causes hemodilution and measurement of hemoglobin or packed cell volume yields a subnormal result; this is known as "spurious" or "pseudo" anemia and occurs in third trimester of pregnancy (due to rise in plasma volume), splenomegaly (due to pooling of red cells in spleen), congestive cardiac failure (due to fluid retention), and paraproteinemias (rise in globulins).

As most of the volume of a red cell is occupied by hemoglobin, any measurement of a patient's total red cell volume (i.e. hematocrit or PCV) is equivalent to hemoglobin determination. Therefore, hemoglobin and hematocrit levels of a patient move together and either can be used interchangeably for diagnosis of anemia. However, red cell count does not always fall with reduction in hemoglobin/hematocrit level (e.g. low hemoglobin or hematocrit in thalassemia minor is associated with raised red cell count) and therefore is not reliable for diagnosis of anemia.

Determination of Hemoglobin Concentration

Various methods are available for estimation of hemoglobin (Table 2.2). Out of these, **cyanmethemoglobin method is the most accurate** and is recommended by the International Committee for Standardization in Haematology. In this method a specified amount of blood is mixed with a solution containing potassium ferricyanide and potassium cyanide (Drabkin's solution); potassium ferricyanide converts hemoglobin to methemoglobin while methemoglobin combines with potassium cyanide to form cyanmethemoglobin. Most forms of hemoglobin's present in blood (e.g. oxyhemoglobin, carboxyhemoglobin, methemoglobin, etc.) except sulfhemoglobin are completely converted to a single compound, cyanmethemoglobin. After completion of the reaction, absorbance of the solution is measured in a spectrophotometer at 540 nm. To obtain the hemoglobin concentration of the unknown sample, its absorbance is compared with that of the standard cyanmethemoglobin solution the hemoglobin concentration of which is known. The absorbance can be converted to hemoglobin concentration by using a formula or from previously constructed calibration graph or table.

Chapter 2: Approach to Diagnosis of Anemias

Table 2.2: Methods for the estimation of hemoglobin.

Colorimetric methods

Color comparison is made between the known standard and the test sample, either visually or by photoelectric colorimeter
• *Visual methods*
  – **Tallqvist blotting paper method:** Highly inaccurate and now obsolete
  – **Sahli's acid hematin method:** Inaccurate
  – **WHO hemoglobin color scale:** Simple, inexpensive, and reliable; especially suitable for those laboratories where photoelectric colorimeter is not available
• *Methods using photoelectric colorimeter*
  – **Cyanmethemoglobin method:** Most accurate and recommended method
  – **Oxyhemoglobin method:** Reliable method; however, no stable standard is available
  – **Alkaline hematin method:** Accurate method

Gasometric method
Oxygen-carrying capacity of blood is measured in Van Slyke apparatus; not suitable for routine use
Chemical method
Iron content of blood is measured and value of hemoglobin is calculated indirectly; tedious and time-consuming method
Specific gravity method
Simple, rapid, and inexpensive method in which a rough estimate of hemoglobin is obtained from specific gravity of blood; used for mass screening like selection of blood donors.

Anemia can be graded according to hemoglobin concentration as shown in Box 2.1.

Determination of Packed Cell Volume (PCV/Hematocrit)

Packed cell volume is the volume of packed red cells obtained after centrifugation of a sample of anticoagulated venous or capillary blood. It is expressed either as a percentage of volume of whole blood or as a decimal fraction.

Uses of PCV are: (i) detection of anemia and polycythemia; PCV is normally about three times the hemoglobin concentration when the latter is expressed in g/dL (Box 2.2); (ii) calculation of red cell indices, such as mean cell volume (MCV) and mean cell hemoglobin concentration (MCHC); (iii) checking the accuracy of hemoglobin value.

Box 2.1: Grading of anemia.
- Mild: Hemoglobin from lower limit of normal to 10.0 g/dL
- Moderate: 10.0–7.0 g/dL
- Severe: <7.0 g/dL

Box 2.2: Rule of 3.
- Red cell count in millions/mm^3 × 3 = Hemoglobin in g/dL
- Hemoglobin in g/dL × 3 = PCV in %
- Rule of 3 is used as a mathematical check by clinicians and technologists
- Rule of 3 applies mainly to normocytic normochromic specimens

There are two methods for determining PCV—macromethod (Wintrobe method) and micromethod (microhematocrit method):

1. **Wintrobe method:** Anticoagulated whole blood is centrifuged in a Wintrobe tube at 2300 G for 30 minutes to pack the red cells. The level of the column of the red cells is directly read from the tube. Wintrobe tube is 110 mm in length with 3 mm internal bore is marked at every 1 mm up to 100 and has a capacity for about 1 mL of blood. After centrifugation, three layers can be distinguished—a column of straw-colored plasma at the top, a thin grayish layer of white cells and platelets in the middle ("buffy layer"), and a column of

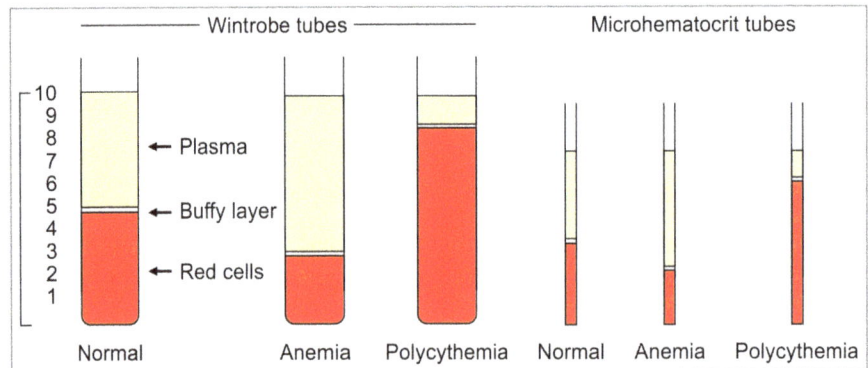

Fig. 2.1: Packed cell volume showing comparison of normal, anemic, and polycythemic blood samples; Red: Column of red cells; Gray: Buffy coat layer; Yellow: Column of plasma.

red cells at the bottom (Fig. 2.1). Sometimes additional information can be derived by observing the color of the plasma (pink in hemolysis, yellow in the presence of jaundice, colorless in iron deficiency anemia) and the thickness of the buffy layer (thick buffy layer indicates leukocytosis, thrombocytosis, or leukemia). Smears can also be prepared from the buffy coat layer for demonstration of blast cells and for malaria parasites (if they are few in number in blood).

2. *Microhematocrit method:* This method is simple, rapid, and needs only a small quantity of blood. Micromethod, however, requires microhematocrit centrifuge (or table top centrifuge with microhematocrit head) and capillary hematocrit tubes (75 mm long with a 1 mm bore). Two types of capillary hematocrit tubes are available: Anticoagulated (coated with heparin so that capillary blood can be directly collected) and plain (without anticoagulant so that anticoagulated blood is needed). The capillary tube is filled about three-fourth with blood, sealed a tone end, and centrifuged in a microhematocrit centrifuge at high speed for 5 minutes. The result is derived by using microhematocrit tube reading device or an arithmetic graph paper.

Determining the Cause of Anemia

When the presence of anemia is established, the next step is to determine the cause of anemia. Various causes of anemia are listed in Table 2.3. Main causes of anemia in India are shown in Box 2.3. Ascertaining the underlying cause of anemia requires correlation of clinical findings with results of laboratory investigations.

Clinical Evaluation

The symptoms and signs in an anemic patient may result from anemia *per se* and the underlying disorder causing anemia. The **symptoms and signs of anemia** include easy fatigability, effort dyspnea, tachycardia, and pallor. In severe cases, congestive cardiac failure can develop. The associated symptomatology may point toward the probable diagnosis and suggest the direction for laboratory investigation. A **history of chronic blood loss**, such as menorrhagia or hemorrhoids suggests iron deficiency as the cause of anemia. Anemia manifesting during **pregnancy** is usually nutritional due to deficiency of folate and iron. An intense and abnormal desire to eat strange substances, such as starch or earth (pica) is a peculiar feature of iron

Table 2.3: Etiological classification of anemia.

Anemias due to impaired red cell production

1. Anemias due to deficiency of nutrients
   - Iron deficiency anemia
   - Megaloblastic anemia due to deficiency of folate or vitamin B_{12}
2. Anemia of chronic disease
3. Sideroblastic anemia
4. Aplastic anemia and related disorders
5. Anemia of chronic renal disease
6. Anemia of liver disease
7. Anemia in endocrine disorders
8. Myelophthisic anemia (anemia due to replacement of marrow by metastatic carcinoma, leukemia, lymphoma, infections, storage disorders, etc.)
9. Congenital dyserythropoietic anemia

Anemias due to excessive red cell destruction (Hemolytic anemia)

Abnormality intrinsic to red cells	Abnormality extrinsic to red cells
1. **Defects in red cell membrane** – Hereditary spherocytosis – Hereditary elliptocytosis	1. **Immune hemolytic anemias** – Autoimmune – Alloimmune – Drug-induced
2. **Defects in hemoglobin** – Quantitative: Thalassemias – Qualitative: Sickle-cell disease; Hemoglobin D, E, or C disease	2. **Mechanical hemolytic anemia** – Microangiopathic – Cardiac – March hemoglobinuria
3. **Defects in enzymes** – Glucose-6-phosphate dehydrogenase deficiency – Pyruvate kinase deficiency	3. **Direct action of physical, chemical, or infectious agents**
	4. **Hypersplenism**

Anemias due to excess blood loss

Box 2.3: Important causes of anemia in India.

- Nutritional deficiency: Iron, folate, less commonly vitamin B_{12}
- Infections: Tuberculosis, malaria, kala-azar, HIV infection/AIDS, hookworm
- Inherited anemias: Thalassemias, sickle cell disorders, glucose-6-phosphate dehydrogenase deficiency
- Blood loss: Obstetrical problems

---

deficiency. When a **chronic alcoholic** presents with anemia, etiological considerations include vitamin B_{12} and folate deficiency, iron deficiency secondary to bleeding, chronic liver disease, and sideroblastic anemia. History of malabsorption, such as in celiac disease and tropical sprue indicates combined deficiency of folate, vitamin B_{12}, and iron. Drugs can cause various types of anemias, such as hypoplastic anemia (e.g. cytotoxic drugs, chloramphenicol, and phenylbutazone), megaloblastic anemia (e.g. methotrexate, trimethoprim, anticonvulsants), iron deficiency anemia (e.g. aspirin secondary to gastric blood loss), and hemolytic anemia (e.g. antimalarials, penicillins, methyldopa). A detailed drug history is therefore essential. A history of jaundice or gallstones in the patient and in a close relative may point toward inherited hemolytic anemia. In some cases, **primary underlying disease** may be responsible for anemia, for example, collagen vascular disease, malignancy, chronic infection, acquired

> **Box 2.4:** Prevalence of hereditary hemolytic anemia.
> - β-thalassemias: Mediterranean countries, Africa, Middle East, India (North India especially in Sindhis, Bhanushalis, Lohanas, Jains), Pakistan, South-East Asia
> - α-thalassemias: Southeast Asia
> - Sickle cell disorders: Africa, Middle East, Central and Southern India
> - Hemoglobin D disease: North India (Punjab)
> - Hemoglobin E disease: South-East Asia, East India (Bengal, Assam)
> - Hereditary spherocytosis: Northern European descent
> - Glucose-6-phosphate dehydrogenase (G6PD) deficiency: Africa, Middle East, India (especially in Parsees)

immunodeficiency syndrome, cirrhosis of liver, chronic renal disease, or endocrine disorder. Sometimes population studies conducted in the past can provide valuable information regarding the **prevalent form of anemia in a geographic area or in a particular community**. This applies particularly to sickle cell anemia, thalassemia, and glucose-6-phosphate dehydrogenase (G6PD) deficiency (Box 2.4).

Laboratory Evaluation

Initial investigations to define the underlying cause of anemia include examination of peripheral blood smear, reticulocyte count, and red cell indices. Depending on the results of these studies further specialized laboratory procedures may be carried out to arrive at a definitive diagnosis, such as bone marrow examination, determination of serum iron and total iron binding capacity, hemoglobin electrophoresis, etc.

Examination of peripheral blood smear: Peripheral blood smear or film provides important information regarding the underlying cause of anemia. Peripheral blood smear is prepared by spreading a drop of capillary or venous blood across a glass slide and staining it with a Romanowsky stain. A well-made blood film should show three zones—thick area or the "head," "body," and the thin portion or the "tail" of the smear. The smear should be smooth and uniform in appearance with gradual transition from thick to thin portion. It should not cover the entire area of the slide.

The blood film should be examined in an orderly manner under low and high powers and oil immersion lens for red cell morphology, presence of nucleated red cells, approximate number of white blood cells, differential leukocyte counts, abnormal white blood cells, parasites, and adequacy of platelets. Valuable information regarding the cause of anemia can be obtained by observing the red cell morphology (Box 2.5 and Fig. 2.2).

> The most important single test to determine the cause of anemia is peripheral blood smear. It provides information in the form of: (1) morphologic abnormalities (of red cells, white cells, and platelets) which are indicative of a particular diagnosis or differential diagnosis, and (2) confirmation of values generated by hematology analyzer (complete blood count) and identification of any spurious results.

Reticulocyte count: Reticulocytes are young red cells that contain RNA remnants. RNA stains with supravital dyes, such as brilliant cresyl blue or new methylene blue with formation of blue precipitates of granules or filaments (Fig. 2.3). After staining, smears are made on a glass slide, reticulocytes are counted among 1,000 red cells, and the result is expressed as a percentage.

> **Box 2.5:** Red cell terminology.
>
> - *Normocytic normochromic:* Red cells with normal size and color (i.e. normal hemoglobin content); 7–8 μ size; pink with small area of central pallor (1/3rd the diameter of red cell)
> - *Anisocytosis:* Significant variation in size of red cells
> - *Poikilocytosis:* Significant variation in shape of red cells; both aniso- and poikilocytosis are nonspecific features of a variety of anemias
> - *Microcytic hypochromic:* Red cells smaller than normal with increased area of central pallor due to deficiency of hemoglobin
> - *Macrocytic:* Red cells larger in size than normal; may be round or oval
> - *Sickle cells:* Elongated and narrow cells with one or both ends curved and pointed
> - *Spherocytes:* Small and densely staining red cells without central area of pallor
> - *Target cells:* Cells with accumulation of hemoglobin in center and periphery with clear intervening area producing a bull's eye or target-like appearance
> - *Schistocytes:* Irregular fragmented cells appearing as helmet-shaped and triangular
> - *Burr cells:* Cells with many spiny, small, regularly spaced projections on surface
> - *Tear drop red cells:* Cells with a tapering drop-like shape
> - *Polychromatic red cells:* Slightly larger red cells with faint blue-gray tint due to presence of ribosomal RNA
> - *Basophilic stippling (punctate basophilia):* Presence of fine (megaloblastic anemia) or coarse (lead poisoning) purple-blue granules (representing ribosomal aggregates) in red cells
> - *Howell-Jolly bodies:* Round, purple nuclear remnants in red cells
> - *Rouleaux:* Arrangement of red cells like a stack of coins
> - *Dimorphic red cells:* Presence of two different populations of red cells, e.g. macrocytic and hypochromic, normocytic and hypochromic, etc. Seen in sideroblastic anemia, partially treated anemia, myelodysplasia, and postblood transfusion

Reticulocyte count is performed to assess erythropoietic activity of the bone marrow in a case of anemia. In anemia due to decreased red cell production or ineffective erythropoiesis, reticulocyte count is low. In anemia with effective red cell production, reticulocyte count is high.
Measures of reticulocytes: Reticulocyte count can be expressed in various ways as follows:
1. **Reticulocyte count:** This is the number of reticulocytes counted amongst 1,000 red cells and expressed as percentage.

$$\text{Reticulocyte count} = \frac{\text{Reticulocytes counted}}{\text{Number of red cells}} \times 100$$

   In adults and children, the normal reticulocyte count is 0.5–2.5%. In newborns, reticulocyte count is 2–5%.
2. **Corrected reticulocyte count:** This is the reticulocyte count corrected for the degree of anemia.

$$\text{Corrected reticulocyte count} = \frac{\text{Reticulocyte count} \times \text{PCV of patient in \%}}{\text{Average PCV for age}}$$

3. **Absolute reticulocyte count:** This is the number of reticulocytes in 1 mm^3 of blood.
   Absolute reticulocyte count = Reticulocyte percentage × Red cell count in million/mm^3
   Normal absolute reticulocyte count is 50,000–100,000/mm^3.
4. **Reticulocyte production index:** After their formation in bone marrow, the reticulocytes normally spend about 2 days in bone marrow and 1 day in peripheral blood before they become fully mature red cells. However in severe hemolytic anemia and acute blood loss,

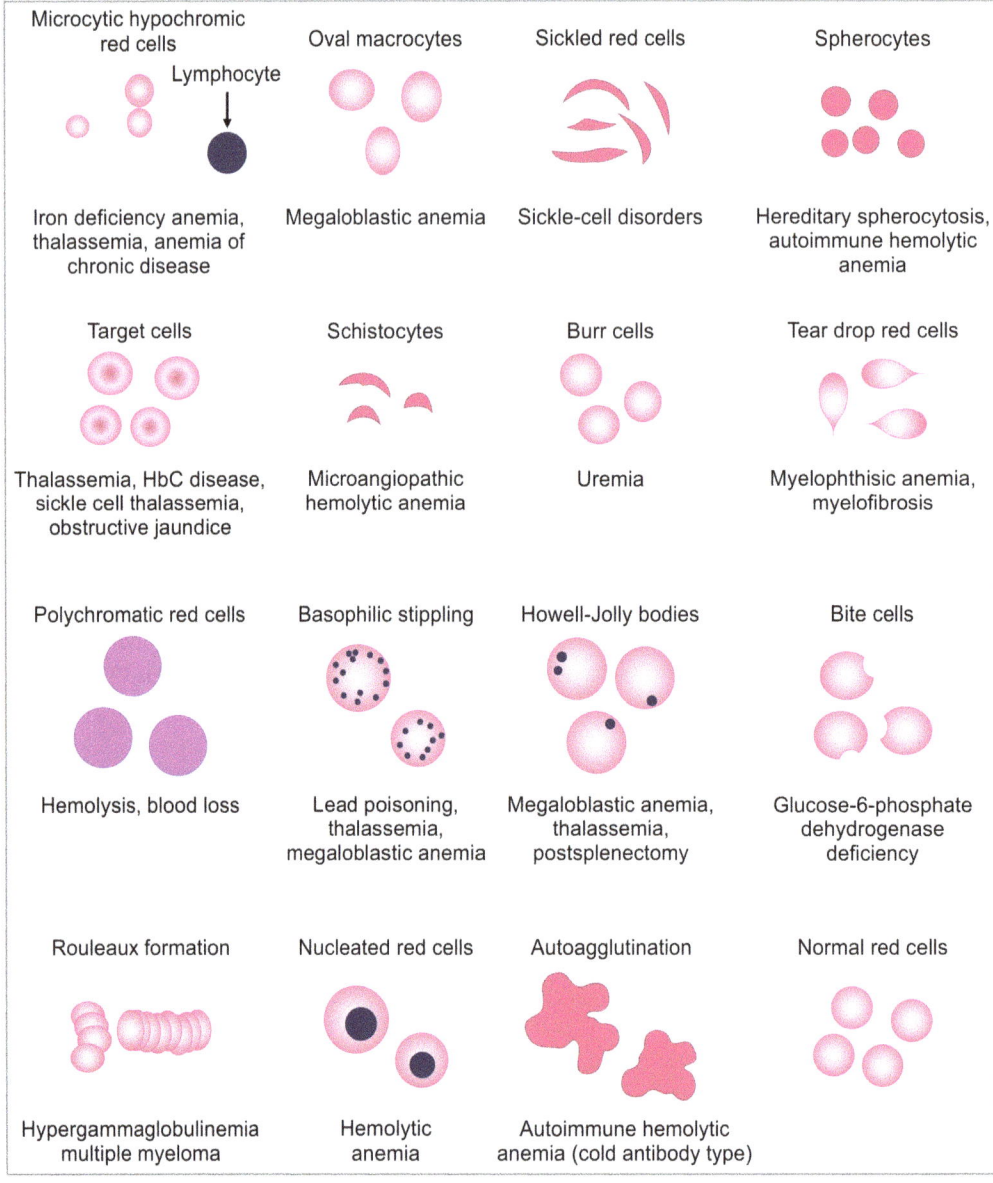

Fig. 2.2: Morphological abnormalities of red cells in different types of anemias; size of red cells is compared with the nucleus of a small lymphocyte (7 μ).

reticulocytes are released prematurely in peripheral circulation where they require more time (2 days) for maturation. This results in doubling of reticulocytes in blood. In such cases to avoid the overestimation of daily red cell production and to get idea about actual erythropoietic activity, reticulocyte production index is derived

$$\text{Reticulocyte production index} = \frac{\text{Corrected reticulocyte count}}{\text{Maturation time in days}}$$

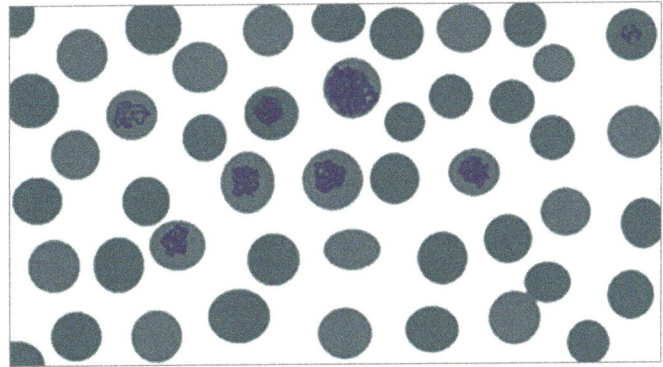

Fig. 2.3: Reticulocytes stained with a supravital stain: Following supravital staining, any non-nucleated red cell containing two or more granules of blue-stained material is considered as a reticulocyte; the blue-stained material represents ribosomal RNA and is more in immature reticulocytes.

Maturation times in days according to PCV are:
- PCV >40%   : 1.0
- PCV 30–40% : 1.5
- PCV 20–30% : 2.0
- PCV >20%   : 2.5

Reticulocytes should ideally be reported as absolute count or as corrected reticulocyte count for proper assessment of bone marrow response (low or appropriate) to anemia. For example, a reticulocyte count of 1% in a patient with 42% PCV and a reticulocyte count of 1% in another patient with 20% PCV may both appear to be normal. However, when corrected for PCV, the corrected reticulocyte counts are respectively 0.9% (normal, indicating normal erythropoietic activity) and 0.3% (low, indicating inadequate erythropoietic activity).

Causes of reticulocytosis:
- Acute blood loss
- Hemolytic anemia
- Response to specific therapy in nutritional anemia.

Causes of reticulocytopenia:
- Deficient red cell production:
  - Iron deficiency anemia
  - Anemia of chronic disease
  - Aplastic anemia
  - Anemia due to marrow infiltration (leukemia, lymphoma, metastatic cancer).
- Ineffective erythropoiesis: Megaloblastic anemia, thalassemia, sideroblastic anemia, congenital dyserythropoietic anemia, myelodysplastic syndrome.

Ineffective erythropoiesis is characterized by failure of production of mature red cells despite erythroid hyperplasia in bone marrow; this is due to destruction of defective erythroid precursors in bone marrow. Although unconjugated bilirubin and serum lactate dehydrogenase are elevated in hemolytic anemia and ineffective erythropoiesis, reticulocyte count is low in ineffective erythropoiesis and raised in hemolytic anemias. Serum LDH levels are markedly increased (often above 1,000 units/mL) in megaloblastic anemia (as compared to hemolytic anemia) due to intramedullary destruction of erythroid precursors (which contain more LDH as compared to red cells).

Some automated hematology analyzers measure reticulocyte count and other additional reticulocyte parameters as follows:

Reticulocyte count: Various fluorescent dyes can combine with RNA of reticulocytes; the fluorescence then is counted in a flow cytometer. More immature reticulocytes fluorescence more strongly as they contain more RNA.

Immature reticulocyte fraction (IRF): This parameter assesses reticulocyte maturity level based on RNA content (intensity of staining). In anemia, low IRF is an early sign of deficient red cell production. Following specific replacement therapy for nutritional anemia, it increases earlier than reticulocyte count and hemoglobin level and thus is an early indicator of therapeutic response. Following hematopoietic stem cell transplantation, an increase in IRF is an early marker of stem cell engraftment.

Reticulocyte hemoglobin content (CHr): Reticulocyte hemoglobin content is a parameter that estimates hemoglobinization of most recently produced red cells. Low CHr (<28 pg) is a marker for early diagnosis of iron deficiency. A raised CHr is an early sign of response to iron therapy (similar to IRF).

Classification of anemia according to the reticulocyte response is presented in Table 2.4.

> Best test for evaluation of pathophysiologic mechanism of anemia is reticulocyte count. It is the most relevant investigation in the initial evaluation of macrocytic and normocytic anemias.

Red cell indices: Red cell indices are helpful in the morphological classification of anemia (Table 2.5). They are derived from the values of red cell count, hemoglobin (Hb) concentration, and PCV. Red cell indices obtained by manual methods are often inaccurate. Electronic hematology cell analyzers more reliably perform them.

The normal ranges of red cell indices in adults are as follows:

MCV = 80–100 fl
MCH = 27–32 pg
MCHC = 32–36 g/dL

1. **Mean corpuscular volume (MCV):** MCV represents the average volume of a single red cell. It is expressed in femtoliters or fl ($1 \text{ fl} = 10^{-15}$ liters). MCV is performed manually as follows:

$$\text{MCV (in fl)} = \frac{\text{Packed cell volume in \%}}{\text{Red cell count in milion per mm}^3} \times 10$$

Table 2.4: Classification of anemia according to the reticulocyte response.

Reticulocyte response	Reticulocyte production index (Absolute reticulocyte count)	Causes
1. Appropriate for the degree of anemia	≥2% (>100,000/μL)	Hyperproliferative anemia (blood loss, hemolytic anemia)
2. Inappropriately low for the degree of anemia	<2% (<75,000/μL)	Hypoproliferative anemia (iron deficiency anemia, megaloblastic anemia, anemia of chronic disease, thalassemia, endocrine diseases, sideroblastic anemia, aplastic anemia, myelodysplasia)

Table 2.5: Morphological classification of anemia.

Macrocytic anemia (MCV >100 fl)	Microcytic anemia (MCV <80 fl)	Normocytic anemia (MCV 80–100 fl)
Megaloblastic anemia	Iron deficiency anemia	Reticulocyte production—normal
Nonmegaloblastic anemia	Thalassemias	• Recent blood loss
• Liver disease	Sideroblastic anemia	• Hemolytic anemia
• Hemolytic anemia	Anemia of chronic disease	Reticulocyte production—deficient
• Alcoholism		• Aplastic anemia
• Myelodysplastic syndrome		• Myelophthisic anemia
• Hypothyroidism		• Chronic renal failure
		• Anemia of chronic disease
		• Hypothyroidism

Anemias are classified as normocytic, microcytic, and macrocytic on the basis of MCV. Since MCV measures average cell volume, it may be normal even though there is marked variation in size of red cells (anisocytosis). Some hematology cell analyzers measure this degree of variation in size of red cells as red cell distribution width or RDW.

2. **Mean corpuscular hemoglobin (MCH):** This is the average amount of hemoglobin in each red cell. It is expressed in picograms or pg (1 pg = 10^{-12} gram) and is derived manually from the following formula:

$$\text{MCH (in pg)} = \frac{\text{Hemoglobin (g/dL)}}{\text{Red cell count in milion/mm}^3} \times 10$$

Low MCH is found in microcytic hypochromic anemia, while high MCH in macrocytic anemia.

3. **Mean corpuscular hemoglobin concentration (MCHC):** This represents the average concentration of hemoglobin in a given volume of packed red cells. It is expressed in g/dL and calculated as follows:

$$\text{MCHC (in g/dL)} = \frac{\text{Hb (g/dL)}}{\text{PCV (\%)}} \times 10$$

Low MCHC occurs in microcytic hypochromic anemia. An increase in MCHC occurs in hereditary spherocytosis.

4. **Red cell distribution width (RDW):** RDW is the degree of variation of red cell size and can be determined on some blood cell analyzers. This parameter may sometimes be helpful for distinguishing iron deficiency anemia from β-thalassemia minor (low MCV with high RDW: Iron deficiency anemia; low MCV with normal RDW: β-thalassemia minor). Amongst macrocytic anemias, RDW is elevated in megaloblastic anemia and is normal in myelodysplastic syndrome.

Apart from morphological categorization of anemia, red cell indices are also helpful in differentiating mild iron deficiency anemia from thalassemia trait. In microcytic hypochromic anemia of iron deficiency, MCV, MCH, and MCHC are low. In thalassemia, MCV and MCH are low but MCHC is normal; target cells and basophilic stippling may also be present on peripheral blood smear. In severe anemia, peripheral blood smear is sufficiently characteristic and red cell indices do not provide additional information. **The red cell indices are mainly helpful in detecting mild or early red cell abnormalities.**

Sometimes in a nonanemic individual, increase or decrease of MCV is detected on a routine hemogram on electronic cell counters. This mandates further investigations, as elevation of MCV is an early indicator of deficiency of folate or vitamin B_{12}, myelodysplastic syndrome, and aplastic anemia. Decreased MCV without anemia occurs in thalassemia trait.

Differential diagnosis of anemias based on MCV and RDW is given in Table 2.6.

Based on findings of complete blood count, a simplified approach for diagnosis of anemia is presented in Figure 2.4.

Role of bone marrow examination in evaluation of anemia: Bone marrow examination is not required for definitive diagnosis in all cases of anemia. Bone marrow examination is especially helpful in anemia with low reticulocyte count like aplastic anemia, myelophthisic anemia

Table 2.6: Differential diagnosis of anemia based on MCV and RDW.

MCV	RDW	Causes
1. Low	Normal	Thalassemia carrier, anemia of chronic disease
2. Low	High	Iron deficiency anemia, hemoglobin H disease, sickle-cell-β thalassemia
3. High	Normal	Myelodysplastic syndrome, aplastic anemia
4. High	High	Megaloblastic anemia, immune hemolytic anemia
5. Normal	Normal	Anemia of chronic disease, sickle cell trait, hereditary spherocytosis
6. Normal	High	Early iron deficiency or megaloblastic anemia, sideroblastic anemia, myelofibrosis, sickle cell anemia

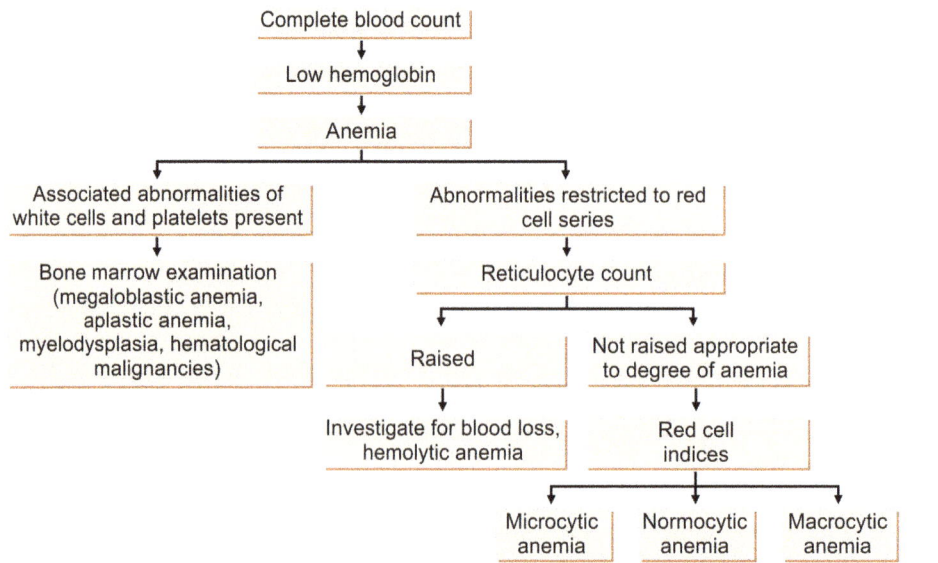

Fig. 2.4: A simplified approach for evaluation of anemia based on complete blood count.

(marrow infiltration by leukemia, metastatic deposits, granulomas), and myelofibrosis. Selective depletion of erythroid series is seen in red cell aplasia and renal disease. Bone marrow examination can be done for evaluation of iron stores for diagnosis of iron deficiency anemia or to distinguish it from anemia of chronic disease; however, availability of simple tests like serum iron, TIBC, and serum ferritin have obviated the need for bone marrow iron stain. Bone marrow is essential for demonstration of ringed sideroblasts in myelodysplastic syndrome and in sideroblastic anemia.

CLASSIFICATION OF ANEMIA INTO THREE MORPHOLOGICAL TYPES

With the help of the information gained from the clinical data and these basic laboratory studies, further investigations can be undertaken to define the underlying cause of anemia.

Morphological classification of anemia into any one of three types (macrocytic, microcytic, or normocytic) is the starting point for investigation of cause of any anemia. However, it is necessary to be aware of certain exceptions as follows: (1) initially, iron deficiency anemia is normocytic, (2) hemolytic anemia, which is usually normocytic, can be macrocytic due to marked reticulocytosis, and (3) deficiency of both folate/vitamin B_{12} and iron causes normocytic anemia. It is also necessary to exclude spurious macrocytosis due to rouleaux formation or red cell agglutination on hematology analyzer.

Evaluation of Macrocytic Anemias

In macrocytic anemia MCV is greater than 100 fl. In most cases, various causes of macrocytic anemia can be differentiated on the basis of reticulocyte count and examinations of peripheral blood smear and bone marrow (Fig. 2.5).

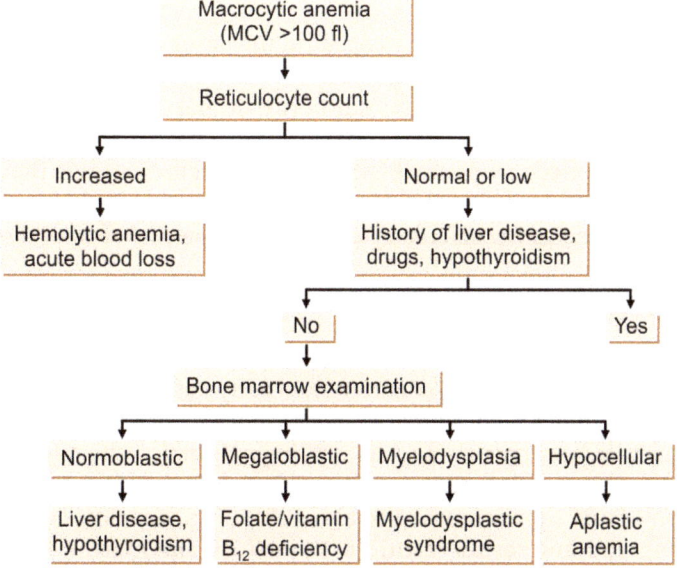

Fig. 2.5: Evaluation of macrocytic anemia.

Two types of macrocytosis can be distinguished on blood smear: round and oval. Their causes are listed in Box 2.6.

Typical features of megaloblastic anemia due to deficiency of vitamin B_{12} or folate are—(1) peripheral blood smear: Macrocytic anemia, leukopenia, and thrombocytopenia (pancytopenia); marked anisopoikilocytosis (variation in size and shape of red cells); Howell-Jolly bodies; and hypersegmented neutrophils (five or more lobes in more than 5% neutrophils); (2) Bone marrow examination: Bone marrow examination confirms the diagnosis of megaloblastic anemia. It shows ineffective erythropoiesis (increase in early erythroid precursors due to premature destruction of more mature erythroid cells resulting in anemia), megaloblasts with nuclear cytoplasmic asynchrony (nuclear chromatin is open or sieve-like while cytoplasm shows hemoglobinization), and presence of giant bands and metamyelocytes. The distinction between folate and vitamin B_{12} deficiencies is based on estimation of serum and red cell folate and serum vitamin B_{12}. Therapeutic trial can also be given to distinguish between the two deficiencies (see chapter on megaloblastic anemias).

Reticulocytosis in hemolytic anemias is another cause of macrocytosis. As reticulocytes are larger than mature red cells, MCV is increased. Chronic extravascular hemolysis is associated with mild icterus, variable splenomegaly, and unconjugated hyperbilirubinemia. Peripheral smear shows polychromatic cells and normoblasts. Intravascular destruction of red cells is associated with hemoglobinemia, hemoglobinuria, and hemosiderinuria.

Macrocytosis in liver disease is uniform, round, and is associated with target cells and abnormal liver function tests.

Most patients with myelodysplastic syndrome are elderly and have bi- or pancytopenia. Bone marrow examination reveals dysmyelopoiesis and sometimes abnormal localization of immature precursors.

In alcoholic patients, macrocytosis can occur in the absence of megaloblastic marrow or alcoholic cirrhosis. The mechanism is unknown.

Macrocytosis also occurs in pregnancy, newborns, during cytotoxic chemotherapy and in aplastic anemia.

Sometimes, spurious macrocytosis on hematology analyzers can result from cold agglutinins in blood (due to clumping of red cells, which appear larger), hyperglycemia, or very high leukocyte count (due to counting of leukocytes in red cell channel of analyzers).

Box 2.6: Oval and round macrocytosis..

- Oval macrocytosis: Megaloblastic anemia due to deficiency of folate or vitamin B_{12}, drug therapy (hydroxyurea, zidovudine, chemotherapy), myelodysplasia
- Round macrocytosis: Alcoholism, liver disease, hypothyroidism

Evaluation of Microcytic Hypochromic Anemia

Causes of microcytic hypochromic anemia are listed in Table 2.5. The most common cause of microcytic hypochromic anemia is iron deficiency. In early stages of iron deficiency, the red cell morphology is normal (normocytic and normochromic). With progressive fall in hemoglobin concentration, anemia becomes microcytic and hypochromic. The degree of reduction in MCV and MCHC is proportional to the severity of anemia. The biochemical parameters of iron deficiency are low serum iron, increased total iron binding capacity (TIBC), low transferrin saturation (<15%), and low serum ferritin (<12 μg/L). Bone marrow examination shows micronormoblastic erythropoiesis and on Prussian blue staining absence of stainable iron.

In β-thalassemia major, severe anemia develops during first few years of life that requires regular blood transfusion therapy. Hepatosplenomegaly is present. Peripheral blood smear shows marked anisopoikilocytosis, severe microcytosis and hypochromia, frequent target cells, basophilic stippling, and normoblasts. Hemoglobin electrophoresis shows predominance of HbF.

In β-thalassemia minor, anemia is either absent or mild and peripheral blood smear shows prominent red cell abnormalities, such as microcytosis, hypochromia, basophilic stippling, and target cells. Hemoglobin electrophoresis typically shows increase in HbA2 (3.5–7%). The laboratory findings that are predictive of thalassemia trait in a case of microcytic anemia are (1) coarse basophilic stippling on blood smear, (2) increased red cell count, (3) normal RDW, (4) Mentzer index (MCV÷RBC count) less than 12, and (5) high serum iron along with normal TIBC. Diagnosis of thalassemia is highly suggestive in the presence of raised Hb2 by HPLC in appropriate ethnic group. Definitive diagnosis is based on molecular testing for the presence of mutation.

Sideroblastic anemia exhibits dimorphic population of red blood cells in peripheral blood (normocytic normochromic and microcytic hypochromic) and ringed sideroblasts in bone marrow.

Patient may be evaluated for anemia of chronic disease if there is a history of chronic inflammation, chronic infection, or malignant disease. The anemia is usually mild to moderate, serum iron and total iron binding capacity are reduced, serum ferritin is elevated, bone marrow morphology is normal and storage iron in marrow is normal or increased. Erythrocyte sedimentation rate is raised and does not correspond with the degree of anemia.

A scheme for evaluation of microcytic hypochromic anemia is presented in Figure 2.6.

Evaluation of Normocytic Normochromic Anemia

Depending upon bone marrow erythropoietic activity, normocytic anemias are divided into two types (Fig. 2.7 and Table 2.5):

Normocytic anemias with increased reticulocyte count—Two possible causes are acute blood loss and hemolysis.
1. *Acute posthemorrhagic anemia:* Acute blood loss can occur either externally or internally (e.g. hemothorax, fracture of hip). Significant blood loss occurring rapidly over a short period of time causes acute blood loss anemia.

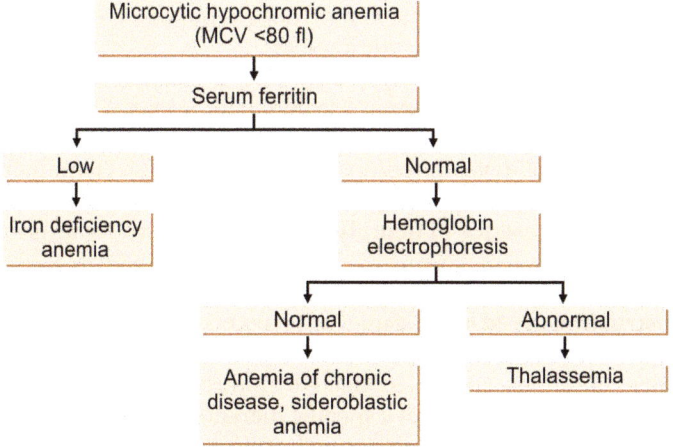

Fig. 2.6: Evaluation of microcytic hypochromic anemia.

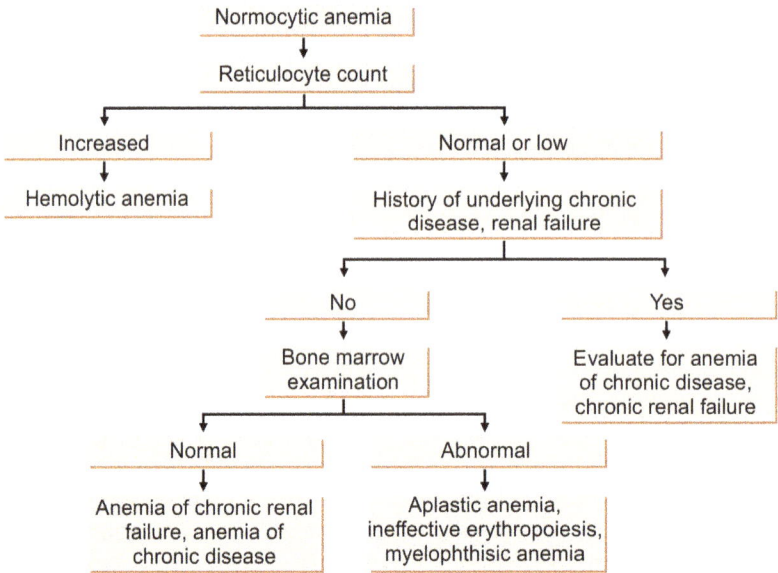

Fig. 2.7: Evaluation of normocytic anemia.

After hemorrhage, to compensate for hypovolemia, there is an increase in plasma volume due to movement of fluid from extravascular sites. This causes hemodilution and fall in hematocrit and hemoglobin levels. Anemia does not become evident for 1–3 days after hemorrhage due to the time needed for restoration of plasma volume. Acute post hemorrhagic anemia is normocytic and normochromic. Stimulation of bone marrow by erythropoietin causes erythroid hyperplasia. Reticulocytosis begins about 3 days after the episode and reaches its peak around 9 to 10 days. During this period, nucleated red cells may appear in peripheral blood. Thrombocytosis and neutrophilic leukocytosis with mild shift to left (i.e. increase in immature white blood cells) are common findings. If hemorrhage is internal, destruction of extravasated red cells and catabolism of heme cause increase in serum bilirubin. If internal hemorrhage is not detected, these findings may be misinterpreted as indicative of hemolytic anemia.

2. *Hemolytic anemia:* Once the possibility of blood loss is ruled out, hemolytic anemia is the prime consideration. Hemolytic anemias are due to increased rate of red cell destruction. When the red cell destruction is balanced by increased red cell production by the bone marrow, anemia may not develop (compensated hemolysis). Hemolytic anemia results when the bone marrow is unable to compensate for the increased rate of red cell destruction.

Tests to establish the presence of hemolysis: Various laboratory tests are used to detect hemolysis.

Red cell destruction can occur either extra or intravascularly (Figs. 2.8 and 2.9 and Table 2.7). **Extravascular destruction of red cells** by macrophages occurs mostly in spleen and liver. This leads to unconjugated hyperbilirubinemia. Increased level of serum unconjugated bilirubin also occurs in other conditions, such as ineffective erythropoiesis, internal hemorrhage, and certain liver disorders. It is, therefore, not a specific marker of hemolysis.

Serum lactate dehydrogenase level rises due to the release of the enzyme from the hemolyzed red cells. Raised levels of lactate dehydrogenase are also observed in megaloblastic anemia,

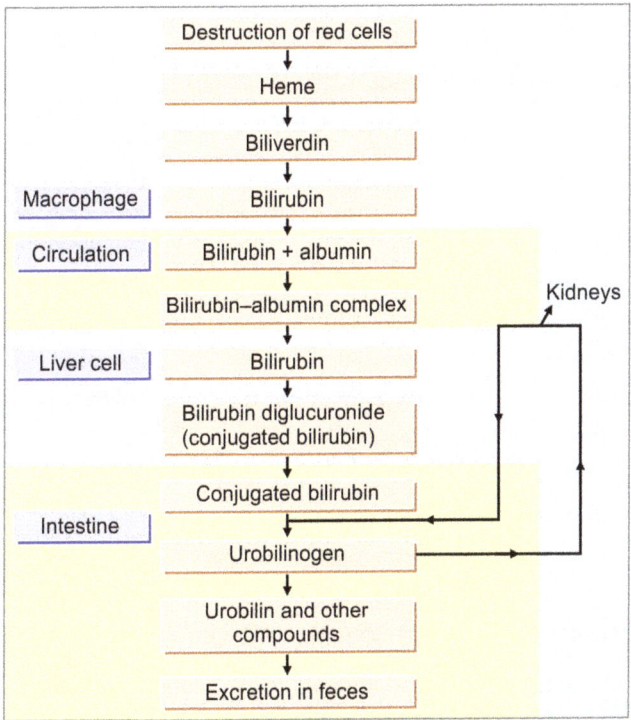

Fig. 2.8: Mechanism of extravascular hemolysis in macrophages of reticuloendothelial system with formation of bilirubin.

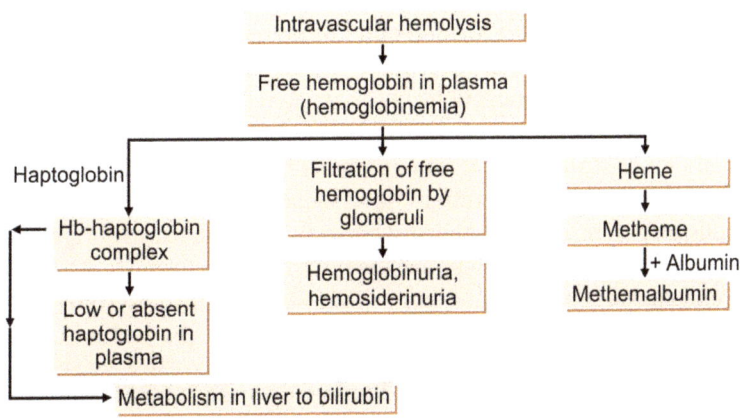

Fig. 2.9: Intravascular hemolysis.

hematologic malignancies, infarction of various organs, and skeletal muscle disorders. Thus increased lactate dehydrogenase alone is not a reliable marker of hemolysis.

Intravascular hemolysis causes release of hemoglobin in circulation. Free hemoglobin combines with haptoglobin in plasma and this complex is then cleared from the circulation by hepatocytes. This causes reduction in the level of plasma haptoglobin. Low plasma haptoglobin levels also occur in extravascular hemolysis, megaloblastic anemia, and liver diseases. Being an acute phase reactant, plasma haptoglobin rises in inflammatory and neoplastic diseases.

Table 2.7: Comparison of extravascular and intravascular hemolysis.

Parameter	Intravascular hemolysis	Extravascular hemolysis
1. Site of hemolysis	Within circulation	Macrophages of spleen, liver, bone marrow, etc.
2. Causes	Blackwater fever, incompatible blood transfusion, PNH, PCH	Hemoglobinopathies, hereditary hemolytic anemias, autoimmune hemolytic anemia
3. Splenomegaly	Absent	Present
4. Reticulocyte count	Increased	Increased
5. Indirect serum bilirubin	Increased	Increased
6. Plasma hemoglobin	Markedly increased	Mild to moderately increased
7. Hemoglobin in urine	Present	Absent
8. Hemosiderin in urine	Present	Absent
9. Methemalbumin (Schumm's test)	Positive	Negative
10. Serum haptoglobin	Decreased	Decreased
11. Serum LDH	Increased	Increased

(PNH: paroxysmal nocturnal hemoglobinuria; PCH: paroxysmal cold hemoglobinuria; LDH: lactate dehydrogenase)

Free hemoglobin (hemoglobinemia) appears in circulation once the plasma haptoglobin disappears. Free heme can bind albumin, leading to the formation of methemalbumin (methemalbuminemia). Methemalbumin can be detected by Schumm's test (detection of distinctive absorption band of methemalbumin at 558 nm on spectrophotometry). Free hemoglobin is also excreted by the kidneys resulting in hemoglobinuria. Benzidine or orthotoluidine test can be used for detection of hemoglobin in urine. Some quantity of hemoglobin in glomerular filtrate is absorbed by renal tubular epithelial cells and stored as ferritin or hemosiderin. Shedding of such cells in urine results in hemosiderinuria which can be demonstrated by iron stain.

Excessive red cell destruction causes compensatory erythroid hyperplasia in the bone marrow. Enhanced erythropoietic activity is associated with reticulocytosis, presence of nucleated red cells, and increased numbers of white cells and platelets in peripheral blood. Young red cells with ribosomal remnants are known as polychromatic cells on Romanowsky stained smears and as reticulocytes when stained supravitally with brilliant cresyl blue or new methylene blue. Polychromatic cells are slightly larger than mature red cells and have a faint blue-gray tint due to the presence of residual RNA. Staining of hemoglobin with acid dyes and staining of RNA with basic dyes produces polychromasia. These signs of accelerated erythropoiesis are also seen in acute blood loss anemia and recovery phase of nutritional anemias. Features common to all hemolytic anemias are presented in Box 2.7.

Box 2.7: Features common to all hemolytic anemias.
- Clinical: Pallor, mild jaundice
- Laboratory:
  a. Biochemical: Increased unconjugated serum bilirubin, increased lactate dehydrogenase, decreased or absent serum haptoglobin
  b. Hematological: Increased reticulocyte count, polychromasia on blood smear, erythroid hyperplasia in bone marrow

No single test is specific for hemolysis and therefore a combination of laboratory tests is usually obtained to document the presence of hemolysis. Hemolytic anemia is characterized by features of (1) accelerated red cell destruction, and (2) accelerated erythropoiesis in bone marrow.

1. Laboratory features of accelerated red cell destruction:
   - Increased unconjugated (indirect) serum bilirubin (usually <5.0 mg/dL)
   - Increased serum lactate dehydrogenase due to release from hemolysed red cells
   - Decreased serum haptoglobin: Hemoglobin entering plasma binds to haptoglobin and hemoglobin-haptoglobin complex is removed by hepatocytes
   - Features of intravascular red cell destruction: Hemoglobinemia, hemoglobinuria, hemosiderinuria, methemalbuminemia.
2. Laboratory features of accelerated erythropoiesis:
   - Reticulocytosis
   - Polychromatophilia on blood smear
   - Erythroid hyperplasia in bone marrow.

Tests to determine the cause of hemolysis: Various causes of hemolytic anemia are listed in Table 2.3. Once the presence of hemolysis is established, further work-up is guided by the clinical information and peripheral smear findings (e.g. sickled forms, spherocytes). Some of the laboratory tests used for demonstrating the cause of hemolysis are—hemoglobin electrophoresis (for abnormal hemoglobins), test for glucose-6-phosphate dehydrogenase deficiency, osmotic fragility test for hereditary spherocytosis, antiglobulin (Coombs') test for immune hemolysis, isopropanol precipitation test for unstable hemoglobins, Ham's test for paroxysmal nocturnal hemoglobinuria, etc. These tests are discussed in respective chapters.

Approach to diagnosis of hemolytic anemia involves establishing the presence of hemolysis followed by determination of the cause of hemolytic anemia (Figs. 2.10 and 2.11).

Normocytic anemias with reduced reticulocyte count: This type of anemia results from hypoproliferation in the bone marrow. Peripheral blood smear shows pancytopenia with relative predominance of lymphocytes in aplastic anemia. Leukoerythroblastic picture is a characteristic feature of myelophthisic anemia.

In both these conditions, bone marrow examination is essential for diagnosis. In renal failure, anemia of chronic disorders, and hypothyroidism, clinical manifestations and ancillary laboratory studies (e.g. renal function tests) are helpful in establishing the diagnosis.

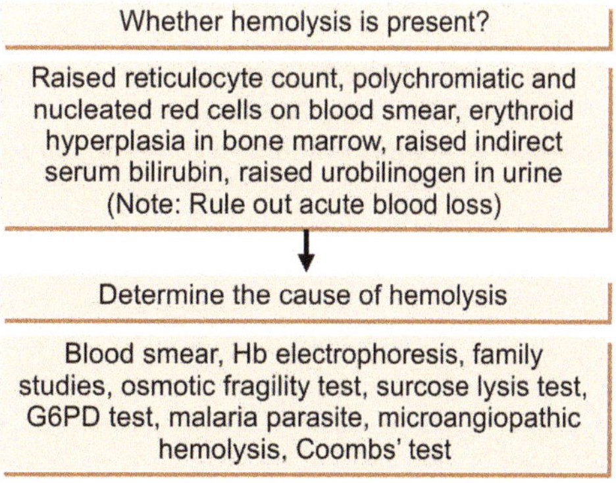

Whether hemolysis is present?
Raised reticulocyte count, polychromiatic and nucleated red cells on blood smear, erythroid hyperplasia in bone marrow, raised indirect serum bilirubin, raised urobilinogen in urine (Note: Rule out acute blood loss)
↓
Determine the cause of hemolysis
Blood smear, Hb electrophoresis, family studies, osmotic fragility test, surcose lysis test, G6PD test, malaria parasite, microangiopathic hemolysis, Coombs' test

Fig. 2.10: Evaluation of hemolytic anemia.

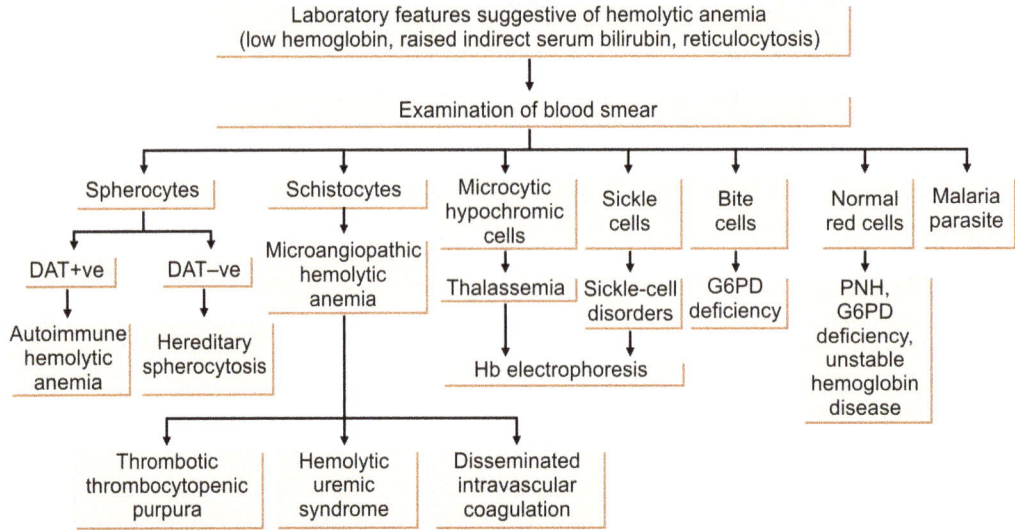

Fig. 2.11: A simplified approach to diagnosis of hemolytic anemia.
(DAT: directantiglobulin test; G6PD: glucose-6-phosphate dehydrogenase; PNH: paroxysmal nocturnal hemoglobinuria; hb: hemoglobin).

BIBLIOGRAPHY

1. Colon-Otero G, Menke D, Hook CC. A practical approach to the differential diagnosis and evaluation of the adult patient with macrocytic anemia. Med Clin North Am. 1992;76:581-97.
2. Hermiston ML, Mentzer WC. A practical approach to the evaluation of the anemic child. Pediatr Clin N Am. 2002;49:877-91.
3. Hoffman R, Benz EJ, Shattil SJ, et al. Hematology. Basic Principles and Practice. 5th edition. Philadelphia. Churchill Livingstone Elsevier; 2008.
4. Lindenbaum J. Hematologic diseeses. An approach to the anemias. In Wyngaarden JB, Smith LH, Bennett JC (Eds.): Cecil Textbook of Medicine, 19th edition. Philadelphia. WB Saunders Co; 1992. pp. 822-31.
5. Massey AC. Microcytic anemia. Differential diagnosis and management of iron deficiency anemia. Med Clin North Am. 1992;76:549-66.
6. Tefferi A. Anemia in adults: A contemporary approach to diagnosis. Mayo Clin Proc. 2003;78:1274-80.

CHAPTER 3

Anemias due to Impaired Red Cell Production

IRON DEFICIENCY ANEMIA

Deficiency of iron is the most common cause of anemia worldwide. Iron deficiency is a state of low total body iron content. Iron deficiency anemia develops when body iron stores are depleted, level of circulating iron is reduced, and there is insufficient iron available for erythropoiesis.

NORMAL IRON METABOLISM

Normal iron metabolism is diagrammatically represented in Figure 3.1.

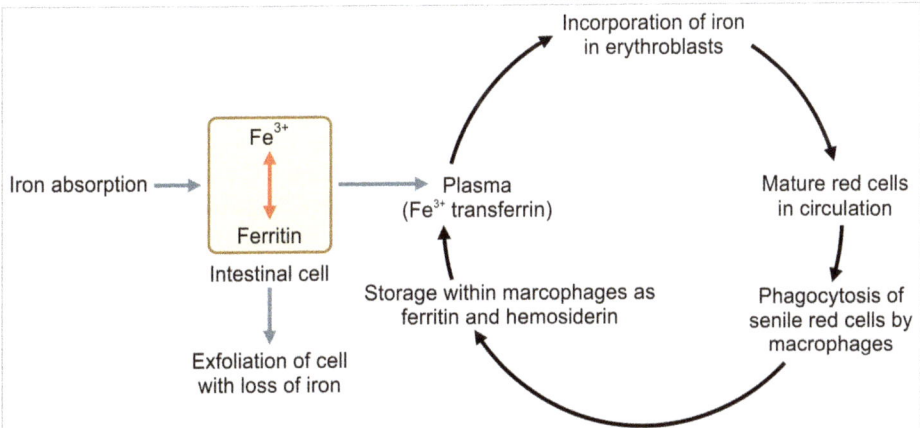

Fig. 3.1: Normal iron metabolism. After absorption iron binds with transferrin and is transported to various tissues. In the bone marrow, iron is internalized by erythroblasts to form heme. Some iron is also stored as ferritin and such erythroblasts containing ferritin aggregates are called sideroblasts. Macrophages contain ferritin and hemosiderin derived mostly from catabolism of senescent red cells. Macrophage iron can be mobilized to circulating iron when required. Iron is lost from desquamation of intestinal cells.

Iron Requirements

Normally, in adult males only a small quantity of iron is lost by exfoliation of epithelial cells from gastrointestinal and urinary tracts and skin. This loss is about 1 mg per day, which needs to be matched by absorption of similar quantity of iron from food. Iron requirement is increased during adolescence due to growth. In females, iron need (and vulnerability to iron deficiency) is greater due to menstrual blood loss and increased demand for iron by the fetus during pregnancy.

The daily iron requirement, which varies according to the age and sex, is shown in Box 3.1.

The normal daily diet (western) of an adult contains about 10 to 20 mg of iron. **To balance the daily iron loss of 1 mg, about 10% of the daily iron intake is absorbed.** Iron absorption is augmented in the presence of iron deficiency and decreased in conditions associated with iron overload. Women absorb more iron as compared to men due to increased iron demand caused by menstrual blood loss and pregnancy.

Body iron compartments are shown in Box 3.2.

> **Box 3.1:** Daily iron requirements.
> - Infants up to 4 months: 0.5 mg
> - Infants 5–12 months and children: 1 mg
> - Menstruating women: 3 mg
> - Pregnancy: 3–4 mg
> - Adult men and postmenopausal women: 1 mg

> **Box 3.2:** Body iron compartments.
> - Total body iron: 50 mg/kg body weight in males; 40 mg/kg body weight in females
> - Hemoglobin iron: 65%
> - Storage iron (ferritin, hemosiderin): 30%
> - Transport iron (transferrin-bound iron): 1%
> - Tissue iron (myoglobin, enzymes): 4%

Dietary Sources of Iron

The main sources are meats, eggs, and green leafy vegetables. Milk is a poor source of iron.

Absorption of Iron

Iron absorption mostly occurs in duodenum and upper jejunum. Absorption is in ferrous form.

Meat contains heme iron about one-fourth of which is directly absorbed by intestinal epithelial cells. The exact mechanism of absorption of heme iron is not well understood. After cellular uptake, heme is broken down and iron is released in the cytoplasm.

Green vegetables contain inorganic iron only 1 to 2% of which is absorbed. The absorption is usually in the ferrous form. In contrast to heme, iron absorption of inorganic iron is affected by certain substances in the diet, i.e. tannates, phytates, phosphates, and certain drugs (antacids, proton pump inhibitors, tetracyclines) retard absorption while ascorbate and amino acids facilitate absorption.

Iron absorption mainly occurs in epithelial cells lining the villi close to gastroduodenal junction. Low pH of gastroduodenal contents facilitates dissolution of ingested iron. Ferric iron (Fe^{3+}) is converted to ferrous form (Fe^{2+}) by an enzyme (a ferric reductase called duodenal cytochrome b or DCYTB) located along the brush border of the epithelial cells. Iron is transported from the apical cell surface into the cell by DMT1 (divalent metal transporter 1). Inside the cell iron is either stored as ferritin (which is lost when enterocyte is exfoliated) or is transported to plasma. Iron is released from the cell through ferroportin 1 at the basolateral surface in Fe^{2+} state. Ferroportin 1 is the only known cellular exporter of iron. Hepcidin regulates expression of ferroportin and is the central regulator of iron metabolism (Fig. 3.2). In plasma, iron is converted back to Fe^{3+} state by a copper-containing enzyme (hephaestin) located on the basal border of the enterocyte or by circulating ceruloplasmin. Fe^{3+} then combines with plasma transferrin and is transported to various body tissues.

Body iron stores and rate of erythropoiesis regulate iron absorption. Iron absorption is stimulated by ineffective erythropoiesis (as occurs in thalassemia). Summary of proteins involved in iron absorption is presented in Box 3.3.

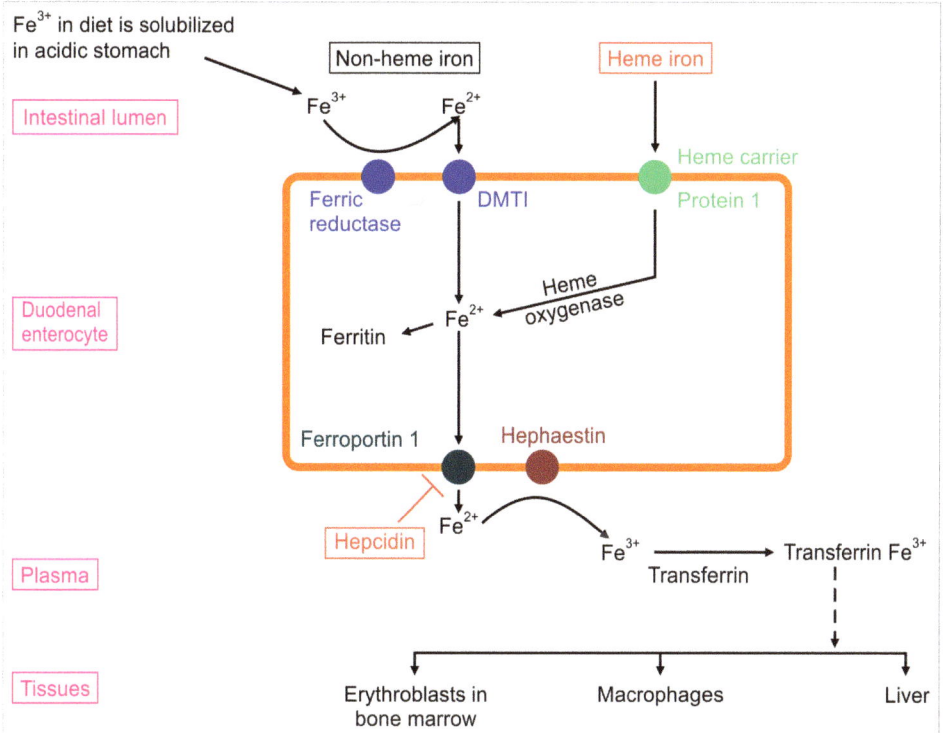

Fig. 3.2: Mechanism of iron absorption.

Box 3.3: Proteins involved in iron absorption.

- **Divalent metal transporter 1 (DMT1):** Protein located on apical surface of duodenal enterocytes that transports ferrous iron (Fe^{2+}) from intestinal lumen to cytosol.
- **Ferroportin 1:** Cellular iron exporter protein expressed on enterocytes (basolateral surface), macrophages, hepatocytes, and placenta; it is inactivated by hepcidin; mutation in *FPN1* gene is associated with hemochromatosis type IV.
- **Hepcidin:** A small peptide hormone produced by liver that is a key regulator of iron absorption and recycling by controlling ferroportin; hepcidin synthesis is increased by inflammation and iron overload, and inhibited by iron deficiency, increased erythropoietic activity, and hypoxia. It is encoded by *HAMP* gene (19q13) mutation of which causes type II or juvenile hemochromatosis.
- **Hephaestin:** A transmembrane protein that transports dietary iron from duodenal enterocytes to circulation; it converts Fe^{2+} iron to Fe^{3+} form.

Transport of Iron

After absorption, iron is transported in plasma by transferrin. Transferrin is a glycoprotein that is produced in the liver. A molecule of transferrin can carry two atoms of iron. If only one binding site of transferrin is occupied by iron, it is known as monoferric transferrin; if both sites are occupied it is termed as diferric transferrin (or holotransferrin). **The iron-binding sites of all the circulating transferrin constitute the total iron binding capacity (TIBC). Usually, about 30% of the iron binding sites are occupied by iron.**

Transferrin carries iron to the erythroblasts in the bone marrow and other cells in the body. Iron is required for production of hemoglobin by erythroid cells. Transferrin binds to specific receptors (transferrin receptor 1 or TfR1) on the surface of the erythroblasts and is internalized by endocytosis along with the receptor. A specialized endosome containing transferrin receptor with attached transferrin is formed. A proton pump increases the pH within the endosome that causes release of iron into the cytoplasm. Transferrin devoid of iron (apotransferrin) and transferrin receptor are returned back to the cell surface for further cycles of iron transport and uptake (Fig. 3.3). Each transferrin receptor 1 can bind two molecules of transferrin.

With maturation of erythroid cells, the extracellular portion of TfR1 is released from the cell surface into the circulation. The concentration of these cleaved receptors, called serum or

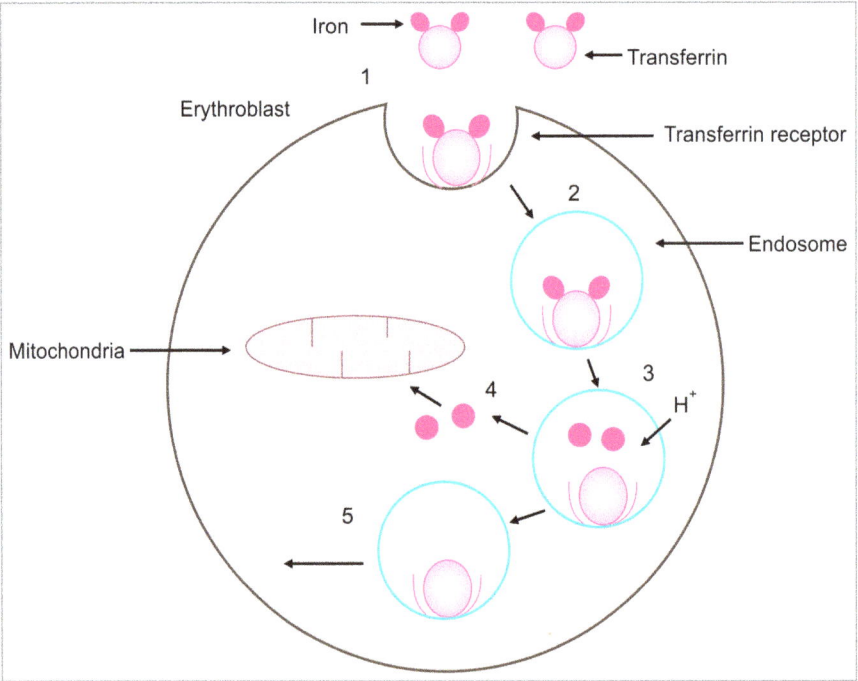

Fig. 3.3: Uptake of iron in erythroblasts. (1) Binding of transferrin to transferrin receptor on cell surface. (2) Transferrin-transferrin receptor complex is internalized by endocytosis with formation of endosome. (3) Inside the endosome, pH is raised by proton pump which causes release of iron molecule from transferrin. (4) Iron is released in cytoplasm and reaches mitochondria where it is inserted into protoporphyrin ring to form heme. (5) Apotransferrin (transferrin devoid of iron) and transferrin receptor are returned back to cell surface for further cycles of iron uptake and delivery.

soluble transferrin receptor (sTfR), is proportional to the erythroid mass. If erythropoiesis is increased, concentration of sTfR in plasma increases.

Incorporation of Iron in Erythroid Precursors

Once inside the cytoplasm of erythroid precursors, iron is inserted into protoporphyrin to form heme. This reaction occurs in the mitochondria of erythroid precursors and is mediated by the enzyme ferrochelatase. Iron is also stored as ferritin in lysosomes of erythroblasts. Erythroblasts which contain aggregates of ferritin are known as sideroblasts. Sideroblasts constitute about 25 to 30% of nucleated red cells in bone marrow.

Storage of Iron

Storage iron is of two types: ferritin and hemosiderin. Storage iron is present within hepatocytes and in macrophages of liver, spleen, and bone marrow.

1. Ferritin consists of a protein shell and an iron core. The protein portion is known as apoferritin that is spherical in shape. The central core of apoferritin consists of numerous (up to 4500) ferric oxyhydroxide molecules. Ferritin is water-soluble and is readily mobilized for hemoglobin synthesis when required. A small amount of ferritin enters circulation through active secretion or cell lysis, and represents serum ferritin. **A direct relationship exists between amount of circulating ferritin and body iron stores** (1 ng/mL of serum ferritin corresponds with approximately 8 mg of storage iron). Serum ferritin concentration decreases to less than 12 µg/L in iron deficiency anemia and increases in iron overload disorders.
2. Hemosiderin represents aggregations of ferritin from which most of the protein (apoferritin) portion has been removed. Normally, hemosiderin is stored in cells of mononuclear phagocyte system in bone marrow, liver, and spleen. Hemosiderin is water insoluble and is less easily available for hemoglobin synthesis. Hemosiderin appears as a golden-brown, coarsely granular pigment when stained with hematoxylin and eosin. Prussian blue reaction is used for demonstration of hemosiderin in bone marrow. Lack of stainable iron in the bone marrow is a diagnostic feature of iron deficiency anemia.

CAUSES OF IRON DEFICIENCY ANEMIA

Causes of iron deficiency can be broadly classified into four groups: inadequate dietary intake, defective absorption, excessive loss of iron, and increased requirements (Box 3.4).

> **Box 3.4:** Causes of iron deficiency anemia.
>
> - Inadequate dietary intake of iron
> - Defective absorption of iron—subtotal gastrectomy, celiac disease, *Helicobacter pylori* gastritis, antacids, proton pump inhibitors, bariatric surgery in obesity
> - Excessive loss of iron—gastrointestinal bleeding (e.g. esophageal varices, hiatus hernia, peptic ulcer, gastritis, Meckel's diverticulum, Crohn's disease, ulcerative colitis, hookworm infestation, various neoplasms especially carcinoma of colon, marathon runners); uterine bleeding (menorrhagia); urinary tract bleeding (hematuria, hemoglobinuria); respiratory tract bleeding (hemoptysis); bleeding disorders
> - Increased requirements for iron—pregnancy, infancy, adolescents

In **infants and children** (especially 6–18 months of age), iron deficiency usually results from poor dietary intake. In **adult males,** iron deficiency occurs usually secondary to chronic blood loss particularly from gastrointestinal tract. In **women of reproductive age group,** iron deficiency is usually the result of menstrual disorders and pregnancy (Box 3.5).

Box 3.5: High risk of iron deficiency anemia.
- Pregnancy
- Women of reproductive age group
- Children <5 years
- Adolescents
- Elderly

Genetic forms of iron deficiency anemia: Many genetic or hereditary forms of iron deficiency anemia are described, which are exceedingly rare. These are caused by autosomal recessive mutations in genes like *SLC11A2* (encodes DMT1, a transmembrane iron transporter), *TF* (encodes transferrin, an iron-binding protein in plasma), CP (encodes ceruloplasmin, a plasma ferroxidase), *GLRX5* (encodes glutaredoxin 5, an enzyme involved in iron-sulfur cluster biogenesis) and *TMPRSS6* (encodes Matriptase-2, a hepcidin suppressor). They cause microcytic hypochromic anemia and are associated with normal or increased body iron stores.

Iron-refractory iron deficiency anemia (IRIDA): This is a recently described hereditary recessive microcytic anemia which does not respond to oral iron therapy. It is caused by mutations in gene *TMPRSS6* that encodes matriptase-2 (MT-2). Normally, production of hepcidin is downregulated by MT-2. In IRIDA, high levels of hepcidin prevent iron absorption and release. This condition partially responds to parenteral iron therapy.

CLINICAL FEATURES

General Clinical Features of Anemia

Patients may present with nonspecific symptoms and signs of anemia such as weakness, easy fatigability, breathlessness on exertion, tachycardia, and systolic heart murmur.

Clinical Features Related to Iron Deficiency

One of the characteristic symptoms of iron deficiency anemia is **pica**. It refers to an abnormal and intense desire to eat strange substances such as clay (geophagia), paint, cardboard, coal, ice (pagophagia), starch (amylophagia), etc. Clinical manifestations due to epithelial abnormalities in mouth, tongue, nails, hypopharynx, and stomach are frequent (due to loss of enzymes that contain iron). These include atrophic glossitis (smooth, red tongue due to atrophy of papillae), angular stomatitis (ulceration or fissuring at angles of mouth), dysphagia, esophageal web, achlorhydria, and gastritis. The fingernails become brittle, lusterless, and flat; in advanced cases their shape changes from normal convex to concave (koilonychias).

The association of iron deficiency anemia, dysphagia, and glossitis is known as Plummer-Vinson (or Patterson-Kelly) syndrome. This syndrome is rare, but is associated with increased risk of postcricoid carcinoma.

Some symptoms are increasingly being recognized in females who are nonanemic but have depleted iron stores like fatigue, cold intolerance, restless leg syndrome, and hair loss (scalp alopecia).

Clinical Features due to Underlying Cause of Iron Deficiency

There may be bleeding from gastrointestinal tract, menorrhagia, poor diet in small children and adolescents, alteration of bowel habits (in adults with colon cancer), etc.

LABORATORY FEATURES

Sequence of events in iron deficiency is presented first followed by various laboratory investigations.

There are three stages in the development of iron deficiency anemia (Box 3.6 and Fig. 3.4)—depletion of iron stores, reduction in circulating iron with iron-deficient erythropoiesis, and development of iron deficiency anemia. (1) The first event in iron deficiency is exhaustion of iron stores and reduction in serum ferritin concentration (<12 µg/L). There is absence of stainable iron in the bone marrow. (2) After depletion of iron stores, the circulating iron level falls and the level of transferrin devoid of iron increases. This manifests as decreased serum iron and transferrin saturation and increased TIBC. This leads to insufficient availability of iron for erythropoiesis. As iron is not available for incorporation into porphyrin ring, zinc (an alternative protoporphyrin ligand) is incorporated in its place with formation of zinc protoporphyrin. This causes increased level of zinc protoporphyrin (ZPP) in the cells. (3) If the state of iron deficiency persists then anemia develops. To start with anemia is normocytic and normochromic. This is followed by appearance of microcytic red cells. The last stage of iron deficiency is microcytic hypochromic anemia with mean cell volume (MCV) less than 80 fl and Mean corpuscular hemoglobin concentration (MCHC) less than 30 g%.

Box 3.6: Stages in the development of iron deficiency anemia.

Depletion of iron stores → Decrease in transport iron with reduced availability of iron for erythropoiesis → Normocytic normochromic anemia → Microcytic anemia → Microcytic hypochromic anemia

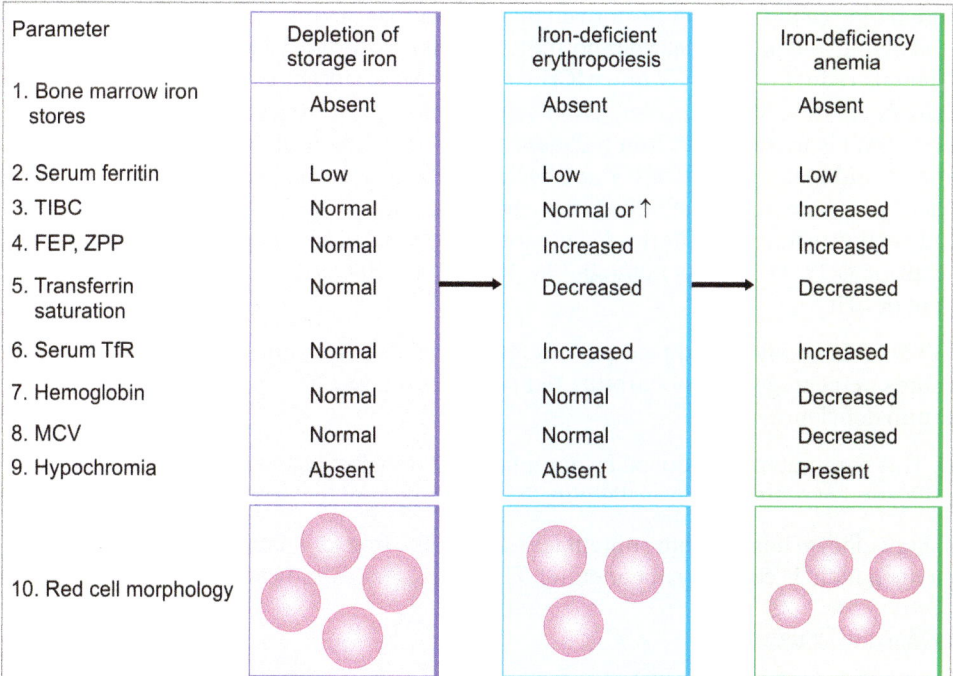

Parameter	Depletion of storage iron	Iron-deficient erythropoiesis	Iron-deficiency anemia
1. Bone marrow iron stores	Absent	Absent	Absent
2. Serum ferritin	Low	Low	Low
3. TIBC	Normal	Normal or ↑	Increased
4. FEP, ZPP	Normal	Increased	Increased
5. Transferrin saturation	Normal	Decreased	Decreased
6. Serum TfR	Normal	Increased	Increased
7. Hemoglobin	Normal	Normal	Decreased
8. MCV	Normal	Normal	Decreased
9. Hypochromia	Absent	Absent	Present
10. Red cell morphology			

Fig. 3.4: Stages in the development of iron deficiency anemia. Microcytic hypochromic anemia is the late stage of iron deficiency.
(TIBC: Total iron binding capacity; FEP: free erythrocyte protoporphyrin; ZPP: Zinc protoporphyrin; TfR: transferrin receptor; MCV: Mean cell volume).

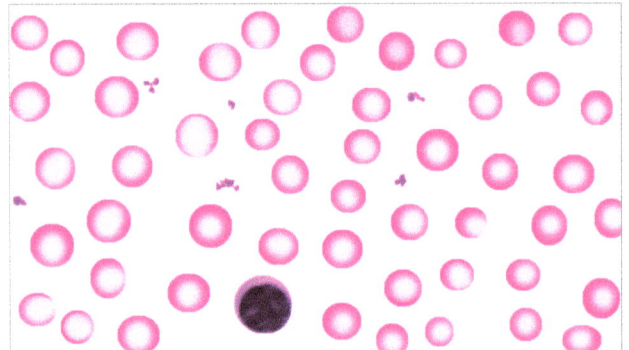

Fig. 3.5: Peripheral blood smear in iron deficiency anemia. Compare the size of red cells with the nucleus of a small lymphocyte.

Peripheral Blood Examination

Initially, anemia is normocytic and normochromic. Later, the red cells show **microcytosis and hypochromia**. The red cells often show variation in size and shape along with elongated cells and **pencil cells**. The white cell count may be normal or mildly decreased. Platelets are often increased, especially in the presence of blood loss (Fig. 3.5).

Red Cell Indices

Although red cell indices may be derived manually after obtaining values of hemoglobin level, red cell count, and packed cell volume, they are best measured by electronic cell counters.

There is reduction of MCV and MCH with degree of reduction being proportional to the severity of anemia. MCHC is reduced in severe or long-standing cases. Red cell distribution width (RDW) is increased in iron deficiency anemia, while in thalassemia minor it is often normal. Combination of low MCV and high RDW is one of the best screening tests for iron deficiency anemia. Newer parameters have been introduced on some hematology analyzers for early detection of functional iron deficiency or iron-restricted erythropoiesis: (1) %hypochromic red cells or %HYPO, (2) low hemoglobin density or LHD, and (3) reticulocyte hemoglobin content or CHr.

% HYPO: This newly introduced parameter is available on some hematology analyzers; it measures percentage of hypochromic red cells (normally <6%). It is helpful for detection of early iron deficiency.

LHD: This parameter is produced by mathematical transformation of MCHC and is useful for identification of reduced iron availability; it has been found to correlate with % HYPO.

CHr: Reticulocyte hemoglobin content falls during the iron-deficient erythropoiesis stage (i.e. when the patient is clinically not anemic). Thus, it is an early indicator of iron deficiency.

Bone Marrow Examination

In iron deficiency anemia, erythropoiesis is micronormoblastic. The micronormoblasts are smaller than normal with reduced amount of cytoplasm that is vacuolated and has ragged cell borders. Hemoglobinization of cytoplasm is defective. These changes are best seen in polychromatic erythroblasts. Granulocytic and megakaryocytic lines are normal. Special stain

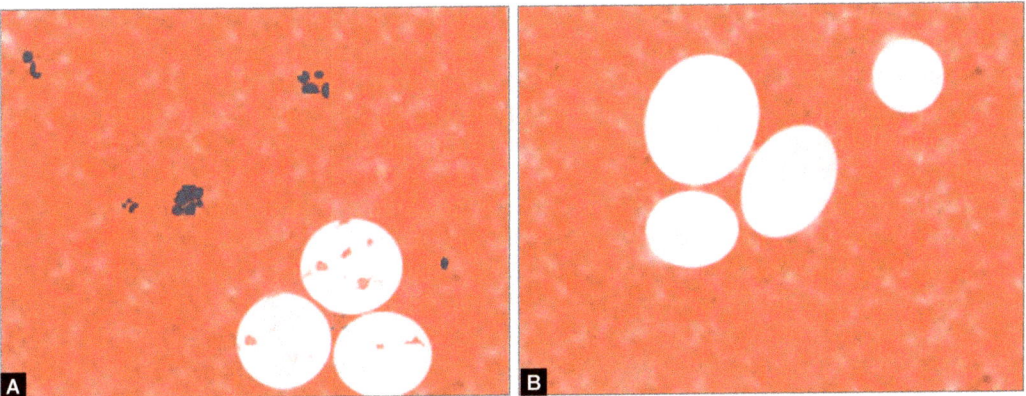

Figs. 3.6A and B: Prussian blue stain on bone marrow aspiration smear: (A) Normal; (B) Iron deficiency anemia.

for iron (Perl's Prussian blue) on bone marrow smears reveals absence of hemosiderin in macrophages and absent or markedly reduced sideroblasts. **Absence of stainable iron in the bone marrow on Perl's Prussian blue reaction is a specific and a reliable test for diagnosis of iron deficiency anemia (Figs. 3.6A and B).**

Serum Ferritin

There is a **direct correlation between amount of storage iron and serum ferritin level** and therefore estimation of serum ferritin is commonly employed for diagnosis of iron deficiency and iron overload. A total of 1 µg/L of plasma ferritin represents about 8 to 10 mg of storage iron. Normal level of serum ferritin varies between 15 and 300 µg/L. Values below 12 µg/L strongly indicate lack of storage iron. Usefulness of this assay, however, is limited by the nonspecific increase in concentration in inflammation, neoplastic disorders, and liver disease.

Serum ferritin is an acute phase reactant. If iron deficiency anemia is associated with these conditions (as is the case in most hospitalized patients), then its diagnosis may require (i) therapeutic trial of iron, (ii) assay of serum transferrin receptor or (iii) demonstration of lack of stainable iron in the bone marrow (Box 3.7). In such cases, in addition, low serum iron and increased TIBC indicate iron deficiency.

Serum Iron, TIBC, and Percent Transferrin Saturation

Alteration in these measurements occurs after depletion of storage iron and are thus normal in early stage.

Box 3.7: Serum ferritin.

- Most sensitive and specific test for diagnosis of iron deficiency anemia. Serum ferritin decreases even before the appearance of anemia
- Serum ferritin correlates with body iron stores (1 µg/L serum ferritin ≈ 10 mg storage iron)
- Serum ferritin <12 µg/L is highly specific for diagnosis of iron deficiency anemia
- Not suitable for diagnosing iron deficiency in patients with concomitant inflammatory, neoplastic, or liver disorder since serum ferritin is an acute phase reactant. Thus, normal serum ferritin does not exclude iron deficiency.

The normal serum iron level is 50 to 150 µg/dL with values in women being slightly lower. In addition to iron deficiency anemia, serum iron levels are also low in chronic inflammation and malignancies. In iron deficiency anemia, serum iron is usually <50 µg/dL. This test is affected by many variables and values should be interpreted along with other tests. Serum iron level shows diurnal variation with highest levels in the morning. Serum iron reflects Fe^{3+} bound to transferrin.

TIBC (normal range 300–400 µg/dL), which reflects amount of transferrin in circulation, is increased in iron deficiency anemia (>400 µg/dL) and reduced in chronic infections.

Serum iron is always measured along with TIBC to calculate transferrin saturation. If serum iron and TIBC are normal, iron deficiency is excluded. If serum iron is very low and TIBC is raised, diagnosis of iron deficiency is confirmed. Low serum iron and low TIBC indicate anemia of chronic disease. With high serum iron and normal TIBC, thalassemia should be considered.

Transferrin saturation is the ratio of serum iron to total iron binding capacity expressed as a percentage and indicates proportion of transferrin to which iron is bound. The average normal value is 30% (normal range is 20–55%). In iron deficiency anemia, transferrin saturation is less than 15%.

$$\% \text{ transferrin saturation} = \frac{\text{Serum iron} \times 100}{\text{TIBC}}$$

Soluble Transferrin Receptor (TfR) Assay

Serum transferrin receptors are derived from proteolysis of cell membrane transferrin receptors during red cell maturation. Level of soluble TfR in serum correlates with the number of cellular transferrin receptors. In iron deficiency anemia, transferrin receptors on erythroid cells increase in number and therefore their serum level also increases. In iron deficiency, elevation of serum TfR follows depletion of iron stores. Unlike serum ferritin, serum TfR is not an acute phase reactant. Therefore, its estimation can be helpful in differentiating iron deficiency anemia from anemia of chronic disease and in diagnosing iron deficiency anemia in patients with chronic inflammation. In patients with iron deficiency anemia, mean serum TfR is more than twice that of normal individuals. In anemia of chronic disease, mean serum TfR level is almost similar to that of normal individuals.

Serum TfR-ferritin index (serum TfR/log ferritin) can detect subclinical iron deficiency (depletion of iron stores) in healthy individuals.

Serum TfR is also elevated in conditions with increased erythropoietic activity (e.g. hemolytic anemias).

Erythrocyte Protoporphyrin

Combination of protoporphyrin with iron to form heme occurs in the mitochondria of erythroid precursors. In iron deficiency anemia, this combination fails to occur; an alternative ligand in the form of zinc is inserted in the protoporphyrin ring with the formation of zinc protoporphyrin (ZPP). Increased level of ZPP occurs in iron deficiency anemia, anemia of chronic disease, thalassemia and lead poisoning. ZPP becomes elevated when iron stores are depleted before the development of anemia and thus can be used as a screening test for detection of early stage of iron deficiency. Determination of ZPP can be applied to large-scale screening of iron deficiency in public health surveys. ZPP can also be used for differentiation of iron deficiency from thalassemia since elevation of ZPP is three to four times more in iron

> **Box 3.8:** Diagnosis of iron deficiency anemia.
>
> - Low hemoglobin and packed cell volume
> - Low MCV, MCH, and MCHC
> - Raised RDW
> - Microcytic hypochromic red cells on blood smear (in late stage)
> - Low serum ferritin
> - Low serum iron and transferrin saturation, and increased TIBC
> - Increased soluble transferrin receptor
> - Bone marrow: Micronormoblasts, absence of stainable iron
>
> *Note:* Combination of MCV, RDW, transferrin saturation, TIBC, serum TfR, and serum ferritin is adequate to assess iron stores in early stage of iron deficiency and in anemia of chronic disease, and eliminates the need for expensive and invasive bone marrow examination.

deficiency as compared to the later. Combination of elevated ZPP with raised RDW is strongly suggestive of iron deficiency since RDW is normal in thalassemia.

Diagnostic laboratory features of IDA are shown in Box 3.8.

Investigations to Define Underlying Cause of Iron Deficiency

This may be obvious (e.g. bleeding) or may require tests such as GIT work-up especially in adults (test for fecal occult blood, endoscopy or radiology, gastric biopsy for *Helicobacter pylori* or atrophic gastritis), pelvic ultrasound in females (if menorrhagia is present), stool examination for hookworm, etc.

> Diagnosis of iron deficiency anemia *perse* is not sufficient in itself. It is essential to search for and treat the underlying cause. In adults, cause of iron deficiency anemia should always be investigated to avoid missing occult gastrointestinal malignancy.

DIFFERENTIAL DIAGNOSIS

Thalassemia Minor

Although both iron deficiency anemia and thalassemia minor show microcytic and hypochromic red cells, presence of target cells, polychromatic cells, and basophilic stippling on blood smear suggest the diagnosis of thalassemia minor. Red cell count is normal or raised in thalassemia minor while it is reduced in iron deficiency anemia. In thalassemia, although red cell abnormalities are prominent anemia is mild or absent. In iron deficiency anemia, red cell changes correlate with severity of anemia. MCV and MCH are markedly reduced as compared to the degree of anemia in thalassemia minor. A typical feature of thalassemia minor on hemoglobin electrophoresis is increased proportion of HbA2 (>3.5%). Bone marrow examination for iron stores also distinguishes the two conditions.

Differentiation of iron deficiency anemia from thalassemia minor is important as continued iron therapy in the latter condition can cause iron overload.

Anemia of Chronic Disease

In anemia of chronic disease, there is defective release of iron from storage sites in reticuloendothelial cells. This leads to insufficient availability of iron for erythropoiesis despite

Table 3.1: Differential diagnosis of iron deficiency anemia.

Parameter	Iron deficiency anemia	Anemia of chronic disease	β thalassemia
1. MCV	Decreased	Normal or decreased	Markedly decreased
2. RDW	Increased	Increased or normal	Increased or normal
3. Red cell morphology	Microcytic hypochromic, pencil cells, anisocytosis	Normocytic normochromic or microcytic hypochromic	Microcytic hypochromic, basophilic stippling, target cells, polychromasia
4. Red cell count	Decreased	Decreased	Normal
5. Serum iron	Decreased	Decreased	Normal
6. TIBC	Increased	Decreased	Normal
7. Transferrin saturation	Decreased	Decreased or normal	Normal or increased
8. FEP	Increased	Increased	Normal
9. Serum TfR	Increased	Normal	Increased
10. Serum ferritin	Decreased	Increased or normal	Normal
11. Hb electrophoresis	Normal	Normal	HbA2 >3.5%
12. Marrow hemosiderin	Low or absent	Normal or increased	Normal

(MCV: mean cell volume; RDW: red cell distribution width; TIBC: total iron binding capacity; FEP: free erythrocyte protoporphyrin; TfR: transferrin receptor 1)

normal iron stores. Anemia of chronic disease is usually normocytic and normochromic but in some cases it is microcytic and hypochromic. Presence of underlying chronic disease, raised ESR not proportional to reduction in hemoglobin concentration, low serum iron and low TIBC, increased serum ferritin, and normal or increased bone marrow storage iron are helpful in arriving at the correct diagnosis.

Sideroblastic Anemia

Sideroblastic anemia may be hereditary or acquired. Typically, the peripheral blood smear shows two types of red cells—normocytic normochromic and microcytic hypochromic (dimorphic anemia). Bone marrow examination (Prussian blue stain for iron) reveals increased or normal storage iron with ringed sideroblasts.

Differential diagnosis of iron deficiency anemia is presented in Table 3.1.

TREATMENT OF IRON DEFICIENCY ANEMIA

Treatment consists of administration of iron and correction of underlying cause of blood loss (such as worm infestation, bleeding from any site). Either oral or parenteral iron preparation can be used. Rise in hemoglobin is similar with both routes.

Oral iron therapy is preferable as it is safer and cheaper than parenteral therapy.

Ferrous sulfate is the preferred preparation. One tablet of ferrous sulfate (200 mg) contains 60 mg of elemental iron. The usual dose is 1 tablet thrice daily.

Following initiation of therapy, reticulocytosis develops within 3 to 7 days and peaks (to 8–10%) between the 8th and 10th day. This is followed by a gradual rise in hemoglobin. Hemoglobin should rise by 1 g/dL (or packed cell volume by 3%) in 4 weeks (known as response to iron therapy). Reticulocyte hemoglobin content (CHr) begins to increase much before the rise of reticulocyte count and hemoglobin concentration. About 6 to 8 weeks are needed for restoration of hemoglobin level. Treatment is continued for further 4 months (total duration of therapy 6 months) to replace body iron stores. Adverse effects of oral iron are vomiting, constipation, diarrhea, and abdominal pain.

Causes of poor response to iron replacement therapy are patient noncompliance, inadequate dosage, malabsorption, continued excess bleeding, coexistent vitamin B_{12}/folate deficiency, concurrent infectious, inflammatory, or neoplastic disease, iron-refractory iron deficiency anemia, and wrong diagnosis.

Indications for parenteral iron therapy are gastrointestinal intolerance to oral iron, advanced stage of pregnancy with moderate to severe anemia, noncooperative patient, and malabsorption of oral iron.

Other indications for parenteral iron are severe anemia with short time to surgery and patients with chronic renal disease who are receiving erythropoietin.

Intravenous iron preparations are of two main types: (1) single dose formulations: iron dextran (low molecular weight), ferumoxytol, ferric carboxymaltose, iron isomaltoside; (2) iron salts that are given in multiple doses: ferrous gluconate, iron sucrose. Iron dextran can be given as a single-dose infusion, but there is a risk of severe life-threatening anaphylactic reaction. A hypersensitivity test is necessary prior to injection of iron dextran. Other side effects of iron dextran are local pain, fever, joint pains, skin rashes, enlargement of lymph nodes, and enlargement of spleen. Iron sucrose is a safe form of parenteral iron but cannot be given as a single-dose infusion. It is given in two to three divided doses every 2 to 3 days to avoid acute iron toxicity.

The amount of iron needed by the patient is derived from the following formula:
Body weight (kg) × 2.3 × (Ideal haemoglobin − Patient's haemoglobin in g/dL) + 500 mg or 1000 mg (for storage iron)

MEGALOBLASTIC ANEMIAS

The megaloblastic anemias are characterized by defective synthesis of deoxyribonucleic acid (DNA) in all proliferating cells. They most commonly result from lack of folic acid or vitamin (vit) B_{12}.

NORMAL VITAMIN B_{12} METABOLISM

Vitamin B_{12} is composed of (i) a corrin nucleus which has four pyrrole rings bound to a central cobalt atom, and (ii) a 5, 6 dimethylbenzimidazole group which is attached to the corrin ring and to the central cobalt atom. The important cobalamins that are distinguished according to the ligand attached to the central cobalt atom are: cyanocobalamin, hydroxocobalamin, adenosylcobalamin, and methylcobalamin. The terms cobalamin and vitamin B_{12} are often used interchangeably.

Sources of Vitamin B_{12}

Liver, dairy products, and sea fish are the major sources. Although bacteria in the large intestine synthesize vitamin B_{12}, it cannot be absorbed from this site. Minimum need of vitamin B_{12} for an adult is 1 to 4 μg/day.

Absorption of Vitamin B_{12}

Vitamin B_{12} is absorbed by two mechanisms—active and passive. About 75% of vitamin B_{12} in the food is absorbed by active mechanism, which requires the presence of intrinsic factor (IF). Intrinsic factor is a glycoprotein produced by parietal cells of gastric mucosa in response to presence of food in the stomach, similar to secretion of acid (vagal and hormonal stimulation). In passive mechanism, absorption occurs by diffusion and works when pharmacologic doses of vitamin B_{12} are ingested; only about 1% of this amount is absorbed by diffusion.

After entering into the stomach, vitamin B_{12} is freed from proteins by the action of pepsin at low pH. Vitamin B_{12} binds to a haptocorrin (previously called as R-binder) secreted in saliva and gastric juice. The haptocorrin-B_{12} complex is resistant to degradation by hydrochloric acid in the stomach. Along with food, haptocorrin-B12 complexes are carried to the duodenum where pancreatic proteases release B_{12} from haptocorrin. Free B_{12} rapidly binds to IF to form IF-B_{12} complex. This complex, which is protease resistant, is transported to the terminal part of ileum where receptors for IF are present on the epithelial cells. These receptors are composed of a complex of two proteins: *cub*ilin and *am*nionless (collectively called as cubam). Dysfunction of cubam due to mutation in either cubulin or amnionless produces megaloblastic anemia with proteinuria, also called as Imerslund-Gräsbeck syndrome. After binding to these receptors, the IF-B_{12} complex is internalized into the ileal mucosal cell along with the receptor. Inside the cell, IF is degraded, B12 attaches to another transport protein called transcobalamin II (TC II), and the receptor is carried back to the surface of the cell for another cycle of IF-B12.

The B_{12}-TC II complex is released into the portal circulation from where it is carried to various organs (Fig. 3.7).

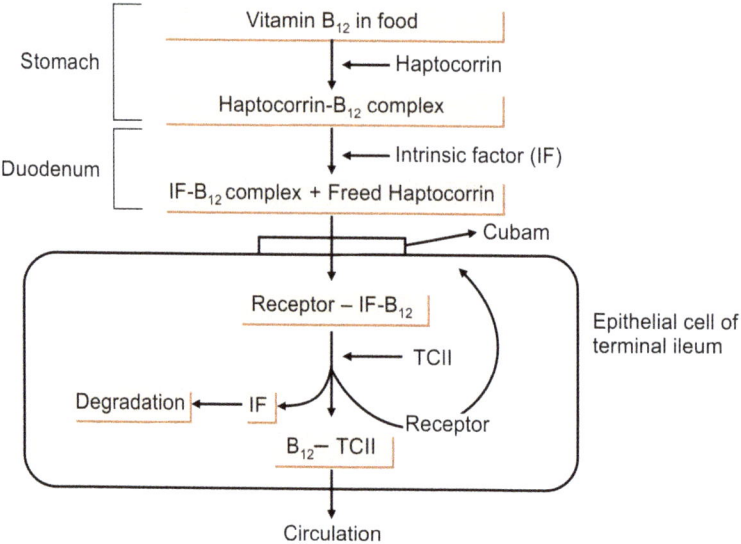

Fig. 3.7: Absorption of vitamin B_{12}

Transport of Vitamin B_{12}

The two vitamin B_{12}-binding proteins in plasma are transcobalamin or TC (previously known as transcobalamin II) and haptocorrins (previously known as transcobalamin I and transcobalamin III); the circulating haptocorrins belong to the same family of gastric haptocorrins.

TC is vitamin B_{12} (which is newly absorbed) transport protein that is synthesized by different types of cells such as liver cells, enterocytes, macrophages, and hematopoietic cells. After absorption, vitamin B_{12} circulates bound to TC and is carried to various organs and tissues, especially liver, bone marrow, and other dividing cells. After binding to specific cell surface receptor for TC, the B_{12}-TC complex is taken inside the cell. TC is destroyed and B_{12} is freed. Congenital absence of TC causes a severe megaloblastic anemia in infancy; however, vitamin B_{12} level in blood is normal.

Haptocorrins are synthesized by cells of organs that secrete them and also by granulocytes. Majority of vitamin B_{12} in circulation (80%) is bound to haptocorrins; this is so because newly absorbed vitamin B_{12} bound to TC is rapidly transported to various tissues, while transport of haptocorrin-B_{12} complex needs more time. Haptocorrins are raised in circulation in myeloproliferative neoplasms, since they are produced by granulocytes.

Storage Sites

The total amount of vitamin B_{12} in the body is 2 to 5 mg (adequate for 3 years). The major site of storage is the liver; other sites are heart and kidneys. Normal daily requirement is 3 to 5 µg of vitamin B_{12}.

Vitamin B_{12} is excreted through the bile and shedding of intestinal epithelial cells. Most of the excreted vitamin B_{12} is again absorbed in the intestine (enterohepatic circulation).

Functions of Vitamin B_{12}

Synthesis of Methionine from Homocysteine

This reaction is mediated by the enzyme methyl tetrahydrofolate homocysteine methyltransferase and requires a cofactor methylcobalamin. During this reaction, methyl tetrahydrofolate (methyl FH4) is converted to tetrahydrofolate (FH4). FH4 is necessary for the formation of methylene FH4 that is a cofactor in the synthesis of deoxythymidine monophosphate (dTMP) from deoxyuridine monophosphate (dUMP). dTMP is required for DNA synthesis (Fig. 3.8).

The "methyltetrahydrofolate trap" hypothesis has been proposed to explain the cause of impaired DNA synthesis in vitamin B_{12} deficiency. According to this hypothesis, deficiency of methylcobalamin leads to impaired conversion of methyl FH4 to FH4. Methylene FH4 required for the synthesis of dTMP is thus not generated, as most of the folate remain strapped as methyl FH4. This ultimately leads to defective synthesis of DNA.

Conversion of Methylmalonyl-CoA to Succinyl-CoA

This reaction requires adenosylcobalamin and methylmalonyl-CoA mutase. Deficiency of vitamin B_{12} is associated with increased levels of methylmalonate and propionate. It is thought that this causes synthesis of abnormal myelin lipids with consequent myelin degeneration and neurological abnormalities.

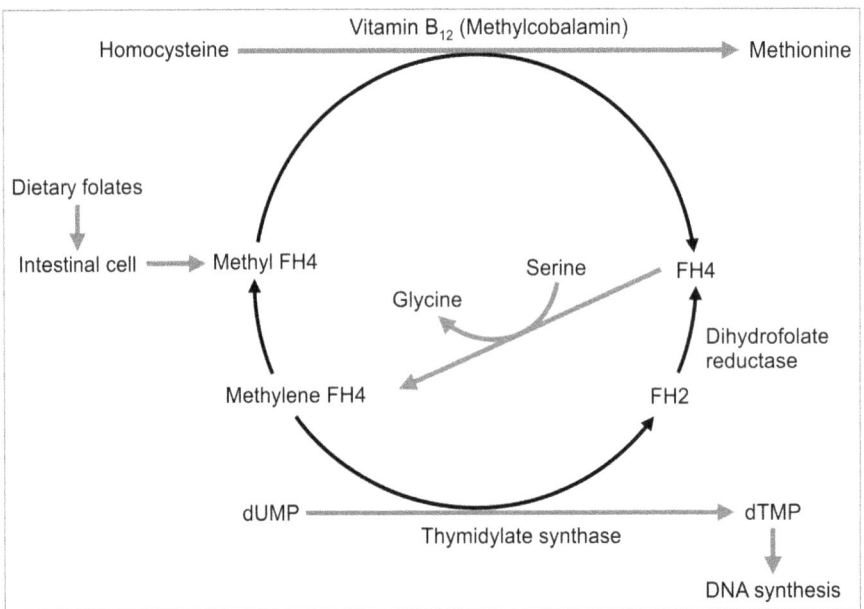

Fig. 3.8: Role of vitamin B12 and folate in synthesis of DNA. 5,10-methylene FH4 is formed when the carbon side chain of serine is transferred to FH4. This carbon is then transferred to dUMP to form dTMP. During this reaction, 5,10-methylene FH4 is oxidized to FH2, which is again reduced back to FH4 by dihydrofolate reductase. Also, methyl group is transferred from 5-methyl FH4 to form methionine from homocysteine that requires vitamin B12 as a cofactor. FH4 is generated during this reaction. Deficiency of vitamin B12 leads to failure of methylation of homocysteine and accumulation of substrate 5-methyl FH4, called as methyl folate trap. The trap results because conversion of 5,10-methylene FH4 to 5-methyl FH4 is irreversible. This intracellular deficiency of FH4 leads to inadequate one carbon transfer metabolism and eventually deficiency of DNA synthesis.
(FH4: Tetrahydrofolate; FH2: Dihydrofolate; dUMP: Deoxyuridylate monophosphate; dTMP: Deoxythymidylate monophosphate)

NORMAL FOLATE METABOLISM

The chemical name for folic acid is pteroylmonoglutamic acid. Folic acid is present in nature mostly as polyglutamates. Conversion of polyglutamate to tetrahydrofolate (the active form) is necessary for folate to participate in metabolic reactions.

1. **Sources of folate:** The major sources are green leafy vegetables, fruits, and liver. Folate is easily destroyed by boiling or heating foods in large amounts of water and most of folate in foods can be lost in this manner.
   The average daily requirement for an adult is about 400 µg. The requirement is more during pregnancy and in children during growth and in other conditions with rapid cell turnover like hemolytic anemias.
   In developed countries, supplementation of flour with folate is carried out.
2. **Absorption:** Dietary folates (polyglutamates) are hydrolyzed to monoglutamates at intestinal brush borders. Absorption of monoglutamates into intestinal epithelial cells (proximal jejunum) is facilitated by luminal surface proton-coupled folate transporter (PCFT). Inside the enterocytes, folate is rapidly converted to methyl tetrahydrofolate.
3. **Transport:** Folate is released in portal circulation as methyltetrahydrofolate and is transported to various tissues. In circulation, two-thirds of methyltetrahydrofolate is

bound to folate-binding protein including albumin and one-third circulates freely. Cellular uptake of methyltetrahydrofolate occurs by two mechanisms: (a) High-affinity folate receptors (FR-α and FR-β) bind and internalize methyltetrahydrofolate through endocytosis. Proton-coupled folate transporter exports folate from endosomes into cytoplasm of cells, across placenta to fetus, and across choroid plexus into CSF. (b) Reduced folate carriers have low affinity but high capacity for methyltetrahydrofolate. If folate level is very high in circulation (supraphysiologic), passive diffusion across cell membrane can occur.

4. **Storage:** Liver is the main site of storage where it is stored mainly as methyltetrahydrofolate polyglutamate. The total amount of folate in the body is about 12–28 mg that is adequate to meet the folate requirements for 3 to 6 months if folate is discontinued from the diet.

5. **Functions of folate:** The major biological action of tetrahydrofolate is to transfer single carbon substituents (e.g. methylene, methyl, or formyl groups) to different compounds. The metabolic reactions in which FH4 acts as a one-carbon donor or acceptor are:
   a. *Synthesis of thymidylate from uridylate:* This is biologically the most important reaction mediated by folate since it is necessary for synthesis of DNA (Fig. 3.8). Lack of tetrahydrofolate leads to diminished synthesis of dTMP and consequently of DNA leading to megaloblastic anemia. In this reaction, methylation of deoxyuridylate monophosphate (dUMP) to deoxythymidylate monophosphate (dTMP) is mediated by methylene tetrahydrofolate. Deoxythymidylate monophosphate or dTMP is the precursor of deoxythymidylate triphosphate (dTTP) which is necessary for DNA synthesis. Dihydrofolate (FH2) formed during this process is reduced by FH2 reductase to tetrahydrofolate (FH4) which then re-enters the cycle.
   b. Synthesis of methionine from homocysteine.
   c. Synthesis of purines.
   d. Histidine catabolism: Deficiency of folate leads to failure to metabolize formiminoglutamic acid (FIGlu), a product of histidine catabolism. As a result, folate deficiency is associated with excessive excretion of FIGlu in urine.

GENERAL MORPHOLOGICAL FEATURES OF MEGALOBLASTIC ANEMIA

Following morphological abnormalities are common to both vitamin B_{12} and folate deficiency. Although they are present in all proliferating cells in the body, they are particularly evident in cells of the hematopoietic system (Figs. 3.9 and 3.10).

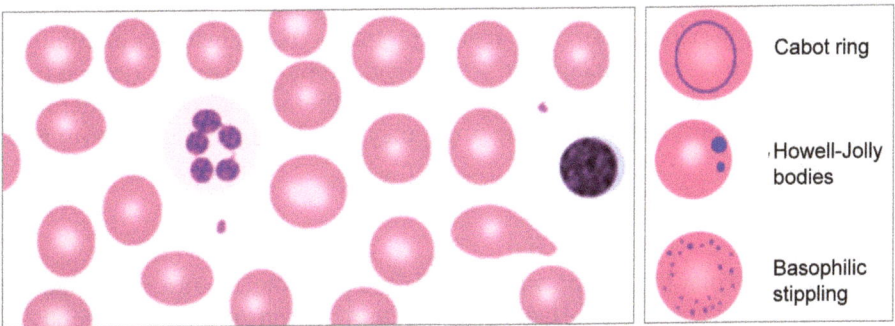

Fig. 3.9: Peripheral blood in megaloblastic anemia showing oval macrocytes, and a hypersegmented neutrophil. A small lymphocyte is shown for comparison of size with red cells. Panel on right shows some morphological abnormalities seen in severe megaloblastic anemia.

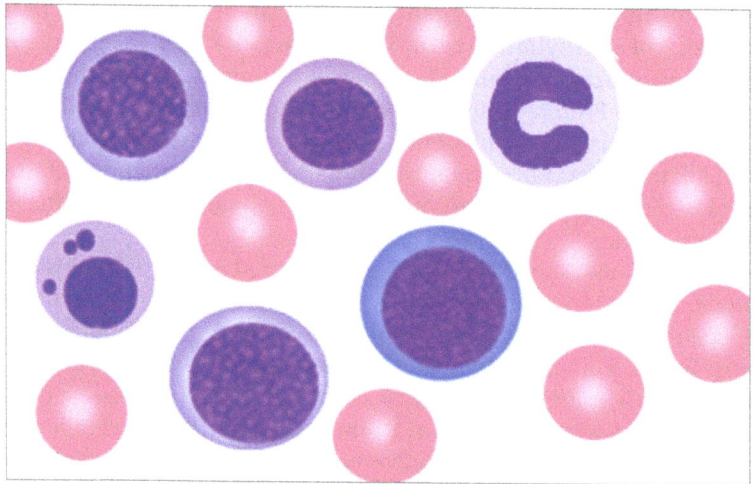

Fig. 3.10: Bone marrow in megaloblastic anemia. Five megaloblasts and one giant band form are seen. Howell-Jolly bodies are seen in the orthochromatic megaloblast.

Peripheral Blood

Megaloblastic anemia affects all the three lineages (red cells, leukocytes, and platelets) and there may be pancytopenia.

Red Cells

Red blood cells are characteristically large and oval (oval macrocytosis) and normochromic. In vitamin B_{12} or folate deficiency, macrocytosis is the earliest sign and can be detected even before the onset of anemia. Hematology analyzers best detect early macrocytosis (raised mean cell volume). Mean cell hemoglobin is increased (due to large cell volume), while mean cell hemoglobin concentration is normal. Macrocytosis may precede the development of anemia especially in pernicious anemia by several months or even years. Mean cell volume can be normal in megaloblastic anemia if there is coexistent iron deficiency, chronic inflammation, thalassemia, or chronic renal failure. In severe anemia, in addition to macrocytosis, marked anisopoikilocytosis (variation in size and shape of red cells), basophilic stippling, Howell-Jolly bodies, and Cabot's rings may also be found. Late or intermediate erythroblasts with fine, open nuclear chromatin (megaloblasts) may be seen in peripheral blood in severe anemia.

(*Note:* Macrocytosis also occurs in alcoholism, hepatic disease, hemolytic states, hypothyroidism and following treatment with chemotherapeutic drugs. Macrocytosis is a normal finding in newborns and during pregnancy. In all these cases however marrow is normoblastic.)

White Cells

Total leukocyte count may be normal or decreased (due to absolute neutropenia). Leukopenia is more marked in severe anemia. Hypersegmentation of neutrophils is one of the earliest signs of megaloblastic hematopoiesis and can be detected even in the absence of anemia. Normally, there are two to three nuclear lobes in a segmented neutrophil. In megaloblastic state, nuclear lobes increase in number. Hypersegmentation of neutrophils is said to be present when more than 5% of neutrophils show five or more lobes or one neutrophil with six or more lobes. Hypersegmented neutrophils tend to be larger in size. Hypersegmentation also occurs in uremia and as a congenital abnormality.

Platelets

In severe anemia, thrombocytopenia is usual. Platelet count, however, does not usually fall below 100,000/μL. Morphologic abnormalities of platelets in the form of giant platelets can occur, especially if platelet count is low. In advanced cases, bleeding time may be abnormal and sometimes purpura can occur.

Neurologic manifestations of vitamin B_{12} deficiency can occur even in the absence of anemia; in such cases, the diagnostic clues are provided by macrocytosis and hypersegmentation of neutrophils in peripheral blood.

Bone Marrow

Bone marrow is hypercellular with up to three-fold increase in erythropoiesis. The term "megaloblast" was coined by Ehrlich for large erythroblasts with abnormal chromatin that were seen in pernicious anemia. In megaloblastic anemia, DNA synthesis is impaired, while RNA synthesis is unaffected. Cell division is restricted due to nuclear immaturity but cytoplasmic components (especially haemoglobin) are synthesized excessively in between cell divisions. Cells therefore become enlarged in size. Megaloblastic features are present in all erythroid precursors. Megaloblasts are named according to the corresponding stage of normoblast-promegaloblast, and early, intermediate, and late megaloblasts. Morphologic differences between megaloblasts and normoblasts are outlined below:
1. Cell and nuclear size and amount of cytoplasm are increased in megaloblasts.
2. The nuclear chromatin of megaloblasts is sieve-like or stippled (open) which can be well appreciated at polychromatic stage. Howell-Jolly bodies are common (Fig. 3.10).
3. The nuclear maturation (progressive condensation of nuclear chromatin) falls behind cytoplasmic maturation (hemoglobinization). This is known as nuclear-cytoplasmic asynchrony or dissociation.
4. Early precursors of erythroid series (promegaloblasts and early megaloblasts) are increased in number in bone marrow as compared to more mature precursors (intermediate and late megaloblasts). This is known as maturation arrest.
5. Mitotic activity is increased.

Megaloblastic changes are better appreciated in polychromatic erythroblast stage in which cytoplasm is blue-pink in color (due to combination of hemoglobin with RNA), while the nuclear chromatin is open and sieve-like.

Granulocytic series also displays megaloblastic changes. Most prominent changes are seen in metamyelocytes that are large (giant metamyelocytes) with horseshoe-shaped nuclei and finer nuclear chromatin, and in band forms. Giant metamyelocytes with open chromatin are virtually diagnostic.

Megakaryocytes are often large with multiple nuclear lobes and paucity of cytoplasmic granules.

Ineffective erythropoiesis: Although bone marrow shows erythroid hyperplasia, reticulocyte count is low indicating ineffective erythropoiesis. Deficiency of folate/vitamin B_{12} leads to inability to convert dUMP to dTMP, the precursor of dTTP. This causes phosphorylation of dUMP to dUTP, which is erroneously incorporated into DNA. This defect is recognized by DNA repair mechanism which attempts to replace uridine with thymidine. However, due to lack of dTTP, the attempt fails and DNA fragmentation and cell apoptosis occur. This is evident as increased lactate dehydrogenase, increased serum bilirubin, and pancytopenia.

Need for bone marrow examination in megaloblastic anemia: Although the bone marrow examination was done in the past for confirmation of megaloblastic nature of macrocytic anemia, it has been replaced by estimation of serum folate and serum B_{12} assays. Bone marrow examination is considered necessary in macrocytic anemia if (1) serum folate and vitamin B_{12} are normal or equivocal, (2) response to vitamin replacement is absent or inadequate, or (3) blood smear shows abnormal cells suggestive of myelodysplastic syndrome.

CAUSES OF MEGALOBLASTIC ANEMIA

Etiology of megaloblastic anemia can be divided into three broad groups: I. Deficiency of folate; II. Deficiency of vitamin B_{12}; and III. Miscellaneous causes.

Most common cause of megaloblastic anemia is deficiency of either folate or vitamin B_{12}. It is worthnoting that vitamin B_{12} deficiency most frequently results from defective absorption of the vitamin while folate deficiency is most commonly due to inadequate dietary intake.

About 3 to 5 years are required for development of vitamin B_{12} deficiency after abrupt cessation of availability of vitamin B_{12}; for folate deficiency, this period is about 3 to 4 months. This time interval is related to the daily requirement and the size of the storage compartment.

Severe deficiency of vitamin B_{12} can result secondarily in decreased absorption of folate, and vice versa. This is so because severe lack of either folate or vitamin B_{12} is associated with atrophy of rapidly dividing small intestinal epithelial cells and malabsorption.

Incidence of vitamin B_{12} is increasing because of (1) increased use of proton pump inhibitors and of metformin, (2) fortification of foods with folate in developed countries, (3) increasing rate of gastric bypass surgery, and (4) rise in elderly population who are more likely to have deficient absorption of vitamin B_{12}.

Deficiency of Folate

Causes of Folate Deficiency

These are listed in Box 3.9.

Insufficient intake: **The most common cause of folate deficiency is poor dietary intake.** The major etiological factor in tropical countries is grossly inadequate intake of green leafy vegetables and animal proteins. This is most commonly seen in elderly and poor people. Improper cooking methods also contribute to the loss of dietary folate.

Folic acid deficiency is very common in **alcoholics** because most of the calories in them are provided by alcohol. Alcohol also interferes with metabolism and probably absorption of folate.

Box 3.9: Causes of folate deficiency.

1. **Insufficient dietary intake**—poor diet with lack of green vegetables, chronic alcoholics, prolonged parenteral nutrition.
2. **Deficient absorption**—malabsorption syndromes such as celiac disease or tropical sprue.
3. **Increased demand**—pregnancy, increased cell turnover (hemolytic anemia, neoplasia).
4. **Drugs**—Trimethoprim, methotrexate, sulfasalazine, anticonvulsants.

It should be noted that apart from folate deficiency, macrocytosis in alcoholics might result from other causes such as direct toxic effect of alcohol on erythroid cells, reticulocytosis secondary to gastrointestinal bleeding or alcohol withdrawal, or hepatic disorder.

Prolonged parenteral fluid therapy in ill patients without vitamin supplements can cause acute megaloblastic anemia (see later).

Deficient absorption: **Celiac disease (also called as non-tropical sprue)** is due to immunological reaction to gliadin (a product of gluten). Gluten and gliadin are proteins, which are present in certain cereals. Histologically, there is atrophy of villi in proximal portion of small intestine with consequent loss of absorptive area.

Patient presents clinically with weight loss and steatorrhea. There is impaired absorption of folate, iron, and other nutrients. D-xylose test for deficient absorption, histopathology, and improvement after diet devoid of gluten are helpful in arriving at the correct diagnosis. Therapy involves gluten-free diet and treatment of associated nutritional deficiencies.

Tropical sprue is endemic in India, West Indies, and Southeast Asia. Infection by enterotoxigenic *Escherichia coli* has been implicated. Tropical sprue affects distal portion of the small intestine. Features of tropical and nontropical sprue resemble each other. Inability to deconjugate polyglutamates in the intestine impairs absorption of folate. Due to affection of terminal ileum, vitamin B_{12} deficiency is also usually present. Treatment consists of administration of folic acid, vitamin B_{12}, and broad-spectrum antibiotics.

Increased demand: Shunting of folate to the fetus causes up to five times increase in folate requirements during **pregnancy**. Megaloblastic anemia of folate deficiency usually develops during the last trimester. To meet the increased demand and to prevent folate deficiency, pregnant women are routinely given 1 mg folic acid per day. Increased incidence of premature labor, placental abruption, pre-eclampsia, and neural tube defects in fetus has been reported in folate-deficient pregnant women.

Cell turnover and consequently folate requirements are increased in hemolytic states. Patients with myeloproliferative disorders, exfoliative skin disorders, and malignancies also have increased folate requirements.

Clinical Features

Clinical manifestations are related to the severity of anemia and are nonspecific. The common features are pallor and mild icterus (due to ineffective erythropoiesis). Angular stomatitis and glossitis may be present. Cardiac failure can occur in severe cases.

Deficiency of either folate or vitamin B_{12} is associated with increased levels of homocysteine in blood. Hyperhomocysteinemia has been linked with increased risk of thrombosis. Severe nutritional deficiency of vitamin B_{12} or folate causes megaloblastic anemia whereas milder deficiencies are associated with increased cardiovascular risk. Insufficient folate during early pregnancy is implicated in the development of neural tube defects in the fetus.

Laboratory Features

Morphologic abnormalities in peripheral blood and bone marrow have been considered earlier. Examination of bone marrow is not indicated in megaloblastic anemia if diagnosis is unequivocal (from clinical features, blood studies, and vitamin assays).

Estimation of serum folate, red cell folate, and serum vitamin B_{12}: These measurements help in establishing the diagnosis and in differentiating folate and vitamin B_{12} deficiencies from one another. There are different methods of assaying these parameters—microbiological, immunmetric, and radioisotopic. Microbiological assays have now largely been replaced by automated methods using immunometric or radioisotope techniques.

Reduction in serum folate level (<4 µg/L) is an early indicator of folate deficiency. However, low values are also obtained in normal subjects when recent dietary intake is low in folate content. In vitamin B_{12} deficiency, serum folate level is normal or increased in most patients and reduced in a minority of patients. Raised serum folate in vitamin B_{12} deficiency represents accumulation of 5-methyltetrahydrofolate ("folate trap").

Folate is incorporated within red cells during erythropoiesis and its level remains constant throughout the life span of red cells. A low red cell folate indicates megaloblastic anemia due to folate deficiency. About 50% of patients with vitamin B_{12} deficiency also have reduced red cell folate levels.

Serum vitamin B_{12} levels are thought to reflect tissue stores. Serum vitamin B_{12} levels are reduced in megaloblastic anemia due to vitamin B_{12} deficiency; however, low values are also obtained in about 30% of patients with folate deficiency.

Thus in folate deficiency both serum and red cell folate are usually markedly reduced while serum vitamin B_{12} is either normal or mildly decreased. In vitamin B_{12} deficiency, serum vitamin B_{12} and red cell folate are depressed, while serum folate is normal or increased. In combined folate and vitamin B_{12} deficiency, all the values are low (Table 3.2).

Methylmalonic acid (MMA) and homocysteine in serum: See under vitamin B_{12} deficiency.

Formiminoglutamate (FIGlu) excretion test: FIGlu is excreted in excessive amounts in folate deficiency. In this test, 15 g oral dose of histidine is given to the patient and urinary excretion of FIGlu is measured spectrophotometrically. Excessive excretion of FIGlu also occurs in vitamin B_{12} deficiency.

Therapeutic trial: Therapeutic trial may be undertaken if nature of deficiency is not evident from clinical data and facilities for vitamin assays are not available. Therapeutic trial should not be undertaken if the patient is having severe anemia, congestive heart failure, angina, neurological manifestations, bleeding tendencies due to thrombocytopenia, or pregnancy. After obtaining baseline hemoglobin/hematocrit levels and reticulocyte count, patient is given folic acid 200 µg orally or vitamin B_{12} 1 to 2 µg IM every day for 10 days. Reticulocytosis beginning on 3rd day and reaching maximum on 6th or 7th day is the optimal response. If such hematologic response is not obtained or if the response is only partial, then the other vitamin is tried. Suboptimal response to one vitamin may be due to combined deficiency of vitamin B_{12} and folate, concomitant deficiency of iron, or presence of complicating infectious or inflammatory disease.

Other feature: Mild increase in indirect serum bilirubin and urinary urobilinogen reflects ineffective erythropoiesis (hemolysis of megaloblasts in marrow). Serum lactate dehydrogenase is also increased due partly to destruction of megaloblasts which contain high concentration of lactate dehydrogenase (LDH); this increase is roughly proportional to the degree of anemia.

Markedly raised serum LDH is an important laboratory determinant of megaloblastic anemia; in hemolytic anemia, serum LDH is mildly to moderately raised.

See Figure 3.11 for diagnostic approach to megaloblastic anemias.

The diagnostic approach involves three steps:
1. Demonstration of presence of megaloblastic anemia
2. Distinguishing between vitamin B_{12} and folate deficiency
3. Determining the underlying cause of deficiency

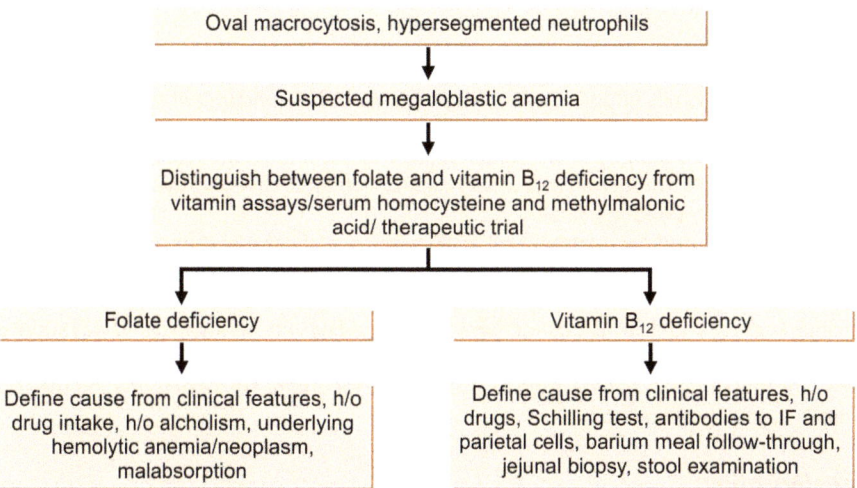

Fig. 3.11: Laboratory diagnosis of megaloblastic anemia. Serum vitmine B_{12} <150 pg/mL or serum folate <4 µg/L are indicative of vitamin B_{12} or folate deficiency, respectively. Serum vitmine B_{12} >400 pg/mL excludes vitamin B_{12} deficiency. If serum vitamin B_{12} level is borderline (150–400 pg/mL), assays for serum methylmalonic acid and serum homocysteine are indicated. In vitamin B_{12} deficiency, both are elevated, while only serum homocysteine is raised in folate deficiency. If there is a strong clinical suspicion of vitamin deficiency and the test results are not contributory, a therapeutic trial with vitamin B_{12} is used.

Treatment of Folate Deficiency

Megaloblastic anemia should never be treated empirically with folic acid alone unless vitamin B_{12} levels are normal. Folate deficiency is treated by 1 to 5 mg folic acid per day orally. Duration of therapy depends on underlying cause. Therapy should be continued until complete hematological recovery is obtained. In patients with chronic hemolysis or malabsorption, long-term folate therapy is required.

Treatment with higher doses of folate may partially improve the anemia of vitamin B_{12} deficiency but not the neurological complications. More dangerously, it can precipitate subacute combined degeneration of spinal cord. Therefore, before beginning therapy, vitamin assays should be obtained. If therapy is urgently required then blood samples are first drawn for assays and then both vitamins are administered. Depending upon the vitamin that is deficient, relevant investigations can be carried out to identify the cause of the deficiency.

For prevention of neural tube defects in the fetus, administration of folate must begin at conception since neural tube closes around 3 weeks.

Deficiency of Vitamin B_{12}

Causes of Vitamin B_{12} Deficiency

These are listed in Box 3.10.

Insufficient intake: This is a very rare cause of vitamin B_{12} deficiency. It has been reported in rigid vegetarians (vegans) who do not even take milk and other dairy products.

Box 3.10: Causes of vitamin B_{12} deficiency.

1. **Insufficient dietary intake:** Strict vegetarians ("vegans")
2. **Deficient absorption:** Pernicious anemia, total or partial gastrectomy, prolonged use of proton pump inhibitors or H_2 receptor blockers, metformin, diseases of small intestine, fish tapeworm infestation.

Box 3.11: Pernicious anemia—Historical aspects.

- The disease was called as "pernicious" in old days because it was invariably fatal.
- First described by Thomas Addison, an English physician, in 1849 and therefore also called as Addison's anemia.
- George Minot, William Murphy, and George Whipple jointly shared the Nobel Prize for Physiology or Medicine in 1934 for introduction of raw liver diet for the successful treatment of pernicious anemia, which was previously uniformly fatal.
- Liver extracts were used for treatment till 1948, when specific therapeutic agent (vitamin B12) was isolated
- William B Castle coined the terms "Intrinsic factor" (which was absent in stomachs of persons of pernicious anemia) and "Extrinsic factor" (which corrected pernicious anemia and was supplied in the diet) in the late 1920s. Extrinsic factor was later identified as vitamin B_{12}.
- In 1964, Dorothy Hodgkin was awarded the Nobel Prize for Chemistry for determining the structure of vitamin B_{12} using crystallography.

Deficient absorption:

1. *Pernicious anemia:* This is the most common cause of reduced intestinal absorption of vitamin B_{12}. Historical features are presented in Box 3.11.
   This disease occurs in middle and older age groups. (Median age at diagnosis is 60 years.) Usual presentation is with anemia. It is an autoimmune disease characterized by chronic atrophic gastritis, failure of secretion of intrinsic factor, and vitamin B_{12} deficiency.
   Gastric atrophy is associated with presence of autoantibodies against intrinsic factor and parietal cells. Pathologic changes are infiltration by mononuclear cells in submucosa and lamina propria of fundus and body of stomach, progressive loss of parietal and chief cells, and their replacement by intestinal type mucous cells. Deficiency of intrinsic factor results from destruction of parietal cells and blocking of vitamin B_{12} binding to intrinsic factor by autoantibodies present in gastric juice. Complete absence of intrinsic factor causes failure of absorption of vitamin B_{12} and megaloblastic anemia. Neurological complications of vitamin B_{12} deficiency may develop. There is association with other autoimmune disorders such as Graves' disease, vitiligo, Hashimoto's thyroiditis, insulin dependent diabetes mellitus, primary hyperparathyroidism, Addison's disease, and myasthenia gravis.
   In addition to morphological signs of megaloblastic anemia in peripheral blood and bone marrow and reduced serum vitamin B_{12} levels, other laboratory features of pernicious anemia include abnormal Schilling test (see later), pentagastrin-fast achlorhydria, and anti-IF and antiparietal cell antibodies in serum. Autoantibodies (IgG) to parietal cells occur in 90% of patients, but are not specific since they also occur in 15% of normal individuals. Antibodies to IF occur in 50% of patients and are diagnostic. These antibodies can also be detected in gastric juice.
   Patients with pernicious anemia have increased risk of gastric cancer and should have regular follow-up examinations by gastric endoscopy. Complete blood count and thyroid function tests should be done annually.
2. *Gastrectomy:* Total gastrectomy is invariably followed by megaloblastic anemia secondary to vitamin B_{12} deficiency as it removes the site of synthesis of intrinsic factor. These patients should be given prophylactic vitamin B_{12} after surgery. Patients with partial gastrectomy need regular follow-up after surgery for early detection of vitamin B_{12} deficiency.
3. *Diseases of the small intestine:* Diseases of small intestine (e.g. tuberculosis, Whipple's disease, blind loop syndrome) or its resection may interfere with absorption of vitamin B_{12} that occurs in terminal ileum.

In blind loop syndrome, stasis of small intestinal contents (e.g. by diverticulum or stricture) may predispose to bacterial colonization and proliferation. Utilization of most of the ingested vitamin B_{12} by bacteria may lead to reduced or nonavailability of vitamin B_{12} for absorption. Treatment consists of parenteral vitamin B_{12}, broad-spectrum antibiotics, and surgical correction of the abnormality.

4. *Infestation by fish tapeworm:* Infestation by fish tapeworm *Diphyllobothrium latum*, due to ingestion of inadequately cooked fish, is observed in Scandinavian countries and the Soviet Republic. The worm produces vitamin B_{12} deficiency by competing with the host for vitamin B_{12} in food. Diagnosis is made by demonstration of ova in stool examination. The infestation can be eradicated by administering niclosamide.

Clinical Features

Clinical features include manifestations of anemia, mild icterus and sometimes neurologic changes. (Neurologic involvement does not occur in folate deficiency.) In vitamin B_{12} deficiency, neurological involvement can occur in the form of:

- Peripheral neuropathy (paresthesiae and numbness)
- Subacute combined degeneration of spinal cord: Classically, vitamin B_{12} deficiency produces degeneration of posterior and lateral columns of spinal cord. This causes loss of position and vibration sense and sensory ataxia. Two signs are commonly elicited: (1) Lhermitte sign (flexion of head causes electric shock-like sensation spreading downwards), and (2) Romberg's sign (inability to maintain body balance with eyes closed and feet close together).
- Cerebral changes (personality changes, dementia, and psychosis). Severe psychotic manifestations due to vitamin B_{12} deficiency is called as "megaloblastic madness."
- In elderly persons, vitamin B_{12} deficiency can present as a neurologic or psychiatric disease without anemia or hematologic changes. Neurological abnormalities are irreversible in late stages and therefore prompt recognition and treatment of deficiency of vitamin B_{12} is necessary.

Patients with vitamin B_{12} deficiency can present with only neurological abnormalities without macrocytosis or anemia (especially in the elderly); however, in such cases, bone marrow examination reveals megaloblastic changes.

Laboratory Features

Morphologic features of megaloblastic anemia in peripheral blood and bone marrow have been outlined earlier. Examination of bone marrow is not indicated in megaloblastic anemia if diagnosis is unequivocal (from clinical features, blood studies, and vitamin assays).

Serum vitamin B_{12} assay: See laboratory features of folate deficiency. Serum vitamin B_{12} < 150 pg/mL strongly suggests deficiency, while level > 400 pg/mL usually rules out deficiency.

Serum holotranscobalamin: This is a subfraction of cobalamin and is a marker of early vitamin B_{12} deficiency.

Methylmalonic acid (MMA) and homocysteine in serum: As outlined earlier, vitamin B_{12} is a coenzyme for two reactions: (1) synthesis of methionine from homocysteine, and (2) conversion of methylmalonyl-CoA to succinyl-CoA. The first reaction also requires methyltetrahydrofolate; therefore homocysteine metabolism is affected by either vitamin B_{12} or folate deficiency and homocysteine is elevated in either vitamin B_{12} or folate deficiency.

When the later reaction (conversion of methylmalonyl-CoA to succinyl-CoA) is blocked, methylmalonic acid accumulates in tissues and serum; elevation of serum MMA is specific for vitamin B_{12} deficiency. Measurement of serum methylmalonic acid and serum homocysteine are more sensitive for detection of vitamin B_{12} deficiency than estimation of vitamin B_{12}. They are raised early in tissue deficiency even before the appearance of hematological changes. Estimation of both MMA and homocysteine is helpful in differentiating vitamin B_{12} deficiency from folate deficiency. In vitamin B_{12} deficiency, both are elevated. In folate deficiency, homocysteine is raised, while MMA is normal. Raised serum MMA level is considered as the single most sensitive and specific test for detection of vitmin B_{12} deficiency.

Schilling test: This test is used for **evaluation of absorption of vitamin B_{12} in the gastrointestinal tract.** The test can be performed in two parts—part I and part II.

Part I: In part I of the test, 0.5 to 1 µg of radiolabeled vitamin B_{12} is given orally. After 2 hours, an intramuscular dose (1000 µg) of unlabeled vitamin B_{12} is given. This dose saturates vitamin B_{12}-binding sites of transcobalamin I and II and displaces any bound radiolabeled vitamin B_{12} thus permitting urinary excretion of absorbed radiolabeled vitamin B_{12}. Radioactivity is measured in subsequently collected 24 hour urine sample and expressed as a percentage of total oral dose.

In normal persons, more than 7% of the oral dose of vitamin B_{12} is excreted in urine. If excretion is less than normal it indicates impaired absorption, which may be due to either lack of intrinsic factor or small intestinal malabsorption. Part II of the test is performed if result of part I is abnormal.

Part II: In part II, patient is orally administered radiolabeled vitamin B_{12} along with intrinsic factor while the remainder of the test is carried out as in part I. If excretion becomes normal, it indicates lack of intrinsic factor. If excretion remains below normal defective absorption in the small intestine is the probable cause.

Abnormal result in part I that is corrected in part II of the test occurs in pernicious anemia. If both parts yield abnormal results, it indicates malabsorption in small intestine; however, such result is also obtained when renal excretion is impaired due to chronic renal disease, commercial intrinsic factor is ineffective or is inactivated by antibodies in stomach, and when absorption of vitamin B_{12} is impaired due to atrophy of ileal epithelial cells secondary to severe vitamin B_{12}/folate deficiency. The large parenteral dose of nonradiolabeled vitamin B_{12} in Schilling test is therapeutic and alters the blood levels of the vitamin. Therefore, blood samples for vitamin B_{12} assay should be obtained before Schilling test is performed.

Thus in short (1) reduced vitamin B_{12} absorption corrected by IF occurs in pernicious anemia and gastrectomy, and (2) reduced vitamin B_{12} absorption not corrected by IF occurs in diseases of terminal ileum and ileal resection (Box 3.12).

Box 3.12: Interpretation of Schilling test.
- **Stage I Normal:** Dietary deficiency
- **Stage I Abnormal, Stage II Normal:** Pernicious anemia, gastrectomy
- **Stage I Abnormal, Stage II Abnormal:** Ileal disease

Disadvantages of Schilling test:
- Test is tedious and complicated
- It is difficult to procure radiolabeled vitamin B_{12}
- Test results are affected by renal function and collection of urine
- Much of the test's relevance is lost due to recent evidence that oral vitamin B_{12} is as effective as parenteral vitamin B_{12} in the treatment of pernicious anemia.

Schilling test has become obsolete and as yet there is no replacement test. Currently, the only test for diagnosis of pernicious anemia is detection of circulating anti intrinsic factor antibodies; however, although the test is highly specific, it has only 60% sensitivity.

Table 3.2: Differences between vitamin B_{12} and folate deficiency.

Parameter	Vitamin B_{12} deficiency	Folate deficiency
1. Prevalence	Less common	More common
2. Minimum daily requirement of nutrient	1–4 µg	400 µg
3. Effect of cooking on nutrient	No effect	Readily destroyed
4. Time interval between onset of deprivation and manifestations	2–5 years	Few weeks to months
5. Usual cause	Inadequate absorption	Inadequate intake or increased demand
6. Peripheral neuropathy	May be present	Absent
7. Serum vitamin B_{12}	Low	Normal
8. Serum folate	Normal or increased	Low
9. Red cell folate	Low	Low
10. Serum homocysteine	Raised	Raised
11. Serum methylmalonic acid	Raised	Normal

Intrinsic factor antibodies in serum: Detection of anti-IF antibodies in serum is diagnostic of pernicious anemia.

Therapeutic trial: See laboratory features of folate deficiency.

See Figure 3.11 for diagnostic approach to megaloblastic anemias. Differences between vitamin B_{12} deficiency and folate deficiency are outlined in Table 3.2.

For specific diagnosis of vitamin B_{12} or folate deficiency, less expensive and widely available tests like serum vitamin B_{12} and serum folate should be used initially; the results should be interpreted in the context of clinical and hematological features. If results are not definitive (serum vitamin B_{12} 150–400 pg/mL) and clinical/hematological feature are suggestive of deficiency, more expensive tests like serum MMA and homocystine are advised.

Treatment of Vitamin B_{12} Deficiency

In vitamin B_{12} deficiency, administration of only folate will partially correct megaloblastic anemia; however, neurological disease is precipitated. Therefore, it is necessary to exclude vitamin B_{12} deficiency before beginning folate therapy. Megaloblastic anemia should never be empirically treated with folate alone. Both vitamins (1 mg cyanocobalamin and 1–5 mg folate per day) are administered in severely ill patients after withdrawing blood samples for vitamin assays. The aims of vitamin B_{12} replacement therapy are correction of hematocrit, to improve neurological abnormalities, and to refill storage pools. Initial therapy consists of 1 mg of cyanocobalamin intramuscular or subcutaneous every day for 1 week. This is followed by dosage of 1 mg twice weekly (second week), 1 mg per week for 4 weeks, and then 1 mg per month for life.

An alternative mechanism independent of IF exists for absorption of vitamin B_{12}. If large amount of vitamin B_{12} is given orally, about 1% of this dose is absorbed. According to some recent observations, oral vitamin B_{12} has been shown to be as effective as parenteral vitamin B_{12} in the treatment of pernicious anemia. For those patients who refuse monthly parenteral vitamin B_{12}, oral vitamin B_{12} (1-2 mg/day as tablets) can be given.

After initiation of therapy, reticulocyte count begins to increase around 3rd day, reaches peak on 6th or 7th day, and gradually returns to normal by the end of 3rd week. By 24 hours, subjective feeling of well-being develops and erythropoies is becomes normoblastic. Hematocrit steadily rises and normalizes in about 1 to 2 months.

Sudden and severe hypokalemia can occur immediately after initiation of therapy which may be rapidly fatal (due to cardiac arrhythmias) if untreated. Acute fall in blood potassium level is thought to be due to internalization of potassium by proliferating cells.

Blood transfusion is indicated in severely anemic symptomatic patients or inpatients with congestive cardiac failure. In such cases, one unit of packed red cells may be transfused slowly in view of the risk of circulatory overload.

Miscellaneous Causes of Megaloblastic Anemia

Drugs

Drug ingestion is a common cause of megaloblastic anemia, only next in frequency to deficiency of folate or vitamin B_{12}. Methotrexate, and to a lesser extent trimethoprim, pentamidine and pyrimethamine are inhibitors of dihydrofolate reductase, an enzyme required for regeneration of tetrahydrofolate from dihydrofolate. Antimetabolites such as 6-mercaptopurine and 5-fluorouracil inhibit the synthesis of DNA directly. These drugs initially produce mild megaloblastic anemia, which is eventually followed by marrow hypoplasia if the drug is not discontinued. Some other drugs causing megaloblastic anemia are cytosine arabinoside, hydroxyurea, zidovudine, antiepileptics, oral contraceptives, and nitrous oxide.

Hematologic Disorders

Megaloblastic features are present in erythroid series in myelodysplastic syndrome and erythroleukemia. In myelodysplastic syndrome, dysplastic features are present in all the three cell lines (erythroid, granulocytic, and megakaryocytic) along with ringed sideroblasts, increased numbers of immature granulocytic precursors, and abnormal localization of blasts in bone marrow. In erythroleukemia, aside from megaloblastic features, erythroblasts are bizarre looking, erythroblastosis is commonly present in peripheral blood, and myeloblasts are increased in bone marrow.

Acute Megaloblastic Anemia

In this condition, there is a sudden and rapid development of megaloblastosis in bone marrow that may be fatal. Nitrous oxide anesthesia, and total parenteral nutrition without vitamin supplementation in critically ill patients are the usual causes. The patient rapidly develops thrombocytopenia or leucopenia or both but anemia is lacking. Bone marrow shows typical megaloblastic features. Administration of folate and vitamin B_{12} is effective.

Congenital Defects of Metabolism

Congenital defects of metabolism involving either folate or vitamin B_{12} are rare.

Causes of nonmegaloblastic macrocytosis: Macrocytosis due to megaloblastic anemia should be differentiated from nonmegaloblastic (or normoblastic) macrocytosis. Conditions associated with nonmegaloblastic macrocytosis and their causes include
- Alcoholism: Direct toxic effect of alcohol on erythroid precursors, poor intake of dietary folates, associated liver disease
- Liver disease: Increased red cell membrane lipids
- Hemolysis or posthemorrhagic anemia: Increased reticulocytes which are larger than red cells
- Hypothyroidism: Mechanism of macrocytosis unknown
- Aplastic anemia: Mechanism of macrocytosis unknown
- Spurious macrocytosis: False elevation of mean cell volume on hematology analyzers due to cold agglutinins, hyperglycemia, or very high leukocyte count.

APLASTIC ANEMIA AND RELATED DISORDERS

Aplastic anemia is a disorder of hematopoiesis in which there are pancytopenia in peripheral blood and decreased cellularity of bone marrow. By definition, there is no abnormal infiltrate (leukemic, cancerous, or other) or increase in reticulin in bone marrow. Aplastic anemia is uncommon in the West; it is more common in East Asia and other developing countries. There are two peaks of presentation of acquired aplastic anemia: one between 15 and 25 years of age and the other in patients > 60 years. Causes of aplastic anemia are listed in Table 3.3.

ACQUIRED APLASTIC ANEMIA

Causes

Approximately two-thirds cases of aplastic anemia are idiopathic. Drugs and chemicals commonly associated with aplastic anemia are listed in Table 3.4. The most often implicated drugs are gold salts, penicillamine, indomethacin, diclofenac, anticonvulsants, and ticlopidine.

Benzene is used as a commercial solvent in many industries. Hematological alterations induced by benzene are hypoplasia of bone marrow, hemolysis, lymphocytopenia, hyperplasia of bone marrow, and acute myeloid leukemia (AML).

Table 3.3: Causes of aplastic anemia.

Acquired	Constitutional
1. Idiopathic	1. Fanconi anemia
2. Drugs and chemicals	2. Dyskeratosis congenita
3. Ionizing radiation	3. Schwachman-Diamond syndrome
4. Infectious diseases: viral hepatitis, cytomegalovirus, Epstein-Barr virus	4. Diamond-Blackfan anemia
5. Paroxysmal nocturnal hemoglobinuria	5. Congenital amegakaryocytic thrombocytopenia
6. Graft vs host disease	
7. Pregnancy	

Table 3.4: Common drugs and toxins implicated in the etiology of aplastic anemia.

Drugs	Chemicals
A. Dose-dependent action—Cytotoxic drugs B. Idiosyncratic action • Antibacterials (Sulphonamides, Chloramphenicol) • Anti-inflammatory drugs (Phenylbutazone, Indomethacin, Piroxicam, Diclofenac, Naproxen) • Antirheumatics (Gold, Penicillamine) • Antiepileptics (Phenytoin, Carbamazepine) • Antithyroids • Tranquilizers (Chlorpromazine) • Others—Furosemide, Allopurinol, Ticlopidine	• Benzene • Insecticides (Organophosphates, organochlorines) • Pentachlorophenol (an antibacterial, fungicide, and a wood-preservative)

Bone marrow injury caused by cytotoxic drugs is dose-dependent and transient, being reversible after discontinuation of the drug. In some persons, pancytopenia with marrow aplasia develops as an idiosyncratic reaction to certain drugs that are normally tolerated by majority of individuals. The idiosyncratic reactions are not dose-dependent, may develop after discontinuation of the drug, and may be irreversible and life-threatening. Chloramphenicol causes two patterns of bone marrow damage—dose-dependent reversible hematopoietic suppression in about 50% of individuals and idiosyncratic aplastic anemia in a small number of individuals.

The dose-dependent reversible hematopoietic suppression is a more common side effect of chloramphenicol. Usually, there is reduction of erythroid precursors that manifests as anemia and reticulocytopenia. Less frequently, there is suppression of granulocytic and megakaryocytic series. Bone marrow examination shows reduction of erythroid precursors, vacuolization of nucleus and cytoplasm in premature cells of erythroid and granulocytic series and ringed sideroblasts. Serum iron level is characteristically raised. These changes occur with prolonged high-dose therapy with chloramphenicol and are reversible on cessation of the drug. However, continued administration in high dosage may lead to aplastic anemia. The pathogenesis of this toxic effect appears to be direct inhibition of proliferation and differentiation of precursor cells in bone marrow. More important side effect of chloramphenicol is the development of idiosyncratic aplastic anemia. It probably occurs due to irreversible genetic damage to the hematopoietic stem cells. It is thought that there is a genetic susceptibility of stem cells to chloramphenicol-induced DNA damage. Patient develops severe pancytopenia and bone marrow failure, which is often life-threatening. This is not related to the dose or duration of therapy and is reported to occur in 1:11,500 to 1:40,000 persons taking the drug. Aplastic anemia may occur days or even weeks after cessation of the drug. Chloramphenicol should be avoided if safer alternative drugs are available and its use for trivial indications should be discouraged.

Bone marrow aplasia has been reported to occur rarely following hepatitis.

Serological markers against the known viral agents are often negative. Aplastic anemia develops about 2 to 3 months following the episode of hepatitis. Posthepatitis aplastic anemia is often severe and life-threatening.

There is a strong association between paroxysmal nocturnal hemoglobinuria (PNH) and aplastic anemia. Aplastic anemia precedes or follows PNH in a significant proportion of patients.

Transfusion of whole blood to immunodeficient children may lead to aplastic anemia. This is probably due to immune-mediated destruction of marrow stem cells by immunocompetent donor lymphocytes (graft-versus-host disease).

Pathogenesis

Three main mechanisms are proposed for pathophysiology of acquired aplastic anemia: damage to hematopoietic stem cells by autoimmune mechanism, inherent stem cell defect, and defective bone marrow microenvironment.

1. Inhibition of hematopoiesis by immunological mechanisms (autoimmunity): This is the major mechanism in the pathophysiology of acquired aplastic anemia. Immune-mediated suppression of hematopoiesis is thought to underlie majority of cases of aplastic **anemia. Response to immunosuppressive therapy supports this concept. Activated T lymphocytes produce cytokines such as** γ **interferon and tumor necrosis factor** α–(TNF-α), which have been shown to suppress the growth of hematopoietic stem cells in vitro. It is thought that hematopoietic stem cells are first antigenically altered by exposure to the causative agent which is followed by cellular immune response. In addition, Fas receptors on hematopoietic stem cells are upregulated by TNF-α leading to apoptosis of stem cells (Fig. 3.12).

2. Defective hematopoietic stem cells: Hematopoietic stem cells and progenitor cells are reduced in number and grow poorly on stroma.

   Shortened telomeres have been observed in cases of aplastic anemia. Telomeres are two ends of chromosomes which shorten with each cell division. Telomere length is normally maintained by the enzyme telomerase. Mutations in telomerase-related genes (e.g. telomerase reverse transcriptase or TERT, telomerase RNA template or TERC) cause shortening of telomeres, reduced proliferation of hematopoietic stem cells, and apoptosis. Short telomeres have been observed in congenital aplastic anemias (dyskeratosis congenita) and in some acquired aplastic anemias. Short telomeres are also associated with predisposition to malignant neoplasms (as observed in some cases of aplastic anemia).

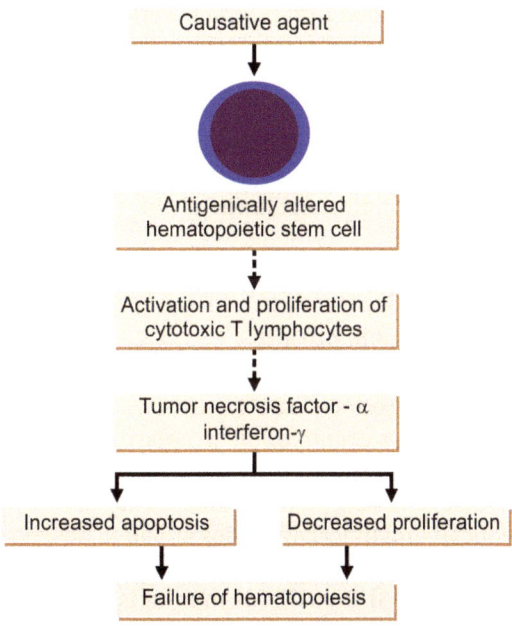

Fig. 3.12: Pathogenesis of immune-mediated acquired aplastic anemia. Antigenically altered hematopoietic stem cells are recognized by cytotoxic T lymphocytes which secrete tumor necrosis factor-α (TNF-α) and interferon-γ (IFN-γ). Both TNF-α and IFN-γ are potent inhibitors of hematopoietic stem cells. Also, Fas receptors on stem cells are upregulated by TNF-α leading to their apoptosis. In addition, cytotoxic T cells can cause direct damage to stem cells.

3. Defective hematopoietic microenvironment that is not able to sustain normal hematopoiesis has been reported in a proportion of patients.

Certain chemical, physical, and viral agents can cause direct damage to bone marrow or hematopoietic stem cells. This can cause either stem cell loss by direct toxicity, failure of microenvironment, or immune-mediated suppression of hematopoiesis. Some individuals are possibly genetically more susceptible to these agents.

Clinical Features

Aplastic anemia presents with signs and symptoms related to pancytopenia. Bleeding is due to thrombocytopenia and may occur in the form of petechiae, ecchymoses, or nasal or gastrointestinal bleeding. Neutropenia is associated with infections. Weakness, easy fatigability, pallor, and breathlessness are related to anemia. **In aplastic anemia, lymph nodes, liver, or spleen are not enlarged. If enlarged, diagnosis other than aplastic anemia should be considered.**

Laboratory Features

Tests to Establish the Diagnosis of Aplastic Anemia

Peripheral blood examination: Peripheral blood shows pancytopenia. Anemia is a constant feature and red cells are usually normocytic and normochromic. Sometimes red cells are mildly macrocytic. The reticulocyte count is low as compared to the degree of reduction in hemoglobin concentration. Granulocytes and monocytes are reduced. If neutrophils are less than 200/cmm, risk of infections is significantly increased.

Predominant white cells in the peripheral blood are lymphocytes. Thrombocytopenia is a consistent finding. Spontaneous bleeding usually occurs when the platelet count is less than 20,000/cmm.

Aplastic anemia is diagnosed if any two of the following are present in peripheral blood (BCSH, 2003):
- Hemoglobin <10 g/dL
- Neutrophil count <1,500/cmm
- Platelet count <50,000/cmm

Bone marrow examination: In aplastic anemia, bone marrow fragments are easily obtained by aspiration. In severe cases, cellularity of the marrow is markedly decreased with most of the particles showing predominance of fat cells. Erythroid and myeloid precursor cells are markedly reduced and megakaryocytes are often absent. The surviving erythroid precursors may show megaloblastic features. The predominant cells of white cell series are lymphocytes and plasma cells (Fig. 3.13). Even if bone marrow is hypocellular, at places small foci of active hematopoiesis are often present. Aspirate from such areas may thus appear normocellular. Therefore, repeated marrow aspirations are sometimes necessary to make the diagnosis of aplastic anemia.

Trephine biopsy (at least 2 cm) is essential to assess overall cellularity and morphology of remaining hematopoietic cells, and to rule out abnormal cellular infiltrate and increased reticulin. Biopsy shows hypocellularity with predominance of fat cells and sparse hematopoietic elements.

It is necessary to assess severity of aplastic anemia from blood and marrow findings. In severe aplastic anemia, there is marked hypocellularity of bone marrow and severe depletion of normal hematopoietic cells.

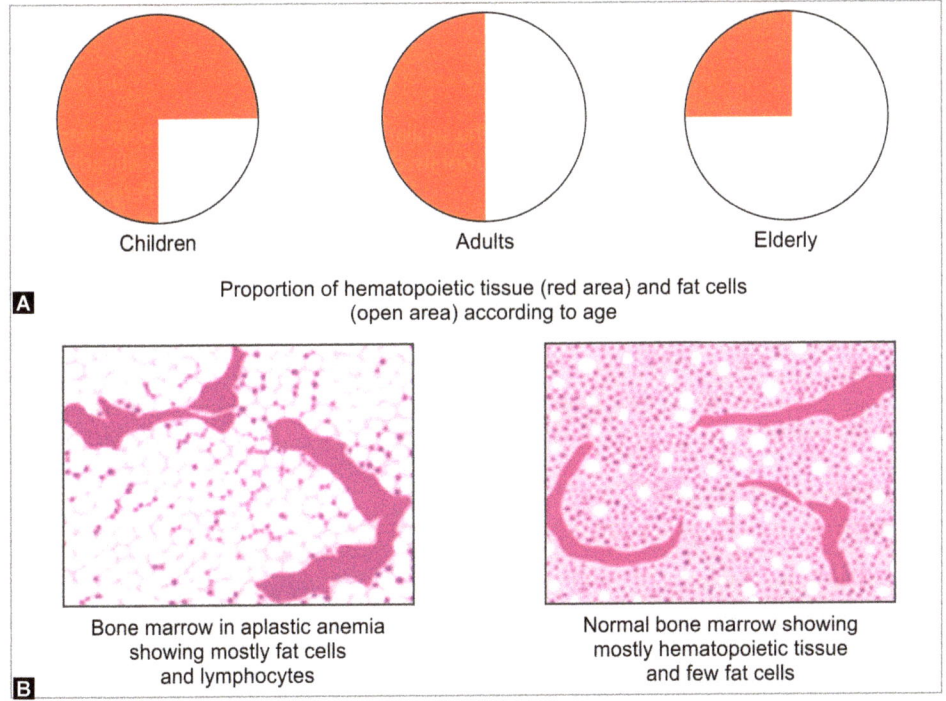

Figs. 3.13A and B: Bone marrow cellularity. (A) Normal proportion of hematopoietic and fat cells according to age; (B) Comparison of normal and aplastic bone marrow.

There is marked cytopenia in peripheral blood predisposing the patient to serious infections and bleeding. Defining such patients has therapeutic implications (Table 3.5).

Tests to Determine Cause of Aplastic Anemia

- Tests for inherited bone marrow failure syndromes: Chromosomal fragility test (Fanconi's anemia), Telomere length measurement (dyskeratosis congenita), Fecal examination for pancreatic elastase and serum pancreatic lipase (exocrine pancreatic dysfunction) and mutation analysis (Shwachman-Diamond syndrome)
- Tests for paroxysmal nocturnal hemoglobinuria: Flow cytometry for CD55 and CD59, Fluorescein-labelled proaerolysin (FLAER)
- Liver function tests and viral hepatitis studies: Transaminases, Serum bilirubin, Tests for hepatitis viruses (hepatitis A, hepatitis B, hepatitis C, hepatitis D, hepatitis E), Epstein Barr virus, Cytomegalovirus
- Tests for autoantibodies: Antinuclear and anti-DNA antibodies for detection of systemic lupus erythematosus.

Diagnosis of aplastic anemia is based on peripheral blood and bone marrow examination. In all cases, it is necessary to exclude underlying cause of aplastic anemia especially inherited bone marrow failure syndromes and paroxysmal nocturnal hemoglobinuria.

Table 3.5: Grading of aplastic anemia.

Severe aplastic anemia (SAA) (Camitta et al, 1976)	Very severe aplastic anemia (VSAA) (Bacigalupo et al, 1988)	Nonsevere aplastic anemia
Peripheral blood Any two of the following: • Neutrophils <500/cmm • Platelets <20,000/cmm • Reticulocytes (corrected for PCV) <1% AND **Bone marrow** Any one of the following: • Marrow cellularity <25% • Marrow cellularity 25–50% with <30% hematopoietic cells	Criteria similar to SAA except neutrophils <200/cmm	• Bone marrow cellularity <25% • Peripheral blood cytopenia not meeting the criteria for SAA

Table 3.6: Causes of pancytopenia.

Pancytopenia with hypocellular marrow	Pancytopenia with cellular marrow
1. Acquired aplastic anemia	1. Megaloblastic anemia
2. Inherited bone marrow failure syndromes (Fanconi anemia, dyskeratosis congenita, Schwachman-Diamond syndrome, congenital amegakaryocytic thrombocytopenia)	2. Storage disorders
3. Hypocellular myelodysplastic syndrome	3. Paroxysmal nocturnal hemoglobinuria
4. Hypocellular acute leukemia	4. Hypersplenism
5. Paroxysmal nocturnal hemoglobinuria	5. Acute leukemia
6. Hairy cell leukemia	6. Myelodysplastic syndrome
7. Lymphoma	7. Lymphoma
8. Myelofibrosis	8. Autoimmune disorders
9. Mycobacterial infections	9. Overwhelming infections
10. Gelatinous transformation of bone marrow	10. Hemophagocytosis syndrome

Differential Diagnosis

Differential diagnosis of aplastic anemia includes disorders causing pancytopenia (anemia + leucopenia + thrombocytopenia). Disorders associated with pancytopenia are listed in Table 3.6.

Fanconi anemia and dyskeratosis congenita occur in younger age and are associated with physical anomalies. Diagnosis of Fanconi anemia is based on chromosomal breakage induced by mitomycin C or diepoxybutane. Dyskeratosis congenita is a telomere disorder in which telomere length is less than first percentile.

Clinically, patients with hematological malignancies usually have enlargement of lymph nodes, spleen or liver and in patients with metastatic carcinoma, primary tumor may be evident. Bone marrow examination shows the presence of abnormal cells.

Hypersplenism is characterized by enlargement of spleen, peripheral blood cytopenia, and normal or hypercellular bone marrow. Underlying cause of splenomegaly may be evident.

Pancytopenia is a common feature of megaloblastic anemia. Diagnosis however is readily evident from macrocytosis and hypersegmented neutrophils in peripheral blood and megaloblastic erythropoiesis in bone marrow.

Differentiation of hypoplastic anemia from hypocellular MDS can be difficult. Dysgranulocytic and dysmegakaryocytic features in peripheral blood and bone marrow, and abnormal cytogenetic analysis favor the latter condition. (Dyserythropoietic features are seen in MDS as well as aplastic anemia.) The distinction between hypocellular MDS and hypocellular AML rests on the percentage of blasts in bone marrow.

Diagnosis of PNH is based on demonstration of abnormal sensitivity of red cells to complement (Ham's test) or flow cytometric analysis for CD55 or CD59 antigens.

For systemic lupus erythematosus, tests for antinuclear antibody and for anti-DNA antibody are done.

Gelatinous transformation of bone marrow (syn: serous degeneration, serous atrophy) is characterized by replacement of hematopoietic cells and fat cells in bone marrow by amorphous extracellular matrix. Its causes are (1) cachexia due to chronic debilitating illnesses like AIDS, cancer, tuberculosis, etc.; (2) anorexia nervosa; and (3) acute infections with multiorgan failure. There is a variable cytopenia in peripheral blood. Bone marrow examination shows deposition of pink, granular, amorphous matrix material replacing fat and hematopoietic tissue (Fig. 3.14). Matrix material is composed of acid mucopolysaccharides and stains positively with PAS and alcian blue (acid pH).

Hemophagocytosis syndrome (syn: hemophagocytic lymphohistiocytosis) is a potentially fatal disorder characterized by pancytopenia, phagocytosis of hematopoietic cells and their progeny (Figs. 3.14A and B), hepatosplenomegaly, and lymphadenopathy. Jaundice, hypofibrinogenemia, and hypertriglyceridemia are usual.

The main histopathologic feature is lymphohistiocytic proliferation in spleen, liver, lymph nodes, and bone marrow. There is no specific laboratory test for diagnosis. The syndrome may be acquired (secondary to cancer, infections, autoimmune disorders) or familial (autosomal recessive).

Treatment

Other causes of bone marrow failure syndromes like Fanconi anemia, paroxysmal nocturnal hemoglobinuria, toxic or postviral aplasia, hypocellular myelodysplastic syndrome, etc. should

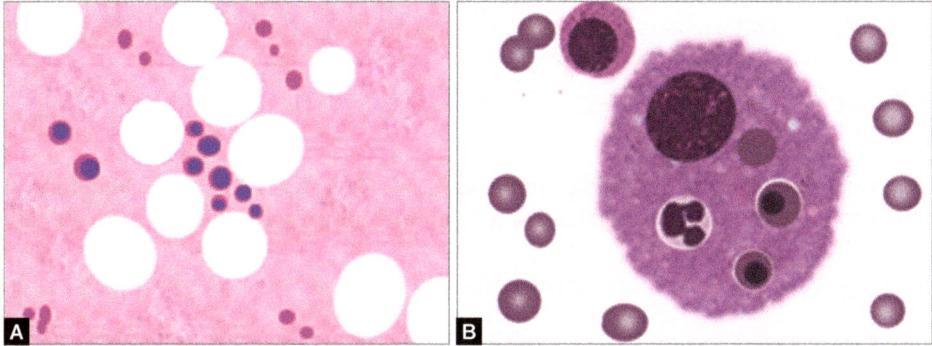

Figs. 3.14A and B: (A) Gelatinous transformation of bone marrow showing replacement of marrow by pink amorphous material; (B) Hemophagocytosis syndrome showing a macrophage with ingested neutrophil, nucleated red cells, and mature red cell.

be excluded before starting therapy. There are two methods of treatment in severe aplastic anemia—(1) allogeneic hematopoietic stem cell transplantation that attempts to achieve cure, and (2) immunosuppressive therapy to bring about remission. In patients with less severe aplastic anemia, the major form of therapy is supportive in the hope of achieving spontaneous recovery.

Hematopoietic Stem Cell Transplantation (HSCT)

This is the ideal treatment in young patients (<40 years) with severe and very severe aplastic anemia if HLA-matched sibling donor is available; cure rate in these patients is 75 to 90%. If HLA-matched sibling donor is not readily available, immunosuppressive therapy is the next option. If there is no response to immunosuppression, the next step is unrelated donor or partial HLA-matched transplantation.

Patients more than 40 years of age are more likely to develop serious complications such as graft-versus-host disease and tolerate them poorly; in these patients treatment of first choice is immunosuppressive therapy (horse antithymocyte globulin and cyclosporine).

Prospective candidates for hematopoietic stem cell transplantation should not be transfused with blood or blood products as far as possible (especially from family members if donor is a sibling) to avoid the risk of alloimmunization and graft rejection.

Immunosuppressive Therapy

It is thought that a large number of cases of aplastic anemia are caused by immunological mechanisms. Activated suppressor T cells have been shown to inhibit hematopoiesis.

Antilymphocyte (or antithymocyte) globulin (ALG or ATG) therapy, which is an antibody against T lymphocytes, probably acts by reducing these suppressor cells. ATG is usually combined with cyclosporine that suppresses the immune system. This is usually given to patients with severe aplastic anemia who do not have HLA-matched sibling donor for HSCT and to all other patients of aplastic anemia. About 30% of patients achieve complete remission while hematopoietic recovery is only partial in majority of patients. Late relapse occurs in some patients. Clonal hematopoietic disorders like paroxysmal nocturnal hemoglobinuria, myelodysplasia, or acute myeloid leukemia can emerge after a few years.

Patients who fail to respond to immunosuppressive therapy after 6 months are said to have refractory aplastic anemia.

> Major side effect of HSCT is graft-vs-host disease, while main side effect of immunosuppressive therapy is higher rate of relapse and development of PNH, AML, or myelodysplasia after a few years.

Androgens

Androgens stimulate erythropoiesis in bone marrow. They may be of some benefit in those patients who fail to show desired response to immunosuppressive therapy and who are not suitable for HSCT.

Eltrombopag

Eltrombopag is a thrombopoietin receptor agonist that has been found to stimulate stem cells and is used in refractory aplastic anemia.

Supportive Measures

Packed red cells should be given when anemia becomes symptomatic. Platelet transfusions are indicated in the presence of bleeding due to thrombocytopenia and prophylactically when platelet count falls below 20,000/cmm. Usefulness of granulocyte transfusions is minimal and the chief form of treatment in neutropenia with infection is antibiotics. Infections should be investigated particularly for opportunistic organisms and vigorously treated.

Prognosis

In the past majority of patients with severe aplastic anemia used to die within 1 year of diagnosis. Now many patients undergoing marrow transplant can hope to achieve cure; however, a proportion of these patients will develop serious complications such as graft-versus-host disease, infections, or graft rejection. Patients receiving immunosuppressive therapy can achieve complete or partial remission; long-term sequelae in these patients are recurrence or evolution of a clonal hematopoietic disorder such as PNH, MDS, or AML.

With supportive therapy, some patients with moderately severe aplastic anemia can achieve spontaneous remission.

Approach to management of aplastic anemia is shown in Figure 3.15.

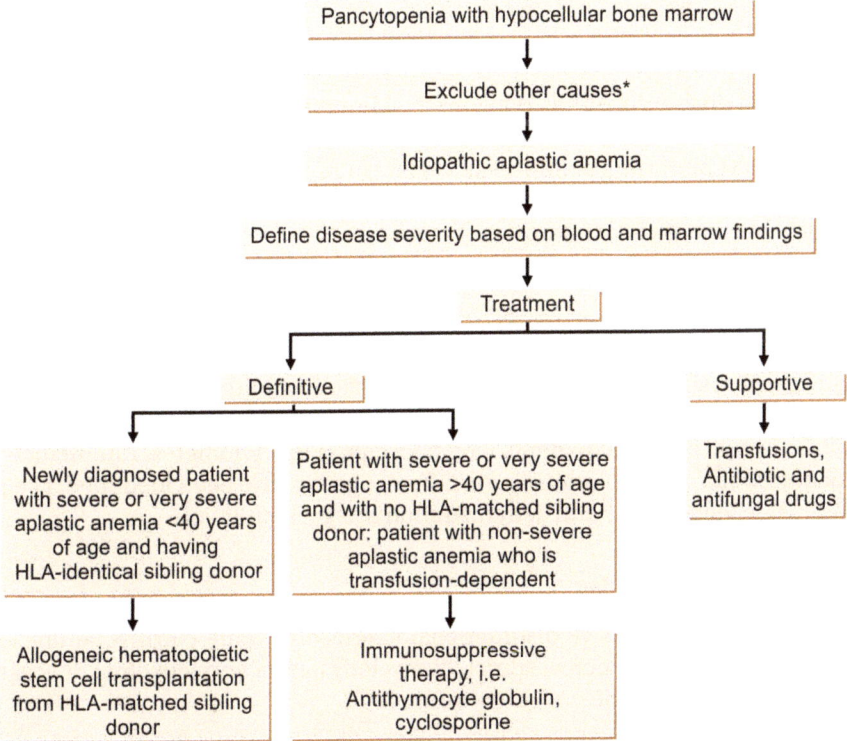

Fig. 3.15: Approach to management of aplastic anemia.
*Systemic lupus erythematosus, hypocellular myelodysplastic syndrome/acute leukemia, myelofibrosis, mycobacterial infections, gelatinous transformation, paroxysmal nocturnal hemoglobinuria, inherited bone marrow failure syndromes

CONSTITUTIONAL APLASTIC ANEMIA

Inherited bone marrow failure syndromes are a heterogeneous group of disorders characterized by bone marrow failure and somatic abnormalities. They are listed in Table 3.3. Bone marrow failure may involve all cell lines or a single lineage. Presentation is usually in childhood but may sometimes be in adults.

Fanconi's Anemia

This is a rare disorder with autosomal recessive mode of inheritance, first described in 1927 by a Swiss pediatrician Guido Fanconi. It is associated with short stature, microcephaly, microphthalmia, microstomia, renal aplasia, café au lait spots, generalized hyperpigmentation of skin, mental retardation and hypoplasia of thumbs and of radii. Hypoplastic anemia develops usually during 5 to 10 years of age. Clinical presentation of Fanconi's anemia is markedly heterogeneous. In some patients, congenital anomalies are absent.

This disease can result from mutations in any one of 15 different genes. Majority of are due to mutations in *FANCA*, *FANCC*, or *FANCG* genes.

Cells have increased susceptibility to spontaneous chromosomal breakage. The screening test is chromosomal breakage test (incubation of peripheral blood lymphocytes with diepoxybutane or mitomycin causes chromosomal breaks which can be seen on karyotyping). Definitive diagnosis is made by mutation analysis.

Patients are at increased risk of myelodysplastic syndrome, acute myeloid leukemia, and solid cancers.

Treatment with anabolic steroids is followed by improvement but side-effects (secondary sexual changes in boys, virilization in girls, hepatic complications like cholestasis, peliosis hepatis, carcinoma) limit the usefulness of this form of therapy in children. Bone marrow transplantation with marrow obtained from nonaffected, HLA-identical sibling donor can establish normal hematopoiesis in most cases.

Dyskeratosis Congenita

This is an inherited bone marrow failure syndrome with diagnostic triad of abnormal skin pigmentation, nail dystrophy, and mucosal leukoplakia. In addition to marrow aplasia, other features are pulmonary fibrosis, liver disease, neurologic and eye abnormalities, and increased predisposition to cancer. These patients have short germ line telomeres. Inheritance may be X-linked or autosomal, and mutations in six different genes have been identified. Diagnosis is based on telomere length assay and demonstration of a gene mutation.

Schwachman-Diamond Syndrome

This is a rare autosomal recessive disorder characterized by bone marrow failure, exocrine pancreatic insufficiency, and increased risk of myelodysplasia and leukemia. It is caused by biallelic mutations in *SBDS* gene on chromosome 7.

Diamond-Blackfan Anemia

This is a rare autosomal dominant disorder presenting in first year of life with congenital anomalies, severe macrocytic anemia, reticulocytopenia, and selective depletion of erythroid precursors in bone marrow. Red cells show elevated fetal hemoglobin and increased erythrocyte adenosine deaminase activity. It is caused by mutations in ribosomal protein genes. Some cases evolve into aplastic anemia. The disease should be distinguished from transient erythroblastopenia of childhood in which recovery occurs within 5 to 10 weeks.

Congenital Amegakaryocytic Thrombocytopenia

This is an autosomal recessive disorder caused by mutations in thrombopoietin (TPO) receptor gene (MPL). It presents at birth with severe thrombocytopenia and absence of megakaryocytes in bone marrow. About 50% of patients develop aplastic anemia by the age of 5 years. There are no specific congenital malformations.

PURE RED CELL APLASIA

This is characterized by selective depletion of erythroid precursors in the bone marrow with consequent severe normocytic normochromic anemia and reticulocytopenia.

Production of leucocytes and platelets is normal. Diagnostic criteria for pure red cell aplasia are (1) severe anemia, (2) reticulocyte count < 1%, and (3) normocellular marrow with mature erythroblasts < 0.5%. Pure red cell aplasia (PRCA) may be divided into two types—constitutional and acquired. Acquired type is further subdivided into primary and secondary forms.

Constitutional Pure Red Cell Aplasia (Diamond-Blackfan Syndrome)

This is considered above.

Acquired Pure Red Cell Aplasia

PRCA occurring during the course of chronic hemolytic anemias in children (such as sickle-cell anemia, thalassemia, glucose-6-phosphate dehydrogenase deficiency) has been designated as aplastic crisis. The receptor for this virus is P blood group antigen. Parvo virus B19 is implicated which has a selective cytopathic effect on erythroid precursors. Patients develop a sudden worsening of their anemia associated with reticulocytopenia, and depletion of erythroid precursors in bone marrow. PRCA is transient with recovery usually occurring in 1 to 2 weeks when antibodies against the virus appear. In normal persons cytopathic effect of the virus on erythroid precursors does not manifest as anemia due to the long life-span of red cells and the transient effect of the virus. In immunocompromised persons, B19 parvo virus causes chronic PRCA since antibody response against the virus is deficient. It may also be associated with thymoma, collagen vascular disorders, myasthenia gravis, chronic lymphocytic leukemia, large granular lymphocytic leukemia, and 5q-myelodysplastic syndrome.

In children PRCA is mostly a self-limited disease while in adults it follows a chronic course. Although immunosuppressive therapy can induce remission, relapses are frequent.

ANEMIA OF CHRONIC DISORDERS

The anemia of chronic disorders (ACD) occurs in chronic infections, or inflammatory or neoplastic diseases. It is also called as anemia of inflammation. Anemia is normocytic normochromic or microcytic hypochromic and serum iron level is low even though storage iron is adequate.

Table 3.7: Diseases associated with ACD.

Chronic inflammation	Chronic infections	Neoplasms
• Rheumatoid arthritis	• Tuberculosis	• Carcinoma
• Systemic lupus erythematosus	• Urinary tract infections	• Lymphoma
• Crohn's disease	• Bacterial endocarditis	• Myeloma
	• Deep-seated abscess	
	• Pneumonia	

Anemia of chronic disorders is the most frequent form of anemia in hospitalized patients (occurs in 50% of hospitalized patients).

"Big 3" groups of diseases associated with ACD are inflammation, infection, and neoplasm. Diseases associated with anemia of chronic disease are listed in Table 3.7.

PATHOGENESIS

Pathogenesis is not clear. Three mechanisms have been proposed—decreased red cell survival, decreased red cell production to compensate for shortened red cell survival, and impairment of iron metabolism (Fig. 3.16).

Decreased Red Cell Survival

Red cell survival is mildly shortened. It is thought that disorders associated with ACD enhance the phagocytic activity of macrophages. These activated macrophages are sensitive to slight alterations in red cells and cause their premature destruction.

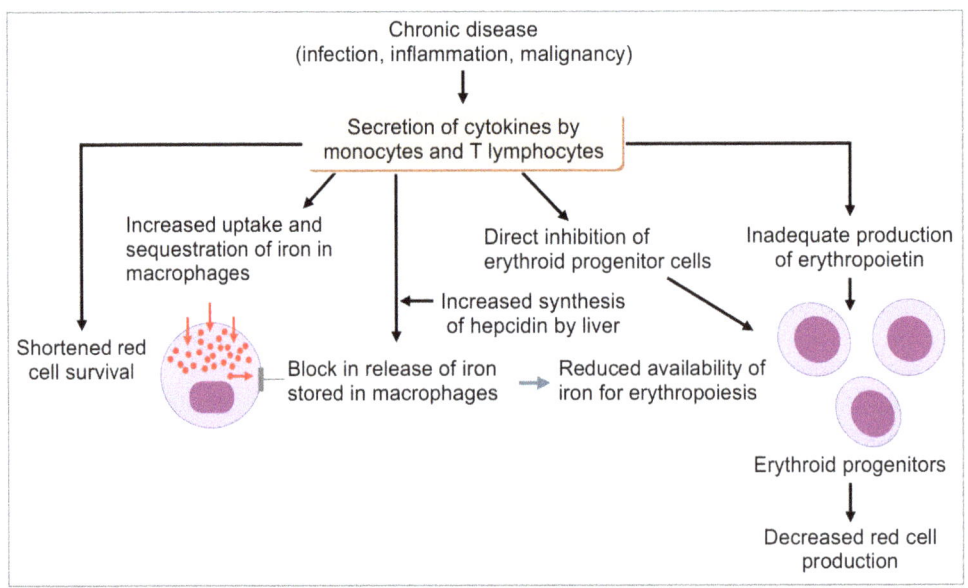

Fig. 3.16: Mechanisms underlying anemia of chronic disease.

Decreased Red Cell Production

This is related to the inappropriately low erythropoietin production for the degree of anemia. Block in the release of iron for erythropoiesis from storages sites also plays a role.

Impairment of Iron Metabolism

In ACD, amount of storage iron in macrophages of reticuloendothelial system is adequate. However the release of iron from macrophages is inhibited. This leads to hypoferremia (low serum iron) and less iron is made available to erythroid precursors in bone marrow. This causes iron-deficient erythropoiesis despite sufficient storage iron.

Cytokines released from activated monocytes and T lymphocytes contribute to anemia of chronic disease. Interleukin-6 induces hepcidin synthesis in liver which in turn binds to ferroportin and inactivates it. The resulting sequestration of iron limits availability of iron for erythropoiesis. Certain cytokines also inhibit erythropoietin release from kidneys and also directly inhibit proliferation of erythroid progenitors.

Inflammatory cytokines, particularly interleukin-1 and TNF play a central role in pathogenesis of ACD.

CLINICAL FEATURES

Signs and symptoms are those of primary disease. Anemia is often mild and nonprogressive. Anemia develops during first 1 to 2 months of illness. There is a rough correlation between severity of disease and degree of anemia.

LABORATORY FEATURES

Anemia is mild to moderate (hemoglobin rarely falls below 8–9 g/dL) and is most commonly normocytic and normochronic; less commonly, it is microcytic and hypochromic (particularly in rheumatoid arthritis). Reticulocyte count is not increased in proportion with the degree of anemia.

Decrease in serum iron is a consistent feature and can be detected even before the appearance of anemia. Total iron-binding capacity is decreased. Serum ferritin is normal or raised. As serum ferritin is nonspecifically raised in inflammation (even in the presence of iron deficiency), estimation of serum soluble transferrin receptor and soluble transferrin receptor/serum ferritin index have been advocated for diagnosis (Table 3.8).

Erythrocyte sedimentation rate is increased.

Bone marrow examination shows normal morphology. A characteristic feature is normal or increased storage iron as demonstrated by Prussian blue reaction.

Free erythrocyte protoporphyrin is raised, as there is no sufficient iron available to form heme.

Alterations in leucocytes and platelets are related to the underlying disease. Diagnostic features of anemia of chronic disease are shown in Box 3.13.

Section 2: Disorders of Red Blood Cells (Anemias)

Table 3.8: Differences between iron deficiency anemia and anemia of chronic disease.

Parameter	Iron deficiency anemia	Anemia of chronic disease
1. Degree of anemia	Variable	Mild
2. Presence of underlying disease	±	Infection, inflammation, neoplasm
3. Mean cell volume	Reduced	Normal or reduced
4. Serum iron	Reduced	Reduced or normal
5. Transferrin saturation	Reduced	Reduced or normal
6. TIBC	Increased	Reduced
7. Serum ferritin	Reduced	Increased or normal
8. Serum transferrin receptor	Increased	Normal
9. Serum transferrin receptor/Serum ferritin index	High	Low
10. Bone marrow storage iron	Reduced or absent	Normal or increased

Box 3.13: Diagnosis of anemia of chronic disease.

- Evidence of chronic disease (raised erythrocyte sedimentation rate, C-reactive protein)
- Mild to moderate anemia; red cells normocytic normochromic (in late stage, microcytic hypochromic)
- Low serum iron, low TIBC, low transferrin saturation
- Serum ferritin: Normal or increased
- Serum transferrin receptor/log ferritin ratio <1
- Serum hepcidin: High

DIFFERENTIAL DIAGNOSIS

Differentiation of ACD from IDA is given in Table 3.8. As disorders associated with ACD can cause anemia by other mechanisms such as bleeding, drug-induced hematopoietic suppression, excessive red cell destruction, or infiltration of marrow, these causative factors should be excluded. Anemias due to renal, liver, or endocrine failure do not come under ACD.

TREATMENT

Iron or vitamin therapy is not indicated in ACD. Effective treatment of underlying disease leads to correction of anemia. In some cases, administration of recombinant erythropoietin has been found to cause resolution of anemia of chronic disease.

SIDEROBLASTIC ANEMIA

SIDEROBLASTS

Sideroblasts are erythroblasts-containing aggregates of iron, which are demonstrable by Prussian blue reaction. There are three types of sideroblasts—type I, type II, and type III (Fig. 3.17).

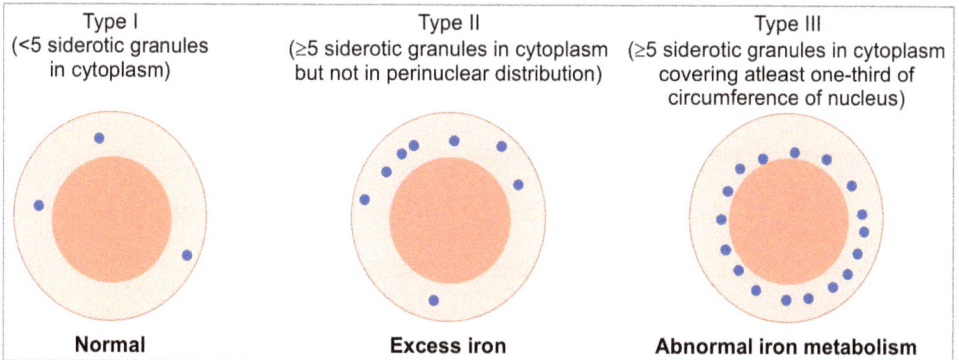

Fig. 3.17: Types of sideroblasts. Blue-colored iron granules are seen in erythroblasts (as seen with Prussian blue staining).

In type I (normal) sideroblasts, iron-containing (siderotic) granules are cytoplasmic, small, and few in number and represent aggregates of ferritin. Such sideroblasts constitute 30 to 50% of erythroblasts in bone marrow in normal subjects. They are reduced in iron deficiency and anemia of chronic disease. The number of sideroblasts in marrow corresponds with percent transferrin saturation.

Type II and type III sideroblasts are abnormal. In type II sideroblasts, iron-containing granules in cytoplasm are numerous and large. They are observed in hemolytic states and iron overload. In type III or ringed sideroblasts, nonferritin iron is deposited in mitochondria that are located around the nucleus. In ringed sideroblasts, iron-containing granules are large, multiple, and are distributed in the form of a partial or complete ring surrounding the nucleus. They are present in sideroblastic anemias. Sideroblastic anemia is diagnosed if ringed sideroblasts are ≥ 15% of marrow erythroblasts.

TYPES AND CAUSES

Sideroblastic anemias are characterized by dimorphic or microcytic hypochromic anemia, ringed sideroblasts in bone marrow (Figs. 3.18A and B), and ineffective erythropoiesis.

Causes of sideroblastic anemia are shown in Box 3.14.

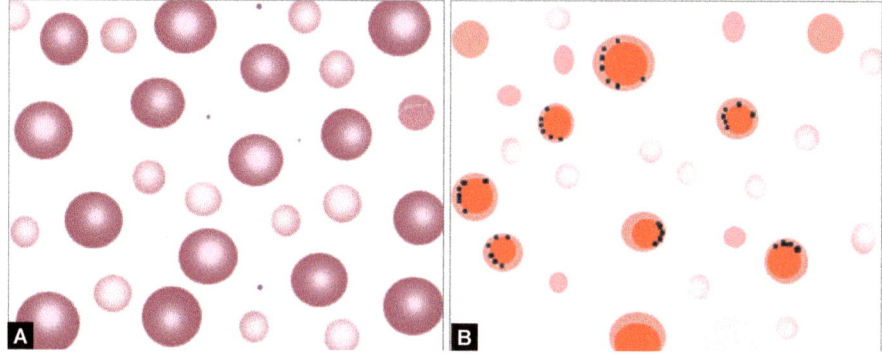

Figs. 3.18A and B: (A) Peripheral blood smear in sideroblastic anemia showing dimorphic population of red cells (one normocytic normochromic and other microcytic hypochromic). (B) Bone marrow aspiration smear stained with iron stain showing ringed sideroblasts containing blue-stained granules of iron in perinuclear distribution.

> **Box 3.14:** Causes of sideroblastic anemia.

- **Hereditary: X-linked, autosomal recessive**
- **Acquired**
  - Primary
    » Refractory anemia with ringed sideroblasts
  - Secondary
    » Hematologic malignancies—myeloproliferative disorders, multiple myeloma, acute myeloid leukemia-M6 type
    » Drugs—isoniazid, pyrazinamide, cycloserine, chloramphenicol
    » Alcoholism
    » Lead poisoning
    » Other—collagen disorders, carcinoma

PATHOGENESIS

Pathogenesis is not clear; impaired heme synthesis in mitochondria appears to play a significant role. The taking up of iron by erythroblasts is regulated partially by intracellular heme concentration. Defective heme synthesis is associated with increased iron uptake due to the feedback mechanism. Protoporphyrin link-up with iron fails to occur owing to reduced availability of the former and excess iron is deposited in mitochondria.

Hereditary Sideroblastic Anemia

The mode of transmission is usually X-linked. There is reduced activity of delta aminolevulinic acid synthetase, an enzyme in the heme biosynthetic pathway. Patients present in childhood or early adult life with anemia. Features of iron overload are often present. Anemia is moderate to severe and may be microcytic hypochromic or dimorphic (mixture of normocytic normochromic and microcytic hypochromic red cells). Serum iron and percent transferrin saturation are increased. Bone marrow shows erythroid hyperplasia and numerous ringed sideroblasts. Some cases partially respond to pyridoxine given in high doses.

Primary Acquired Sideroblastic Anemia

This is refractory anemia with ringed sideroblasts (RARS), a form of myelodysplasia. It occurs in middle-aged or elderly subjects. Anemia is typically dimorphic (microcytic hypochromic and macrocytic). Morphologic abnormalities of neutrophils like Pelger-Huet cells and hypogranular forms are seen. Bone marrow shows variable megaloblastic maturation and dyshematopoietic features. Prussian blue stain for iron reveals increased storage iron and ringed sideroblasts. Clonal chromosomal abnormalities may be detected. Progression to acute myeloid leukemia occurs in about 1 to 2% of patients.

Secondary Acquired Sideroblastic Anemia

Sideroblastic anemia can occur in severe alcoholics who have malnutrition and deficiency of folate. Morphologic abnormalities are dimorphic anemia in peripheral blood and megaloblastic erythropoiesis, vacuolization of erythroblasts, and ringed sideroblasts in bone marrow.

Lead poisoning (plumbism) in adults usually follows industrial inhalation of fumes while in children (often 1–3 years of age) eating of flakes of lead-based paint is the usual cause. The clinical manifestations in adults include abdominal colic and motor neuropathy. In children, it is associated with low IQ, lack of concentration, hyperactivity, and impairment of growth and development. Anemia is mild to moderate and is usually normocytic and slightly hypochromic. Basophilic stippling can be striking but is not regularly observed. Stippling is due to aggregation of ribosomes, which are not removed owing to lead-induced deficiency of 5' nucleotidase. Bone marrow reveals erythroid predominance and ringed sideroblasts. The mechanism of anemia in lead poisoning is not clear. Lead inhibits several enzymes involved in heme synthesis including ALA dehydratase and heme synthetase (ferrochelatase). This causes raised levels of free erythrocyte protoporphyrin (in the form of zinc protoporphyrin) and there is increased urinary excretion of coproporphyrin and delta-amino-levulinic acid. Apart from defective heme synthesis, there is also some hemolytic component in lead poisoning due to direct injury to red cell membrane. Several studies suggest that lead poisoning does not result in microcytic hypochromic anemia; presence of such anemia in plumbism is due to the presence of coexistence of iron deficiency due to other cause or due to inheritance of α-thalassemia trait. Presence of both iron deficiency and lead poisoning in children can be serious since more lead is absorbed due to iron deficiency and more amount of ferrochelatase is inhibited. Screening for plumbism should be done by direct lead measurement; zinc protoporphyrin is not recommended since it is increased late and it cannot differentiate between iron deficiency and thalassemia if lead deficiency is also present. Treatment consists of administering EDTA.

ANEMIA OF CHRONIC RENAL FAILURE

Anemia is a common feature of chronic renal failure (CRF). It refers to anemia resulting from impaired endocrine and excretory functions of kidney.

PATHOGENESIS

Following mechanisms are involved in the causation of anemia of CRF:

Loss of Endocrine Function of Kidney

Failure to synthesize erythropoietin plays a major role.

Loss of Excretory Function of Kidney

Inhibition of Erythropoiesis

Retention of toxic products and azotemia exert direct inhibitory effect on proliferation and differentiation of erythroid precursor cells.

Shortening of Red Cell Survival

The activity of hexose monophosphate shunt has been found to be impaired in CRF. This may make hemoglobin prone to oxidant damage by drugs or chemicals. Activity of the ATPase which fuels the Na⁺-K⁺ pump of the membrane is also subnormal. Both these functional changes may cause shortening of red cell life-span or hemolysis. The nature of the toxic substance causing these metabolic changes is unknown.

Other factors such as bleeding (secondary to defective platelet function) and microangiopathic hemolytic anemia (due to deposition of fibrin in arterioles in some renal diseases) may aggravate the anemia in chronic renal disease but they are not directly responsible for "anemia of CRF."

CLINICAL AND LABORATORY FEATURES

Usually, signs and symptoms of chronic renal failure predominate and anemia is discovered incidentally. Rarely, manifestations of renal failure are minimal and patient presents with anemia. Degree of anemia roughly corresponds with the level of blood urea nitrogen (BUN); the greater concentration of blood urea nitrogen is associated with more severe anemia. The anemia is typically normocytic and normochromic with normal reticulocyte count. Burr cells (red cells with many tiny regularly placed projections on surface) are frequent (Fig. 3.19). Platelet function is defective due to uremia (prolonged bleeding time and impaired platelet aggregation with epinephrine, ADP, and collagen). Bone marrow appears normocellular with normal maturation sequence and there is no or only slight compensatory erythroid hyperplasia in response to anemia. Concentration of erythropoietin is lower as compared to the degree of anemia.

TREATMENT

Some improvement in anemia occurs with hemodialysis. Renal transplantation is followed by rapid correction of anemia. The effect of androgens (which increase release of erythropoietin

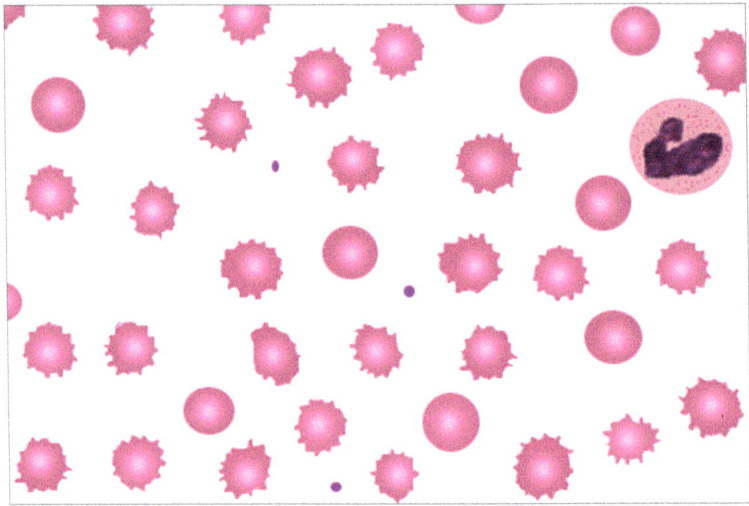

Fig. 3.19: Blood smear in chronic renal failure showing numerous burr cells (echinocytes).

from kidneys and also directly stimulate erythropoiesis) is partial in correcting anemia. Recombinant human erythropoietin has proved to be remarkably effective in anemia of CRF and is now the treatment of choice.

ANEMIA OF LIVER DISEASE

"Anemia of liver disease," which occurs in majority of patients with chronic liver disease, is caused by reduced red cell life-span and impaired red cell production.

The cause of premature red cell destruction is not known but may be related to congestive splenomegaly. Red cell production in chronic liver disease is inadequate for the degree of anemia. The red cell abnormalities in peripheral blood include round macrocytosis and target cells. Target cells have increased cholesterol and lecithin in the membrane.

Erythropoiesis is normoblastic or macronormoblastic; macronormoblasts are large cells with normal chromatin pattern. Improvement in liver function corrects "anemia of liver disease." Apart from "anemia of liver disease," other causes of anemia in liver disorders are:
1. Iron deficiency anemia due to blood loss from anatomical lesions such as esophageal varices or bleeding secondary to coagulation factor abnormalities;
2. Acute blood loss anemia secondary to gastrointestinal hemorrhage;
3. Spur cell anemia—Some patients with severe chronic liver disease develop spur cell hemolytic anemia. Spur cells are red cells with spikes on their surface. Spur cells have increased amount of membrane cholesterol, are rigid, and are prematurely destroyed in the spleen.
4. Megaloblastic anemia due to nutritional folate deficiency in alcoholics;
5. Hypersplenism; and
6. Aplastic anemia in viral hepatitis.

MYELOPHTHISIC ANEMIA

Extensive involvement of bone marrow by neoplastic, infectious, and metabolic (storage) diseases may produce myelophthisic anemia. The peripheral blood prominently shows nucleated red cells and immature myeloid cells such as metamyelocytes, myelocytes, promyelocytes, or even myeloblasts. This peripheral blood picture is called as leucoerythroblastosis (Fig. 3.20). Underlying disease dominates the clinical presentation. Causes of myelophthisic anemia are listed in Box 3.15.

Anemia is normocytic normochromic and mild to moderate. Tear drop red cells is a characteristic feature. Total leukocyte count is normal, low, or raised. Platelets may be normal or reduced.

Bone marrow biopsy is necessary in all cases for definitive diagnosis. Treatment consists of management of the underlying disorder.

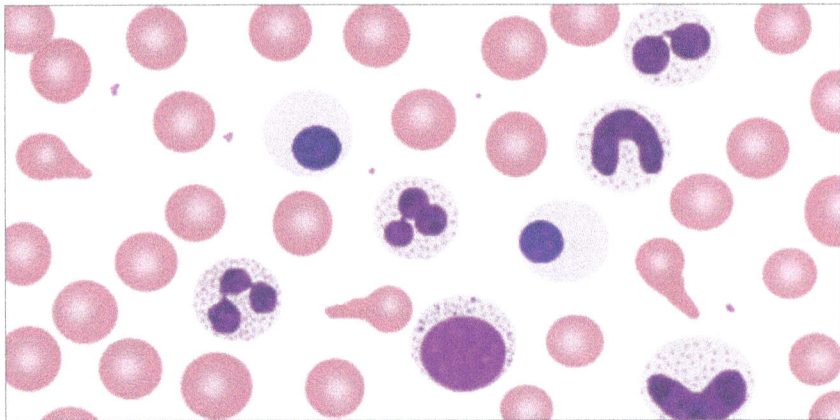

Fig. 3.20: Leukoerythroblastic blood picture showing immature white and red blood cells in peripheral blood. Tear drop red cells are also present.

Box 3.15: Diseases causing myelophthisic anemia.

- Malignant diseases
  - **Hematological:** Acute and chronic leukemias, myeloproliferative disorders, multiple myeloma
  - **Nonhematological diseases metastatic to marrow:** Carcinomas of lung, breast, prostate, stomach, etc.
- **Lipid storage diseases:** Gaucher's disease, Niemann-Pick disease
- **Disseminated infectious diseases:** Military tuberculosis

CONGENITAL DYSERYTHROPOIETIC ANEMIAS

Congenital dyserythropoietic anemias (CDA) are rare inherited anemias. The features of CDA are (i) dyserythropoiesis especially presence of erythroblasts with multiple nuclei in bone marrow, (ii) ineffective erythropoiesis, and (iii) presentation usually in infancy or childhood (usually > 10 years) with anemia, splenomegaly and mildly increased indirect serum bilirubin. Morphologic abnormalities in the bone marrow are limited to the erythroid series. There is excessive deposition of iron in tissues. Three types of CDA are distinguished—I, II, and III. Types I and II have autosomal recessive mode of inheritance, while type III is dominantly inherited. Table 3.9 lists salient features of three main types of CDA. Additional variants have been described that need further characterization (types IV, V, VI, and VII).

Anemia with dyserythropoiesis also occurs in association with megaloblastic anemia, thalassemia, congenital hemolytic anemias, certain infections, alcoholism, drugs, myelodysplasia, and acute myeloid leukemia. However, in CDA, dyserythropoiesis is primary and inborn.

Table 3.9: Congenital dyserythropoietic anemias.

	Feature	Congenital dyserythropoietic anemia type 1	Congenital dyserythropoietic anemia type 2	Congenital dyserythropoietic anemia type 3
1.	Inheritance	Autosomal recessive	Autosomal recessive	Autosomal dominant
2.	Location of gene involved	15q15.1-q15.3 (*CDAN1*)	20q11.2	15q22
3.	Age at presentation	In-utero with hydrops, neonatal, childhood or adolescence	5–30 years (average 18–20 years)	Not available
4.	Physical examination	Splenomegaly	Jaundice, splenomegaly, hepatogemaly	-
5.	Iron overload	Present	Present	Absent
6.	Anemia	Mild to moderate	Mild to moderate	Mild
7.	Mean cell volume (MCV)	Raised	Normal or mildly increased	Normal or mildly increased
8.	RDW	Raised	Raised	Raised
9.	Blood smear	Anisopoikilocytosis with punctuate basophilia	Anisopoikilocytosis with punctuate basophilia	Anisopoikilocytosis with punctuate basophilia
10.	Bone marrow erythroblasts	Megaloblastic, binucleation (<10%), chromatin bridges between nuclei of pairs of erythroblasts	Binucleation (10-35%) of late polychromatic erythroblasts	Multinuclearity, gigantoblasts
11.	Electron microscopy	Spongy nuclei (Swiss-cheese), invasion of nuclei by cytoplasm	Excess cisternae of endoplasmic reticulum parallel to plasma membrane (double membrane)	Intranuclear clefts, cytoplasmic precipitates
12.	Ham test	Negative	Positive	Negative
13.	Anti-i hemagglutination	Slight	Strong	Variable
14.	SDS-PAGE	Normal	Abnormal migration (faster) of band 3	Normal
15.	Molecular diagnosis	CDAN1	SEC23B	KIF23

(*Source:* Kawthalkar SM. Essentials of Clinical Pathology, second edition, M/s Jaypee Brothers Medical Publishers, India, page 281, 2018).

CDA TYPE I

Peripheral blood shows macrocytosis. Bone marrow shows marked erythroid hyperplasia. Morphologic alterations in erythroblasts include megaloblast-like or spongy nuclear chromatin, erythroblasts with incompletely separated nuclei, binucleated erythroblasts, and internuclear chromatin bridges between two erythroblasts.

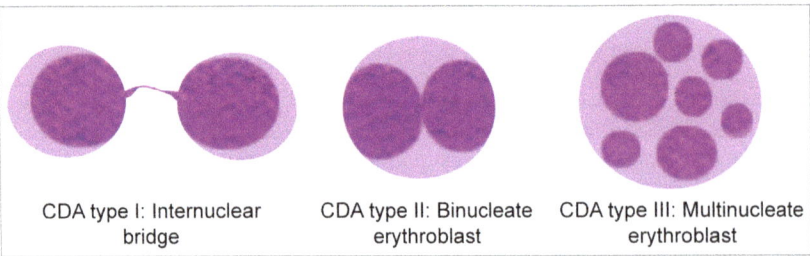

Fig. 3.21: Abnormalities of erythroblasts in congenital dyserythropoietic anemias.

CDA TYPE II

This is the most frequent type and is also known as HEMPAS (hereditary erythroblastic multinuclearity with positive acidified serum test). Normocytic normochromic anemia is frequent.

Bone marrow shows binucleate and multinucleate erythroblasts, pleuripolar mitoses, and karyorrhexis.

The red cells in HEMPAS are hemolyzed by acidified normal sera and are thus similar in this character to red cells of paroxysmal nocturnal hemoglobinuria (PNH). However, lysis of red cells in PNH in acidified serum test is due to abnormal sensitivity to complement, and all sera will cause lyses. In HEMPAS, there is a unique antigen on the surface of the red cells known as "HEMPAS" antigen which reacts with complement-fixing IgM antibody; only those sera which contain significant amount of anti-HEMPAS antibody cause lysis of red cells.

Cold-reacting anti-I and anti-i antibodies react strongly with HEMPAS cells. Splenectomy is followed by some improvement.

CDA TYPE III

This is the rarest type. It is characterized by red cell macrocytosis in peripheral blood and giant erythroblasts in the bone marrow with multinuclearity (up to 12 nuclei may be present) (Fig. 3.21).

BIBLIOGRAPHY

1. Andrews NC. Disorders of iron metabolism. N Engl J Med. 1999;341:1986-95.
2. Appelbaum FR, Fefer A. The pathogenesis of aplastic anaemia. Semin Hematol. 1981;4:241-57.
3. Bacigalupo A, Hows JM, Gluckman E, et al. Bone marrow transplantation (BMT) versus immunosuppression for the treatment of severe aplastic anaemia (SAA):A report of EBMT SAA Working Party. Br J Hematol. 1988;70:177-82.
4. Beris P, Miescher PA. Hematological complications of infectious agents. Semin Hematol. 1988;25: 123-39.
5. Bottomley SS, Muller-Eberhard V. Pathophysiology of hemesynthesis. Semin Hematol. 1988;25: 282-302.
6. British Committee for Standards in Haematology (BCSH) General Haematology Task Force:Guidelines for the diagnosis and management of acquired aplastic anaemia. Br J Haematol. 2003;123:782-801.

7. Brittenham GM, et al. Clinical consequences of new insights in the pathophysiology of disorders of iron and heme metabolism. American Society of Hematology Education Programme Book. Hematology; 2000.
8. Camitta BM, Donall Thomas E, Nathan DG, et al. A prospective study of androgens and bone marrow transplantation for treatment of severe aplastic anemia. Blood. 1979;53:505-14.
9. Camitta BM, Storb R, Donall Thomas E. Aplastic anemia:Pathogenesis, diagnosis, treatment, and prognosis. N Engl J Med. 1982;306:645-52, 712-18.
10. Cartwright GE, Deiss A. Sideroblasts, siderocytes, and sideroblastic anemia. N Engl J Med. 1970;292:185-93.
11. Cartwright GE. The anemia of chronic disorders. Semin Hematol. 1966;3:351-75.
12. Chanarin I. Megaloblastic anaemia, cobalamin, and folate. J Clin Pathol. 1987;40:978-84.
13. Chanarin I. The Megaloblastic Anemias, 2nd edn. Oxford. Blackwell Scientific Publications; 1979.
14. Cook JD. Clinical evaluation of iron deficiency. Semin Hematol. 1982;14:6-18.
15. Cook JD. Iron methodology—An overview. In Methods in Hematology. Vol 1. Cook JD (Ed):Iron. New York. Churchill Livingstone. 1980.
16. Daughety MM, DeLoughery TG:Unusual anemias. Med Clin N Am. 2017;101:417-29.
17. Deloughery TG. Iron deficiency anemia. Med Clin N Am. 2017;101:319-32.
18. Dessypris EN. The biology of pure red cell aplasia. Semin Hematol. 1991;28:275-84.
19. Eschbach JW, Egrie JC, Downing MR, et al. Correction of the anemia of end-stage renal disease with recombinant human erythropoietin. Results of a combined phase I and II clinical trial. N Engl J Med. 1987;316:73-78.
20. Finch C. Regulators of iron balance in humans. Blood. 1994;84:1697-1702.
21. Ganz T:Hepcidin and iron regulation, 10 years later. Blood. 2011; 117:4425-43.
22. Gluckman E, Marmont A, Speck B, et al. Immunosuppressive treatment of aplastic anemia as an alternative treatment for bone marrow transplantation. Semin Hematol. 1984;21:11-19.
23. Goddard AF, McIntyre AS, Scott BB. Guidelines for the management of iron deficiency anemia. Gut. 2000;46 (Suppl IV):iv1-iv5.
24. Goodnough LT, Nemeth E, Ganz T. Detection, evaluation, and management of iron-restricted erythropoiesis. Blood. 2010;116:4754-61.
25. Gordon-Smith EC, Rutherford TR. Fanconi anemia:Constitutional aplastic anemia. Semin Hematol. 1991;28:104-12.
26. Goudsmit R, Beckers D, DeBruijne JI, et al. Congenital dyserythropoietic anaemia type III. Br J Haematol. 1972;23:97-105.
27. Green R, Dwyre DM:Evaluation of macrocytic anemias. Semin Hematol. 2015; 52:279-86.
28. Herbert V. Biology of disease: Megaloblastic anaemias. Lab Invest. 1985;52:3-19.
29. Hines JD, Grasso JA. The sideroblastic anemias. Semin Hematol. 1970;7:86-105.
30. Horne III MK. Iron deficiency. In Bethesda handbook of clinical hematology. 2nd edn. Rodgers GP, Young NS (Eds):Philadelphia. Lippincott Williams & Wilkins. 2010.
31. Kumar V, Abbas AK, Fausto N, et al. Robbins and Cotran pathologic basis of disease, 8th edn. Philadelphia. Saunders Elsevier; 2010.
32. Lee GR. The anemia of chronic disease. Semin Hematol. 1983;20: 61-80.
33. Lewis SM, Nelson DA, Pitcher CS. Clinical and ultrastructural aspects of congenital dyswerythropoietic anemia type I. Br J Hematol; 1972;23:113-19.
34. Marsh JCW, Ball SE, Cavenagh J, et al. Writing Group British Committee for Standards in Haematology:Guidelines for the diagnosis and management of aplastic anaemia. Br J Haematol; 2009; 147:47-70.
35. Means Jr. RT, Krantz SB. Progress in understanding the pathogenesis of the anemia of chronic disease. Blood; 1992;80:1639-47.
36. Mufti GJ, Bennett JM, Goasguen J, et al. Diagnosis and classification of myelodysplastic syndrome:International Working Group on morphology of myelodysplastic syndrome (IWGM-MDS) consensus proposals for the definition and enumeration of myeloblasts and ring sideroblasts. Hematologica. 2008;93:1712-17.

37. Nissen C. The pathophysiology of aplastic anemia. Semin Hematol. 1991;28:313-8.
38. Oh RC, Brown DL. Vitamin B_{12} deficiency. Am Fam Physician. 2003;67:979-86.
39. Provan D, Weatherall DJ. Red cells II:Acquired anemias and polycythemia. Lancet. 2000;355:1260-68.
40. Sears DA. Anemia of chronic disease. Med Clin North Am. 1992;76:567-80.
41. Snow CF. Laboratory diagnosis of vitamin B_{12} and folate deficiency:A guide for the primary care physician. Arch Intern Med. 1999;159:1289-98.
42. Speck B. Allogenic bone marrow transplantation for severe aplastic anemia. Semin Hematol. 1991;28:319-21.
43. Stewart FM. Hypoplastic/Aplastic anemia. Role of bone marrow transplantation. Med Clin North Am. 1992;76:683-97.
44. Tischkowitz MD, Hodgson SV. Fanconi anemia. J Med Genetics. 2003;40:1-10.
45. Toh B, van Driel IR, Gleeson PA. Pernicious anemia. N Engl J Med. 1997;337:1441-48.
46. Umbriet J. Iron deficiency:A concise review. Am J Hematol. 2005; 78:225-231.
47. Weiss G, Goodnough LT. Anemia of chronic disease. N Engl J Med. 2005;352:1011-23.
48. Wickramasinghe SN. Dyserythropoiesis and congenital dyserythropoietic anemias. Br J Haematol. 1997;98:785-97.
49. Wong KY, Hug G, Lampkin BC. Congenital dyserythropoietic anemia type II:Ultrastructural and radioautographic studies of blood and bone marrow. Blood. 1972;39:23-30.
50. Young N. Hematologic and hematopoietic consequences of B19 parvovirus infection. Semin Hematol. 1988;25:159-72.
51. Young NS, Scheinberg P, Liu JM. Bone marrow failure syndromes:Acquired and constitutional aplastic anemia, paroxysmal nocturnal hemoglobinuria, pure red blood cell aplasia, and agranulocytosis. In Bethesda Handbook of Clinical Hematology. 2nd edn. Rodgers GP, Young NS (Eds):Philadelphia. Lippincott Williams & Wilkins; 2010.
52. Young NS. Aplastic anemia. Lancet. 1995;346:228-32.

CHAPTER 4

Anemias due to Excessive Red Cell Destruction

DISORDERS OF RED CELL MEMBRANE

Abnormalities in the red cell membrane causing hemolytic anemia are shown in Table 4.1.

Table 4.1: Disorders of red cell membrane associated with hemolytic anemia.

Disorder	Inheritance	Defective gene	Pathophysiology	Red cell morphology
Hereditary spherocytosis	AD (75%), AR (25%)	Ankyrin, spectrin, Band 3, protein 4.2	Defective vertical interaction between cytoskeletal proteins and lipid bilayer	Spherocytes
Hereditary elliptocytosis	AD	Spectrin, protein 4.1	Defective horizontal protein interactions	Elliptocytes (>50%)
Hereditary pyropoikilocytosis	AR	Partial spectrin deficiency	Defective horizontal protein interactions	Poikilocytes (Fragments)
Overhydrated hereditary stomatocytosis (Hereditary hydrocytosis)	AD	Not known	Abnormal permeability to sodium leading to cell swelling	Stomatocytes
Dehydrated hereditary stomatocytosis (Hereditary xerocytosis)	AD	Not known	Loss of intracellular potassium due to increased permeability	Target cells, red cells with hemoglobin puddled at periphery
Southeast Asian ovalocytosis*	AD	Band 3	Red cell membrane rigidity; resistance to *P. falciparum* invasion	Rounded elliptocytes with transverse ridges or longitudinal slit
Acanthocytosis (Abetalipoproteinemia)**	AR	*MTTP* gene	Increase in sphingomyelin in membrane	Acanthocytic red cells

* Not associated with hemolytic anemia
** Acanthocytosis is also seen in McLeod phenotype and neuroacanthocytosis syndromes.

HEREDITARY SPHEROCYTOSIS

Hereditary spherocytosis (HS) is a congenital hemolytic disorder characterized by an inherited defect in the red cell membrane cytoskeleton leading to the formation of spherocytic red cells. Spherocytes, being less deformable than normal red cells, are trapped and destroyed in the spleen. Spherocytes have reduced surface area to volume ratio and are osmotically fragile. Although most common mode of inheritance is autosomal dominant, autosomal recessive transmission occurs in some cases. HS occurs in all races but has a high prevalence in people of northern European descent (1:5000). In our country, HS is found mainly in North India.

ETIOPATHOGENESIS

The Basic Lesion

Normally, lipid bilayer of the red cell membrane is anchored to the underlying skeleton by two major linkages. The first linkage involves interaction of ankyrin with spectrin in skeleton and band 3 in the bilayer. The second attachment between skeleton and bilayer is provided by glycophorin C and protein 4.1 (see Fig. 1.13, Chapter 1). Deficiency in any of these interactions causes weakening of contact between lipid bilayer and skeleton. As a result, areas of the lipid bilayer, which are not directly supported by the underlying skeleton, are lost from the cells in the form of small lipid vesicles. This causes decrease in surface area of red cell relative to volume with resultant spherocyte formation.

HS may result from deficiency of following skeletal proteins—spectrin, ankyrin, band 3, and protein 4.2. In the usual autosomal dominant type of HS, mutation in ankyrin (*ANK1*) gene is most common followed by mutation in β spectrin (*SPTB*), band 3 (*SLC4A1 or EPB3*), α spectrin (*SPTA*), and protein 4.2 or paladin (*EPB42*) genes.

Red Cell Destruction by Spleen

Spherocytes are more rigid and less deformable than normal red cells. This nondeformability prevents the passage of spherocytes from the splenic cords into the splenic sinuses through the slit-like narrow openings. They are retained in the splenic cords for unduly long time. In the splenic cords, red cells encounter unsuitable environment in the form of low glucose and reduced pH. Metabolic deprivation of red cells accentuates membrane loss with release of small vesicles and increase in spherical shape of red cells. Cellular dehydration occurs due to loss of potassium from the red cells. Some of the red cells may escape into the circulation where they appear as dense microspherocytes on blood films. This small population of microspherocytes is osmotically most fragile. Most of the spherocytes are, however, retained in the red pulp where they are destroyed by macrophages. Red cells that escape are retrapped by spleen and phagocytosed (Fig. 4.1).

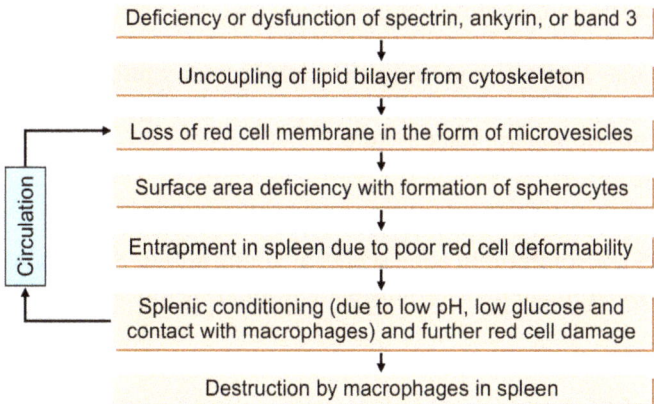

Fig. 4.1: Pathogenesis of hemolysis in hereditary spherocytosis.

INHERITANCE

Most of the cases exhibit autosomal dominant pattern of inheritance, while recessive transmission is less common. Usually, dominant inheritance is associated with mild to moderate disease while recessively inherited spherocytosis is associated with severe hemolysis.

CLINICAL FEATURES

Heterogeneity

The clinical presentation is markedly heterogeneous. Majority of patients present in childhood with mild to moderate anemia, intermittent jaundice, and enlarged spleen. Some other member of the family such as a sibling or a parent is similarly affected.

In some patients clinical features are mild or entirely absent. HS may first be detected while investigating a patient who has gallstones or splenomegaly and minimal or no anemia (well-compensated hemolysis). In still other persons the only abnormality is increased red cell osmotic fragility (OF); such persons come to attention when family members of the affected patient are investigated.

Rarely hereditary spherocytosis may present as a severe hemolytic anemia requiring regular transfusion support.

Exacerbation of Anemia

Sometime the steady course of hereditary spherocytosis is punctuated by episodes of exacerbation of anemia or crises.

In **aplastic crisis**, there is temporary aplasia of erythroid precursors in the bone marrow resulting in sudden worsening of anemia. Infection by human parvovirus has recently been recognized as the cause. Parvovirus B19 selectively infects erythroblasts and transiently suppresses erythropoiesis. Infection by this virus may be asymptomatic or may manifest with fever, chills, bodyache, and facial rash. Transient suppression of erythropoiesis in persons with normal red cell life-span does not manifest as anemia. However, in patients with chronic hemolytic anemia in whom the red cell life-span is markedly shortened, infection is associated with sudden aggravation of anemia, reticulocytopenia, and erythroblastopenia. Treatment consists of transfusion support during the aplastic phase. Increased turnover of erythroid cells due to hemolysis may lead to **megaloblastic crisis** if dietary intake of folate is insufficient. Exacerbation of hemolysis (**hemolytic crisis**) may occur during intercurrent infection due to hyperplasia of monocyte-macrophage system.

Gallstones

Pigment gallstones are common in adolescents or young adults. Sometimes HS is diagnosed incidentally during investigation of a young patient with gallstones.

Chronic Leg Ulcers

These are present in an occasional patient.

LABORATORY FEATURES

Examination of Peripheral Blood

In most patients anemia is usually mild to moderate. MCHC is increased (>35 g/dL) due to cell dehydration, MCH is normal, while MCV is slightly low. Reticulocytosis is present. MCV is on lower side of normal (despite reticulocytosis). Combination of MCHC (>35.4 g/dL) along with RDW (<14%) and increased percentage of hyperdense or hyperchromic cells (reported by some hematology analyzers have been reported to be indicative of HS.

On blood smear examination, characteristic feature is spherocytosis (Fig. 4.2). A spherocyte is a red cell that is smaller in size, does not have central pallor and appears densely hemoglobinized (hyperchromic).

Some mutations are associated with typical morphological abnormalities of red cells like (1) both spherocytes and acanthocytes (mutation of β spectrin gene), pincer- or mushroom-shaped cells (specific and sensitive for band 3 deficiency), and sphero-ovalocytes and stomatocytes (protein 4.2 deficiency in Japanese).

Spherocytes, however, are not unique to HS and are also prominently seen in other disorders such as immune hemolytic anemias (warm antibody type), ABO hemolytic disease of the newborn, hemolytic transfusion reactions, and burns.

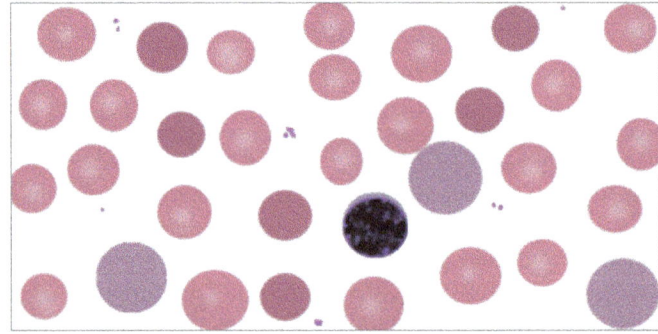

Fig. 4.2: Blood smear in hereditary spherocytosis. Spherocytes are small (compare with small lymphocyte), dense cells with no central pallor. Polychromatic cells are also increased due to hemolysis.

Bone Marrow Examination

This reveals erythroid hyperplasia. Aplastic and megaloblastic crises can be identified by bone marrow examination.

Osmotic Fragility Test

The osmotic fragility (OF) test is the commonly employed screening test for HS. The incubated variant of OF test (see below) is more sensitive than the unincubated test. This test determines susceptibility of red cells to hemolysis when they are subjected to osmotic stress. The red cells are suspended in decreasing concentrations of hypotonic saline solutions and the amount of hemolysis is measured. Water enters the red cells when they are placed in hypotonic saline solution. Due to their biconcave shape, normal red cells can withstand hypotonicity by increasing their volume; beyond a certain limit increase in swelling is not possible, and cells burst by discharging their hemoglobin into the supernatant. Spherocytes have a decreased surface to volume ratio and therefore, they are able to withstand less swelling than normal and are osmotically fragile, i.e. hemolysis occurs in more concentrated solution than normal cells (Fig. 4.3 and Box 4.1). There are various methods of recording results of OF test:

i. Highest concentration of saline at which hemolysis starts (normal 0.50 g/dL NaCl) and the highest concentration of saline at which it is complete (normal 0.30 g/dL of NaCl).
ii. Concentration of saline showing 50% lysis (median corpuscular fragility); normal value is 0.40 to 0.45 g/dL NaCl. Higher value denotes increased fragility.
iii. A graph may be plotted with amount of hemolysis on vertical axis and saline concentrations on horizontal axis. Normal OF curve is sigmoid-shaped. Shift of the curve to the right indicates increased OF.

Limitations of Osmotic Fragility Test

- **Increased OF** is due to spherocytosis, which may result from a variety of causes (HS, immune hemolysis, burns, etc.). Therefore, OF test is not specific for diagnosis of HS.

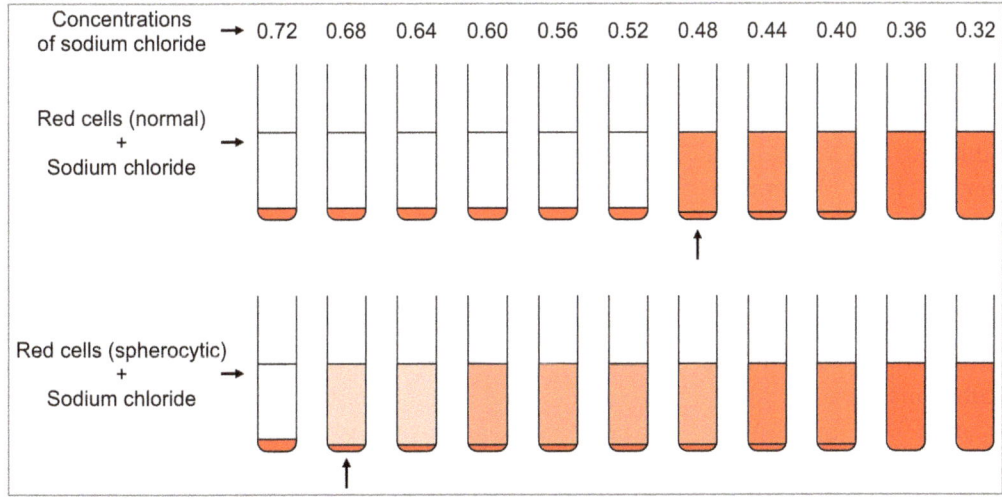

Fig. 4.3: Osmotic fragility test. In hereditary spherocytosis (lower set of tubes), hemolysis starts (up arrow) at a higher saline concentration as compared to normal (upper set of tubes).

> **Box 4.1:** Osmotic fragility test.
> - Measures ability of red cells to take up water when kept in hypotonic saline solutions
> - Due to their biconcave shape, normal red cells take up more water and increase their volume by up to 70% before lysing. Owing to ↑volume to surface area ratio, spherocytes can take up relatively little water and can withstand very little increase in their volume
> - Normally red cells show beginning of hemolysis at 0.5% saline, while spherocytic red cells lyse at higher saline concentration
> - OF is more marked if red cells are incubated at 37°C for 24 hours before the test
> - Test is not diagnostic of HS. Positive result (increased fragility) should be interpreted in the light of clinical and other laboratory features

- OF test is **normal in patients with mild HS** having very few spherocytes in their blood. The sensitivity of the test, however, can be increased by performing the test after incubation of cells at 37°C (see below).
- Test is time-consuming, tedious; and if spherocytes are present on blood smear, adds little to diagnosis.
- **Decreased osmotic fragility** (increased resistance to lysis in hypotonic solutions) is seen in iron deficiency anemia, thalassemia, sickle-cell disease, and liver disease. Therefore, the test is falsely negative in the presence of above disorders.
- OF test cannot distinguish between causes of spherocytosis.

Osmotic Fragility Test after Incubation

Sterile blood is incubated at 37°C for 24 hours followed by determination of OF in hypotonic saline solutions. During incubation, metabolic deprivation of spherocytes occurs (mainly due to decreased concentration of glucose) with resultant membrane destabilization, loss of membrane, and enhancement of spherical shape. Failure of membrane pump with accumulation of sodium and water also plays a role. The sensitivity of the test is thus increased. Incubated OF test may, however, be normal in a small number of patients with HS.

It should be noted that OF is increased in any disorder associated with spherocytosis and is thus not specific for HS. Normal OF test result does not rule out HS as it may be normal in mildly affected patients.

Autohemolysis Test

In this test, blood is incubated at 37°C for 48 hours and the degree of spontaneous hemolysis is noted. The test is performed with and without addition of glucose. Amount of hemolysis is estimated in a colorimeter and the result is expressed as a percent lysis (normal: <4%; with glucose: <0.5%).

Red cells in hereditary spherocytosis are abnormally permeable to sodium probably because of defect in membrane skeleton. Therefore, there is compensatory increase in sodium extrusion by the membrane pump, which thus requires more ATP than normal. During in vitro incubation this causes rapid exhaustion of available red cell ATP and glucose by way of increased glycolysis. Depletion of ATP leads to failure of membrane pump and swelling of red cells as they gain sodium and water. During incubation membrane loss from the red cells is accentuated which increases the volume to surface ratio. Autohemolysis thus, results with smaller red cell volume. Thus during the 48 hours incubation period in this test, glucose exhaustion occurs due to increased utilization and autohemolysis is increased. With the addition of glucose, autohemolysis is corrected to normal levels.

Autohemolysis is also increased in deficiency of a glycolytic enzyme such as pyruvate kinase due to a block in the utilization of glucose. In this case, however, addition of glucose fails to correct the abnormality.

Acidified Glycerol Lysis Time

This test assesses the rate of lysis of red cells and the result is expressed as the length of time needed for 50% lysis ($AGLT_{50}$). Normal blood requires more than 30 minutes for 50% lysis. In HS, the time required for lysis is considerably shortened (25–150 seconds) since spherocytes (due to their high volume to surface area ratio) tolerate swelling for a lesser duration than normal cells. Along with hypotonic saline solution, in the reagent system, glycerol is used which slows the rate of movement of water across the red cell membrane; this allows easier measurement of time required for lysis.

As compared to OF test, this test is simple and rapid. But, it is not diagnostic of hereditary spherocytosis since it is also positive in autoimmune hemolytic anemia, chronic renal insufficiency, leukemias, and during gestation.

Hypertonic Cryohemolysis Test

This recently introduced test is reported to be more specific for diagnosis of HS than OF test. In this test, percent cryohemolysis is observed after transferring cells from 37 to 0°C for 10 minutes. In HS, percent cryohemolysis is more (>20%) as compared to that in normal (3–15%).

Eosin-5-maleimide Binding Test

This is a rapid flow cytometric screening test. Fluorescently labeled eosin-5-maleimide (EMA) binds to band 3 and Rh-related proteins with a 1:1 stoichiometry on red cell membrane. The relative amount of fluorescence correlates with the amount of EMA binding and is analyzed by flow cytometry. Reduced fluorescence intensity of EMA-labeled red cells is observed in HS due to band 3 deficiency, and also in HS associated with spectrin and ankyrin deficiency. The test has high sensitivity and specificity for identification of HS. However, the result is normal in mild HS.

Identification of Deficient Cytoskeletal Protein

It may be possible to identify the deficiency of a specific red cell membrane protein. The usual method consists of sodium dodecylsulfate-polyacrylamide gel electrophoresis of red cell membrane proteins followed by quantitation of separated proteins by densitometric tracing. Deficiencies of spectrin, ankyrin, band 3, protein 4.2, and some other membrane proteins can be identified by this method in majority of patients.

More sensitive method of membrane protein quantitation is radioimmunoassay.

> **Box 4.2:** Diagnosis of hereditary spherocytosis.
> - Presentation in childhood with anemia, jaundice, and splenomegaly
> - Positive family history (autosomal dominant) of jaundice, gallstones, or of splenectomy
> - Spherocytosis on blood smear
> - Reticulocytosis
> - Red cell indices: ↑MCHC, ↓MCV
> - Negative direct antiglobulin test
> - Screening test: OF test, AGLT, cryohemolysis, EMA binding test
> - Confirmatory test: Electrophoretic analysis of red cell membrane proteins (Diagnosis does not require screening test or confirmatory test if other typical features listed above them are present)

DIAGNOSIS OF HEREDITARY SPHEROCYTOSIS

Diagnostic features of HS are shown in Box 4.2.

DIFFERENTIAL DIAGNOSIS

Diagnosis of hereditary spherocytosis is usually easily made on the basis of mild to moderate anemia with spherocytosis, splenomegaly, jaundice, increased OF, and evidence of hereditary spherocytosis in the first-degree relative.

Sometimes anemia is mild or absent and the patient may first present with isolated splenomegaly, gallstones, or "aplastic crisis." Clinical evaluation and examination of blood film for spherocytes are necessary for correct diagnosis.

HS may have to be differentiated from other causes of spherocytosis including autoimmune hemolytic anemia and ABO hemolytic disease of the newborn. Differentiation is made by antiglobulin (Coombs') test and family studies.

TREATMENT

To plan appropriate treatment, it is necessary to grade HS into mild, moderate, and severe forms (based on hemoglobin, reticulocyte count, and serum bilirubin). Treatment of severe HS is **splenectomy**. Splenectomy corrects hemolytic anemia (though underlying skeletal defect and spherocytosis persist) and prevents complications such as gallstones. Although splenectomy is associated with increased life-long risk of sepsis from pneumococci and other encapsulated bacteria, risk is more in children and for this reason splenectomy is deferred until the child is 6 years old and is carried out only if the disease is severe or moderate. The risk of postsplenectomy infections can be reduced by immunizing children with polyvalent pneumococcal, *H. influenzae,* and meningococcal vaccines and by penicillin prophylaxis. Administration of folate is necessary in moderate or severe disease to prevent megaloblastic anemia due to increased erythrocyte turnover.

HEREDITARY DISORDERS OF HEMOGLOBIN

GENERAL FEATURES AND APPROACH TO DIAGNOSIS

Inherited disorders of hemoglobin are the most common genetic disorders in the world. More than 300,000 infants are born every year worldwide with these disorders and many of the affected children die before the age of 5 years. Depending on the nature of genetic defect, they can cause chronic hemolytic anemia or may remain asymptomatic. These disorders are more common in Mediterranean region, Africa, and Southeast Asia. In many countries, they constitute a public health problem.

Classification

These disorders are divided into three broad groups:
1. Hemoglobinopathies
2. Thalassemias
3. Hereditary persistence of fetal hemoglobin (HPFH)

Inherited disorders of hemoglobin due to structural alteration of the globin polypeptide chain are called as **hemoglobinopathies**. Majority of hemoglobinopathies result from substitution of a single amino acid in globin chain due to a point mutation in the β globin gene. The most frequent hemoglobinopathies are HbS, HbC, and HbE. Inherited disorders of hemoglobin due to reduced synthesis of one or more globin chains are known as **thalassemias**. The two common types of thalassemias are α and β. **HPFH** is characterized by failure of normal neonatal switch from hemoglobin F to hemoglobin A.

Both hemoglobinopathies and thalassemias are common in India (Box 4.3 and Table 4.2).

Box 4.3: Hereditary disorders of hemoglobin in India.
- **β thalassemias:** North, West, and East India, with highest prevalence in Sindhis, Punjabis, Gujaratis, and Bengalis
- **HbS:** Central and Southern India
- **HbD:** North India (especially Punjab)
- **HbE:** North East India

Table 4.2: Hereditary disorders of hemoglobin prevalent in India.

Disorder	State	Clinical phenotype
A. Hemoglobinopathies		
HbS	Heterozygous	Asymptomatic
	Homozygous	Severe
HbD^{Punjab}	Heterozygous	Asymptomatic
	Homozygous	Mild
HbE	Heterozygous	Asymptomatic
	Homozygous	Asymptomatic
B. Thalassemias		
β thalassemia minor	Heterozygous	Asymptomatic
β thalassemia major	Homozygous	Severe
C. Double heterozygous states		
HbS/β$^+$ thalassemia		Mild
HbS/β^0 thalassemia		Like sickle-cell anemia
HbS/HbD^{Punjab}		Like sickle-cell anemia
HbE/β thalassemia		Like β thalassemia major
HbD^{Punjab}/β thalassemia		Mild

Geographic distribution of hemoglobinopathies and thalassemias parallels the distribution of *Plasmodium falciparum*. Heterozygotes with these disorders are relatively resistant to *P. falciparum* malaria.

It is predicted that frequency of inherited hemoglobin disorders is likely to increase because of following factors: (1) natural selection of heterozygotes due to protection afforded against malaria, (2) practice of consanguineous marriages in some affected ethnic groups, (3) increased survival of affected patients due to improvements in social conditions and public health, and (4) rapidly increasing population size in general in India.

Correct diagnosis of hemoglobin disorders is essential for proper management, for genetic counseling of prospective parents, and for prenatal diagnosis and decision regarding termination of pregnancy.

Different inherited disorders of hemoglobin are as follows:

Hemoglobinopathies

Hemoglobins with reduced solubility: Some point mutations in the β globin gene cause alteration in the solubility of hemoglobin. In these, a nonpolar amino acid is substituted for a polar one near the surface of the molecule. For example, point mutation GAG→GTG at the 6th codon of β globin gene leads to the formation of sickle hemoglobin (HbS). Upon deoxygenation HbS polymerizes causing formation of sickle cells; these cells are less deformable than normal, cause vascular occlusion and are also phagocytosed in spleen.

Another example is HbC, which is formed by substitution of lysine for glutamic acid at position 6 of globin chain ($β^6$Glu→Lys). Crystallization of HbC increases rigidity of red cells, which are destroyed in spleen.

Unstable hemoglobins: Instability of hemoglobin molecule arises from mutations that interfere with structural relationship between globin chains and heme. Instability results in precipitation of hemoglobin with formation of Heinz bodies that attach to the red cell membrane. The red cells become rigid, and are sequestered and destroyed in the spleen. The unstable hemoglobins are also called as congenital Heinz body hemolytic anemias.

Hemoglobins with low oxygen affinity: Some mutations in globin gene stabilize the hemoglobin in deoxygenated state. There is higher than normal oxygen delivery to the tissues so that oxygen demands are met at a lower hemoglobin concentration ("pseudoanemia"). A large percentage of deoxygenated hemoglobin can cause cyanosis.

Hemoglobins with increased oxygen affinity: An example is Hb Chesapeake in which a mutation at $α_1β_2$ interface stabilizes the hemoglobin in the oxygenated or relaxed state. Oxygen is not released readily to the tissues resulting in tissue hypoxia and compensatory erythrocytosis.

Hemoglobin M: M hemoglobins arise from mutations that stabilize iron of heme in the nonfunctional ferric state. Such hemoglobins are unable to bind oxygen and produce cyanosis.

Structural hemoglobin variants causing phenotype of thalassemia: Some mutations produce an abnormal hemoglobin molecule as well as reduced synthesis of globin chains, e.g. hemoglobin E ($β^{26}$ Glu→Lys) which is associated with the phenotype of β thalassemia.

Nomenclature of hemoglobinopathies: More than 700 hemoglobinopathies have been reported so far. Majority of them are clinically insignificant. Variant hemoglobins are denoted by various methods like letters, name of the place where first discovered, residence of the prepositus, or family name of the index case. The first abnormal hemoglobin discovered was HbS (S for sickle). More systematic nomenclature consists of denoting the type of polypeptide chain, position, and the amino acid substitution, e.g. HbS is denoted by $\beta^{6\,Glu\text{-}Val}$, which represents substitution of valine for glutamic acid at position 6 of β globin chain.

Thalassemias

Molecular lesions in thalassemias cause reduced or absent synthesis of one or more of the globin chains. Imbalance in globin chain synthesis causes precipitation of unpaired globin chains, ineffective erythropoiesis and hemolysis.

Approach to Diagnosis of Disorders of Hemoglobin

Correct diagnosis can be made if a systematic approach is pursued. This consists of obtaining clinical details including patient's ethnic origin and family history, performing few basic hematological investigations, followed by confirmatory studies, which are guided by clinical data and results of baseline studies. Hemoglobin disorders are widely prevalent among certain population groups and knowledge of this may allow one to make an easier diagnosis in a relevant case, e.g. β thalassemias are frequent in Mediterranean areas, Middle East, and in parts of North India; sickle-cell disease is common in tropical Africa and in certain tribes in Central and Southern India.

Presence of a similar disease or a relevant positive laboratory test in a close relative is a strong evidence of hereditary nature of the disease and helps in making the diagnosis in doubtful cases.

Various laboratory tests used in the evaluation of hemoglobin disorders are as follows: (1) Measurement of hemoglobin or hematocrit, red cell count, and red cell indices; (2) examination of blood smear; (3) electrophoretic identification of abnormal hemoglobins—cellulose acetate electrophoresis at alkaline pH, citrate agar electrophoresis at acid pH, (4) high-performance liquid chromatography (HPLC), (5) immunoassay for hemoglobin variants, (6) globin chain electrophoresis; (7) tests for HbS—slide test using reducing agent, solubility test, (8) quantitation of hemoglobin A2, (9) quantitation of hemoglobin F, (10) determination of distribution of HbF in red cells, (11) tests for inclusion bodies, and (12) globin chain synthesis studies (Fig. 4.4 and Box 4.4).

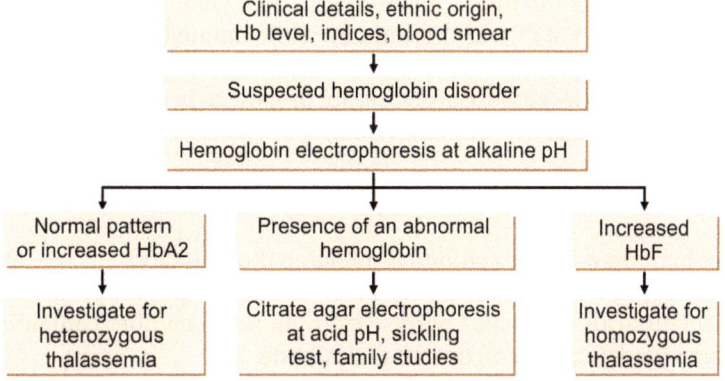

Fig. 4.4: Investigations in inherited disorders of hemoglobin.

> **Box 4.4:** Laboratory diagnosis of disorders of hemoglobin.
>
> **Presumptive diagnosis**
> - Hemoglobin electrophoresis
> - Isoelectric focusing
> - High-performance liquid chromatography
> - Capillary electrophoresis
>
> **Definitive diagnosis**
> - DNA analysis
> - Protein analysis by mass spectrometry

Initial Peripheral Blood Examination

Generally, anemia is severe in homozygous states whereas in heterozygotes, anemia may be mild or absent.

Red cell indices are of critical importance in diagnosis of thalassemias, in which MCV and MCH are characteristically low. Red cell distribution width (RDW, a measure of variation in size of red cells) is increased in iron deficiency anemia, while it is normal in thalassemia. Peripheral blood smear will show characteristic morphologic abnormalities such as: permanently sickled cells (sickle-cell diseases), numerous target cells (hemoglobin C disease), etc.

Hemoglobin Electrophoresis at Alkaline pH

The initial screening test in the evaluation of hemoglobinopathies is electrophoresis at alkaline pH (8.5) using a tris EDTA-borate buffer. Various supporting media are used to achieve separation of hemoglobins such as filter paper, starch gel, or cellulose acetate membranes. Most widely used medium is cellulose acetate because the method is simple, only a small quantity of blood is needed, separation of hemoglobins is rapid, quantitation of different hemoglobins is possible, and strips can be stored permanently.

Principle: The migration of molecules having a net charge in an electric field is known as electrophoresis. The electrical charge of the hemoglobin molecule results from the presence of ionized carboxyl and amino groups. Many amino acid substitutions in the globin chain alter the charge, while some do not. The positive or negative charge and strength of the charge depend on the nature of amino acid substitution and pH of the electrophoretic medium. In an alkaline buffer solution, hemoglobins migrate from cathode (-) to anode (+) and various hemoglobins have different rates of migration due to differences in their charge. Hemoglobins having more positive charge than HbA are nearer the cathode while hemoglobins having more negative charge are nearer the anode in relation to HbA. Identification of different hemoglobins is based on their relative positions on cellulose acetate strip. In some hemoglobinopathies, alteration in charge by different amino acid substitutions is identical with resultant identical electrophoretic migration.

Procedure
1. Red cells are hemolyzed and a solution is prepared (hemolysate).
2. Hemolysate is applied near one end of cellulose acetate strip (point of origin).
3. Cellulose acetate strips are placed in the electrophoresis chamber containing Tris-EDTA-borate buffer with point of origin toward the cathode.
4. Electric current is applied till adequate separation is achieved.

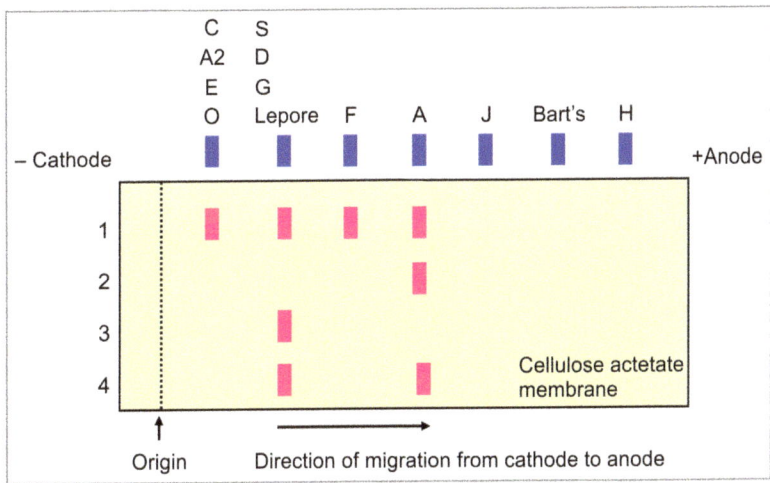

Fig. 4.5: Cellulose acetate electrophoresis at alkaline pH. Lane 1: Control (AFSC); control is prepared by mixing blood from normal infant and persons with sickle-cell trait and HbC trait. Lane 2: AA (Normal person); Lane 3: SS (sickle-cell anemia); and Lane 4: AS (sickle-cell trait). Positions of various hemoglobins are shown at the top of cellulose acetate membrane for comparison.

5. The cellulose acetate strips are removed from the chamber, stained with a protein stain such as Ponceau S, and dried.

The test sample should be compared with a control sample containing known normal and abnormal hemoglobins. Usually, a control sample known to contain hemoglobins A, F, S, and C is always included in every electrophoresis and is applied to each strip next to the test sample.

Relative mobilities of some hemoglobins using cellulose acetate electrophoresis at alkaline pH are shown in Figure 4.5.

Normal electrophoresis pattern in adults is reported as AA. Disorders of hemoglobin cause decrease or absence of HbA, sometimes an increase of HbF and/or HbA2, and sometimes an abnormal hemoglobin. While reporting abnormal hemoglobins, hemoglobin with the highest concentration is written first followed by hemoglobin that is in lesser amount. Thus AC or AS indicate that concentration of HbA is higher than HbC or HbS (i.e. HbC or HbS trait, respectively) while CA or SA denote that amount of HbC or HbS exceeds that of HbA (i.e. HbC-β thalassemia or sickle-cell-β thalassemia).

Electrophoresis at alkaline pH allows provisional identification from cathode to anode of following hemoglobins—C/A2/E/O-Arab, S/D/G/Lepore, F, A, J, Bart's, H. Thus, hemoglobin variants A2, C, E, and O-Arab migrate to the same position on cellulose acetate electrophoresis at alkaline pH. Similarly, hemoglobins S, D, G, and Lepore have identical migration. These comigrating hemoglobins cannot be differentiated from each other only on the basis of cellulose acetate electrophoresis at alkaline pH. For this purpose, a second procedure is needed. Presence of HbS can be confirmed by sickling test using 2% sodium metabisulfite or solubility test. If test for HbS is positive, then idea about genotype is gained by assessing relative proportions of HbA, HbF, and HbS. If proportion of HbA is more than HbS, it indicates AS genotype (sickle-cell trait). If HbS exceeds HbA, then it is indicative of HbS-β$^+$ thalassemia; and complete absence of HbA in the presence of HbS and HbF occurs in sickle-cell anemia and HbS β^0 thalassemia. Family studies are helpful in arriving at the correct diagnosis.

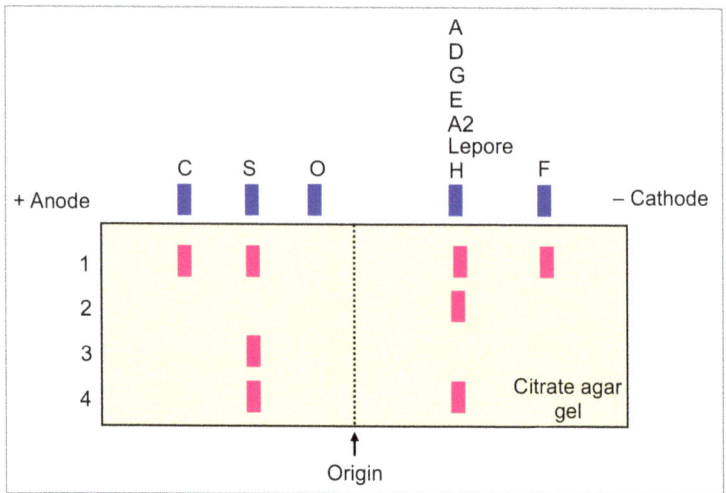

Fig. 4.6: Citrate agar gel electrophoresis at acidic pH. Lane 1: Control (A, F, S, C); Lane 2: AA (normal); Lane 3: SS (sickle-cell anemia); and Lane 4: AS (sickle-cell trait). Positions of various hemoglobins are shown above the agar gel for comparison.

For differentiating other identically migrating hemoglobins, citrate agar electrophoresis at acid pH needs to be performed.

Elevation of HbF or HbA2 in the absence of any abnormal hemoglobin suggests thalassemia. In such cases, alkali denaturation test for quantitation of HbF, estimation of HbA2, and family studies are helpful in making the diagnosis.

Citrate Agar Electrophoresis at Acidic pH

This is a useful method for further characterization of hemoglobin variants after electrophoresis at alkaline pH.

As seen from Figure 4.6, the hemoglobin variants C, S, A, and F migrate to different locations. Citrate agar electrophoresis at acid pH provides separation of hemoglobins that have similar mobilities on cellulose acetate at alkaline pH. Thus HbS can be distinguished from HbD and HbG, and HbC from HbE and HbO-Arab. However, hemoglobin variants D, E, G, Lepore, and H have migration identical to HbA.

In cellulose acetate electrophoresis at alkaline pH, large proportion of HbF can obscure HbS. However, with citrate agar at acid pH, clear separation of HbA and HbS from HbF is obtained. Therefore, citrate agar electrophoresis at acid pH is well suited for neonatal screening of sickle-cell anemia.

High-Performance Liquid Chromatography

This technique is used as a screening test for (1) detection, identification, and quantification of hemoglobin variants, and (2) quantitation of HbA2 and HbF. It is also well suited for neonatal screening since it can detect small amounts of hemoglobin and needs small amount of blood. Various automated HPLC systems are available commercially.

Hemoglobins A, F, S, C, E/A2, D^{Punjab}, O-Arab, and D^{Philadelphia} can be separated and identified with HPLC.

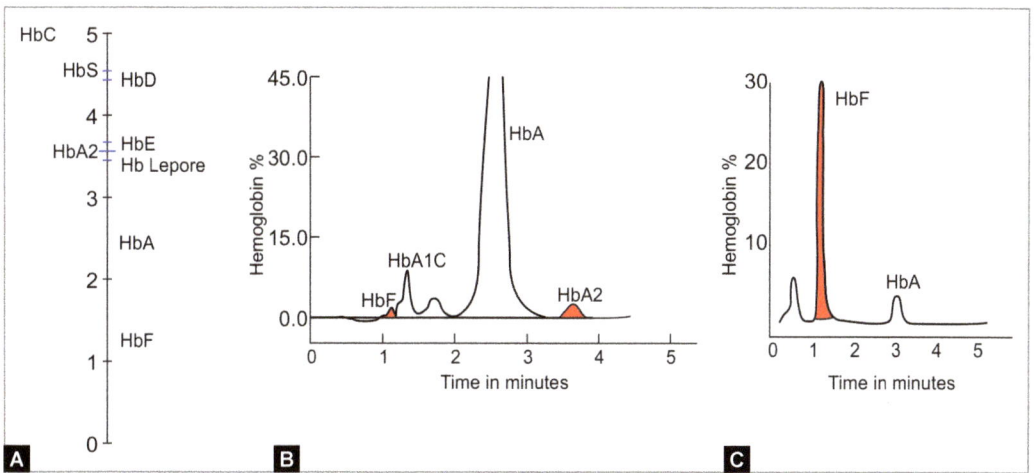

Figs. 4.7A to C: High-performance liquid chromatography: (A) Retention time of various hemoglobins; (B) HPLC in normal adult; (C) HPLC in normal newborn.

In this automated technique, blood sample (hemolysate) is introduced into a column packed with silica gel. Different hemoglobins get adsorbed onto the resin. Elution of different hemoglobins is achieved by changing the pH and ionic strength of the buffer. Hemoglobin fractions are detected as they pass through a detector and recorded by a computer (Figs. 4.7A to C). As compared to electrophoresis, low concentration of HbF and HbA2 can be estimated by HPLC.

Isoelectric focusing: This refers to separation of hemoglobins according to their isoelectric points or pI (i.e. the point at which they do not have a net charge) in an electric field through a pH gradient. Precast polyacrylamide or agarose gels containing ampholytes with varying pI values are available commercially. The ampholytes produce a stable pH gradient (pH 6.0 at anode to pH 8.0 at cathode). When hemolysate is applied near cathode, hemoglobins migrate through the gel and become stationary when their isoelectric points are reached to produce a distinct sharp band. As compared to electrophoresis, the technique has higher resolution and certain hemoglobins which comigrate on cellulose acetate electrophoresis can be separated. However, quantitation of hemoglobin A2 is not possible and the technique is expensive (Figs. 4.8A and B).

Capillary electrophoresis: This is either zone electrophoresis or isoelectric focusing carried out in a capillary tube. The technique is rapid, needs only a small sample, and quantitation is possible.

Immunoassay for Hemoglobin Variants

Commercial kits are available for detection of hemoglobin variants. These assays use monoclonal antibodies against specific hemoglobin variants. Currently, HbS, HbC, HbE, and HbA can be detected by this method.

Globin Chain Electrophoresis

α and β globin chains are separated from each other by the addition of 6 M urea and 2-mercaptoethanol to the buffer. When subjected to electrophoresis these chains migrate

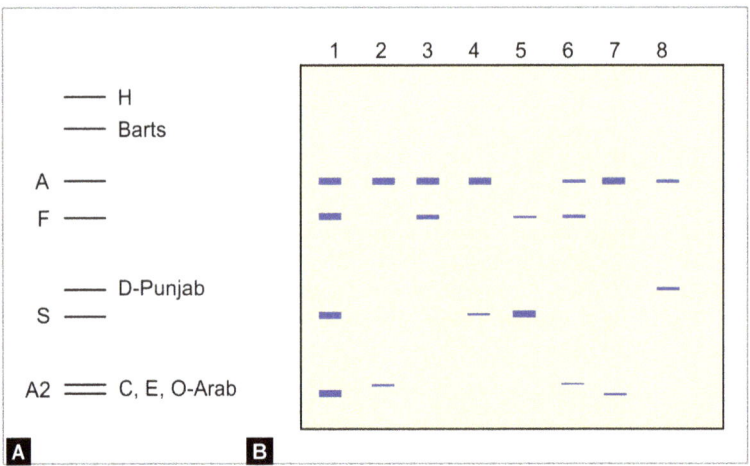

Figs. 4.8A and B: Separation of hemoglobins by isoelectric focusing: (A) Relative mobilities of different hemoglobins on isoelectric focusing; (B) Isoelectric focusing on agar gel. (1) Control: A, F, S, C; (2) Normal AA pattern with A2; (3) Normal newborn: A, F: (4) Sickle-cell trait: A, S; (5) Sickle-cell anemia with SS and increased HbF; (6) β thalassemia trait with A, F, and A2; (7) HbE trait: A, E; and (8) HbD trait: A, D.

differently. The procedure is performed at both acid and alkaline pH and reveals characteristic patterns of migration of abnormal α and β chains.

This method provides a means of identifying abnormal hemoglobin variants that cannot be identified by routine electrophoretic methods (i.e. cellulose acetate at alkaline pH and citrate agar at acid pH). It is especially helpful when variants other than S and C are present and which have identical migration on both cellulose acetate and citrate agar systems.

Tests for Hemoglobin S

Two types of tests are available:
1. *Sickling test:* When red cells containing HbS are subjected to deoxygenation, they become sickle-shaped while cells that do not contain HbS remain normal. Certain reducing chemical agents such as 2% sodium metabisulfite or sodium dithionite can deprive red cells of oxygen.

    Blood and a reducing agent are mixed on a glass slide and a cover slip is placed over it that is sealed with petroleum jelly-paraffin wax mixture. Amount of HbS in red cells and degree of deoxygenation influence the speed and extent of sickling. Sickling is usually evident after 30 minutes; if it is not then the slide is re-examined after allowing it to stand overnight. The sickled cells have minimum of two pointed projections (Fig. 4.9).

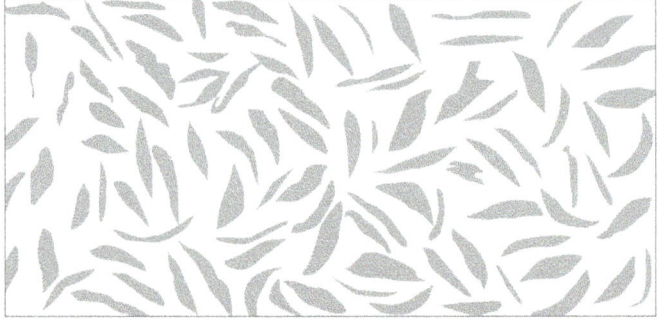

Fig. 4.9: Sickling test (Wet preparation).

Causes of false-negative test
- Inactive, outdated reagents (incomplete reduction of oxygen tension)
- Blood samples containing low proportion of HbS (e.g. young infants, some cases of sickle-cell trait)
- Improper sealing of coverslip (in hot climate).

Causes of false-positive test
- High concentration of sodium metabisulfite
- Carryover from positive sample due to inadequate washing of pipette
- Mistaking crenated red cells for sickled cells.

Limitations of sickling test
- This test simply detects presence of HbS and does not differentiate sickle-cell anemia from sickle-cell trait or other sickling syndromes.
- This test cannot be used for mass screening, as an experienced microscopists required for interpretation.

2. Solubility test: Small amount of blood is added to a solution that contains high-phosphate buffer, a reducing agent (sodium dithionite) and saponin. Red cells are hemolyzed and HbS, if present, is reduced by dithionite. Reduced HbS forms insoluble polymers, which refract light, and solution becomes turbid. A reader scale is held at the back of the tube; in negative test lines will be clearly seen since HbA is soluble in phosphate buffer, while lines will not be seen in positive test due to formation of polymers of HbS (Fig. 4.10). Positive result is also obtained with HbS Travis and HbC Harlem. The solution remains clear in the presence of HbA, HbF, HbC, HbD, HbG, and HbO-Arab.

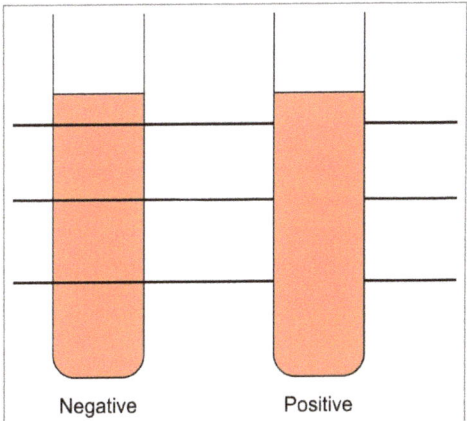

Fig. 4.10: Sickle-cell solubility test. In negative test, lines of the reader scale kept behind the tubes are clearly visible. In positive test, lines are not seen due to turbidity.

For mass scale screening of HbS, solubility test is the most widely used, rapid, reliable, and cost-effective test.

Causes of false-negative test
- Use of old or outdated reagents
- Low concentration of HbS as in young infants or in severe anemia (Solubility test should not be performed in infants <6 months to avoid getting misleading results.)
- Following blood transfusion.

Causes of false-positive test
- Paraproteinemia
- Hyperlipidemia
- Polycythemia
- Leukocytosis

Estimation of HbA2

Normally, HbA2 ($\alpha_2\delta_2$) comprises of only a small proportion (1.5–3.0%) of total hemoglobin in adults. A raised HbA2 (3.5–7%) is a characteristic feature of thalassemia minor. Estimation of HbA2 is also useful for distinguishing sickle-cell anemia (HbA2 < 4%) from sickle-cell β^0 thalassemia (HbA2 > 4%).

In some cases of β thalassemia minor, HbA2 is normal (called as normal HbA2 β thalassemia). When iron deficiency complicates β thalassemia minor, HbA2 is usually normal and therefore, it is not possible to make diagnosis of β thalassemia minor until iron deficiency is adequately treated. HbA2 percentage is normal or low in δβ thalassemia and in α^0 thalassemia trait.

There are two methods for estimation of HbA2: elution from cellulose acetate and microcolumn chromatography. A newer method is HPLC.

Estimation of HbA2 by elution from cellulose acetate: Cellulose acetate electrophoresis at pH 8.9 is carried out to separate HbA2 from other hemoglobins. Zones of HbA2 and of other hemoglobins are cut and eluated separately into different amounts of buffer. Absorbance of HbA2 eluate from remaining hemoglobins is measured in a spectrophotometer and percentage of HbA2 is calculated. This technique, however, is labor-intensive if a large number of samples are to be tested.

Estimation of HbA2 by microcolumn chromatography: In this method, a glass tube or a column is filled with a supporting medium such as anion exchange resin DEAE cellulose and blood sample is introduced into the column. Mixture of hemoglobins gets adsorbed onto the resin. HbA2 is selectively eluted by using a buffer with specific pH and ionic strength. Other hemoglobins are eluted by using a buffer with different pH and ionic strength. Eluted HbA2 and other hemoglobins are spectrophotometrically measured and percentage of HbA2 is calculated.

Estimation of HbA2 by both the above methods is not possible if a hemoglobin variant which comigrates with HbA2 at alkaline pH is present (e.g. HbC, E, or O-Arab).

Estimation of Fetal Hemoglobin

Fetal hemoglobin ($\alpha_2\gamma_2$) is the predominant form of hemoglobin during fetal life. After birth, HbF level gradually falls and is approximately 25% at 1 month, 5% at 6 months, and less than 2% at 1 year. In adults HbF is less than 1%. Significant elevation of HbF usually occurs in β thalassemia major, hereditary persistence of fetal hemoglobin, δβ thalassemia, and sickle-cell disease; quantitation of HbF is usually done in these disorders. Mild elevation occurs during pregnancy and in aplastic anemia, megaloblastic anemia, paroxysmal nocturnal hemoglobinuria, chronic leukemias, and erythroleukemia.

There are various methods for estimation of HbF (If HbF is >2%, it can be recognized usually on electrophoresis). The commonly used method is the Betke method. In this method, a strong alkali (sodium hydroxide) is added to the hemolysate to denature HbA and after a specified time, saturated ammonium sulfate is added. The denatured hemoglobin is precipitated by ammonium sulfate. Fetal hemoglobin resists denaturation and remains in solution. The amount of hemoglobin remaining in solution (i.e. undenatured hemoglobin or HbF) is measured spectrophotometrically and is calculated as the percentage of the total hemoglobin. Betke's method is reliable for estimation of 2 to 40% of HbF. For higher levels of HbF, method of Jonxis and Visser can be used. In this method, rate of alkali denaturation is measured in a spectrophotometer and extrapolated back to zero time to get the amount of HbF. Other methods are radioimmunoassay and HPLC.

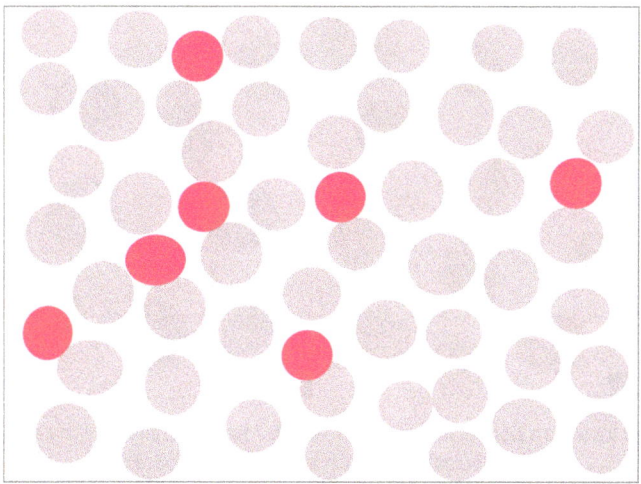

Fig. 4.11: Acid elution test for intercellular distribution of HbF. Red cells containing HbF are dark while those without HbF are pale and empty.

Intercellular Distribution of HbF

Test for cellular distribution of HbF is employed to distinguish hereditary persistence of fetal hemoglobin (HPFH) from δβ thalassemias. In HPFH, HbF is distributed evenly in all the red cells (pancellular distribution) whereas in δβ thalassemias only some of the red cells contain HbF (heterocellular distribution).

The method most commonly employed for evaluation of cellular distribution of HbF is acid elution test of Kleihauer–Betke. In this test, fresh blood films on glass slides are fixed with ethanol. HbA is readily eluted from red cells by acid solution, while HbF resists acid-elution and remains within the cells. After staining, cells containing large amount of HbF appear dark, while cells with no HbF appear unstained and empty ("ghosts"). The acid elution test was originally employed to confirm and quantitate fetomaternal hemorrhage by detecting fetal red cells in maternal circulation (Fig. 4.11).

Tests for Inclusion Bodies

Following types of inclusions are detected in hemoglobinopathies (Figs. 4.12A and B):

HbH inclusions: Due to the redox action of certain dyes (brilliant cresyl blue) HbH may be precipitated in mature or nucleated red cells as multiple, small, ragged inclusions. They are seen in Hb Bart's hydrops fetalis syndrome, HbH disease, and α thalassemia carrier states.

In splenectomized patients with HbH disease, preformed HbH inclusions can be detected when peripheral blood is incubated with methyl violet.

α chain inclusions: α chain inclusions in homozygous β thalassemia are seen only in nucleated red cells in bone marrow, but after splenectomy they are also seen in peripheral blood. Peripheral blood or bone marrow sample is incubated with methyl violet, films are prepared and observed under microscope. α chain inclusions appear as single, ragged structures closely attached to the nucleus.

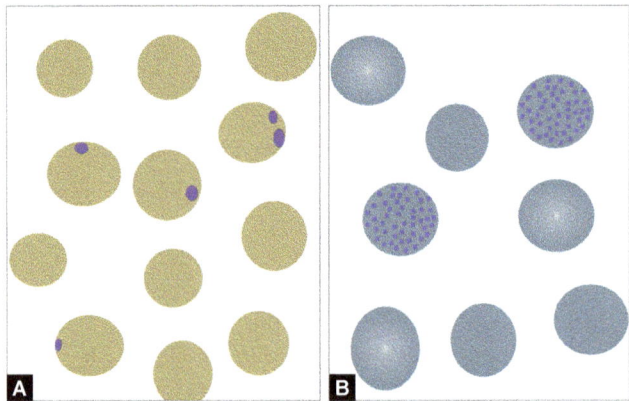

Figs. 4.12A and B: Inclusion bodies in red cells: Heinz bodies (A) stained with crystal violet and HbH inclusions stained with brilliant cresyl blue (B).

Heinz bodies: Heinz bodies are formed by precipitation of denatured hemoglobin, which can be detected after vital staining with methyl violet. They stain deep purple and are usually attached to the cell membrane. Apart from unstable hemoglobin disease they are also seen in glucose-6-phosphate dehydrogenase (G6PD) deficiency after oxidative denaturation of hemoglobin by drugs or chemicals.

Globin Chain Synthesis Studies
Sometimes electrophoretic and other usual hematological studies fail to diagnose thalassemias and in these cases globin chain synthesis ratio may be helpful.

Reticulocytes are capable of globin synthesis. Reticulocyte-enriched red cells (obtained by centrifugation) are incubated in a medium, which contains a radioactive amino acid (usually ^{3}H leucine). The cells are then washed and hemolyzed and globin is extracted with acid-acetone. Globin chains are dissociated by CM-cellulose chromatography and their specific radioactivity is determined by counting in a scintillant. The values are expressed as a ratio of α chain to β chain activity.

Normal α/β ratio is about 1.0. It is reduced in α thalassemia and raised in β thalassemia and is proportional to the severity of defect.

THE THALASSEMIAS

The thalassemias are a heterogeneous group of inherited disorders of hemoglobin characterized by reduced or absent production of one (or rarely more) of the globin chains. They are the commonest single gene disorders in the world.

The disease was termed thalassemia, derived from the Greek word *thalassa* for sea, since it was formerly thought that the disease occurs only in the Mediterranean population. However, the disease is not restricted to the Mediterranean and is distributed widely in other tropical countries. The disease was first described by Thomas Cooley (a pediatrician from Detroit, USA) in 1925. Homozygous β thalassemia or thalassemia major is Cooley anemia. The thalassemias constitute a major public health problem in the countries surrounding the Mediterranean and in the Middle and the Far East. Lack of standard medical care and of regular and safe blood supply in some countries is associated with considerable morbidity and mortality from thalassemias.

Classification of Thalassemias

The classification of thalassemias is based on (1) the type of globin chain that is deficiently synthesized, (2) clinical expression of the disease, or (3) transfusion requirements.

- **Classification according to the type of globin chain which is deficiently synthesized:** The two most common types are α (alpha) and β (beta) thalassemias. Less common types are δβ (delta-beta) thalassemia and γδβ (gamma-delta-beta) thalassemia.
- **Classification according to clinical severity:** β **thalassemias** have been clinically classified on the basis of severity of anemia into three types—thalassemia major, thalassemia intermedia, and thalassemia minor. Patients with severe transfusion-dependent anemia are said to have thalassemia major. In thalassemia minor, affected individuals are usually asymptomatic with mild or no anemia in spite of prominent red cell abnormalities in peripheral blood. Thalassemia intermedia is characterized by intermediate degree of severity of anemia that does not require regular blood transfusions. Each of these clinical types is genetically diverse. Clinical types of α **thalassemia** are Hb Bart's hydrops fetalis syndrome, HbH disease, thalassemia trait, and silent carrier.
- **Classification based on regular transfusion requirements:** Recently, a new clinical classification has been proposed based on requirement of regular transfusion therapy. According to this classification, thalassemias are divided into two main types: nontransfusion-dependent thalassemia (NTDT) and transfusion-dependent thalassemia (TDT).
    - Nontransfusion-dependent thalassemias (NTDT):
        - Transfusions not required: Thalassemia minor (β-thalassemia trait, α-thalassemia trait)
        - Transfusion occasionally or intermittently required: Thalassemia intermedia (β-thalassemia intermedia, mild or moderate HbE/β thalassemia, HbH disease)
    - Transfusion-dependent thalassemia (TDT): Lifelong, regular transfusions required (β thalassemia major, severe HbE/β thalassemia).

Molecular Basis of Thalassemias

Molecular lesions in thalassemias are complex. Of the two common types, majority of β thalassemias are caused by point mutations, while most of the α thalassemias result from gene deletions.

β Thalassemias

There is a single β globin locus on each chromosome (number 11) and as humans are diploid there are two β genes. Normal structures of globin genes and globin synthesis have been considered earlier (see chapter on "Overview of physiology of blood").

β thalassemias are classified into two major types: $β^0$ thalassemia and $β^+$ thalassemia. $β^0$ thalassemia is characterized by complete absence of β chain synthesis (complete deficiency of β chains) while in $β^+$ thalassemia β chain synthesis is reduced but not completely lacking (partial deficiency of β chains). Usually, individuals having one normal and one abnormal β globin gene have β thalassemia minor while persons in whom both β globin genes are abnormal have β thalassemia major.

β thalassemia displays marked genetic heterogeneity with more than 200 molecular lesions having been reported; these may be silent, mild causing relative reduction in β chain synthesis ($β^+$), or severe causing complete absence of β chain production ($β^0$). It has been observed, however, that in a particular population (e.g. Asian Indians, Mediterranean, Southeast Asian, American Blacks, etc.). Only a few β thalassemia mutations are consistently and commonly found and account for 90% of the abnormal β thalassemia genes (Box 4.5). Mutations frequent in Asian Indians are illustrated in Figure 4.13 and also shown in Box 4.6.

Box 4.5: Common mutations causing β thalassemia in different ethnic groups.

Asian Indians
- IVS-1 position 5 (G→C) Consensus splice site mutation
- 619 bp deletion
- Codon 8/9+G Frameshift mutation
- IVS-1 position 1 (G→T) Splice junction mutation
- Codons 41/42 (–TTCT) Frameshift mutation

Southeast Asians
- IVS-2 position 654 (C→T) Cryptic splice site mutation
- Codons 41/42 (–TTCT) Frameshift mutation
- –28 A→G Promoter mutation
- Codon 17 A→T Nonsense codon mutation

Mediterranean
- Codon 39 (CAG→TAG) Nonsense codon mutation
- IVS-1 position 1 (G→A) Splice junction mutation
- IVS-1 position 110 (G→A) Cryptic splice site mutation
- IVS-1 position 6 (T→C) Consensus splice site mutation
- IVS-2 position 745 (C→G) Cryptic splice site mutation

African American
- –88 (C→T) Promoter mutation
- –29 (A→G) Promoter mutation
- Poly-A (AATAAA→AACAAA) RNA cleavage poly-A signal mutation

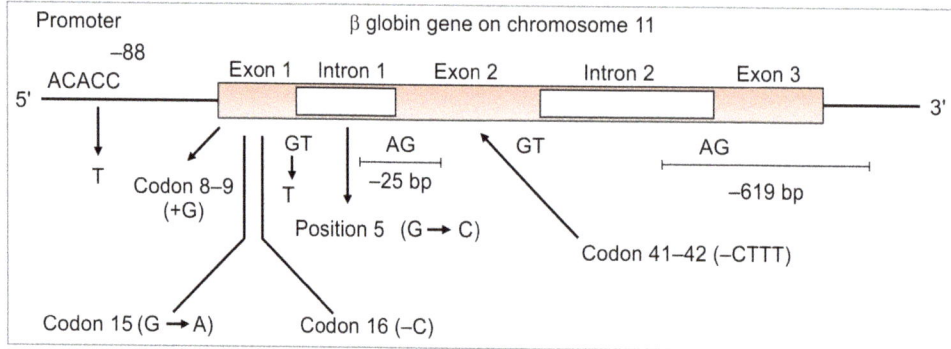

Fig. 4.13: Schematic representation of β thalassemia mutations frequently observed in Asian Indians.

Box 4.6: Common β thalassemia mutations in India.
- Intron 1 position 5 (G→C)
- 619 base pair deletion
- Intron 1 position 1 (G→T)
- Frameshift mutation in codon 8–9 (+G)
- Frameshift mutation in codon 41–42 (–CTTT)
- Codon 15 (G→A)

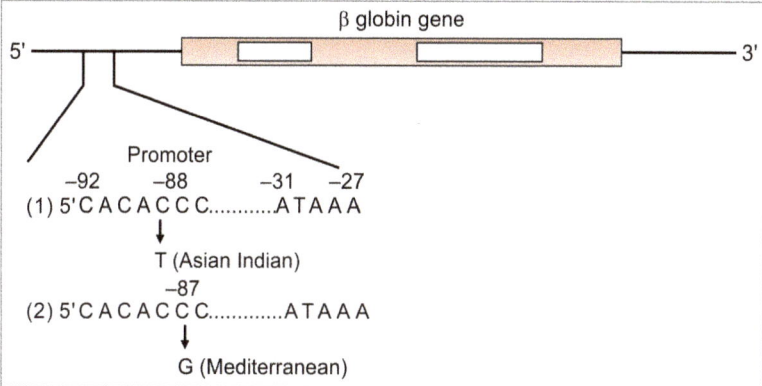

Fig. 4.14: Two examples of mutations affecting transcription in selected population groups are shown. Arrows indicate sites where one base is substituted by another (–88C→T and –87C→G). By convention, nucleotides that are located 5′ to the gene are given minus number from the transcription start nucleotide. Both these mutations cause β⁺ thalassemia.

A brief outline of mutations causing β thalassemia is given below.

Mutations which affect transcription: Initiation and rate of transcription are regulated by the promoter region which is located immediately in front (upstream or 5' end) of globin genes. Two highly conserved sequences in the promoter region, ATAAA and CACACCC, appear to be essential for efficient initiation of transcription of the β globin gene. Mutations affecting these promoter sequences cause reduction in globin gene transcription. As some amount of β globin is produced, patients develop β⁺ thalassemia. Some of the mutations that affect transcription are shown in Figure 4.14.

Mutations that affect splicing of RNA: Mutations that cause abnormal splicing are very common. Majority of them occur within introns but some of them affect exons.

Splicing mutations may alter the normal splice junction or may create alternative splice sites at abnormal locations.

Mutations altering normal splice junction: The GT and AG dinucleotides at the start (5' splice site) and the end (3' splice site) of introns, respectively, are obligatory for normal splicing. If mutations alter these splice sites then splicing fails to occur resulting in absence of β globin synthesis and formation of β⁰ thalassemia alleles (Fig. 4.15).

Mutations creating alternate splicing sites at abnormal locations. They occur in introns or exons. A mutation in intron or exon produces an alternate splicing site so that some of the messenger RNAs are spliced at mutant site and some are spliced at normal site. As shown in Figure 4.16, a mutation G→A at position 110 of intron 1 produces a new active splicing site AG. It has been shown in this case that 90% of splicing occurs at newly created abnormal site and about 10% at normal site. This results in severe β⁺ thalassemia as abnormal splicing predominates.

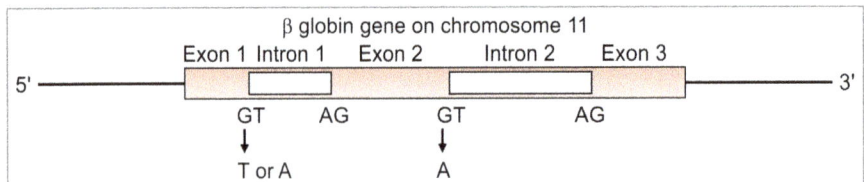

Fig. 4.15: Mutations that alter normal splice junctions. Arrows indicate substitutions that alter the normal splice site. The mutations illustrated are intron 1 position 1 G→T (Asian Indians), intron 1 position 1 G→A (Mediterranean), and intron 2 position 1 G→A. All these mutations cause β⁰ thalassemia.

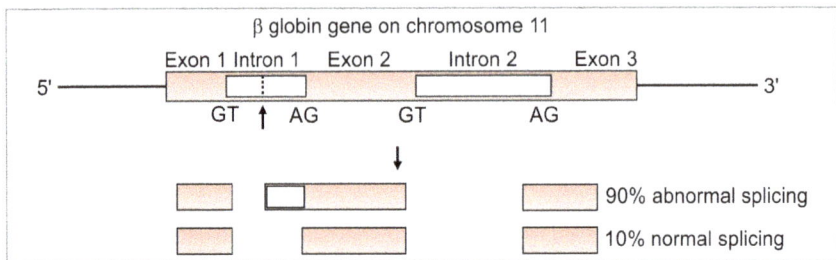

Fig. 4.16: Mutation creating alternate splicing site in intron 1. Arrow (↑) shows mutant splicing site in intron 1 due to substitution G→A at position 110.

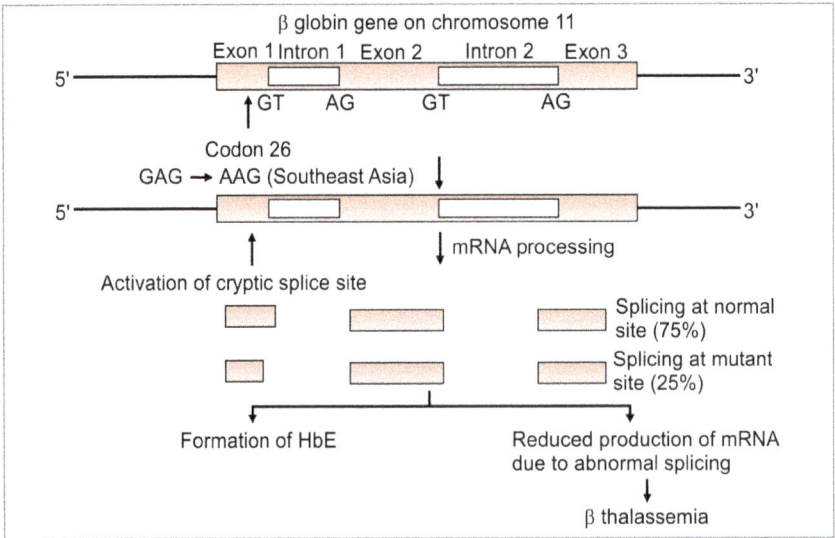

Fig. 4.17: Activation of cryptic splice site in exon 1 by mutation G→A in codon 26. This substitution causes (1) formation of an abnormal hemoglobin HbE, and (2) alteration of sequence in exon 1 which activates a cryptic splice site.

Mutations in exons may also activate cryptic splice sites. An example is substitution G to A in codon 26 (GAG→AAG) of exon 1. This mutation has two effects: activation of cryptic splice site and formation of abnormal hemoglobin, HbE. A cryptic splice site is one, which resembles to some extent the normal splice site but is not used normally for splicing. A mutation in the cryptic site makes it an active splice site. Normal splicing of mRNA containing the G to A substitution in codon 26 of exon 1 leads to the formation of the abnormal hemoglobin, HbE. This mutation is associated with reduced production of mRNA (Fig. 4.17).

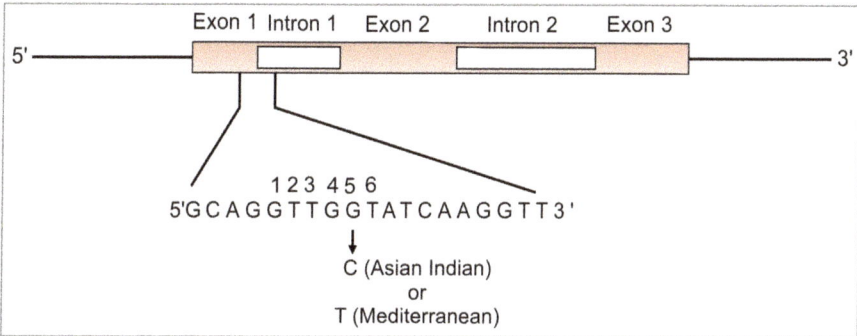

Fig. 4.18: Two mutations affecting consensus sequence shown are: (1) intron 1 position 5 (G→C) and (2) intron 1 position 5 (G→T). They cause β⁰ thalassemia.

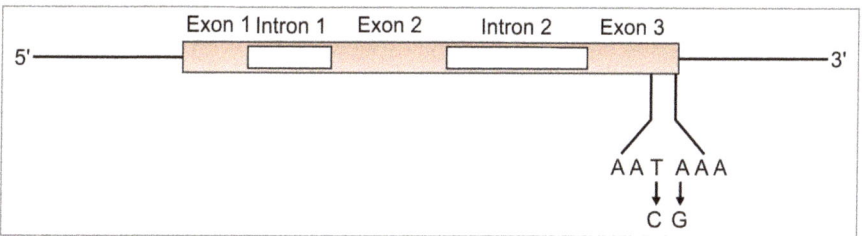

Fig. 4.19: Polyadenylation mutations.

Mutations affecting consensus sequences: Apart from AG and GT dinucleotides, sequences surrounding the intron-exon boundaries are markedly similar.

These sequences are highly conserved during evolution and are known as consensus sequences. Mutations in consensus sequences produce β thalassemia of variable severity (Fig. 4.18).

Polyadenylation mutations: Mutations in polyadenylation sequence AATAAA at the 3' end of the globin gene are associated with β⁺ thalassemia (Fig. 4.19).

Mutations which lead to the formation of the chain termination codon: UAA, UAG, and UGA are chain-termination codons in β globin mRNA. Substitution of a single nucleotide in the coding sequence to create chain termination codon (nonsense mutation) will interrupt the translation of mRNA. This will generate nonfunctional fragments of β globin and cause β⁰ thalassemia (Fig. 4.20).

Frameshift mutations: Reading frame comprises of sequentially arranged triplets of three bases. Each triplet codes for a specific amino acid. Mutations that delete or insert one, two, or more than three bases cause alteration in the sequence of the reading frame. This results in the formation of incorrect amino acids and secondly, at some place in the sequence, chain termination codon is formed which stops translation at that place (Fig. 4.21). These mutations cause β⁰ thalassemia.

Deletions: 619-base pair deletion of the β globin gene is common in Asian Indians. It removes part of intron 2, exon 3, and some sequences 3' to the globin gene (Fig. 4.22). This deletion causes β⁰ thalassemia in the homozygous state. Apart from this, gene deletions are rare in β thalassemias.

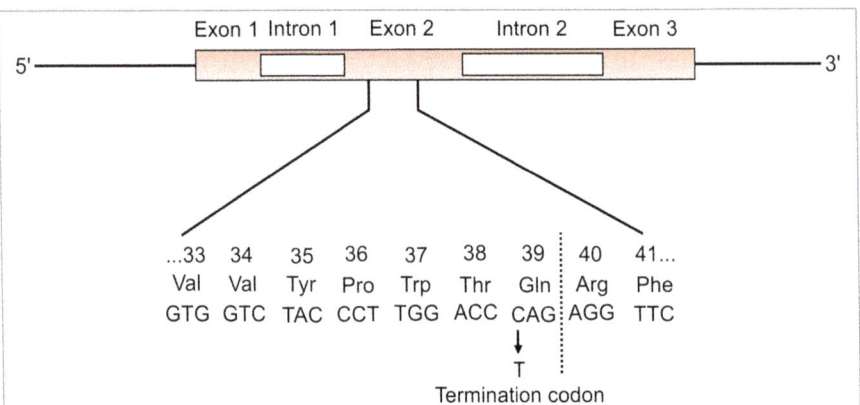

Fig. 4.20: Mutation to termination codon. Nonsense mutation in codon 39 (C→T) prevalent in Mediterranean population is shown. This mutation causes formation of a stop codon TAG (UAG in mRNA) at the 39th codon which leads to premature termination of translation.

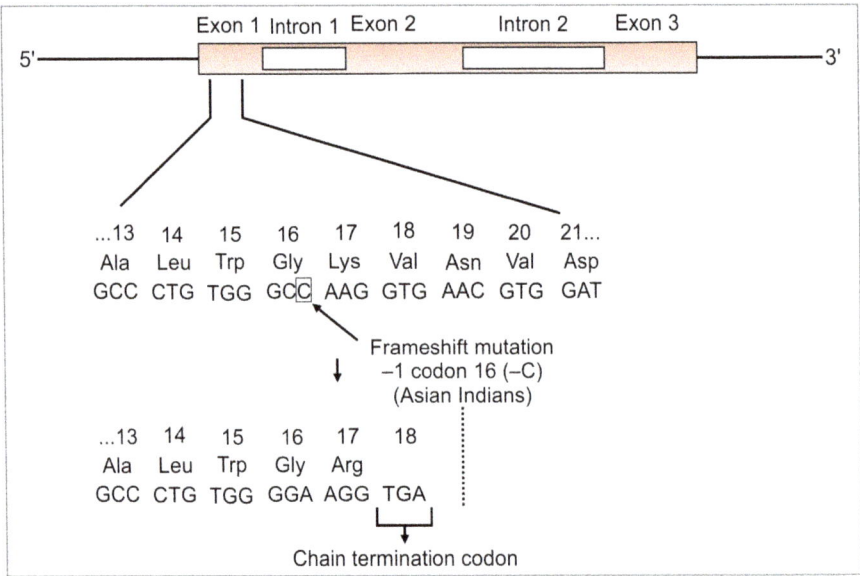

Fig. 4.21: Frameshift mutation in codon 16. A deletion C in codon 16 alters the reading frame and also creates a chain termination codon prematurely at codon 18.

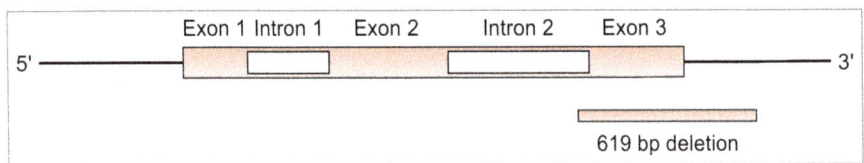

Fig. 4.22: The Indian 619 bp deletion.

Dominant thalassemia: Recently, mutations have been identified in exon 3 of β globin gene that cause production of unstable globin chains. Unstable globin chains and unpaired chains precipitate in erythroblasts in bone marrow that leads to their premature destruction. This causes disease expression even in heterozygous state; this is called as **dominant thalassemia.**

α Thalassemias

There are two α gene loci on each chromosome 16 and since humans are diploid there are four α genes. The normal α globin haplotype is αα and the normal genotype is written as αα/αα.

α thalassemias are classified into two types—$α^0$ and $α^+$ thalassemias. In a^0 thalassemia, there is total absence of α chain synthesis from one chromosome, while in $α^+$ thalassemia α chain synthesis from one chromosome is decreased but not absent.

More than 120 mutations have been reported to cause α thalassemia. Most cases of α thalassemias result from gene deletions. Deletions which remove both α genes cause complete absence of α chain production from the affected chromosome ($α^0$ thalassemia). They are particularly common in Southeast Asia. Hydrops fetalis and HbH disease are largely restricted to Southeast Asia because of prevalence of cis α gene deletions (αα/—). Deletion of one α globin gene out of the two is associated with $α^+$ thalassemia. However, $α^+$ thalassemias also result from mutations of α globin genes (nondeletional $α^+$ thalassemia). In rare cases, deletions affecting upstream enhancer elements [depicted as ($αα^T$)] despite normal α genes cause α thalassemia; these deletions always remove MCS-R2 enhancer. Various mutations giving rise to $α^+$ thalassemia include: (1) Mutations which cause aberrant splicing; (2) Mutations of chain terminator codon: Single base substitution in chain terminator codon results in, instead of termination of chain, continuation of translation until another chain terminator codon is encountered. This results in lengthening of α polypeptide chain. Two examples of this are Hb Constant Spring (chain-terminating codon UAA is changed to CAA which codes for glutamine), and Hb Koya Dora (UAA→UCA which codes for serine); (3) Mutations which cause instability of α globin chain after translation. The newly produced α chains are rapidly degraded.

Since individuals in India most often carry αα/α-haplotype ($α^+$), severe forms of α thalassemia are rare.

ATR-X syndrome: A *trans*-acting mutation of *ATRX* gene located on X chromosome causes α thalassemia along with severe mental retardation and dysmorphic facial appearance. *ATRX* gene influences the expression of α globin genes and also some other genes, the mechanism of which is unknown.

Prevalence of Thalassemias

About 1 to 5% of the world population are carriers for thalassemia mutation. Most (90%) of patients with this disorder live in low- to middle-income countries. Due to continuing population migration, the disease is gradually becoming common in developed countries and assuming a global problem.

β thalassemias are prevalent in "β thalassemia belt" which covers Mediterranean region, Africa, Middle East, some areas of India, Pakistan, and Southeast Asia. In India, β thalassemia is more common in certain communities such as Punjabis, Lohanas, Sindhis, Bengalis, Gujaratis, Bhanushalis, and Jains (Box 4.7).

$α^0$ thalassemias are common in Southeast Asia (China, Thailand, Vietnam, Malaysia, the Phillipines), eastern Mediterranean region, and in Middle East; they are uncommon in Africa and India. $α^+$ thalassemia is relatively more common in India.

Box 4.7: Thalassemias in India.
- β thalassemia is frequent; α thalassemia is rare.
- Carrier rate of β thalassemias is about 3% (Average)
- β thalassemia is more prevalent in certain communities from North India

Thalassemias (and sickle-cell disease and G6PD deficiency) are prevalent in those parts of the world where malaria has been common. The high frequency of these disorders in certain areas is probably because heterozygotes are protected against falciparum malaria. According to the theory of "balanced polymorphism," disadvantage of homozygous state is "balanced" by protection afforded to heterozygotes against malaria. Genetic analysis studies suggest that thalassemic mutations have arisen independently in different parts of the world. Due to natural selection of heterozygotes (who are genetically more "fit" because of protection against malaria) these genes have achieved high frequency.

The mean prevalence of β thalassemia heterozygotes in India is reported to be 3.3%. Every year 10,000 to 11,000 children with thalassemia major are born in India (10% of all thalassemics in the world).

HbE/β thalassemia and HbH disease are becoming increasingly more common in many regions of the world due to changing demographics. Clinical phenotype of HbE/β thalassemia resembles either thalassemia major or intermedia. HbE/β thalassemia is the commonest form of severe thalassemia in eastern India, Bangladesh, and Southeast Asia.

Pathogenesis, Clinical Features, and Laboratory Features of Thalassemias

β Thalassemias

There are three clinical forms of β thalassemias—β thalassemia major, β thalassemia intermedia, and β thalassemia minor.

β Thalassemia Major

This was first described by Thomas Cooley in 1925 in children of Italian descent and is also known as Cooley's anemia.

β thalassemia major is the most severe of the β thalassemias and is characterized by severe anemia which requires regular transfusion therapy. It may be produced by following genotypes—β^0/β^0, β^0/β^+, or β^+/β^+.

Pathogenesis

1. *Anemia:* (i) Normal adult hemoglobin is composed of two α and two β globin chains and heme. In β thalassemia major, the underlying genetic defect is responsible for inability of erythroid cells to synthesize adequate amounts of β globin chains. This causes excessive accumulation of free α chains since there are no complementary β chains to form a tetramer. The unbound α chains precipitate within erythroblasts and red cells. These α chain inclusions damage the cell membrane leading to the lysis of erythroblasts and red cells in the bone marrow, i.e. ineffective erythropoiesis (Fig. 4.23). The two major mechanisms responsible for anemia are hemolysis and ineffective erythropoiesis, which in turn result from excess of α chains. α-globin monomers are formed from excess α chains and contain α chain-heme aggregates (α-hemichromes) and reactive oxygen species. These cause hemolysis through (1) membrane damage due to oxidation of protein 4.1 and membrane lipids, and defective assembly of spectrin-actin-band 4.1 in cytoskeleton, and (2) aggregation of band 3 proteins which forms a neoantigen and binds IgG and complement. Ineffective erythropoiesis possibly results from (1) activation of apoptosis and maturation arrest of erythroblasts by reactive oxygen species, and (2) maturation arrest of erythroblasts due to

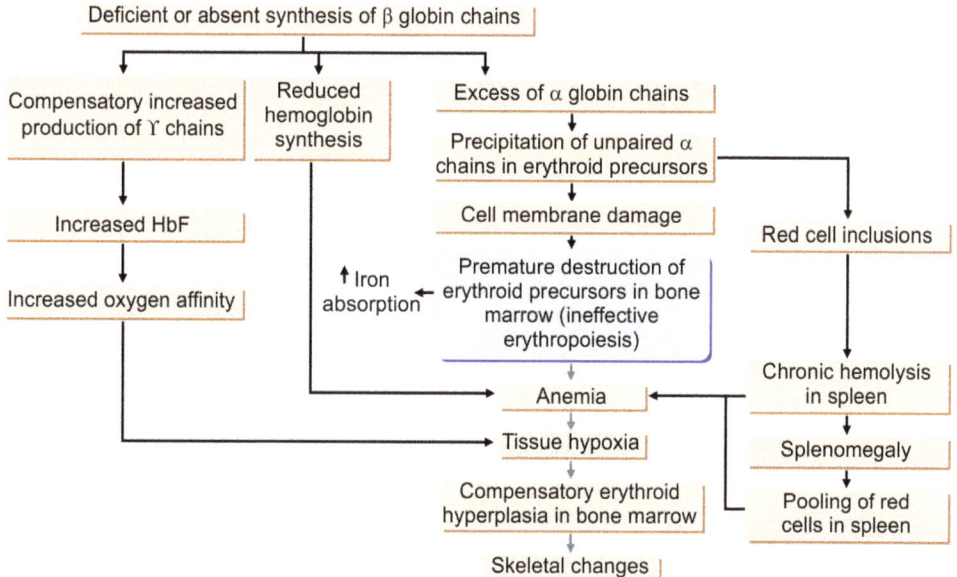

Fig. 4.23: Pathogenesis of β thalassemia major.

degradation of GATA1 by sequestered heat shock protein 70 (due to its direction interaction with free α globin). (ii) The red cells containing α chain aggregates have reduced flexibility and are trapped in the spleen. Removal of inclusions by splenic macrophages damages the red cell membranes; such red cells are ultimately destroyed by macrophages in the spleen and liver. Thus in addition to intramedullary destruction, red cells are also destroyed peripherally in the spleen (hemolysis). (iii) Reduced synthesis of hemoglobin due to lack of β globin production leads to the formation of microcytic hypochromic red cells. (iv) Excessive peripheral destruction of red cells invariably leads to splenomegaly. Pooling of considerable proportion of red cells within large spleen further aggravates the anemia. (v) Hemoglobin F is the predominant hemoglobin in β thalassemia major and is due to increased proliferation of cells capable of synthesizing γ chains. HbF does not release oxygen as readily to the tissues as HbA since it poorly binds 2,3-diphosphoglycerate and thus exacerbates tissue hypoxia.
2. *Skeletal changes:* Severe anemia and tissue hypoxia stimulate erythropoietic drive and cause extreme bone marrow hyperplasia. Expansion of hyperactive bone marrow causes weakening and deformities of skull and of facial bones. Thinning of cortex may lead to pathological fractures.
3. *Iron overload:* Iron absorption from the intestine is increased in β thalassemia major due to ineffective erythropoiesis. Chronic regular blood transfusion therapy markedly increases the iron accumulation and causes iron overload (Fig. 4.24). Iron overload may damage parenchymal cells of various organs such as pancreas (diabetes mellitus), liver (cirrhosis), gonads (infertility), and heart (arrhythmias and heart failure).

Clinical Features

Switch from the synthesis of HbF ($\alpha_2\gamma_2$) to HbA ($\alpha_2\beta_2$) occurs after birth and therefore anemia develops insidiously during infancy (i.e. around 6 months of age) and gradually becomes

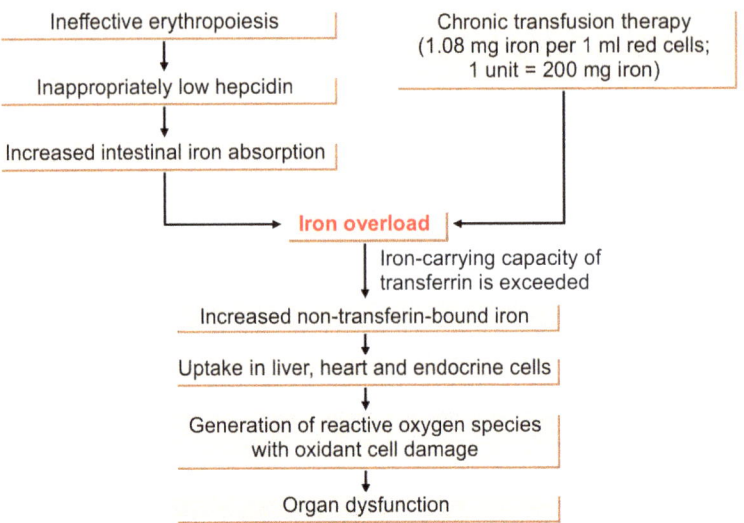

Fig. 4.24: Pathogenesis of iron overload in β thalassemia major.

worse. Typically, children with β thalassemia major present with severe anemia, failure to thrive, retarded growth, hepatosplenomegaly, and skeletal and facial changes. Frontal bossing and overgrowth of maxilla produce thalassemic or "chipmunk" facies. Various radiological changes have been described such as widening of diploe of the skull, "hair on end" appearance, widening of medullary cavity and thinning of cortex of long bones, and pathological fractures. Other radiologic changes include broad ribs with "rib-within-rib" appearance, squaring of vertebral bodies, and shortening of long bones. Osteoporosis [(reduced bone mineral density) is usual and results from defective osteoblastic activity and increased osteoclast activation (mediated by receptor activator of nuclear factor κB ligand (RANKL)/osteoprotegerin pathway)]. Osteoporosis is responsible for frequent fractures following minor trauma. These children suffer from repeated infections; raised serum iron level that favors bacterial proliferation has been implicated. Folate deficiency commonly develops due to increased erythroid turnover. Other complications are hypersplenism, and manifestations related to foci of extramedullary hematopoiesis compressing vital structures, such as spinal cord. Untreated patients usually die from anemia or infections before 5 years of age. Early institution of regular blood transfusion therapy is associated with normal growth and development during the first decade of life. However, iron overload gradually develops during adolescence. Manifestations of iron overload include growth retardation, hyperpigmentation of skin, hepatocellular damage with cirrhosis, insulin-dependent diabetes mellitus, gonadal dysfunction (delayed or absent pubertal development), hypoparathyroidism, hypothyroidism and cardiac failure. Most of the patients die by the end of the 20 or 30 years of life from refractory heart failure and arrhythmias. Chronic transfusion therapy is also associated with risk of transmission of viral infections such as human immunodeficiency virus (HIV), and hepatitis B and C viruses (HBV and HCV).

There is increased risk of thrombosis in patients with β thalassemia intermedia (and also in β thalassemia major, α thalassemia syndromes, and hemoglobin E/β thalassemia). This is thought to result from exposure of phosphatidylserine and other negatively charged lipids on cell membranes of defective erythrocytes which activate coagulation, platelets, and endothelial

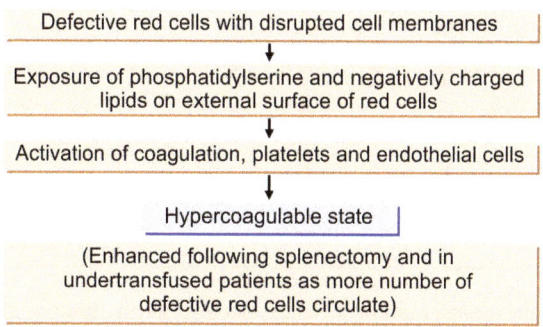

Fig. 4.25: Pathogenesis of hypercoagulability state in β thalassemia.

cells. The risk is more in nontransfused or undertransfused patients and in splenectomized patients (as more numbers of defective red cells are in circulation). Thromboembolic events include stroke, pulmonary embolism, deep vein thrombosis, and portal vein thrombosis (Fig. 4.25).

Laboratory Features

1. *Peripheral blood examination:* Patient presents with severe anemia with hemoglobin concentration between 2 and 6 g/dL. Anemia is typically microcytic and hypochromic. On peripheral blood smear examination, red blood cells show marked anisopoikilocytosis, severe hypochromia, plenty of target cells, Howell-Jolly bodies, basophilic stippling, and nucleated red cells (Fig. 4.26).
   Reticulocytosis is modest (5–15%), but is less as compared to the degree of anemia.
   The reason for this is ineffective erythropoiesis. Leukocytes and platelets are usually unremarkable.
2. *Test for inclusion bodies:* Aggregates of unpaired α-chains within erythroblasts in bone marrow may be detected with supravital (methyl violet) staining. After splenectomy they are also demonstrated in red cells in peripheral blood.
3. *Hemoglobin electrophoresis:* This characteristically shows elevated HbF (10–98%) (Fig. 4.27). HbA_2 may be normal or increased. In homozygous $β^0$ thalassemia, HbA is completely lacking, while in $β^0/β^+$ and $β^+/β^+$ thalassemias, some amount of HbA is present.

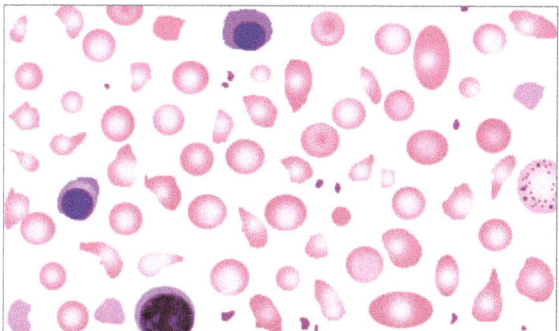

Fig. 4.26: Blood smear in thalassemia major showing microcytic hypochromic red cells, nucleated red cells, anisopoikilocytosis, target cells, basophilic stippling, and polychromasia.

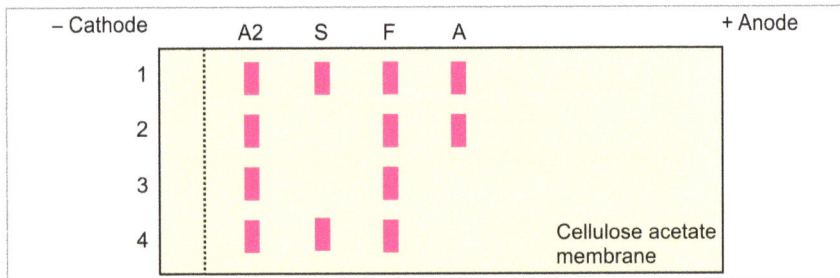

Fig. 4.27: Diagrammatic representation of typical electrophoresis findings in β thalassemia minor (Lane 2), β thalassemia major (Lane 3), and sickle-cell β thalassemia (Lane 4). Lane 1 is control.

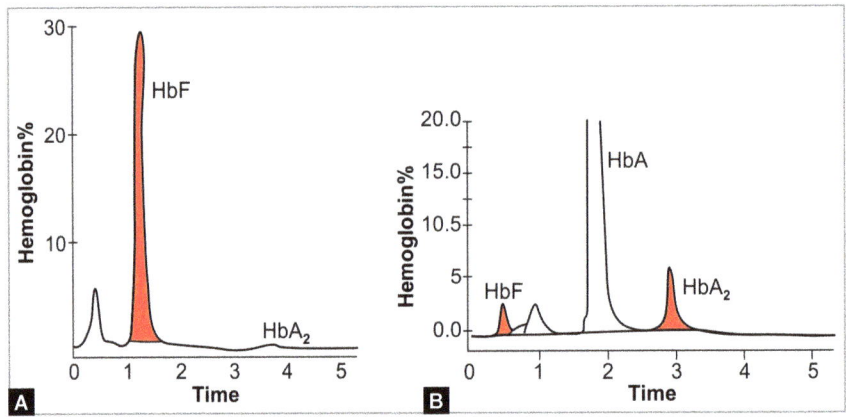

Figs. 4.28A and B: High-performance liquid chromatography findings in (A) β thalassemia major; and (B) β thalassemia minor.

4. *Other investigations:* **Bone marrow examination** shows severe erythroid hyperplasia. Storage iron is increased. **Acid elution test** reveals heterogeneous distribution of HbF in red cells.
Unconjugated serum bilirubin and serum iron are increased while osmotic fragility of red cells is decreased.
HPLC findings in thalassemia major and minor are shown in Figures 4.28A and B.

β Thalassemia Minor

This is the heterozygous carrier state of β thalassemia characterized by little or no anemia but prominent morphologic changes of red cells. It results when a person inherits normal β gene from one parent and either $β^0$ or $β^+$ thalassemia allele from the other. Degree of imbalance of globin chain synthesis and ineffective erythropoiesis are much less as compared to thalassemia major. These patients are usually asymptomatic but may develop anemia during demanding situations such as infections or pregnancy.

Detection of β thalassemia minor is essential for genetic counseling and to distinguish it from iron deficiency anemia. Long-term administration of iron in these patients can cause iron overload and organ damage.

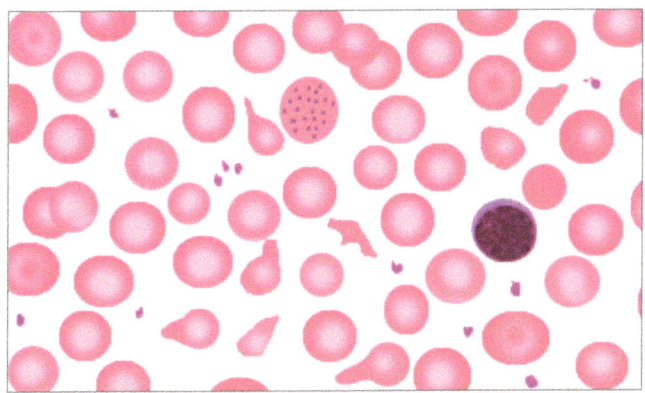

Fig. 4.29: Blood smear in thalassemia minor. Anisopoikilocytosis with microcytic hypochromic red cells and basophilic stippling are seen.

Laboratory features: Hemoglobin level is either normal or mildly decreased and is generally not less than 9.0 g/dL. Red blood cells characteristically show reduced MCV (<70 fl) and reduced MCH (<25 pg). Determination of red cell indices is a commonly employed method for detection of β thalassemia trait in population screening. MCHC is normal. Red cell count is increased. Reticulocyte count and serum bilirubin are slightly elevated.

Morphologic abnormalities of red cells are striking and consist of target cells, basophilic stippling, microcytosis, and hypochromia (Fig. 4.29).

OF test shows resistance to hemolysis. Single tube OF test is frequently done to identify heterozygotes of β thalassemia (see population screening of thalassemias and Fig. 4.31).

A characteristic laboratory feature of β thalassemia minor is elevation of HbA_2 (3.5-7.0%). HbF may be mildly increased. Definitive diagnosis of β thalassemia minor is based on HPLC (which quantitates HbA_2) or Hb electrophoresis.

Differential diagnosis: The major differential diagnosis is **iron deficiency anemia** since both exhibit microcytic and hypochromic red cells. This is considered in chapter on iron deficiency anemia. Another differential diagnosis is α thalassemia trait which cannot be distinguished from β thalassemia minor on the basis of cell counts and blood smear.

Typical clinical and laboratory features of β thalassemias are summarized in Table 4.3.

Inheritance of β Thalassemia with Structural Hemoglobinopathies

The inheritance of β thalassemia with structural β globin variants is common. Sickle-cell β thalassemia is considered below.

Sickle-cell β thalassemia (Micro-drepanocytic disease): This disorder occurs when one β gene carries HbS mutation and the other gene carries β thalassemia mutation (double heterozygous state). It is commonly observed in West Africa, the Mediterranean countries, and India. Clinical manifestations are decided by whether the β thalassemia gene inherited is $β^0$ or $β^+$.

i. *Sickle-cell $β^0$ thalassemia:* Clinical manifestations resemble sickle-cell anemia except splenomegaly that persists into adult life. (In sickle-cell anemia, spleen characteristically undergoes autoinfarction and is usually not palpable beyond childhood.)

Table 4.3: Typical clinical and laboratory features in β thalassemias.

Type	Genotype	Anemia	Red cell morphology	Hb electrophoresis	Clinical features
β thalassemia minor	β/β⁺, β/β⁰	Absent or mild (Hb > 10 g/dL)	Microcytic hypochromic; target cells, basophilic stippling	HbA$_2$ >3.5%; HbF <10%	Asymptomatic
β thalassemia intermedia	β⁺/β⁺, dβ/δβ, β⁰/δβ; interaction of β⁰/β⁰ or β⁺/β⁺ with α thalassemia	Moderate (Hb 7–10 g/dL)	Similar to major, but with less severe changes	HbF (10–95%); absent or little HbA; HbA$_2$ normal or raised	Onset at a later age than major; splenomegaly +; not transfusion-dependent
β thalassemia major	β⁰/β⁰, β⁰/β⁺, β⁺/β⁺, β⁰/HbE, β⁺/HbE	Severe (Hb <7 g/dL)	Severe anisopoikilocytosis, microcytosis, hypochromia, many target cells, basophilic stippling, many nucleated red cells	HbF (10–95%); absent or little HbA; HbA$_2$ normal or raised	Onset in infancy; splenomegaly+++; marked skeletal changes; transfusion-dependent

Peripheral blood smear shows features of both sickle-cell anemia and thalassemia such as sickle cells, microcytic and hypochromic cells, and target cells. MCV and MCH are decreased.

On hemoglobin electrophoresis, HbS is the predominant hemoglobin (70–80%), HbA is absent, and HbA$_2$ (3–5%), and HbF (10–20%) are elevated (see Fig. 4.27). Diagnosis is confirmed by demonstrating that one parent has sickle-cell trait and the other has β thalassemia trait.

HPLC or hemoglobin electrophoresis cannot differentiate between sickle cell anemia and sickle cell-β⁰ thalassemia since HbA is absent in both conditions. Distinction is based on low MCV and MCH in the later and family studies.

ii. *Sickle-cell β⁺ thalassemia:* Two clinical phenotypes are distinguished—severe and mild.

Severe form of sickle-cell β⁺ thalassemia occurs in Mediterranean countries and clinical picture bears resemblance to sickle-cell anemia. Red cell morphology is typical of thalassemia. Hemoglobin electrophoresis shows HbS as the major component, some HbA, and mildly raised HbF and HbA$_2$.

Mild sickle-cell β⁺ thalassemia occurs predominantly in Africa and resembles sickle-cell trait. In sickle-cell β⁺ thalassemia, HbS is always more than HbA, while reverse is true for sickle-cell trait.

Diagnosis is confirmed by family studies (one parent with sickle-cell trait and the other with β thalassemia minor).

α Thalassemias

Humans have four α globin genes, two on each chromosome 16. Defect in any one of the α globin genes produces α thalassemia. Defect may occur in one, two, three, or all four α globin genes with progressive deficiency of α chain production. Since α chains are present in both fetal and adult hemoglobins, α thalassemia manifests in both fetal and adult lives. In Punjab, 12% of the population has α^+ thalassemia. α^0 thalassemia alleles are rare in India.

There are three main clinical forms of α thalassemias—Hemoglobin Bart's hydrops fetalis syndrome, hemoglobin H disease, and α thalassemia carrier state.

Hemoglobin Bart's Hydrops Fetalis Syndrome

This is the most severe form of α thalassemia and results from homozygous state for α^0 thalassemia (- -/- -). Since α^0 thalassemia alleles are prevalent in South East Asia and in eastern Mediterranean countries (Italy, Greece, Cyprus), hydrops fetalis is common in these regions.

Absolute deficiency of α chains in fetal life leads to excess of γ chains that form tetramers (γ_4) or Hb Bart's in fetal red cells. Tetramers of γ chains are more stable than aggregates of α chains in β thalassemia and therefore, ineffective erythropoiesis is less marked in α thalassemia. Red cell destruction in spleen and reduced hemoglobin synthesis contribute to anemia. Hb Bart's is a high oxygen affinity hemoglobin and causes severe tissue hypoxia.

Infants with this disease are either stillborn or die soon after birth. They are severely anemic, and have massive anasarca and hepatosplenomegaly.

The blood film shows severe anisopoikilocytosis, microcytosis, and erythroblastosis. Hemoglobin level is 5 to 8 g/dL. Large amount of Hb Bart's (approximately 80%) is present in cord blood. Both HbA and HbF are absent since no α chains are synthesized. Globin chain synthesis studies demonstrate complete absence of α chain synthesis (α/β ratio of 0). Both the parents are obligatory carriers of a^0 thalassemia.

Hemoglobin H Disease

HbH disease most commonly develops when both α^0 and α^+ thalassemias are inherited (- -/-α), i.e. there is deletion of three α genes.

Due to marked deficiency of α chain synthesis, tetramers of β chains (β_4) are formed (HbH). They are more stable and more soluble than tetramers of α chains found in β thalassemia; ineffective erythropoiesis is therefore not a significant factor in the genesis of anemia. β chain tetramers precipitate in older red cells and form red cell inclusions; these red cells are destroyed in spleen. HbH is high oxygen affinity hemoglobin and does not readily deliver oxygen to the tissues thus contributing to tissue hypoxia.

These patients have anemia (hemoglobin 7–10 g/dL), icterus, and hepatosplenomegaly. Transfusions are usually not needed. Blood film shows anisopoikilocytosis, hypochromia, microcytes, and target cells. When blood is incubated with an oxidizing dye such as brilliant cresyl blue, inclusion bodies are formed due to precipitation of HbH. If spleen has been removed, preformed HbH inclusions can be shown with methyl violet.

Cord blood of the newborns shows 10 to 40% of Hb Bart's that is slowly replaced by HbH during infancy. In adults, HbH ranges between 5 and 40%. Both Hb Bart's and HbH are fast-migrating hemoglobins at alkaline pH (i.e. they move more rapidly than HbA). Globin chain synthesis studies show α/β ratio of 0.2 to 0.4.

Family study shows that one parent has α^0 thalassemia trait (- -/$\alpha\alpha$), and the other has α^+ thalassemia trait (-$\alpha/\alpha\alpha$).

α Thalassemia Carrier States

These are asymptomatic forms of α thalassemias. They are of two main forms: α^0 thalassemia trait (- -/$\alpha\alpha$) and α^+ thalassemia trait (-$\alpha/\alpha\alpha$).

α^0 thalassemia trait (- -/$\alpha\alpha$): This results from interaction of α^0 thalassemia (- -) with normal haplotype ($\alpha\alpha$). Thus, there is deletion of two α genes. Since it is asymptomatic, this condition is usually detected during routine hematological studies or during family studies of a person suffering from thalassemia.

Persons with this condition have very mild anemia, microcytic and hypochromic red cells, and decreased MCV and MCH. In adults, hemoglobin electrophoresis is normal (although trace amounts of HbH are present, they are not detectable by electrophoresis). HbH inclusions may be detected in very few red cells after a prolonged and exhaustive search. Globin chain synthesis studies reveal a α/β ratio of approximately 0.7.

A total of 5 to 15% of Hb Bart's can be detected by electrophoresis in newborns; it gradually disappears during the first few months of life. α^0 thalassemia trait may be diagnosed in the newborn period by doing electrophoresis for Hb Bart's.

Diagnosis is difficult in adults and depends on the exclusion of other causes of microcytic and hypochromic red cells such as iron deficiency, anemia of chronic disease, sideroblastic anemia, and β thalassemia minor. Family studies and ethnic origin of the person may be helpful. Definitive diagnosis requires globin chain synthesis studies and genetic analysis. These persons carry the risk of having a severely affected child if they marry another carrier.

α^+ thalassemia trait (-$\alpha/\alpha\alpha$): This results from interaction of α^+ thalassemia (-α) with normal haplotype ($\alpha\alpha$). Thus there is deletion of one α gene.

Red cell morphology and indices are normal or there may be a slight decrease in MCV or MCH. HbH is not detectable in adults. Globin chain synthesis studies reveal a slight reduction in α/β chain ratio (0.8) which is difficult to interpret in an individual patient.

In some newborns 1 to 2% of Hb Bart's may be detected while in others it is absent. Thus, it is difficult to diagnose α^+ thalassemia trait in both newborns and adults and the only definitive way is globin gene analysis that will reveal deletion of one α globin gene.

Salient features of α thalassemias are summarized in Table 4.4.

Two unusual forms of α thalassemia are (1) α thalassemia with mental retardation syndromes, and (2) α thalassemia associated with myelodysplastic syndrome.

α thalassemia with mental retardation syndromes: Two syndromes with α thalassemia and mental retardation are recognized: (1) ATR-X syndrome: This is characterized by Hb H disease along with severe mental retardation and a characteristic dysmorphic facial appearance. It results from mutations of a gene on X chromosome. (2) ATR-16 syndrome: In this condition, entire α-globin gene cluster along with adjacent DNA in chromosome 16 is deleted. There are various facial and skeletal abnormalities and mild mental retardation.

α thalassemia associated with myelodysplastic syndrome: Elderly patients with myelodysplastic syndrome rarely develop Hb H disease in the form of severe microcytic hypochromic anemia, anisopoikilocytosis, Hb H inclusions in red cells, and detectable Hb H on electrophoresis or HPLC.

Table 4.4: Typical clinical and laboratory features in α thalassemias.

Type	Genotype	Anemia	Red cell changes	Hb electrophoresis Newborn	Hb electrophoresis Adult	Clinical features
1. Silent carrier	αα/α-	Absent	None	1–2% Hb Bart's	Normal	Asymptomatic
2. α thalassemia trait	α-/α-, αα/--	Absent or mild	Microcytic hypochromic	5–15% Hb Bart's	Normal	Usually asymptomatic
3. HbH disease	α-/--	Moderate	Microcytosis, target cells	20–40% Hb Bart's	HbH	Moderate anemia, hepatosplenomegaly
4. hydrops fetalis	--/--	Severe	Numerous erythroblasts	80–100% Hb Bart's	–	Fatal; death in utero or after birth

Thalassemia Intermedia

Thalassemia intermedia is a disorder the clinical expression of which is intermediate between thalassemia major and thalassemia minor. These patients do not require transfusions or require them only intermittently.

Thalassemia intermedia presents in the later age (i.e. 2–5 years) as compared to thalassemia major. (The age of presentation of thalassemia major is around 6 months.) These patients have chronic hemolytic anemia, splenomegaly, and bone changes; growth and development is usually normal and survival into adulthood is common. Hemoglobin level is in the range of 6 to 9 g/dL. Peripheral blood examination shows thalassemic red cell changes: anisopoikilocytosis, microcytosis, hypochromia, target cells, basophilic stippling, and nucleated red cells. Pattern of hemoglobin electrophoresis depends on underlying genotype.

Thalassemia intermedia is genetically diverse. It can be produced by many different molecular lesions:
1. Inheritance of mild β⁺thalassemia in homozygous state (β⁺/β⁺);
2. Homozygous state for δβ thalassemia (δβ/δβ): δβ thalassemias are characterized by increased synthesis of HbF and therefore homozygous state is milder than β thalassemia major;
3. Inheritance of both β thalassemia and δβ thalassemia;
4. Coinheritance of α and β thalassemias. This causes decrease in the globin chain imbalance;
5. Dominant β⁺ thalassemia trait

Prevention of Thalassemias

Thalassemias constitute a significant public health problem in some countries. In India, the mean prevalence of β thalassemia gene is reported to be 3.3% with a much higher frequency in certain communities. Thousands of thalassemic children are born every year in India. The ideal therapy of thalassemia major consists of regular blood transfusion therapy every 3 to 4 weeks and iron chelation therapy. The cost of such treatment is exorbitant (about Rs. 100,000/- per annum in India) and imposes a considerable strain on economic resources in those countries where thalassemias are widely prevalent. Therefore, prevention of thalassemia should receive high priority.

Various Strategies for Prevention of Thalassemias

1. **Health education:** Education of the people through mass media of communications can create awareness of the disease, its economic load, and desirability of prevention by identifying carriers.
2. **Carrier screening and genetic counseling:** Screening involves identification of heterozygous individuals by some simple tests. Heterozygous persons should not marry another heterozygote for the same gene due to the risk of having affected children. In genetic counseling couples at risk (i.e. when both partners are genetic carriers) are explained various options available such as prenatal diagnosis followed by selective termination of pregnancy and alternative methods of having a child such as artificial insemination, adoption, etc.
3. **Prenatal diagnosis:** Prenatal diagnosis of affected fetus and selective termination of pregnancy is now available at some places. Prenatal diagnosis is carried out in couples who are already having an affected child (retrospective diagnosis) or in couples who are identified as carriers by screening (prospective diagnosis).

Carrier Screening

Screening in thalassemia consists of detection of genetic carriers or heterozygotes by some rapidly applied tests. Screening is done to identify individuals with β thalassemia minor, α^0 thalassemia trait, dβ thalassemia trait, or heterozygous state for abnormal hemoglobins such as Hb Lepore or HbS. For the screening program for the detection of heterozygotes to be successful, following prerequisites should be fulfilled: (i) prevalence of the carrier state should be high in a particular population group; (ii) the screening tests which are employed should be suitable for mass screening; and (iii) facility of genetic counseling and prenatal diagnosis should be available. Heterozygous screening programs have brought about a remarkable decrease in the incidence of thalassemia in some Mediterranean countries (Cyprus and Sardinia).

Screening for the carrier state may be conducted in specific caste groups located in particular geographical areas. Those caste groups that are showing a significant prevalence of a hemoglobinopathy should be identified; this information is also obtained from previous public health surveys. Carrier screening can be done during pregnancy in antenatal clinics, after engagement of couples, or during adolescence. One widely used approach is to screen couples just before marriage or before pregnancy. If one partner is found to be a carrier for abnormal gene, then the other partner should be screened. If both are carriers then prenatal diagnosis should be considered to prevent the birth of a thalassemic child (refer to Fig. 4.37). Screening of pregnant women should be done in first trimester of pregnancy so that prenatal diagnosis by chorionic villus sampling can be offered earlier in pregnancy if required. Limited resources pose an important constraint on large-scale screening program in India.

Commonly employed methods for screening include the following (Fig. 4.30):

Red cell indices: Determination of red cell indices (MCV, MCH) by electronic counters is a reliable method for assessing microcytosis and hypochromia, a characteristic feature of thalassemia traits. In these conditions, MCV is less than 76 fl and MCH is less than 27 pg. In α^+ thalassemia trait, red cell indices may be within normal range.

Single tube OF test: This test can be performed in small routine-work laboratories, where automated hematology analyzer is not available. It is based on the principle that red cells in thalassemia are more resistant to osmotic hemolysis than normal red cells. Since the usual

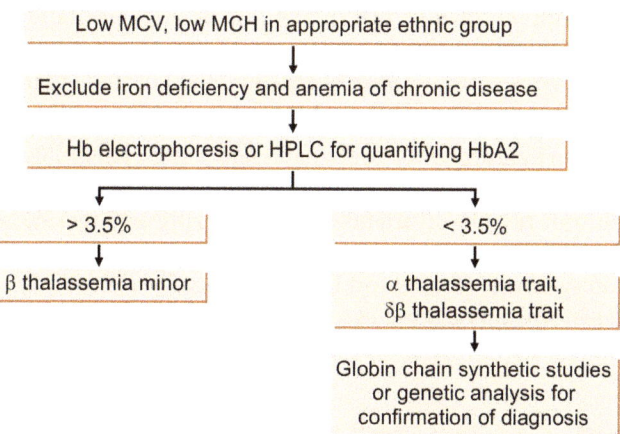

Fig. 4.30: Algorithm for identification of thalassemia carrier state.

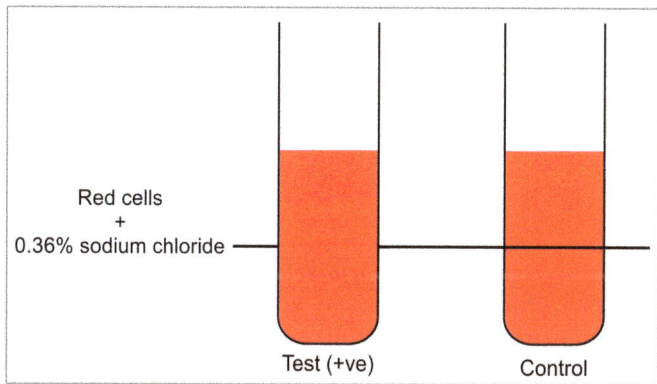

Fig. 4.31: Single tube osmotic fragility test. Normal red cells undergo lysis when suspended in 0.36% sodium chloride and the solution becomes clear (line of reader scale visible), while microcytic hypochromic red cells in thalassemia are resistant to osmotic lysis and solution is turbid (line of reader scale is not visible).

multiple tube osmotic fragility test is cumbersome, single tube OF test has been devised. In this test, red cells are suspended in 0.36% buffered saline and hemolysis is looked for either visually (Fig. 4.31) or in a spectrophotometer. This test, however, is not specific for β thalassemia since positive test is also seen in iron deficiency anemia, sickle-cell trait, and α^0 thalassemia trait. Another measure of resistance to osmotic lysis is **glycerol lysis time** test. This test measures rate of hemolysis of red cells suspended in a solution of glycerol and the result is expressed as the length of time required for 50% lysis. Patients with β thalassemia trait have increased values.

Estimation of HbA2: If red cell indices show reduced MCH and MCV, and if iron deficiency is ruled out, then quantitation of HbA_2 should be carried out. In β thalassemia trait HbA2 is characteristically raised (3.5–7%). If iron deficiency complicates β thalassemia trait, then HbA2 quantitation should be repeated after correction of iron deficiency.

HbA2 level is normal in α thalassemia trait, a specific type of β thalassemia known as "normal HbA2 β thalassemia," δβ thalassemia trait, and Hb Lepore trait. In such cases diagnosis may be suspected when MCV and MCH are reduced and iron status is normal. Definitive diagnosis of carrier state in α thalassemia trait needs globin chain synthesis studies and DNA analysis.

Hemoglobin electrophoresis at alkaline pH: This should be done in all individuals suspected of having thalassemia trait. This identifies any abnormal hemoglobin present such as HbS, C, D, E, or Lepore, and also assesses HbF. Further characterization of some hemoglobin variants can be made by citrate agar electrophoresis at acid pH.

Other tests: HbF, raised in heterozygotes of δβ thalassemia and of hereditary persistence of fetal hemoglobin (HPFH), can be quantitated by alkali denaturation test and its cellular distribution assessed by acid elution test. In δβ thalassemia trait, HbF is 5 to 15% with heterocellular distribution, while in HPFH HbF is 15 to 25% with pancellular distribution. Definitive diagnosis requires globin chain synthesis studies and DNA analysis.

Test for HbH inclusions can be done in α thalassemia trait.

Prenatal Diagnosis

The hemoglobinopathies are the most common genetic disorders in humans and constitute a major public health problem in many countries. Prenatal diagnosis is a cost-effective and sensible approach for their prevention.

Prenatal diagnosis is contemplated when both the prospective parents are identified as thalassemia carriers. It is done to prevent birth of a child with β thalassemia major or Hb Bart's hydrops fetalis syndrome.

There are two major techniques for prenatal diagnosis of thalassemias:
1. **Globin chain synthesis studies (during second trimester of pregnancy** on fetal blood obtained by cordocentesis); and
2. **Fetal DNA analysis (during first trimester of pregnancy** on cells obtained from amniocentesis or chorionic villus biopsy).
1. *Measurement of globin chain synthesis in fetal blood:* This test is done in second trimester of pregnancy because fetal blood can reliably be obtained only after 18 weeks of pregnancy. Fetal blood is aspirated from umbilical cord under ultrasound guidance (cordocentesis). The procedure is as follows:
    i. Fetal blood sample (reticulocyte-enriched fraction) is incubated with radioactive amino acid (^{3}H leucine) which is incorporated in globin chains during *in vitro* globin synthesis.
    ii. Different types of globin chains are separated on CM-cellulose chromatography.
    iii. Amount of radioactivity incorporated in globin chains is measured in a liquid scintillation counter to assess the rate of synthesis of α, β, and γ chains. Whether the fetus is having thalassemia major or minor is decided on the basis of ratio of β chains to γ and α chains.

    As fetal blood sampling can be carried out only after 18 weeks of gestation, there is a prolonged indecisive period and pregnancy termination, if required, is difficult. The risk of procedure-related fetal loss is 3 to 4%.

    This technique is usually reserved for those cases in which DNA diagnosis is not possible, i.e. if nature of genetic defect is not known and linkage analysis cannot be done.

Analysis of fetal DNA: Prenatal diagnosis of hemoglobin disorders is most commonly done by fetal DNA analysis. Fetal DNA can be obtained either by amniocentesis or by chorion villus biopsy. In amniocentesis, 20 to 30 mL of amniotic fluid is aspirated at 14 to 20 weeks of gestation and DNA is extracted from amniotic fluid cells after culture. Risk of fetal loss with amniocentesis is 0.5%. Chorion villus biopsy consists of obtaining a small piece of developing placenta under ultrasound guidance at 8 to 12 weeks of gestation. Transcervical route is commonly used to obtain biopsy and with this approach risk of fetal loss is not significantly increased as compared to amniocentesis. Studies on amniotic fluid cells need to be performed relatively late in pregnancy (second trimester). Chorionic villus biopsy can be obtained at 8 to 12 weeks of gestation (first trimester) and it has become the procedure of choice for obtaining fetal cells for DNA analysis.

The nature of the molecular lesion first needs to be determined in both the members of the couple and in other closely related family members. For this, it is necessary to know the ethnic origin of the couple at risk, as only a few specific mutations are prevalent in a particular community.

Method of DNA analysis for prenatal diagnosis in a given case depends on whether mutation remains known or unknown after family studies (both partners and affected child)—

1. *For known mutations:*
   - Amplification refractory mutation system (ARMS)
   - Dot blot using ASO probes
   - Reverse dot blot hybridization
   - Direct electrophoresis for 619 bp deletion
   - Restriction enzyme analysis of PCR product
2. *For unknown mutations:*
   - Denaturation gradient gel electrophoresis
   - Restriction fragment length polymorphism (RFLP)
   - Direct sequencing of amplified DNA
   - Southern blotting for deletions using specific gene probes.

Techniques of DNA Analysis

For known mutations:

1. *Methods employing DNA amplification:* Polymerase chain reaction (PCR) technology that was introduced in 1985 by Saiki and others has had a remarkable impact on the molecular diagnosis of genetic diseases. PCR can amplify the DNA fragment of interest several million times in a short period. With this technique a specific portion of the patient's DNA can be identified in a few hours even from a very small sample. In PCR, a short segment of DNA (target DNA) is amplified with the help of two primers and a thermostable DNA polymerase. The primers are two short oligonucleotides that hybridize to the sites flanking the region to be amplified. The DNA polymerase is the thermostable Taq polymerase that synthesizes the complementary DNA sequence.

   Each cycle of PCR consists of three steps that are performed at different temperatures (Fig. 4.32):
   a. *Denaturation:* In this step, double-stranded DNA is converted to single-stranded DNA by heating at 94 to 96°C. Heating destroys chemical bonds between base pairs.
   b. *Annealing:* Temperature is lowered to 50 to 55°C and synthetic primers are allowed to bind to complementary sites flanking the region of interest.
   c. *Extension:* The temperature is raised to 72°C. In this step, a thermostable DNA polymerase (Taq polymerase) makes a DNA strand complementary to the DNA that is flanked by the primers. Extension occurs by addition of deoxynucleotides and a copy of the target DNA sequence is made.

Above three steps comprise one cycle and the process is repeated for 25 to 35 cycles. This results in exponential amplification of the target DNA sequence. Amplified DNA is utilized in various methods for diagnosis of genetic defects. These include restriction

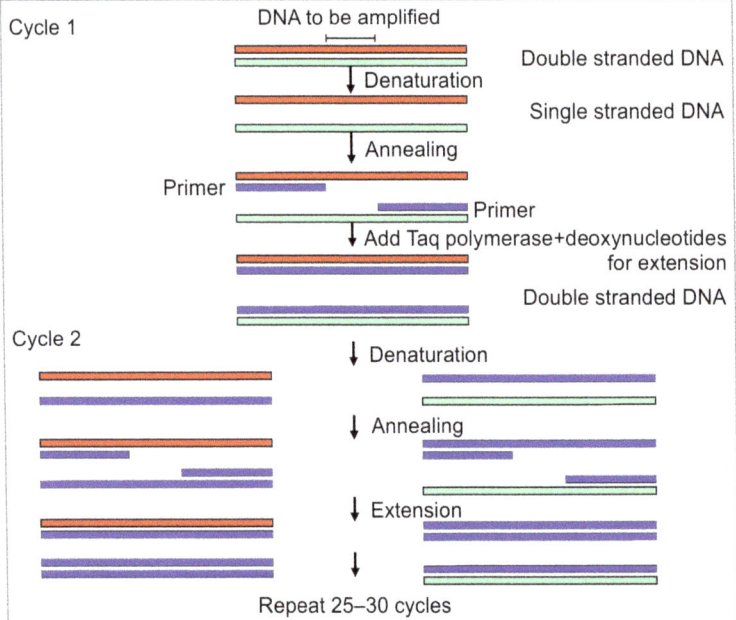

Fig. 4.32: Polymerase chain reaction.

enzyme digestion followed by gel electrophoresis, dot-blot analysis using allele-specific oligonucleotide probes, reverse dot hybridization, and amplification refractory mutation system.

i. *Restriction enzyme digestion and gel electrophoresis:* This method is used when a mutation affects a restriction site for endonuclease enzyme. DNA sequence of interest is amplified by PCR, cleaved with a restriction enzyme, electrophoresed on agarose gel to separate the fragments according to size, stained with ethidium bromide, and observed under ultraviolet light. When a mutation is present, a fragment of a different size is obtained. An example where this approach is used is detection of codon 39 nonsense mutation (CAG→TAG) by *Mae* I restriction analysis. If this mutation is present, then it creates a restriction site and thus a fragment of smaller size is obtained.

ii. *Dot blot analysis with allele-specific oligonucleotide probe:* Many mutations can be detected by this method. Genomic DNA of interest is amplified by PCR, denatured, and applied (dot blotted) on two nylon membranes. Two oligonucleotide probes (each 18–20 bases long), out of which one is complementary to the normal DNA and the other to the abnormal or mutant DNA, are tagged with the radioisotope. After hybridization of one nylon membrane with normal probe and of other with mutant probe, genotype of a person (normal, heterozygous, or homozygous) can be determined (Fig. 4.33). Oligonucleotide probe can be labeled with horse radish peroxidase (instead of radioactive material) that produces a color change after hybridization.

iii. *Reverse dot hybridization:* This is another PCR-based technique for detection of known genetic mutations. In this method, an oligonucleotide probe complimentary to the mutant sequence is fixed onto a nylon membrane while amplified genomic DNA to be tested is hybridized to the membrane. The primers used for amplification of genomic DNA are biotinylated. Therefore, presence of biotin in dots on the membrane indicates hybridization of genomic DNA with mutant oligonucleotide probe.

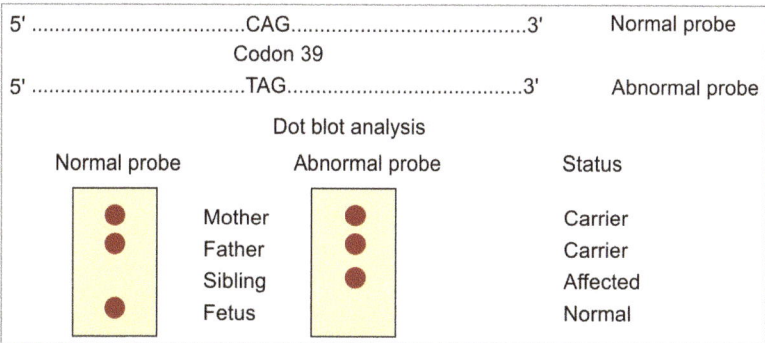

Fig. 4.33: Dot blot analysis showing identification of β⁰ 39 mutation C→T by radio labeled oligonucleotide probes in a family for prenatal diagnosis. The normal probe consists of normal nucleotide sequence (18–20 bases long) with normal codon CAG at position 39 of β globin gene. The abnormal probe has mutant nucleotide sequence TAG at position 39. The substitution C→T at position 39 causes formation of a chain terminator codon and leads to β⁰ thalassemia. Lower part of the figure shows nylon membrane with blotted amplified DNA that is hybridized with normal and abnormal radio labeled probes.

    iv. *Amplification refractory mutation system (ARMS):* This technique, based on PCR technology, makes use of two allele specific oligonucleotide primers one of which is complimentary to normal DNA and the other to the mutant DNA sequence. Annealing and subsequent DNA amplification will occur only when nucleotide sequence of primer is identical to that of genomic DNA. A normal primer will not anneal to mutant DNA sequence and thus extension of primer and DNA amplification will not occur. When mutant primer is used, amplification will occur only in the presence of corresponding mutation in genomic DNA. Gel electrophoresis followed by ethidium bromide staining is used for visualization of amplified DNA.
2. *Direct detection of genetic defect:* Two methods are available: Southern blot and oligonucleotide probe.
    i. *Southern blot analysis:* Large gene deletions can be directly detected by Southern blot analysis. This is applicable to most cases of α thalassemias and a few cases of β thalassemias such as Indian 619 bp deletion. Mutations that alter the recognition site for restriction enzymes can also be detected by this method.
    Principle: DNA is isolated from cells (amniotic or chorionic villus) and is separated into fragments by one or more restriction enzymes. Restriction enzymes are derived from bacteria and recognize a specific sequence of base pairs in DNA and cleave the DNA molecule at sites where this sequence is encountered. Multiple fragments of DNA of varying sizes are formed which migrate according to size when electrophoresed (smaller fragments move more rapidly than the larger ones). These double-stranded DNA fragments are then denatured with a strong base into single strands and then blotted onto nitrocellulose membranes. To identify the fragment of interest, a radioactive complementary DNA probe is then hybridized to the nitrocellulose or nylon membrane. (A probe is a radio labeled DNA sequence used to detect the presence of a complimentary nucleotide sequence in an unknown DNA fragment by molecular hybridization.) The labeled probe and the membrane are then incubated together under conditions that favor the formation of double-stranded DNA molecules. Hybridization will occur if the probe finds a sequence complementary to the DNA to bind on the

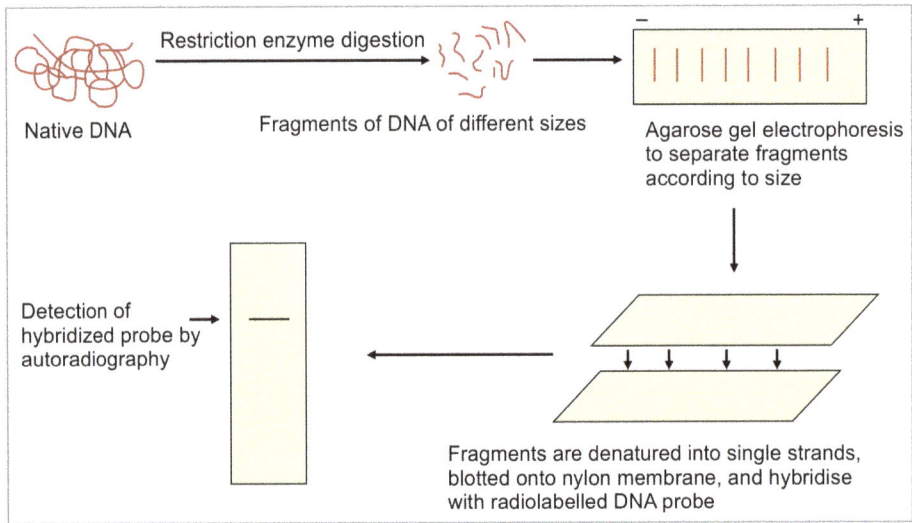

Fig. 4.34: Principle of Southern blot analysis.

nitrocellulose membrane. Since the probe is radioactive, position of the hybridized band can be identified by exposing the membrane to X-ray film (autoradiography) (Fig. 4.34).

This technique was developed by Edwin Southern and hence the name.

This approach is illustrated in prenatal diagnosis of sickle-cell anemia (see Fig. 4.42).

ii. *Oligonucleotide probe analysis:* Majority of point mutations do not change the recognition sequence of restriction enzymes. Here allele-specific oligonucleotide probes may be utilized for direct detection of abnormal genes. The principle of this technique is summarized below:
   a. Two oligonucleotide probes (having 18–20 bases), one normal and another abnormal (mutant), are prepared and are radiolabeled. These probes differ from one another by a single base.
   b. Fetal DNA is subjected to digestion by a restriction enzyme. Agarose gel electrophoresis is carried out to separate the fragments. This separation can be carried out on two agarose gels (one for each probe). Hybridization is carried out with normal and abnormal oligonucleotide probes on the respective, identically run gels. This is followed by autoradiography. Under appropriate conditions, these probes hybridize only to complementary (i.e. perfectly matched) sequences in the DNA. The normal probe will hybridize to normal sequence while the abnormal probe will hybridize to mutant sequence. This approach is illustrated in Figure 4.35.

For unknown mutations:
1. *Restriction fragment length polymorphism (RFLP) analysis:* DNA sequence variations which alter cutting site of a restriction enzyme occur frequently in populations and restriction enzyme pattern of all individuals is not alike. These variations that affect restriction sites and produce fragments of different size after digestion of DNA are known as restriction fragment length polymorphisms (RFLPs). The polymorphic sites can be used as "markers" for genetic diseases if they are closely linked to an abnormal gene and cosegregate in affected families (Fig. 4.36).

Chapter 4: Anemias due to Excessive Red Cell Destruction

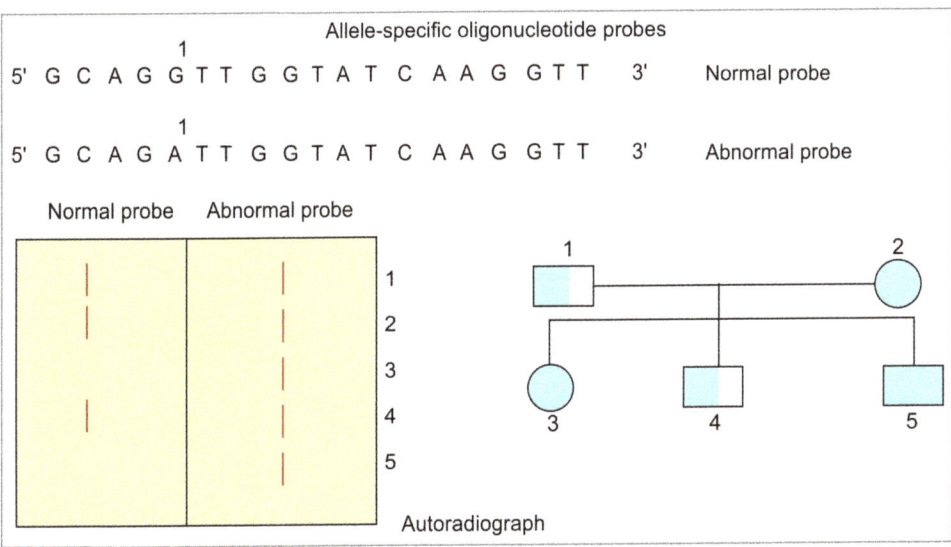

Fig. 4.35: Oligonucleotide probe analysis: Upper part of the figure shows two oligonucleotide probes. The normal probe represents the sequence near the intron 1 of the normal β globin gene. The abnormal probe represents the point mutation G→A at position 1 of the intron 1 (IVS-1 nt1 G→A). This mutation alters the splice junction and causes β⁰ thalassemia. Lower part of the figure shows autoradiogram of gels used for diagnosis of above mutation in a family. Both normal and abnormal probes are yielding positive signals with DNAs of father (1), mother (2), and child (4) and therefore, they are heterozygous for this mutation. DNA from one child (3) is homozygous for the mutation since it is showing hybridization only with the abnormal probe. DNA from the fetus (5) is also homozygous for the mutation and termination of pregnancy is advisable.

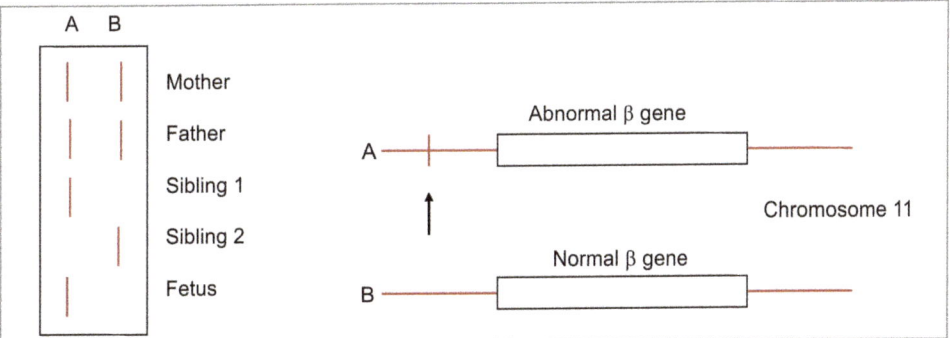

Fig. 4.36: Detection of restriction fragment length polymorphism by Southern blot analysis. Right part of the figure shows two β gene alleles. In the allele A, specific site for restriction enzyme is present (arrow) while in the allele B it is absent. Therefore on Southern blot analysis, the restriction enzyme produces two short fragments in allele A, while the fragment is longer in allele B. In this example (left part of figure), both parents are heterozygous for this polymorphism (AB) and are carriers of β thalassemia gene. Sibling 1 and fetus are homozygous for abnormal β gene (AA) and are affected, while sibling 2 is normal (BB).

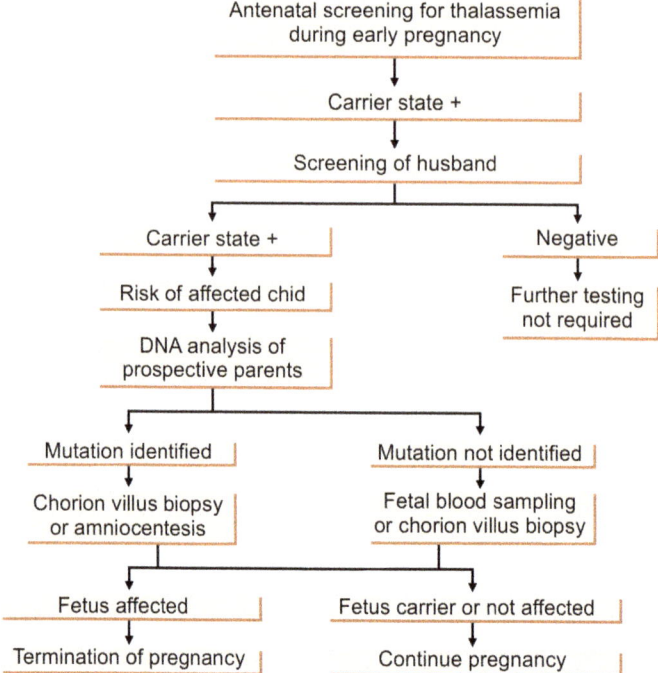

Fig. 4.37: Approach to prenatal diagnosis of thalassemia.

Linkage of the polymorphism to the abnormal gene should be established by studying close family members before attempting prenatal diagnosis. Both the mother and the father should be heterozygous for the polymorphism (i.e. each chromosome should show a different restriction enzyme pattern). The polymorphic site should be closely linked to the abnormal gene so that they are transmitted together during meiosis. If the linkage is not close then the crossing over of chromosomal material between homologous chromosomes during meiosis may "separate" the polymorphic site from the abnormal gene; this will lead to a false negative result in the fetus. General approach to prenatal diagnosis of thalassemia is outlined in Figure 4.37.

Principles of Therapy in Thalassemias

Regular red cell transfusions and chelation therapy for iron overload are the cornerstones of therapy for β thalassemia major. If faithfully followed this treatment allows the thalassemia patients to lead a near-normal life.

β thalassemia major poses a major psychological, financial, and social burden on patients and their families. For them, long-term support is best provided by centers having the necessary expertise in managing these disorders. Societies have been formed by the parents of the affected children that provide guidance and help to newly diagnosed patients.

Blood transfusion: Before the availability of transfusions, patients with β thalassemia major invariably used to die from severe anemia and congestive cardiac failure before 2 years of age. Initially, transfusions were given to thalassemic patients only when their anemia became severely symptomatic. With this "on demand transfusion" therapy, although patients could live up to 15–20 years of age, they remained incapacitated and suffered from complications of chronic anemia and excessive erythroid hyperplasia in bone marrow such as skeletal and facial deformities and hepatosplenomegaly.

"Hypertransfusion program" was then formulated which consisted of regular transfusion therapy so as to maintain the hemoglobin concentration constantly above 9.5 to 10.0 g/dL. This form of therapy radically improved the quality of life of thalassemic patients and is now widely followed. The aim of this therapy is to prevent anemia and hypoxia and to suppress endogenous erythropoiesis. If started early in life hypertransfusion program promotes normal growth and development up to adolescence, prevents disfiguring skeletal deformities as excessive erythropoiesis and consequent marrow expansion are suppressed, limits hepatosplenomegaly by reducing extramedullary hematopoiesis, reduces cardiomegaly by reducing cardiac work, and reduces intestinal iron absorption as endogenous erythropoiesis is suppressed.

Blood transfusion therapy is begun around 6 months of age. Packed red cells should be given. Freshly obtained red cells are preferred to limit *the iron burden* (as each milliliter of red cells contains 1 mg of iron, only viable red cells should be transfused). Patients are transfused with 11 to 14 mL of red cells per kg every 3 to 4 weeks.

Since these patients are totally dependent on chronic blood transfusion therapy, every effort should be made to minimize transfusion-related complications. Saline-washed red cells can be used to avoid sensitization to plasma antigens and leukocyte antigens; leukocyte reduction filters reduce alloimmunization to leukocyte antigens; and the risk of transfusion-transmitted infections is substantially reduced by screening blood for human immunodeficiency virus, hepatitis B and C viruses, and syphilis. Hepatitis B vaccine should be administered to all newly identified patients. Extended red cell typing (atleast for Rh, Duffy, Kidd, and Kell antigens) is performed for all transfusions to prevent alloimmunization.

Currently, it is recommended to maintain a mean hemoglobin level of 12.0 g/dL, with pretransfusion hemoglobin of 9.5 to 10.0 g/dL.

Iron chelation therapy: Iron overload is the major cause of morbidity and death in β thalassemia major. Ineffective erythropoiesis causes increased iron absorption; this is the major factor causing iron overload in undertransfused patients. In regularly transfused patients, main cause of iron burden is repeated blood transfusions.

Iron overload causes damage to parenchymal cells of various organs particularly liver (cirrhosis), endocrine glands (diabetes mellitus, delayed sexual maturation, infertility, hypothyroidism, hypoparathyroidism), and heart (cardiac arrhythmias, congestive cardiac failure).

Iron chelation therapy is usually started at the age of 3 years. The drug employed for the treatment of iron overload is desferrioxamine (DF), an iron chelator that is given along with vitamin C to promote iron excretion. It is preferably administered by infusion pump 25 to 60 mg/kg body weight subcutaneously daily for 12 hours for 5 to 6 days a week. Problems associated with DF therapy include high cost, cumbersome mode of administration, noncompliance, and adverse reactions such as convulsions, coma, cataracts, retinal damage, deafness, impairment of growth, and infections by Yersinia.

Due to high cost and difficulties of administration of DF, oral iron-chelating drug is needed. Deferiprone (1,2-dimethyl-3-hydroxy-pyridin-4-one or L1) appears to be promising and is being extensively used in India. Major side effects are agranulocytosis, arthropathy, and

Table 4.5: Properties of iron-chelating drugs used in thalassemia.

Parameter	Desferrioxamine	Deferiprone	Deferasirox
1. Molecular weight	657 Da	139 Da	373 Da
2. Iron:chelator binding ratio	1:1	1:3	1:2
3. Plasma half-life	20–30 minutes	1.5–3.5 hours	12–18 hours
4. Route of administration	Parenteral (SC/IV)	Oral	Oral
5. Daily dose	25–50 mg/kg 5 days a week	75 mg/kg three times daily	20–30 mg/kg once daily
6. Route of iron excretion	Urine and feces	Urine	Feces
7. Side effects	Impaired vision or hearing, growth retardation	Gastrointestinal upset, arthralgia, agranulocytosis	Gastrointestinal upset, rashes, raised serum creatinine

possible hepatic fibrosis. Another oral iron-chelating drug is deferasirox (DFX). Comparison of three main iron-chelating drugs in the management of thalassemia is presented in Table 4.5.

Assessment of body iron load: Methods for assessing body iron burden are:
1. Serum ferritin: This test is widely available, relatively inexpensive, and repeated measurements are possible. However, serum ferritin is elevated during inflammation, infection, and deficiency of ascorbate. Correlation with total body iron is imprecise.
2. Liver biopsy for quantitation of iron: This is considered as the gold standard as it correlates well with body iron stores. Simultaneous assessment of liver histology (fibrosis, inflammation) is possible. Needle biopsy sample of 1 mg dry weight is adequate for assessment of iron load by atomic absorption spectrometry. The test is invasive with risk of intra-abdominal bleeding. More than 15 mg/g dry weight is associated with high risk of cardiac disease. However, cardiac disease may be present even if liver iron is low.
3. Magnetic resonance imaging (MRI): MRI is gaining popularity for assessment of liver and cardiac iron. The test is noninvasive and correlates well with liver iron and risk of cardiac disease. Currently the method of choice for assessment of iron load is estimation of cardiac iron using T2* MRI technique.
4. Superconducting quantum interference device (SQUID) for liver iron load: This test is very expensive and has very limited availability.

Iron chelation therapy and techniques for monitoring iron burden are expensive and majority of patients with thalassemia major are unable to afford them. In India, only about 5 to 10% of children born with thalassemia receive optimal treatment.

Splenectomy: Indication for splenectomy is transfusion requirement exceeding 180 to 200 mL of packed red cells/kg/year. Due to the risk of sepsis, splenectomy should be avoided before 5 to 6 years of age. Postsplenectomy, pneumococcal, *H. influenzae*, and meningococcal vaccines and penicillin prophylaxis are necessary.

General measures: These include folic acid supplementation, early treatment of intercurrent infections, hormone replacement therapy in endocrine failure, and treatment of cardiac failure. Patients with HbH disease should refrain from antioxidant drugs.

Hematopoietic stem cell transplantation: Regular transfusions and iron chelation therapy have improved the quality of life in thalassemia. Although bone marrow transplantation is associated with significant morbidity and mortality, it is the only form of therapy that can cure the disease. The decision to transplant bone marrow should be based on assessment of risks and benefits in an individual patient. Results are best if hematopoietic stem cell transplantation is carried out in young patients who have not yet developed complications of disease or of treatment.

Experimental forms of therapy: These include:
- Enhancement of HbF production—Currently, hydroxyurea and butyrate are being tried to increase HbF production that will improve hemoglobin level and reduce ineffective erythropoiesis.
- Gene therapy—This consists of introduction of normal gene in stem cells to replace the abnormal gene. Research is in progress for gene therapy.

SICKLE-CELL DISORDERS

Sickle-cell disorders are those conditions in which the red cells become sickle-shaped when they are subjected to low oxygen tension. James Herrick from Chicago first described a case of sickle-cell disease in 1910 in a young black student. Sickle-cell disorders include following conditions:

1. **Sickle-cell diseases (SCD):** Sickled cells are responsible for distinctive clinical manifestations. They can be divided into following types:
    i. *Sickle-cell anemia (SCA):* This is the homozygous state for hemoglobin S (HbSS) that results when the sickle-cell gene (β^S) is inherited from both parents. The genotype is $\beta^S\beta^S$.
    ii. *Sickle-cell β thalassemia:* This is the double heterozygous state in which the sickle-cell gene is inherited from one parent and β thalassemia gene from the other parent. It is divided into two types: Sickle-cell β^0 thalassemia (genotype $\beta^S\beta^0$) in which normal β chain synthesis is completely lacking, and sickle-cell β^+ thalassemia (genotype $\beta^S\beta^+$) in which normal β chain synthesis is partially deficient.
    iii. Combination of hemoglobin S (HbS) with other structural hemoglobin variants can produce a double heterozygous state such as HbSD disease, HbSC disease, HbSO-Arab disease, Hb SE disease, etc.
2. **Sickle-cell trait:** This is the heterozygous carrier state for HbS (HbAS) in which sickle-cell gene is inherited from one parent and gene for HbA from the other. The genotype is $\beta^S\beta$.

Sickle-cell Anemia

Sickle-cell anemia is the most severe form of sickle-cell disease and is the homozygous state for hemoglobin S (HbSS).

Prevalence of HbS

Hemoglobin S is particularly frequent in tropical Africa, Middle East, and Central and Southern India. The global incidence is 300,000 to 400,000 per year. Prevalence in equatorial Africa is thought to be 20%. There is high childhood mortality particularly in Africa and India. HbS has a high prevalence in those parts of the world where malaria is common; this relationship is explained by the theory of balanced polymorphism. Young children with sickle-cell trait develop comparatively mild falciparum malaria. Theory of balanced polymorphism proposes that selective advantage gained by sickle-cell heterozygote (i.e. protection against severe falciparum malaria) is balanced by disadvantage of homozygous state (i.e. sickle-cell anemia). Genetic studies suggest that sickle mutation may have arisen independently in different parts of the world and has achieved high frequency due to natural selection.

Five haplotypes of sickle mutation have been identified by polymorphic sites in five regions: Cameroon, Africa (Senegal, Benin, Bantu), and Arab-India. This suggests that sickle mutations have originated independently in five regions. Sickle-cell anemia in India is milder than African form. This is due to increased HbF production and coinheritance of α thalassemia. Alpha thalassemia occurs in >50% of sickle population in India.

The exact mechanism of protective effect in sickle-cell trait is not known. However, it is possible that red cells infected with *P. falciparum* undergo more rapid sickling owing possibly to decreased intracellular pH caused by parasite's chemical reactions and are phagocytosed readily by macrophages of the reticuloendothelial system.

Pathogenesis

The sickle-cell disorders all result from inheritance of sickle-cell gene that codes for abnormal β globin chain. There is change of a single base A→T in the 6th codon of β globin gene so that there is substitution of thymine for adenine. This in turn results in substitution of valine for glutamic acid at position 6 of β polypeptide chain. The amino acid substitution in HbS is represented as β^6 Glu→Val.

Polymerization of HbS: Polymerization of HbS molecules inside the red cells is responsible for sickling of red cells. When examined ultrastructurally, sickled cells show bundles of fibers aligned along the long axis of the cell or of the pointed projections. Each fiber consists of 14 filaments arranged in pairs. Each filament is made of HbS molecules stacked in a helical manner.

Polymerization results only on deoxygenation. It is a time-dependent process. Initially, HbS molecules aggregate to form a polymer of critical size; this is the rate-limiting nucleation phase. Once a critical polymer is formed, aggregation of additional HbS molecules occurs rapidly to form well-aligned fibers. The time between deoxygenation and formation of the polymer of critical size is known as delay time or lag phase. This has significance when sickling and unsickling occurs due to deoxygenation and oxygenation, respectively, in circulation. Oxygenation in the lungs causes rapid dissociation of aggregated HbS molecules, viscous gel turns into fluid state, and the red cell shape becomes normal (if membrane damage has not occurred.) The red cell remains unsickled in the oxygenated arterial blood. When deoxygenation occurs in capillary circulation, most of the red cells do not sickle since reoxygenation occurs in pulmonary circulation before polymer of sufficient size is formed. However, shortening of delay time (e.g. due to low pH, increased HbS concentration, etc.) will lead to sickling in capillary circulation with resultant vaso-occlusion.

Reversibly and irreversibly sickled cells: Initially, sickling of red cells is reversible. The sickle or holly-leaf shape of red cells conforms to the shape of the polymerized hemoglobin. With oxygenation, polymerized HbS (viscous gel state) returns to depolymerized (fluid-liquid) state. When repeated sickling and unsickling of red cells occurs, membrane is damaged and the red cell shape becomes permanently altered leading to the formation of irreversibly sickled cell; even with reoxygenation, shape of the red cell does not return to normal. Thus in sickle-cells disease, two categories of sickle-cells occur—reversibly sickled and irreversibly sickled (Fig. 4.38).

Reversibly sickled cells are those in which polymerization of HbS and red cell shape alteration can revert back to normal. These cells undergo polymerization and shape change

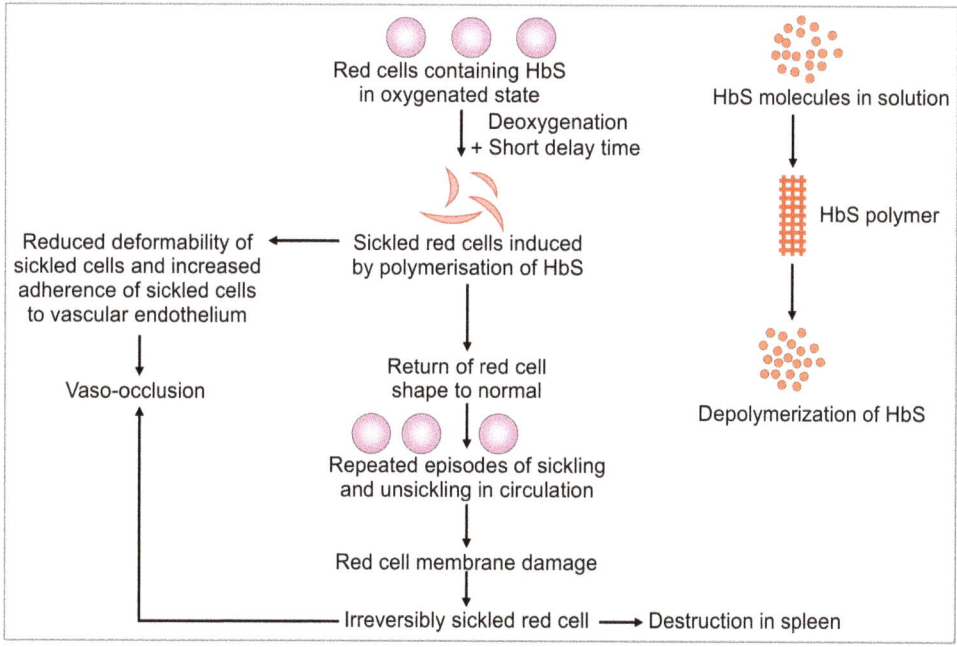

Fig. 4.38: Formation of sickled red cells in circulation.

upon deoxygenation while after reoxygenation in the lungs dissociation of polymers occurs with return of normal cell shape.

In irreversibly sickled cells, red cell shape does not return to normal even after reoxygenation. Although depolymerization occurs upon reoxygenation red cells remain irreversibly sickled. These cells appear on air-dried blood films as elongated cells one or both ends of which are pointed. The membrane of these cells is damaged which precludes the return of cell shape to normal even after reoxygenation and depolymerization of HbS. They have rigid cell membranes and are trapped and destroyed in the spleen. The severity of hemolysis correlates with the number of these cells in circulation.

Factors which influence sickling:
 i. *Intracellular concentration of HbS and of other hemoglobins:* There is a direct relationship between the amount of HbS in the red cell and propensity of red cells to sickle. In sickle-cell trait due to the predominance of HbA in the cell, sickling is prevented unless the oxygen tension is considerably low. In contrast, in red cells of patients with sickle-cell anemia, HbS is the predominant form of hemoglobin (80–90%) and sickling occurs readily.
 HbF does not participate with HbS in sickling process and therefore, infants do not develop manifestations till the time HbF declines to adult values. In Bedouin Arabs of Saudi Arabia and certain tribes of central India, sickle-cell anemia is associated with significant elevation of HbF and a less severe disease. Heterozygotes for HbS and HPFH do not have anemia owing to the high HbF percentage.
 ii. *Association with thalassemias:* In sickle-cell-β^+ thalassemia, due to the presence of HbA the disease is milder. Interaction of α thalassemia with sickle-cell anemia reduces mean corpuscular hemoglobin concentration and hemolysis; however vaso-occlusive crises remain unchanged.

iii. *Interaction with other abnormal hemoglobins:* HbS interacts less readily with HbC or HbD than with other HbS molecules and therefore, persons with HbSC disease or HbSD disease have milder manifestations (as compared to Hb SS disease).
iv. *Coinheritance of hereditary persistence of fetal hemoglobin:* This leads to milder manifestations.
v. *Mean corpuscular hemoglobin concentration (MCHC):* Increased MCHC due to cellular dehydration favors the intermolecular contact between HbS and enhances polymerization. This factor is responsible for sickling of red cells in hyperosmolar milieu of renal medulla.
vi. *Decreased oxygen tension:* The most important determinant affecting sickling is deoxygenation. Amount of hypoxia required to induce sickling depends on the proportion of HbS (HbSS red cells: 40 mm Hg whereas HbAS red cells: 15 mm Hg).
vii. *Temperature:* Cold induces vasoconstriction and increases sickling.
viii. *Low pH:* Decrease in pH (acidosis) increases sickling probably by inducing the deoxy state of hemoglobin.

Polymerization of HbS is promoted in hypoxic, acidotic, and hypertonic environments of spleen and kidney.

Pathogenesis of vaso-occlusion: Following processes contribute to the development of vaso-occlusion in sickle-cell anemia: (1) depletion of nitric oxide by free heme released from hemolysis (leading to alteration in vascular tone, slowing of blood flow, and upregulation of adhesion molecules); (2) adhesion of young deformable red cells to vascular endothelium (promoted by leukocyte activation and inflammatory cytokines released during infection/inflammation); and (3) increased blood viscosity from less deformable red cells and sickled forms.

Clinical Features

Clinical manifestations usually develop around 3 to 4 months of age when the level of HbF falls. Clinical expression of sickle-cell anemia is highly variable. Some patients have a severe disease with early mortality while others experience a near normal life-span with few complications. Main complications are vaso-occlusive crises while anemia itself poses little problem. Anemia of variable degree is present in all patients. It is more severe in SCA and sickle-cell β^0 thalassemia as compared to sickle-cell β^+ thalassemia. Usually, patients adapt well to their anemia. Anemia is aggravated in the presence of folate deficiency, aplastic crisis, and splenic sequestration crisis.

Growth and development: These are considerably impaired in children with sickle-cell anemia.

Splenomegaly: Splenomegaly is present in infants and young children and is caused by reticuloendothelial hyperplasia. In sickle-cell anemia, in later life, spleen becomes small and fibrotic due to repeated splenic infarctions, and is not palpable. Spleen, however, remains palpable in adults in sickle-cell β thalassemia.

Infections: Children (especially < 5 years) with sickle-cell anemia are susceptible to fulminant infections by a variety of organisms especially *Streptococcus pneumoniae* (sepsis, meningitis), *Salmonella* (osteomyelitis), *E. coli, H. influenzae*, and *Shigella*. Increased risk of infections in sickle-cell anemia is due to impairment of splenic phagocytic function or "functional splenectomy."

Vaso-occlusive and hematologic crises: Crises are acute episodic events that interrupt the steady-state course of sickle-cell anemia. They are of two major types: vaso-occlusive and hematologic.
  i. *Vaso-occlusive crises:* Vaso-occlusive crisis is the most prominent manifestation of sickle-cell anemia. It results from obstruction of microcirculation by stiff sickled red cells with ischemia and infarction in the area of distribution of artery. Precipitating factors include infection particularly in children, exposure to cold, and physical and emotional stress; however, in many cases precipitating factor is unidentifiable. Presentation is in the form of sudden onset of severe pain, usually in bones (upper or lower limbs or back), joints, chest, or abdomen. In small children, painful crises usually manifest as "hand foot syndrome" or dactylitis (painful swelling of bones of hand or foot).
  ii. *Hematologic crises:* In hematologic crisis, there is an acute aggravation of anemia that may rapidly lead to cardiac failure and death if untreated. It is of following types:
     a. *Aplastic crisis:* In sickle-cell anemia, red cell life-span is markedly shortened (average 20 days) due to extravascular hemolysis of abnormal red cells. Therefore, any event causing decrease in erythropoiesis will markedly reduce hemoglobin concentration. Aplastic crisis appears to be caused by infection by parvo virus that selectively infects erythroblasts. Suppression of erythropoiesis is usually transient lasting for about 7 to 10 days. Transfusion support is essential during the aplastic phase. On blood smear, features suggestive of aplastic crises are disappearance of polychromatic cells and nucleated red cells. Reticulocyte count is markedly low. White blood cells and platelets are not affected.
     b. *Megaloblastic crisis:* This results from folate deficiency that may develop during intercurrent illness or during pregnancy. Blood smear examination reveals macrocytes and hypersegmented neutrophils.
     c. *Hemolytic ("Hyperhemolytic") crisis:* Increased rate of red cell destruction over the chronic hemolytic state is called as hemolytic crisis. There is a sudden fall in hemoglobin concentration and levels of icterus and reticulocyte count increase. Hemolytic crisis is uncommon and coexistence of G6PD deficiency with superimposed oxidant stress may be responsible in some cases; presence of ghost red cells on blood smear suggests this condition.
     d. *Splenic sequestration crisis:* Sudden and massive accumulation of blood in spleen causes rapid increase in size of spleen over a period of several hours, with abdominal fullness, decrease in circulatory volume, sudden fall of hemoglobin, thrombocytopenia, and circulatory failure. Later, nucleated red cells, polychromatic cells, and reticulocytes increase. This occurs in patients of sickle-cell disease who have splenomegaly, i.e. infants or children (especially 6 months–3 years) with sickle-cell anemia or adults with sickle-cell β thalassemia. Earlier, this was a common cause of death in infants; however, education of parents to detect enlarging spleen, early diagnosis, and early institution of transfusion has decreased mortality. Recurrence can be avoided by removal of spleen.

Strokes: Ischemic stroke is one of the most devastating complications of sickle-cell disease and occurs in small children. Cerebral infarction is more common than hemorrhage. It usually manifests with hemiplegia. Strokes are associated with significant morbidity and mortality. Recurrence of stroke is common. Early detection is now possible with the use of transcranial Doppler ultrasonography (which detects cerebral stenoses preceding stroke). If detected early, exchange transfusion reduces the risk of subsequent stroke and brain damage.

Genitourinary system: Renal abnormalities are common in sickle-cell anemia. Renal medulla is especially vulnerable to ischemic injury due to its hypertonic, acidotic, and anoxic milieu. Impairment of renal concentrating function is a common and the earliest sign of kidney damage. Ischemia of renal medulla with papillary necrosis can develop which manifests with sudden onset of hematuria. A few patients develop proteinuria and nephrotic syndrome. Proteinuria and renal failure are increasing in frequency, as patients with sickle-cell anemia are living longer. In patients with proteinuria due to glomerular sclerosis, administration of angiotensin converting enzyme inhibitor can arrest the progression of disease.

Priapism may be short-lived ("stuttering") or prolonged, painful, and persistent. It is due to obstruction of venous return of corpora cavernosa and is seen in postpubertal males. It may lead to impotence from damage to vascular erectile system.

Pregnancy: During pregnancy there is an increased incidence of spontaneous abortion, prematurity, stillbirth, and intrauterine growth retardation (due to vaso-occlusion of placenta). In the mother, incidence of infections, chest syndrome, and postpartum hemorrhage is increased.

Skeletal system: Apart from vaso-occlusive crises in bone, other skeletal changes in sickle-cell anemia include widening of medullary cavity due to marrow hyperplasia, dactylitis (hand foot syndrome, i.e. digits are painful, tender, and swollen) in small children, avascular necrosis of femoral or humeral heads, and *Salmonella* osteomyelitis.

Respiratory system: Acute onset of fever, cough, wheezing, dyspnoea, pleuritic type of chest pains, and new lung infiltrates involving at least one complete segment on chest radiograph in sickle-cell anemia is called as "acute chest syndrome." It may be caused by fat embolism from infarcted bone marrow, pulmonary edema, or infection, but the differentiation is difficult. Patients typically have low hemoglobin and leukocytosis. It is a common cause of death in children. Repeated attacks may lead to chronic lung disease with fibrosis of lung parenchyma. Pulmonary hypertension and cor pulmonale can occur.

Hepatobiliary system: Hepatic damage may result from hepatic infarctions and transfusion-transmitted hepatitis. A significant percentage of patients have bilirubin gallstones (due to persistent elevation of serum bilirubin from chronic hemolysis). Inheritance of a variant of *UGT1A1* (gene that codes for UDP-glucuronosyl transferase enzyme) that causes Gilbert syndrome increases risk of gallstones.

Iron overload: Iron overload with organ dysfunction can be seen in adults who have been repeatedly transfused.

Skin: Chronic leg ulcers are common around ankles on the medial aspect. They do not heal readily and have a tendency to recur.

Proliferative retinopathy: Proliferative retinopathy due to retinal vascular occlusion is an important complication and is more common in patients with HbSC disease (seen in Africa). Arteriovenous communications and neovascularization may lead to vitreous hemorrhage, detachment of retina, and visual loss.

Laboratory Features

1. **Peripheral blood examination:** Anemia is usually moderate with hemoglobin concentration ranging between 6 and 9 g/dL. Hematocrit derived from hematology analyzers is more reliable since manual packed cell volume is artifactually raised due to

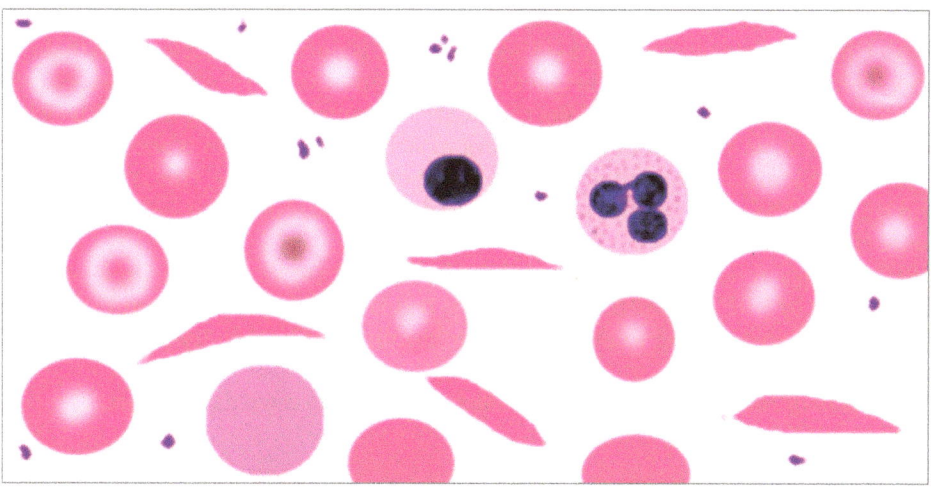

Fig. 4.39: Blood smear in sickle-cell anemia.

excessive plasma trapping by sickled red cells. Anemia is normocytic and normochromic. (In Arabs, hemoglobin is near normal or normal due to very high HbF percentage.) Red cell distribution width is increased. Typical blood smear findings are anisopoikilocytosis, sickle cells (crescent- or sickle-shaped cells with pointed ends), boat-shaped cells (crescent-shaped cells without pointed ends; highly suggestive but not pathognomonic), target cells, polychromatic cells, basophilic stippling, and nucleated red cells. Irreversibly sickled cells make up about 5 to 50% of red cells on the blood smear. Their percentage usually parallels the degree of hemolysis since they have a very short survival time (Fig. 4.39). (Sickle cells are often absent in neonates and are only occasionally seen in adults with high HbF.) Morphologically, irreversibly sickled cells are very dense, crescent- or sickle-shaped with pointed ends and smooth outline without any spicules. Target cells are especially frequent in sickle-cell β thalassemia. Reticulocyte count is increased (typically 10–20%). Mild polymorphonuclear leukocytosis is usual. The platelet count is raised as splenic trapping is lacking or is decreased. Thrombocytopenia occurs during vaso-occlusive crisis.

Features of hyposplenism (Howell–Jolly bodies, Pappenheimer bodies, numerous target cells) are observed after infancy.

Findings during painful crises are increase in leukocyte count, neutrophilia, increase in polychromatic cells, increase in number of sickled red cells (from baseline level), and increase in nucleated red cells.

2. ***Other investigations:*** Erythrocyte sedimentation rate is low despite reduced hemoglobin concentration. This is because of inability of red cells to form rouleaux. Unconjugated serum bilirubin is increased. Factor VIII and fibrinogen levels are raised.
3. ***Identification of HbS:*** Sickle hemoglobin or HbS can be detected by slide test using 2% sodium metabisulfite, solubility test, hemoglobin electrophoresis, and HPLC. These tests have been considered earlier. (See "Hereditary disorders of hemoglobin—General features and approach to diagnosis.") A few comments follow.

Slide test using reducing agent or solubility test merely detect the presence of HbS and cannot distinguish between sickle-cell trait and sickle-cell disease. Diagnosis of the phenotype of the sickle-cell disorder (sickle-cell trait or a particular type of sickle-cell disease) can be made by hemoglobin electrophoresis at alkaline pH using cellulose acetate or by citrate agar electrophoresis at acid pH. In sickle-cell anemia, predominant hemoglobin is HbS (80–95%), HbF is variably increased (5–15%), and HbA2 is normal. In sickle-cell β thalassemia also, HbA is totally absent, but in this condition proportion of HbA2 is increased (>3.5%). Family studies are helpful in making the correct diagnosis (i.e. one parent with sickle-cell trait and the other with β thalassemia trait). In sickle-cell trait, HbA is about 60% and HbS is 40% (HbA is always more than HbS). In sickle-cell β thalassemia, HbS is more than HbA and HbA2 is increased (Fig. 4.40 and Table 4.6). Electrophoresis is also necessary for genetic counseling.

HPLC findings in sickle-cell anemia and sickle-cell trait are shown in Figures 4.41A and B.

4. *Estimation of HbF by alkali denaturation test* is necessary to determine the severity of sickle-cell anemia and to detect the coinheritance of hereditary persistence of fetal hemoglobin (HPFH).
5. *Estimation of HbA2* is required for the diagnosis of sickle-cell β thalassemia.

Differential Diagnosis

1. Sickle cell-β⁰ thalassemia: See under Thalassemia (Inheritance of β thalassemia with structural hemoglobinopathies).
2. Sickle cell-hemoglobin C disease: This compound heterozygous state is seen in West Africa. Clinically, splenomegaly persists in adulthood and retinopathy and ischemic necrosis of bones are common. Blood smear shows numerous irregularly contracted red cells, target

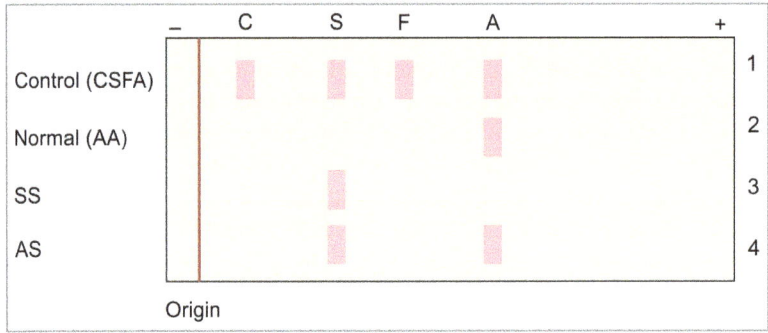

Fig. 4.40: Hemoglobin electrophoresis at alkaline pH. Lane 1: Control; Lane 2: Normal or AA pattern; Lane 3: sickle-cell anemia or SS pattern; and Lane 4: sickle-cell trait or AS pattern.

Table 4.6: Salient features of sickle-cell disorders.

Sickle-cell disease	Genotype	Clinical manifestations	Solubility test	Hb electrophoresis
1. Sickle-cell anemia	β^S/β^S	Moderate to severe anemia; crises	+	HbS predominant; no HbA; HbA_2 normal
2. Sickle-cell β⁰ thalassemia	β^S/β^0	Moderate anemia; splenomegaly persists in adults	+	HbS predominant; no HbA; HbA_2 increased
3. Sickle-cell trait	β^S/β	No anemia	+	HbA > HbS
4. Sickle-cell β⁺ thalassemia	β^S/β^+	Mild anemia	+	HbS > HbA; HbA_2 increased

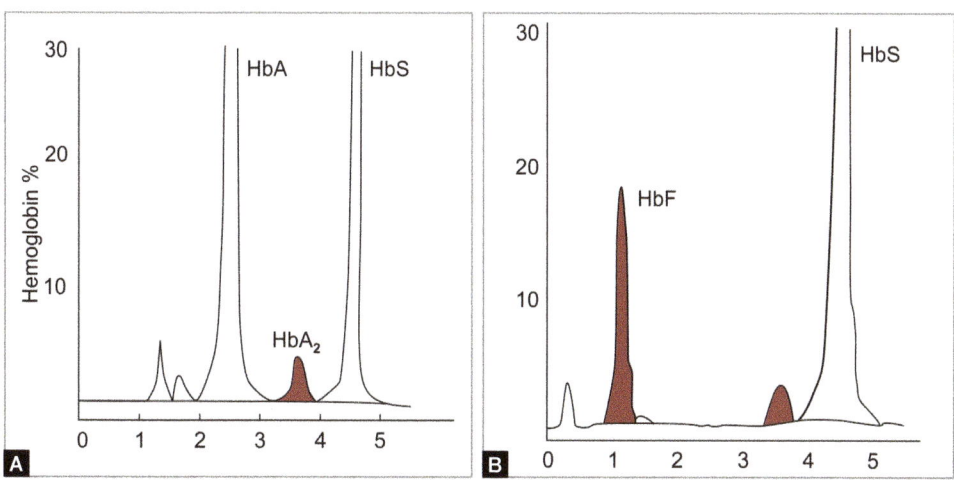

Figs. 4.41A and B: High-performance liquid chromatography in (A) sickle-cell trait and (B) sickle-cell anemia.

cells, and boat-shaped cells. Unusual poikilocytes specifically seen in this condition resemble sickle cells but have straight edges or are angulated or branched. Also, red cells containing Hb C crystals may also be seen. Definitive diagnosis is based on family studies and HPLC or hemoglobin electrophoresis.
3. Sickle cell-hemoglobin D-Punjab: Distinction from sickle cell anemia is based on family studies and HPLC or hemoglobin electrophoresis.
4. Sickle cell-hemoglobin O-Arab
5. Compound heterozygous state for HbS and hereditary persistence of fetal hemoglobin

Neonatal Screening for Sickle-cell Anemia

Screening can be carried out to identify those newborns who will later develop sickle-cell anemia. The rationale behind this approach is that preventive measures can be taken (like penicillin prophylaxis, education of parents, and vaccinations against encapsulated organisms and hepatitis B virus) to avert serious complications and reduce morbidity and mortality in later life. Screening of newborn can be carried out in communities with increased frequency of sickle-cell gene. This approach is used in the USA in African Americans as well as in the UK.

In newborns, solubility test and sodium metabisulfite test cannot be used for screening since concentration of HbS is very small (<10%). Widely used test for this purpose is citrate agar gel electrophoresis at acid pH. Hemolysate from cord blood sample is used. Newborns who will develop sickle-cell anemia show predominance of HbF, some HbS, and absent HbA; those with sickle-cell trait have HbF, HbS, and HbA. HPLC and mass spectrometry are well-suited for mass screening but are expensive.

Prenatal Diagnosis

Mothers from high-risk ethnic group should be screened in early pregnancy for HbS carrier state. If prospective mother as well as father are positive, they should be offered the option of prenatal diagnosis or of newborn screening. Two distinct approaches are available for prenatal diagnosis of sickle-cell anemia: fetal blood analysis and fetal DNA analysis.

Fetal blood analysis: This involves globin chain synthesis studies in fetal blood using CM-cellulose chromatography. Abnormal globin chain is separated from normal globin chain and quantitated. Fetal blood sampling (by cordocentesis) can only be done after 18 weeks of gestation. Apart from prolonged waiting period, risk of procedure-related fetal loss is also comparatively greater.

Fetal DNA analysis: Fetal DNA may be obtained either from amniotic fluid cells or from chorionic villi (see prenatal diagnosis of thalassemias). Chorionic villus biopsy is preferred because, if required, termination of pregnancy can be performed earlier.

Various methods are available for analysis of fetal DNA. Some of them are outlined below. (For details see "Prenatal diagnosis of thalassemias.")

i. *Southern blot analysis:* A restriction enzyme called *Mst* II recognizes three specific sites in normal β globin gene and cleaves DNA at these sites (Fig. 4.42). It produces two fragments of normal β globin gene: one measuring 1.15 kb and the other 0.2 kb. Mutation producing sickle hemoglobin causes a single base change A→T in the 6th codon of β globin gene. This mutation abolishes one cleavage site for *Mst* II in such a manner that only one large fragment 1.35 kb long is produced after *Mst* II digestion. The technique consists of digestion of extracted DNA with *Mst* II followed by separation of fragments according to size by agarose gel electrophoresis. Fragments are denatured and then transferred onto nitrocellulose membrane. Radio labeled 1.15 kb probe complementary to 5' end of normal β globin gene is hybridized. On autoradiography, a single 1.15 kb band indicates normal β globin genes on both homologous chromosomes (β/β), and a single 1.35 kb band indicates

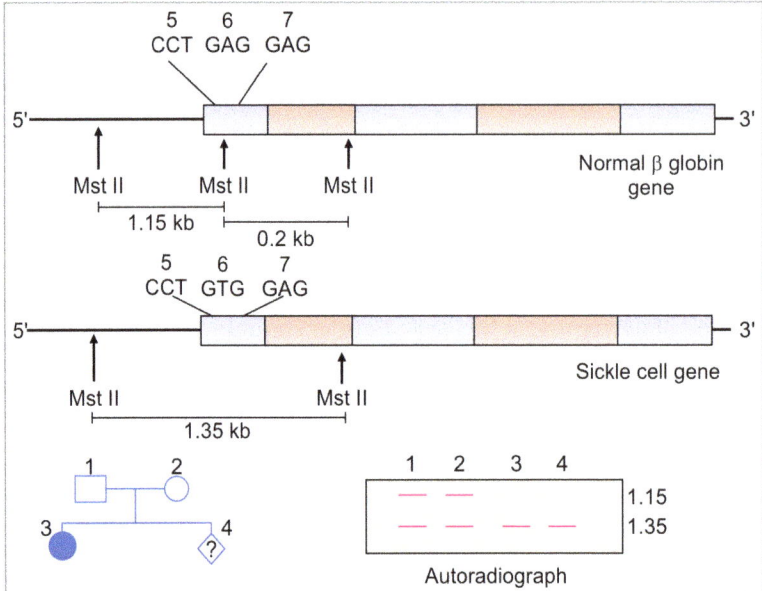

Fig. 4.42: Southern blot analysis of β globin gene using restriction enzyme Mst II. Normal β globin gene has three restriction sites for the enzyme Mst II (arrows on upper part of figure) with production of two fragments 1.15 kb and 0.2 kb. Sickle mutation results in abolition of one restriction site with formation of a large fragment 1.35 kb. Lower part of the figure shows Southern blot analysis. Both father (Lane 1) and mother (Lane 2) are heterozygous for sickle-cell mutation (sickle-cell trait); offspring in Lane 3 is affected, while fetus in Lane 4 also has sickle-cell anemia.

that both β globin genes have sickle mutation (i.e. $β^S/β^S$ or sickle-cell anemia). Presence of both 1.15 kb and 1.35 kb bands indicate heterozygous state for $β^S$ gene (i.e. $β^S/β$ or sickle-cell trait).

ii. *Restriction fragment length polymorphism (RFLP) analysis:* Principle of this technique is already outlined earlier (see "Prenatal diagnosis of thalassemias"). Normal β globin gene is associated with 7.0 kb fragment while $β^S$ gene is associated with 13.0 kb fragment in some populations, when restriction enzyme *Hpa* I is used. This polymorphism can be used to track the presence of $β^S$ gene in a particular family.

iii. Methods employing DNA amplification:
   a. *Direct detection of mutation with restriction enzymes:* The PCR-amplified DNA is digested with a restriction enzyme (such as *Dde* I). Fragments of different size are produced in normal β globin gene and in $β^S$ globin gene as mutation abolishes a cleavage site in the latter.
   b. *Allele-specific oligonucleotide probe analysis:* Two allele-specific probes are synthesized, one complementary to the normal sequence and the other to the abnormal (sickle mutation) sequence. Amplified DNA is dot blotted on to nylon membranes and probes are applied. Hybridization occurs if sequences are complementary to each other.
   c. *Color DNA amplification:* Normal β globin gene primer and mutant ($β^S$) globin gene primer are labeled with different fluorescent dyes. The resulting normal and abnormal amplified gene products are of different colors and can be easily identified.

Preimplantation genetic diagnosis: This is now an established alternative to prenatal diagnosis of sickle cell anemia in couples both of whom are having sickle cell trait.

Treatment

Treatment of sickle-cell anemia is symptomatic and supportive. Patients with sickle-cell disease are best managed at a comprehensive care center that has properly trained multidisciplinary staff; such centers are, however, rarely available. Main treatment modalities in sickle-cell anemia are shown in Box 4.8.

Box 4.8: Main treatment modalities in sickle-cell anemia.
- Penicillin prophylaxis
- Vaccination against *S. pneumoniae*, *H. influenzae*, influenza virus, and hepatitis B virus
- Folate supplementation
- Hydroxyurea
- Transfusion therapy: chronic or partial exchange
- Iron chelation (if iron overload)

1. Measures to prevent crises include early detection and treatment of infections and avoidance of exposure to extreme cold, stress, hypoxia, and dehydration. All infections should be treated intensively. In addition to routine vaccination, all children should be vaccinated against *Streptococcus pneumoniae*, *Neisseria meningitides*, *Haemophilus influenzae* type B, seasonal influenza virus, and hepatitis B virus. Routine penicillin prophylaxis should be initiated in children younger than 5 years.
2. Treatment of vaso-occlusive episode involves relieving pain by analgesics, keeping patient warm, maintaining adequate fluid intake, oxygenation, and treatment of infections. Partial exchange transfusion reduces percentage of sickled cells and improves oxygenation; this may limit organ damage during acute vascular episode.
3. During pregnancy in sickle-cell anemia, due to the increased risk of prematurity and stillbirth in fetus and of maternal vaso-occlusive crisis, close antenatal supervision is

required. Folic acid and iron should be given routinely. Regular blood transfusion therapy has been advocated, but usefulness of this approach is not yet proved.
4. Oral contraceptive pill as a means of family planning should be avoided as it poses increased risk of thrombosis.
5. Exchange transfusion has been advised prior to surgery to reduce the risk of vaso-occlusive episodes by decreasing the percentage of HbS (to less than 30%). During operation, hypoxia, dehydration, circulatory stasis, and exposure to cold should be avoided.
6. Radiographic contrast media cause dehydration of red cells, increase MCHC and precipitate sickling. Exchange transfusion has been recommended prior to cerebral angiography.
7. Cerebrovascular accidents are managed with prompt exchange transfusion during acute episode to reduce HbS to less than 30%. This limits neurologic damage. Following this, regular blood transfusion therapy is started to prevent recurrence of strokes by maintaining this HbS level.
8. Acute chest syndrome: Patients with low oxygen saturation level can benefit from exchange transfusion. Patients are given adequate analgesia, incentive spirometry to prevent further infiltrates, and broad-spectrum antibiotics.
9. Role of transfusion therapy in sickle-cell anemia is summarized in Box 4.9. Regular blood transfusions merely to increase hemoglobin concentration are not indicated since they lead to increase in blood viscosity. Benefits of transfusion include rise in HbA concentration, reduction of HbS concentration through dilution by donor red cells, and temporary suppression of erythropoiesis thereby reducing production of HbS containing red cells. Blood transfusions are indicated in certain situations as follows:
    i. *Packed red cell transfusion* to improve oxygen-carrying capacity is required during symptomatic anemia (i.e. causing breathlessness, impending CCF) aplastic crisis, acute splenic sequestration crisis, etc.

Box 4.9: Blood transfusion in sickle-cell disease.

- In SCD patients, blood for transfusion should be:
    - Matched for Rh (C, D, E) and Kell antigens since they are responsible for most cases of alloimmunization
    - Negative for HbS by sickle solubility test (for correct assessment of sickle-cells post-transfusion)
    - Leukocyte-depleted (to reduce viral transmission and prevent febrile reactions)
- Blood transfusion is not indicated in steady state anemia
- Main complications are hyperviscosity, iron overload in adults from chronic transfusion therapy, transmission of infections, and alloimmunization (usually against C, E, and Kell antigens)
- Acute simple transfusion, i.e. packed red cell transfusion (10–15 mL/kg) is indicated in—
    - Symptomatic anemia
    - Aplastic crisis
    - Splenic sequestration crisis
    - Before surgery
    - Acute ischemic stroke (if exchange transfusion is not readily available)
    - Acute chest syndrome (early)
- Exchange transfusion is indicated in:
    - Acute ischemic stroke
    - Impending stroke
    - Acute chest syndrome (if severe clinical worsening)
- Chronic transfusion is indicated for:
    - Prevention of recurrence of stroke

ii. *Regular chronic transfusion therapy* is employed to reduce the number of HbS containing cells (to less than 40%). This is indicated to prevent recurrence of strokes in cerebrovascular episodes. Role of this form of therapy prior to major surgery and during pregnancy is being investigated.

iii. *Partial exchange transfusion* is indicated during acute or impending attack of cerebrovascular episode or vaso-occlusive episode. Exchange transfusion reduces viscosity, avoids hypervolemia, and improves oxygen-carrying capacity. The purpose behind this therapy is to limit or prevent their reversible organ damage.

10. Hydroxyurea: A mainstay of treatment in sickle-cell anemia is hydroxyurea (now called hydroxycarbamide). It has following benefits in sickle-cell anemia: (a) it increases production of HbF (possibly by enhancing transcription of genes controlling γ-globin chain synthesis) and reduces number and severity of crises (as HbF does not participate with HbF in sickling process, polymerization of HbS is retarded); (b) it reduces white cell count thus causing anti-inflammatory effect; (c) it increases red cell volume and hydration thus reducing sickling and hemolysis; (d) it decreases adhesiveness of red cells and leukocytes; and (e) it releases nitric oxide that causes vasodilatation.

    Hydroxyurea reduces the number of painful crises, transfusion requirements, and incidence of acute chest syndrome. It is indicated in children, adolescents, and adults with sickle-cell anemia who have frequent pain, severe vaso-occlusive events, and severe anemia.

11. Hematopoietic stem cell transplantation is the only form of therapy that can cure the disease. Since it is associated with significant morbidity and mortality, it should be reserved for severely affected patients having HLA-matched sibling donor.

Prognosis

The course of sickle-cell anemia is highly variable. Some patients have relatively mild disease with survival into adulthood while others die during infancy or early childhood from severe disease. Leading causes of death include severe sepsis, cerebrovascular episode, acute chest syndrome, and splenic sequestration crisis.

Measures to improve survival in sickle cell anemia are summarized in Box 4.10.

> **Box 4.10:** Measures to improve survival in sickle-cell anemia.
>
> - Neonatal screening: Identification of affected newborns will lead to parent education, penicillin prophylaxis, and early treatment of infections.
> - Vaccination against *H. influenzae, S. pneumoniae, N. meningitides, H. influenzae,* and hepatitis B virus
> - Early institution of emergency, supportive, or intensive treatment
> - Transcranial Doppler ultrasound for detection of children with increased risk of stroke
> - Administration of blood transfusion/exchange transfusion and hydroxyurea

Sickle-cell Trait

This is the asymptomatic heterozygous state for sickle-cell gene (β^s/β). In sickle-cell trait, HbS comprises around 40% of total hemoglobin, the remaining 60% being HbA. Since HbA is the predominant hemoglobin, it prevents red cells from sickling at low oxygen tensions occurring physiologically. The red cell life-span is normal.

Persons with sickle-cell trait do not have anemia and are usually asymptomatic. However, this condition has genetic importance and also is significant if patient becomes hypoxic. Some clinical abnormalities, however, have been reported to occur in these persons: deficient urine concentrating ability, infarction of spleen and vaso-occlusive crises at high altitudes, and

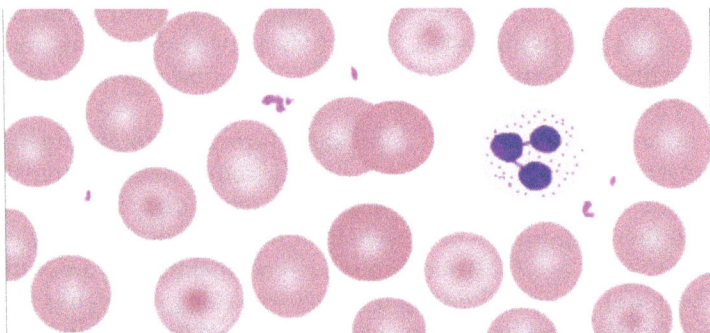

Fig. 4.43: Blood smear in sickle-cell trait showing target cells.

hematuria (renal papillary necrosis). Instances of sudden death have been reported following strenuous exercise.

Few target cells may be present on blood films (Fig. 4.43). Typical sickle cells are not seen; however, few plump cells with pointed ends are often present. Diagnosis requires demonstration of HbS by sodium metabisulfite slide test or solubility test and hemoglobin electrophoresis. Hemoglobin electrophoresis reveals more HbA (60%) than HbS (40%).

No treatment is required and duration of survival of individuals is normal.

DISORDERS OF RED CELL ENZYMES

GLUCOSE-6-PHOSPHATE DEHYDROGENASE DEFICIENCY

Glucose-6-phosphate dehydrogenase (G6PD) deficiency is the most common red cell enzymopathy in humans (affecting about 400 million people worldwide) and is characterized by reduced activity of glucose-6-phosphate dehydrogenase in red cells, and occurrence of hemolysis usually after exposure to oxidant stress (Box 4.11).

More than 400 biochemical variants of G6PD have been identified. The variants are grouped into five classes by World Health Organization Scientific Working Group (Table 4.7).

Box 4.11: Prevalence of G6PD deficiency.

- Very common, with > 7% of the world population having defective gene
- High prevalence in Africa, Middle East, Mediterranean countries, and Asia
- In India, prevalence varies from 0 to 27% in different castes and ethnic groups
- G6PD Mediterranean, G6PD Kerala-Kalyan, and G6PD Orissa are the variants most prevalent in India
- Especially high prevalence in Parsees and Vatalia Prajapatis.

Polymorphic mutations occur with high frequency in malaria-endemic areas (WHO classes II and III) and include G6PD A—(common in Africa) and G6PD Mediterranean (common in Mediterranean countries, Middle East, and India). In such cases, hemolysis develops only following oxidant exposure. **Sporadic mutations** occur anywhere in the world at low frequency and patient develops chronic hemolytic anemia (WHO class I).

The well-known abnormal G6PD variants associated with G6PD deficiency are G6PD A—(prevalent in Africa; 1/2 life 13 days) and G6PD Mediterranean (1/2 life several hours). G6PD variant with normal enzyme activity is G6PD B (1/2 life 60 days). The deficient variants common in India are G6PD Mediterranean, G6PD Kerala-Kalyan, and G6PD Orissa. Normally,

Table 4.7: Variants of G6PD.

Class	G6PD enzyme activity	Clinical manifestations
I	<5% of normal	Rare; chronic congenital nonspherocytic hemolytic anemia
II	<10% of normal	Episodic acute hemolysis induced by oxidant drugs
III	10–60% of normal	Acute self-limited hemolysis following oxidant drugs or infections
IV	60–100% of normal	—
V	Increased	—

enzyme activity decreases with red cell ageing so that young red cells have the highest enzyme activity and older red cells have relatively lower activity. G6PD A-variant enzyme has decreased stability and therefore, deficiency of enzyme in older red cells is more pronounced. In G6PD deficiency associated with G6PDA-variant, oxidant injury causes hemolysis of only older red cells and therefore, hemolytic episode is mild to moderate in severity and self-limited even if oxidant agent is continued. G6PD Mediterranean is a markedly unstable enzyme and its activity is reduced in red cells of all ages. Therefore in these cases oxidant injury is associated with severe, nonself-limited hemolysis.

Pathogenesis of Hemolysis

G6PD enzyme catalyzes the first step in the hexose monophosphate (HMP) shunt. It catalyzes the oxidation of glucose-6-phosphate to 6-phosphogluconate, and simultaneously generates NADPH from NADP. The only source of NADPH in red cells is the HMP shunt, which is dependent on the activity of G6PD enzyme. (HMP shunt produces ribose, which is an essential component of DNA and RNA. Ribose, however, can be produced by other pathways that are not G6PD-dependent.)

In addition to various biosynthetic reactions, NADPH is required for continuous supply of reduced glutathione (GSH). GSH detoxifies harmful hydrogen peroxide or H_2O_2 (an oxidative metabolite) to water with the help of an enzyme, glutathione peroxidase. In G6PD deficiency, sufficient glutathione is not available to remove H_2O_2 (Figs. 4.44A and B). Accumulation of H_2O_2 causes oxidation of free –SH groups of hemoglobin and subsequent denaturation and precipitation of globin chains. This leads to the formation of Heinz bodies that are red cell inclusions bound to red cell membrane and represent precipitated globin. Such red cells are rigid and are trapped in the spleen. Heinz bodies are selectively removed by splenic macrophages ("pitting") with subsequent membrane loss, and formation of spherocytes. Such red cells are susceptible to splenic sequestration and phagocytosis by macrophages. Oxidation of heme also leads to the formation of methemoglobin; its role in hemolysis, however, is unclear.

Apart from extravascular destruction of red cells in spleen, intravascular hemolysis also occurs and is probably caused by peroxidation of membrane lipids by oxidant injury.

Genetics

G6PD deficiency is an X-linked disorder and therefore, occurs exclusively in males. In female heterozygotes, expression is variable. This is because of the process of random inactivation of one X chromosome (lyonization) during embryogenesis. Expression of deficiency in females depends on relative proportions of normal and abnormal chromosomes that are inactivated. Homozygous females showing clinical features of G6PD deficiency have also been reported.

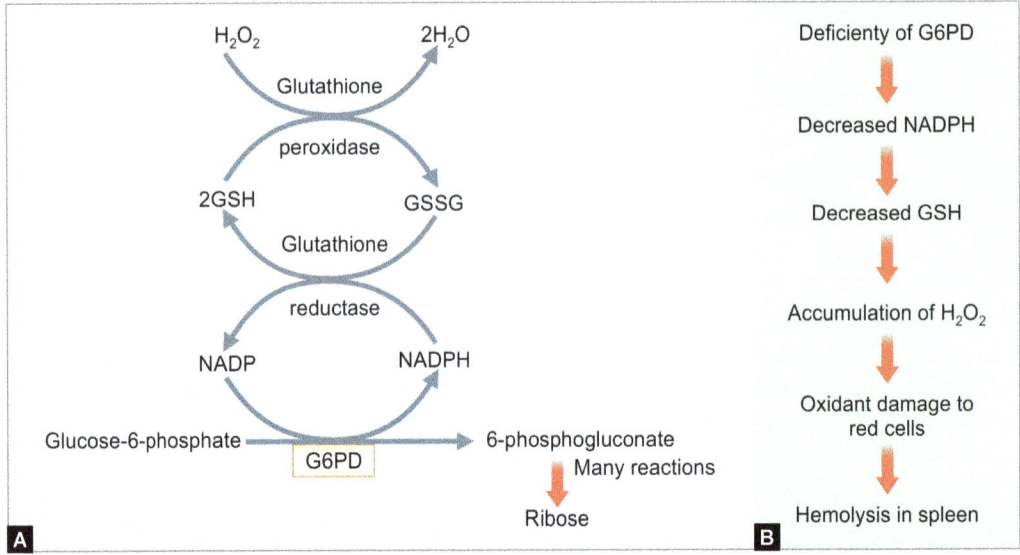

Figs. 4.44A and B: (A) Role of G6PD in detoxification of hydrogen peroxide; (B) Effect of G6PD deficiency.

Malaria and G6PD Deficiency

It has been suggested that high frequency of G6PD deficiency in certain parts of the world is probably related to the protection it affords against *P. falciparum* malaria. This protection is largely limited to the female heterozygotes. African heterozygous females have two populations of red cells: G6PD B (normal) and G6PD A—(deficient)—due to random inactivation of chromosomes during embryogenesis. Growth of the parasite is inhibited in the G6PD-deficient red cells. However, it has been shown that the malaria parasite can adapt to this deficiency by synthesizing its own G6PD enzyme after four to five cycles in G6PD-deficient red cells. Therefore, parasite can grow and develop in hemizygous males (in whom all red cells are G6PD-deficient) after a few cycles. In female heterozygotes, the parasite may invade either G6PD-normal or –deficient red cells during successive cycles. Therefore, stimulus to the parasite to adapt by synthesizing its own G6PD is considerably diminished. This results in decreased parasitemia in female heterozygotes and protection against severe disease.

Clinical Features

In G6PD deficiency, hemolysis usually develops after exposure to oxidant stress, such as drugs (Box 4.12) or infection. There is usually sudden development of pallor, jaundice, and dark-colored urine (due to hemoglobinuria) 1 to 3 days after exposure to the drug. Anemia is most severe around 7 to 10 days following drug ingestion. Hypotension and acute renal failure may develop in severe cases. In class III variant, hemolysis is mild to moderate and self-restricted, i.e. hemolysis ceases even when patient goes on taking the offending drug. This is due to hemolysis of predominantly older red cells, and resistance of younger red cells to oxidant damage. In class II variant, hemolysis is marked, nonself-limited, and may require blood transfusion; this is because young red cells also have severely deficient G6PD activity.

Hemolysis following infection (pneumonia) develops 1 to 2 days after onset of fever and is usually mild.

Box 4.12: Common drugs and chemicals causing hemolysis in G6PD deficiency.

- **Antimalarials: Primaquine**, Chloroquine, Quinacrine, **Pamaquine**
- **Antibacterials:** Sulphacetamide, **Sulphamethoxazole**, Sulphanilamide, Sulphapyridine, **Nalidixic acid, Nitrofurantoin**, Furazolidone, **Dapsone**
- **Analgesics:** Acetanilid, **Aspirin, Phenacetin**
- **Others:** Phenylhydrazine, Ascorbic acid, Vit K (water-soluble), **Methylene blue**, Naphthalene (mothballs), henna compounds (present in hair dyes, tattoos), Chinese herbs, "RUSH" (isobutyl nitrate, amyl nitrate), Rasburicase

Agents marked in bold: Definite risk of hemolysis

Favism (precipitation of hemolysis by ingestion of fava beans) is a unique feature occurring in individuals in Mediterranean and Arab countries. Fava beans contain oxidants that cause hemolysis hours or days following ingestion; it may be fatal.

G6PD deficiency most commonly manifests with neonatal jaundice (Box 4.13). In severe cases, kernicterus and death can occur. It is mainly observed in Asia (including India) and Mediterranean countries.

Individuals with type I variant have chronic hemolytic anemia. It manifests in infancy or childhood with hepatosplenomegaly and jaundice. Hemolysis is chronic and there is no relationship with ingestion of drugs or infections, although hemolysis is enhanced by these causes.

Laboratory Features

Evidence of Hemolysis

During hemolysis, general features of hemolytic anemia are present. Peripheral blood smear shows: polychromasia, fragmented red cells, spherocytes, bite cells (red cells having bitten out margins due to plucking out of precipitated hemoglobin by splenic macrophages), and half-ghost cells (one-half of red cell appears empty, while other half is filled with hemoglobin) (Figs. 4.45A and B). Biochemical investigations reveal unconjugated hyperbilirubinemia, hemoglobinemia, hemoglobinuria (Box 4.14), and decreased or absent haptoglobin.

Box 4.13: Clinical manifestations of G6PD deficiency.

- Neonatal jaundice
- Drug-induced hemolytic anemia
- Chronic hemolytic anemia
- Favism
- Hemolysis following infection

Box 4.14: Causes of hemoglobinuria.

- Glucose-6-phosphate dehydrogenase deficiency
- Blackwater fever
- Paroxysmal nocturnal hemoglobinuria
- Paroxysmal cold hemoglobinuria
- Mismatched blood transfusion
- *Clostridium welchii* infection

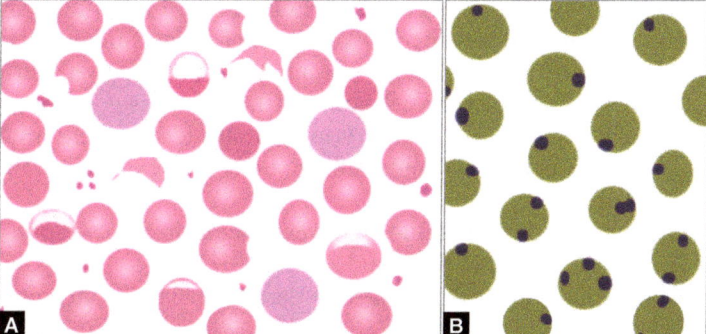

Figs. 4.45A and B: (A) Blood smear: half-ghost cells, bite cells, microspherocytes, fragmented cells, and polychromatic cells; (B) Heinz bodies (supravital staining with crystal violet).

Heinz Bodies

They can be detected after vital staining with methyl violet. They are usually seen immediately following hemolysis. Heinz bodies are deep purple small inclusions attached to red cell membrane. In addition to G6PD deficiency, they are also seen in unstable hemoglobin disease.

Tests for Detection of G6PD Deficiency

Diagnosis rests on demonstration of G6PD deficiency by a qualitative or a quantitative test.

Qualitative or Screening tests: Various screening tests are available. The most widely used, inexpensive, and recommended test is fluorescent spot test.

i. *Fluorescent spot test:* This test is recommended by International Committee for Standardisation in Hematology.

If G6PD is present in the blood sample, it reduces NADP to NADPH. NADPH fluoresces when exposed to ultraviolet light while NADP fails to do so. The method consists of following steps:

1. To the reagent mixture that consists of buffered solution of glucose-6-phosphate, NADP, saponin, and oxidized glutathione (GSSG) whole blood is added. Glucose-6-phosphate is substrate for G6PD; saponin is used for lysis of red cells; and GSSG oxidizes small amount of NADPH formed and thus renders the test more sensitive for the detection of mild G6PD deficiency.
2. A drop (spot) of this mixture is applied on to the filter paper and examined under ultraviolet light.

Following controls should always be run to test the accuracy of results: positive control (known G6PD-deficient sample) and negative control (normal or non-G6PD-deficient sample).

Result: If G6PD is present in the test sample then NADPH is produced from NADP. NADPH fluoresces under ultraviolet light while NADP fails to do so. Presence of fluorescence indicates normal G6PD activity, while absence of fluorescence indicates G6PD deficiency (<20% activity).

This test is simple, specific, and requires only small amount of blood. It is used for diagnosis of G6PD deficiency in individual cases and in population surveys.

Limitations:

1. During attack of hemolysis, this test may yield falsely normal result. This is because during hemolysis, preferentially older red cells (which contain the lowest G6PD activity) are destroyed, and the remaining red cells in circulation have more G6PD activity in comparison. Further, a brisk reticulocyte response follows hemolysis. Reticulocytes have high G6PD activity. Therefore, if screening test is performed during this period, normal or increased G6PD activity will be found. In such a case, screening test should be repeated after a few weeks. Another way is to separate older red cells from blood sample by centrifugation (older red cells settle at the bottom) and the test is performed on these cells.
2. Falsely abnormal test may be obtained in severe anemia from any cause. This is because too few red cells are present in the blood sample.
3. It is difficult to diagnose those female heterozygotes that have small proportion of G6PD-deficient red cells.

ii. *Methemoglobin reduction test:* Sodium nitrite is an oxidant that converts oxyhemoglobin to methemoglobin. Methylene blue is a redox dye that reduces methemoglobin to hemoglobin in G6PD normal red cells but not in G6PD-deficient red cells. [In methemoglobin, iron exists in the oxidized or ferric (Fe^{3+}) state.] Presence of methemoglobinemia imparts brownish color to the blood. Brown color indicates G6PD deficiency; red color indicates normal G6PD activity, while intermediate color indicates heterozygous state.
Limitations: Same as in fluorescent spot test.
iii. *Dye decolorization test:* Hemolysate is incubated with buffered mixture of a dye (such as dichlorophenol indophenol or DPIP), glucose-6-phosphate, and NADP. If G6PD exists in the hemolysate, then it converts NADP to NADPH. NADPH reduces the dye to a colorless compound. In the presence of G6PD deficiency, time taken for dye decolorization is longer. Advantages of this method include: (1) easy detection of heterozygotes, and (2) suitability for large-scale screening since large number of samples can be tested simultaneously.

Quantitative assay of G6PD: This test is available only in reference laboratories. Hemolysate is incubated with glucose-6-phosphate. The rate of reduction of NADP to NADPH depends upon G6PD activity in the lysate. The rate of production of NADPH is measured in a spectrophotometer at 340 nm and G6PD activity is derived.

During acute hemolytic episode, test for G6PD deficiency may yield negative result due to reticulocytosis (since reticulocytes have high G6PD content). In suspected cases, the test should be repeated about 6 weeks after the hemolytic episode.

Tests for Detection of Heterozygotes

Due to the process of random inactivation of one X chromosome during embryogenesis (lyonization), female heterozygotes for G6PD deficiency possess two types of red cells: normal and G6PD-deficient. The proportion of G6PD-deficient and G6PD-normal red cells is therefore variable. When a screening test is performed which utilizes lysate of red cells, or if the proportion of deficient red cells is small then it will give a normal result. Methods that measure enzyme activity in intact red cells are more sensitive in detecting heterozygotes if the proportion of G6PD-deficient red cells is small. Two tests are commonly employed: Methemoglobin elution test and Tetrazolium-linked cytochemical method.

Methemoglobin elution method: Blood is incubated with sodium nitrite, and methylene blue (or preferably nile blue sulfate). Sodium nitrite converts oxyhemoglobin to methemoglobin. Methylene blue (or nile blue sulfate) changes methemoglobin to oxyhemoglobin in G6PD-normal red cells. Potassium cyanide is added which combines with methemoglobin to form methemoglobin cyanide. From this blood, smears are prepared on glass slides. After drying, slides are dipped in a solution of hydrogen peroxide. Hydrogen peroxide elutes (or removes) methemoglobin. The smears are then stained. Red cells containing oxyhemoglobin (i.e. G6PD-normal red cells) take the stain, while red cells from which methemoglobin has been removed (i.e. G6PD-deficient red cells) do not stain and appear as "ghosts."

Tetrazolium-linked cytochemical method: Methemoglobin is formed when sodium nitrite is added to blood. In the presence of normal G6PD activity, nile blue sulfate (a redox dye) converts methemoglobin to oxyhemoglobin; in G6PD-deficient red cells this conversion does not occur. A tetrazolium compound (MTT) is then added. Oxyhemoglobin reduces MTT to form coarse purplish-black granules of monoformazan. MTT is not reduced by methemoglobin. In heterozygotes, two populations of red cells can be distinguished: one containing granules (normal red cells) and one without granules (G6PD-deficient red cells).

Differential Diagnosis

Some cases of unstable hemoglobinopathy resemble G6PD deficiency in causing hemolysis of red cells on exposure to oxidant stress. Diagnosis of unstable hemoglobins requires heat instability test and isopropanol precipitation test.

Treatment

Patients should be instructed to avoid oxidant drugs that precipitate hemolysis. Prompt treatment of infections is essential.

Treatment during hemolytic attack is supportive. Blood transfusion may be indicated in severe cases. Adequate urinary output should be maintained to prevent renal damage due to hemoglobinuria.

IMMUNE HEMOLYTIC ANEMIAS

CLASSIFICATION

Hemolysis due to immune mechanism occurs when antibody and/or complement bind to red cell membrane. In immunologically mediated hemolysis, destruction of red cells usually occurs by type II (cytotoxic) hypersensitivity reaction. The antigen is on the surface of the red cells. The specific antibody in the circulation binds with the antigen. This causes extravascular or intravascular red cell destruction.

Immune hemolytic anemias are classified into three types—autoimmune, iso (or allo-) immune, and drug-induced (Box 4.15).

In autoimmune hemolytic anemia (AIHA), hemolysis occurs when antibodies and/or complement in patient's circulation react with and cause destruction of patient's own red cells. Classification of AIHA (Box 4.16) is based on thermal characteristics of the antibody and presence or absence of underlying disease. In AIHA, autoantibodies may be of IgG, IgM, or IgA class. Generally, IgG and IgM antibodies are, respectively, of warm and cold types; however, in paroxysmal cold hemoglobinuria, IgG antibodies are of cold-reactive type.

Box 4.15: Classification of immune hemolytic anemias.

- Autoimmune: Warm-reactive antibody type, cold-reactive antibody type, transplant-associated
- Alloimmune: Hemolytic disease of fetus and newborn, hemolytic transfusion reaction
- Drug-induced

In alloimmune hemolytic anemia, hemolysis occurs due to reaction between red cells (antigen) from one individual with antibody from another individual. Alloantibodies are usually of IgG class.

> **Box 4.16:** Classification of autoimmune hemolytic anemias.
>
> 1. *Warm antibody type (antibody maximally active at 37°C and mostly IgG)*
>   - Primary (idiopathic)
>   - Secondary:
>   - Autoimmune disorders (e.g. systemic lupus erythematosus)
>   - Neoplastic disorders (lymphoproliferative disorders like chronic lymphocytic leukemia and malignant lymphoma, carcinomas, teratoma)
>   - Drug-induced
>   - Immunodeficiency disorders (acquired immunodeficiency syndrome, hypogammaglobulinemia)
> 2. *Cold antibody type (antibody maximally active at 0 to 4°C)*
>   - Cold agglutinin disease (cold-reactive antibody is IgM)
>   - Primary
>   - Secondary (infections like *Mycoplasma pneumoniae*, Epstein-Barr virus, cytomegalovirus, malaria, etc; Lymphoproliferative disorders; Autoimmune disorders)
>   - Paroxysmal cold hemoglobinuria (cold-reactive antibody is IgG)
>   - Primary
>   - Secondary (Infection by *Treponema pallidum*, viruses)
> 3. *Mixed warm- and cold-antibody type*
> 4. *Transplant-associated hemolytic anemia*
>   - Hematopoietic stem cell transplant (ABO group incompatibility)
>   - Solid organ transplant (Passenger lymphocyte syndrome)

AUTOIMMUNE HEMOLYTIC ANEMIAS DUE TO WARM-REACTING AUTOANTIBODIES

This is the most common form of AIHA. In this type, IgG antibodies or complement (C3b) bind to red cell membrane and are recognized by specific receptors on macrophages. The warm autoantibodies are panagglutinins, i.e. they react with all red cells in the diagnostic red cell panel. Red cells lightly coated with IgG do not activate complement and are trapped and phagocytosed in spleen (since concentration of antibodies on red cells is low and splenic circulation is sluggish). Red cells heavily coated with IgG antibodies activate complement and coated with both IgG and C3b; such red cells are phagocytosed in both liver (fast circulation) and spleen. Macrophages have receptors for both IgG and C3b component of complement. Macrophages may completely phagocytose the red cell or may remove a small part of the membrane; in the latter case, loss of surface area causes formation of a microspherocyte. Some such red cells escape into the circulation and can be recognized on peripheral blood smear. Spherocytes are rigid and are sequestered and destroyed during subsequent passages through spleen (Figs. 4.46A to C). There is a direct relationship between severity of hemolysis and number of spherocytes and with the immunoglobulin subclass of the antibody (IgG1 or IgG3).

Clinical Features

Most patients have mild anemia, icterus, and splenomegaly. Occasionally, onset may be sudden with severe manifestations. In secondary AIHA, clinical features of underlying disease predominate. Association of hemolytic anemia with thrombocytopenia can occur in children and is known as Evans' syndrome.

Section 2: Disorders of Red Blood Cells (Anemias)

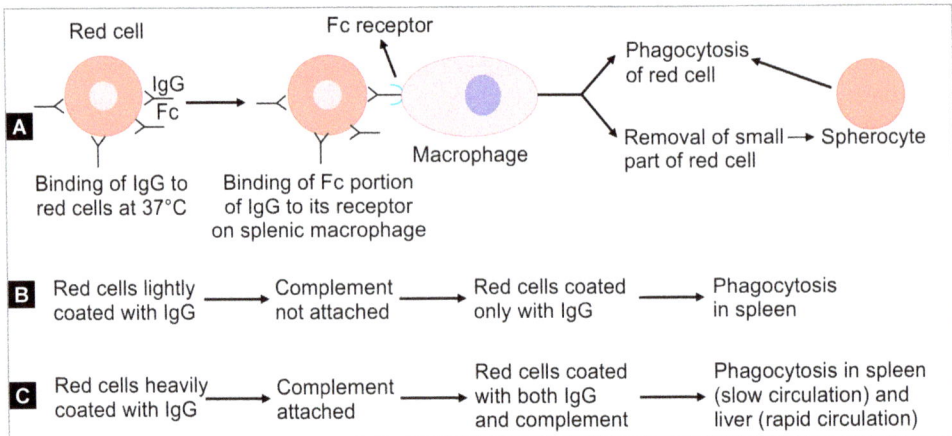

Figs. 4.46A to C: (A) Mechanism of hemolysis in warm-type AIHA; (B) If the concentration of IgG antibodies that are coating red cells is low, then complement is not activated and red cell phagocytosis occurs in spleen where blood flow is sluggish; (C) If the concentration of antibodies coating red cells is high, complement is activated and phagocytosis of red cells occurs in both spleen and liver (fast blood flow) by macrophages which have receptors for both IgG (Fc) and complement (C3b).

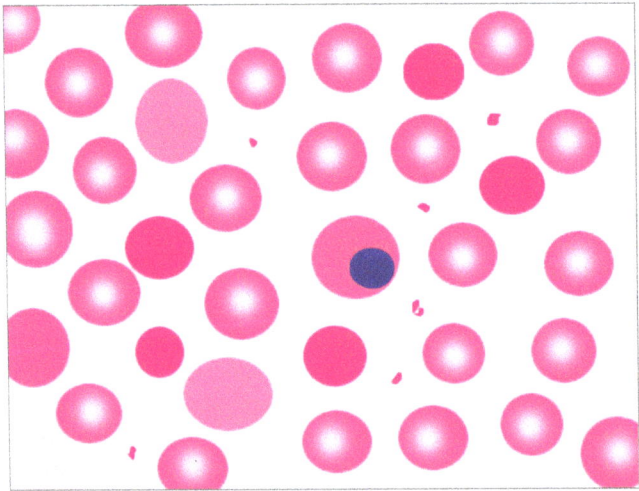

Fig. 4.47: Blood smear in autoimmune hemolytic anemia. Spherocytes, polychromatic cells, and a normoblast are seen.

Laboratory Features

Peripheral blood examination: This shows variable degree of anemia depending on severity of hemolysis, microspherocytosis of red cells, and reticulocytosis. A spherocyte is smaller in size than normal red cell, lacks central area of pallor, and appears densely hemoglobinized. Fragmented red cells, polychromasia, and nucleated red cells may be present (Fig. 4.47). Mild neutrophilic leukocytosis is usual. Platelet count is normal. In the presence of thrombocytopenia, Evans' syndrome should be considered. In this condition, antibodies against both red cells and platelets are present.

Antiglobulin (Coombs') test: This test determines whether hemolysis has an immunological basis. There are two types of antiglobulin test—direct and indirect. Direct antiglobulin test

Chapter 4: Anemias due to Excessive Red Cell Destruction

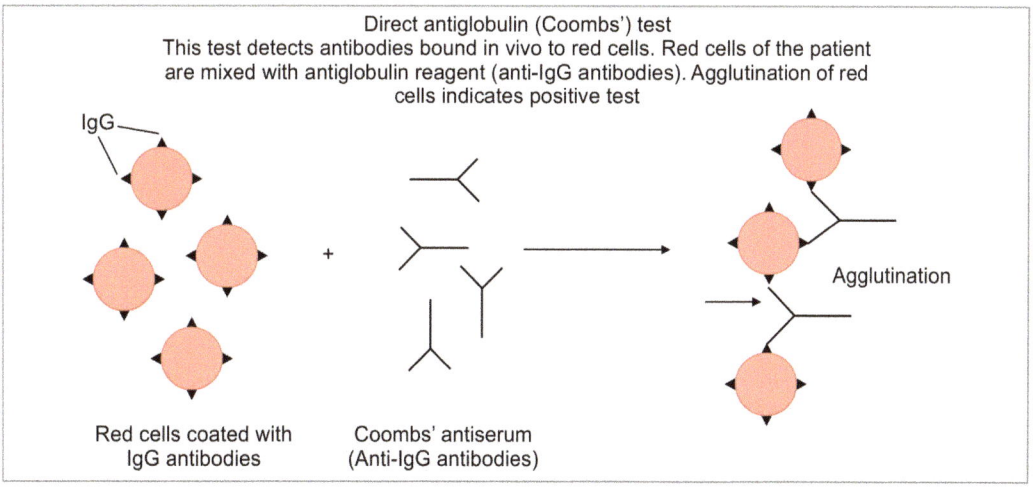

Fig. 4.48: Principle of direct antiglobulin test.

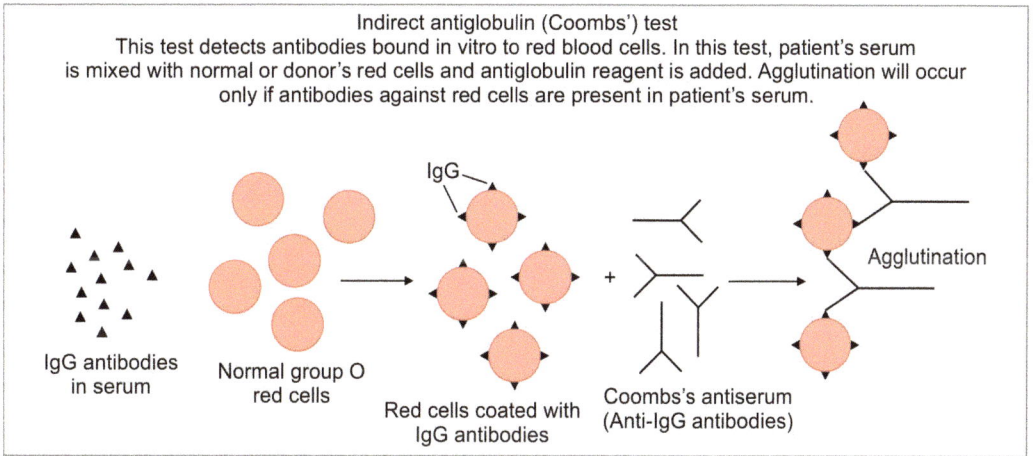

Fig. 4.49: Principle of indirect antiglobulin test.

(DAT) is used to demonstrate antibodies or the complement attached to red cells *in vivo* (Fig. 4.48). Indirect antiglobulin test (IAT) is used to demonstrate the presence of antibodies or complement in serum after sensitizing red cells in vitro (Fig. 4.49).

Diagnosis of warm-type AIHA is based on DAT. Polyspecific antiglobulin reagent consists of anti-IgG as well as anti-C3 antibodies. If red cells have been coated with IgG and/or C3 *in vivo*, then addition of polyspecific antiglobulin reagent will cause agglutination of such red cells (Fig. 4.50). If red cells show agglutination with polyspecific reagent then the test is repeated using monospecific reagents. The monospecific antisera react selectively with anti-IgG or specific complement components and thus the nature of the antibody can be identified. A negative DAT does not rule out the diagnosis of AIHA. Causes of positive DAT are shown in Box 4.17. Antiglobulin antibodies give a positive reaction when about 300 IgG molecules are bound to each red cell; if less, a negative result will be obtained. Tube method for DAT has now been replaced by gel technology or column agglutination which is simple to perform and more reliable (see Chapter 18 "Serologic and microbiologic techniques"). Indirect antiglobulin test is

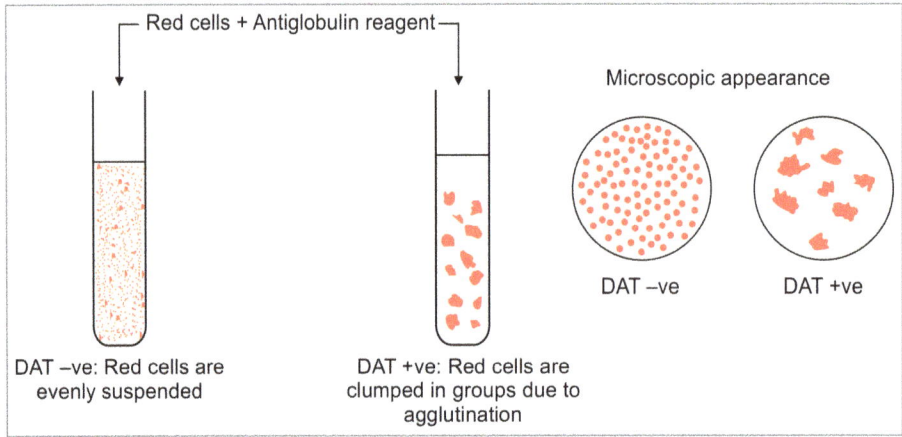

Fig. 4.50: Interpretation of antiglobulin test.

Box 4.17: Causes of positive direct antiglobulin test.
- Autoimmune hemolytic anemia
- Immune hemolytic transfusion reaction (immediate or delayed)
- Hemolytic disease of fetus and newborn
- Drug-induced immune hemolytic anemia
- Hematopoietic stem cell transplantation
- Administration of intravenous immunoglobulin, antilymphocyte globulin, or Rh immunoglobulin

Box 4.18: Laboratory diagnosis of autoimmune hemolytic anemias.
- Evidence of hemolytic anemia: Normocytic or macrocytic anemia, reticulocytosis, decreased serum haptoglobin, increased serum lactate dehydrogenase, increased serum bilirubin (indirect)
- Warm AIHA: Direct antiglobulin test positive with IgG or IgG + C3d
- Cold AIHA: Direct antiglobulin test positive with C3d only
- Primary or secondary AIHA: Clinical features, laboratory tests like bone marrow examination (for lymphoid neoplasms), antinuclear antibody test (autoimmune disorders), CT scan (for solid neoplasm)

usually not required for diagnosis of AIHA (warm or cold types), except for diagnosis of drug-induced immune hemolytic anemia.

Laboratory diagnosis of AIHA is presented in Box 4.18.

Other investigations: Search should be made for underlying disorder. OF of red cells is increased and correlates with number of spherocytes. Unconjugated serum bilirubin is elevated.

Differential Diagnosis

AIHA should be distinguished from hereditary spherocytosis that may present for the first time during adult life (positive family history and negative antiglobulin test), drug induced immune hemolytic anemia (h/o recent drug exposure) and microangiopathic hemolytic anemia (schistocytes, thrombocytopenia, and evidence of intravascular coagulation). Bite by brown recluse spider can cause a severe hemolytic anemia with spherocytes in peripheral blood and positive DAT. Hematopoietic stem cell transplant recipients (who have received ABO- or Rh-incompatible allograft) can develop AIHA due to antibodies produced by immunocompetent memory B lymphocytes from the donor. Alloimmune hemolysis should be suspected in patients with recent history of tansfusion.

Treatment

1. Underlying disease should be found and appropriately treated.
2. Majority of patients respond to corticosteroids (1 mg/kg body weight/day). Steroids inhibit macrophage phagocytosis and reduce synthesis of antibodies by spleen.
3. Splenectomy is indicated when improvement does not occur with corticosteroids. Splenectomy removes the major site of red cell destruction in AIHA.
4. Rituximab (monoclonal antibody against CD20 antigen of B lymphocytes) is another option for unresponsive cases. Other forms of treatment which may be of benefit are azathioprine, cyclophosphamide, and cyclosporine.
5. Blood transfusion: Blood transfusion is given only when absolutely essential. It is difficult to obtain serologically compatible blood because antibody in the patient's serum is a "panagglutinin" and reacts with red cells from most donors. Therefore on cross matching all the blood units are found to be incompatible.

If the patient has developed alloantibody due to previous transfusion or pregnancy then autoantibodies may conceal this alloantibody during cross matching. This may induce hemolytic transfusion reaction in the recipient. For detection of alloantibodies, autoadsorption technique is employed in which autoantibodies in the serum are removed by adsorbing them with patient's own red cells and the serum is then tested for alloantibodies.

If the autoantibody is found to have specificity against a particular blood group antigen, then blood that is deficient in the particular antigen should be used for transfusion. If specificity against a particular antigen is not detected, then a large number of group-specific blood units should be tested and the unit that is most compatible should be transfused. Smallest volume of blood necessary for maintaining oxygen carrying capacity should be transfused at a slow rate.

AUTOIMMUNE HEMOLYTIC ANEMIAS DUE TO COLD-REACTING AUTOANTIBODIES

This is caused by those autoantibodies which react with red cells maximally in cold (0–4°C) and which also retain immunologic reactivity at higher temperatures (30°C). It is of two types—cold agglutinin disease (CAD) and paroxysmal cold hemoglobinuria (PCH). The two types differ from each other in antibody class, nature of the red cell antigen, and clinical features.

Cold Agglutinin Disease

Cold-reactive antibodies or agglutinins are usually of IgM class. Polyclonal IgM cold agglutinins are present in all normal human sera in low titer and are probably formed as a result of immunologic response to infection by certain micro-organisms. Since they are present at low level, they are clinically insignificant. Increased production of polyclonal IgM cold agglutinins occurs in Epstein-Barr virus and mycoplasma infections commonly. Occasionally in large cell lymphoma, monoclonal IgM cold agglutinins are increased. In primary CAD, monoclonal (kappa) IgM cold agglutinins are found in the absence of any underlying disease. It occurs in older persons and some such patients subsequently develop B cell lymphoproliferative disorder.

Most cold agglutinins are directed against I and i antigens on red cells.

The ability of the cold agglutinins to cause significant hemolysis depends on its titer and thermal amplitude (i.e. highest temperature at which antibody can cause red cell agglutination). If the antibody is having high titer and high thermal amplitude, it will cause significant hemolysis.

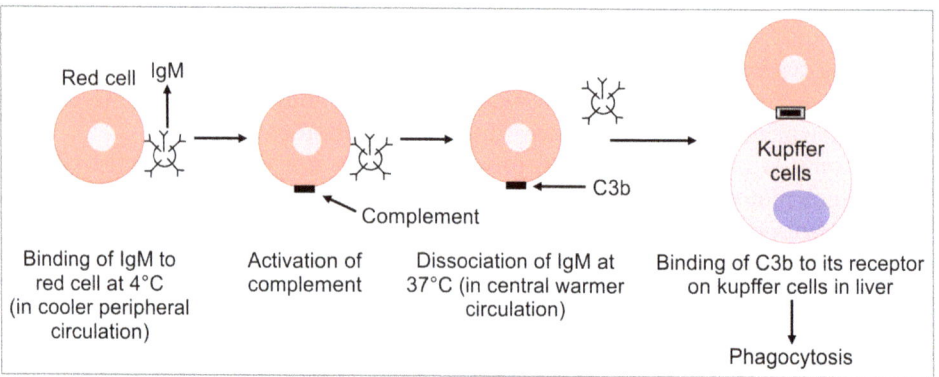

Fig. 4.51: Mechanism of hemolysis in cold-type AIHA (cold agglutinin disease).

In CAD, cold agglutinins having high thermal amplitude react with red cell antigens in cooler peripheral circulation. This leads to (i) aggregation of red cells in peripheral circulation with acrocyanosis and (ii) activation of complement via classical pathway. Complement activation stops at C3b stage due to the presence of regulatory inhibitors on red cell surface. IgM cold agglutinins dissociate from red cells in central warmer circulation, but C3b remains bound to red cells. Hemolysis of C3b-coated red cells occurs mostly in liver (Fig. 4.51). Cell-bound C3b is rapidly converted to C3dg by C3b inactivator. C3dg-coated red cells are resistant to hemolysis since macrophages do not have receptors for C3dg. In addition, complement pathway is terminated once C3dg is formed and membrane attack complex is not generated. Hemolysis in CAD therefore, is of extravascular type, and intravascular hemolysis by membrane attack complex is rare.

Clinical features: In idiopathic and lymphoma-associated CAD, two types of presentation are seen depending on thermal amplitude of the antibody. Autoantibody with high thermal amplitude causes chronic hemolysis; with low thermal amplitude autoantibody acute hemolysis develops during exposure to cold. Raynaud's phenomenon and acrocyanosis may result from blockage of cooler peripheral microvasculature by agglutination of red cells.

CAD associated with infectious disease usually develops 2 to 3 weeks after onset and causes mild and short-lived hemolysis.

Laboratory features: Anemia is commonly mild to moderate but may be severe during acute episode. Presence of cold agglutinins may be suspected from complete blood count on hematology analyzers due to spurious elevation of MCV, MCH, and MCHC by red cell agglutinates; verification is readily done by warming the blood and repeating complete blood count. Autoagglutination of red cells is a characteristic feature. It can be observed on peripheral blood smear (Fig. 4.52) and also in anticoagulated blood kept at room temperature. On warming autoagglutination disappears.

Red blood cell autoagglutination is also observed in paroxysmal cold hemoglobinuria, IgM paraproteinemia, and presence of cold agglutinins in blood.

The DAT employing anticomplement (anti-C3) reagent is positive and detects C3dg-coated red cells.

Cold-reactive autoantibodies agglutinate all red cells and therefore may cause error in blood grouping. For cell grouping blood sample should be kept at 37°C and should be washed with normal saline before testing to remove IgM autoantibodies coating red cells. A diluent

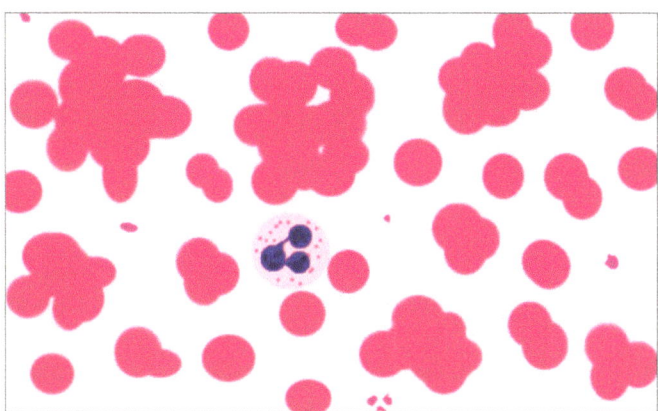

Fig. 4.52: Blood smear showing autoagglutination of red cells.

control (red cells + 6% albumin in saline) must be included. Sometimes, it may be necessary to inactivate IgM molecules by 2 mercaptoethanol before doing cell grouping. Serum grouping is usually done at 37°C or autoadsorbed serum may be employed.

IgM autoantibodies may mask the presence of alloantibody during antibody screening test and cross matching. Alloantibody screening should be carried out at 37°C; red cells should be washed with prewarmed saline and monospecific anti-IgG reagent is used. Agglutination-potentiating reagent (such as albumin) should not be used during the test procedure. Alternatively, autoadsorbed serum may be employed for identification of alloantibody.

Treatment

i. Underlying cause should be identified and treated (e.g. lymphoma).
ii. Exposure to cold should be avoided.
iii. Corticosteroids and splenectomy are not helpful.
iv. In primary disease, mainstay of treatment is rituximab.
v. Plasmapheresis to reduce circulating antibody level is a temporary measure.
vi. Transfused red cells are destroyed by cold antibodies in the same manner as patient's red cells and may sometimes precipitate acute renal failure. Therefore, transfusions should be given only when absolutely essential.

Paroxysmal Cold Hemoglobinuria (PCH)

In this rare type of AIHA, there is a sudden onset of acute intravascular hemolysis with abdominal pain, backache, pallor, and hemoglobinuria. Association with cold is usual but is not always present. Two types of PCH are distinguished: acute and chronic.

(1) Acute PCH: In children the hemolytic episode usually follows a viral infection, is self-limited and is not related to exposure to cold. (2) Chronic PCH: In older people the condition is idiopathic, follows a chronic course and is precipitated by cold. Association with syphilis is nowadays rare.

The antibody is a polyclonal IgG with specificity against P red cell antigen. IgG antibodies react with red cells and bind complement in colder peripheral circulation. On return of red cells to central warmer circulation, IgG antibodies dissociate. Formation of membrane attack complex causes lysis of red cells.

Table 4.8: Differences between warm-type AIHA, cold agglutinin disease, and paroxysmal cold hemoglobinuria.

Parameter	Warm-type AIHA	Cold agglutinin disease	Paroxysmal cold hemoglobinuria
1. Nature of antibody	IgG	IgM	IgG
2. Temperature at which antibody is maximally active	37°C	4°C	4°C
3. Mechanism of hemolysis	Opsonization	Complement-mediated	Complement-mediated
4. Site of hemolysis	Extravascular	Extravascular	Intravascular
5. Blood smear	Spherocytes	Agglutination	Agglutination, spherocytes, erythrophagocytosis
6. Direct antiglobulin test	Positive with IgG or IgG + C3d	Positive with C3d only	Positive with C3d only
7. Donath-Landsteiner test	Negative	Negative	Positive
8. Target red cell antigen	Panagglutinin	I, i	P
9. Underlying diseases	B-lymphoproliferative disorders, autoimmune disorders	B-lymphoproliferative disorders, viral infections	Syphilis, viral infections
10. Main forms of treatment in idiopathic cases	Corticosteroids, splenectomy, rituximab	Protection from cold, rituximab, chlorambucil	Supportive, rituximab

In acute PCH, hemoglobin and red cell count are severely reduced. Blood smear shows small red cell aggregates, spherocytes, prominent erythrophagocytosis by neutrophils, as well as large round vacuoles in neutrophils; occasionally red cell resetting around neutrophilos is seen.

DAT is positive during hemolytic attack due to coating of red cells with C3. Diagnosis is made by Donath–Landsteiner test. In this test, patient's serum (containing IgG antibodies and complement) is incubated with normal red cells in cold (4°C). IgG autoantibodies bind to red cells and cause hemolysis of coated red cells when temperature is raised to 37°C. The IgG autoantibody in PCH is also called as biphasic hemolysin because of this property.

Secondary PCH is self-limited and exposure to cold should be avoided. Steroids and cytotoxic therapy may be of benefit in idiopathic chronic cases.

Differences between warm-type and cold-type AIHA are listed in Table 4.8.

DRUG-INDUCED IMMUNE HEMOLYTIC ANEMIAS

Drug-induced immune hemolytic anemia may result from three mechanisms:
1. Drug adsorption on red cell membrane;
2. Immune complex or "innocent bystander" mechanism;
3. Production of autoantibodies against red cell antigens.

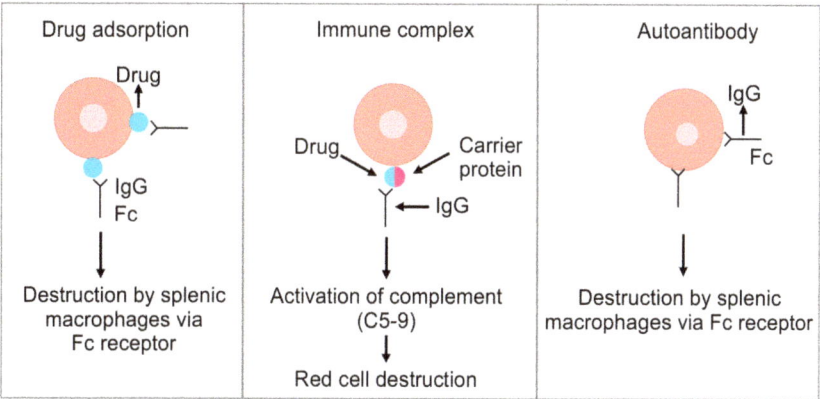

Fig. 4.53: Mechanisms of hemolysis in drug-induced hemolytic anemias.

Box 4.19: Selected drugs causing immune hemolytic anemia.
- Drug adsorption: Penicillin, ampicillin, methicillin, carbenecillin, cephalosporins
- Immune complex: Quinidine, quinine, phenacetin, hydrochlorothiazide, rifampicin, isoniazid
- Autoantibody formation: Methyldopa, mefenamic acid, L-dopa, procainamide, diclofenac, ibuprofen

Mechanisms of hemolysis in drug-induced immune hemolytic anemia are shown in Figure 4.53. Selected drugs causing drug-induced immune hemolytic anemia are shown in Box 4.19.

Drug Adsorption on Red Cell Membrane

When penicillin is given in very high doses, it binds tightly to red cell membrane proteins. If the patient has developed IgG antibody against penicillin, it reacts with the penicillin bound to the red cell membrane. The red cells to which penicillin and its IgG antibody are bound are destroyed by macrophages via Fc receptors (extravascular hemolysis). Although typically seen with penicillin, it also occurs with cephalosporins. Mild to moderate hemolysis of insidious onset usually occurs.

Direct antiglobulin test is positive with anti-IgG reagent. Antibodies in the serum and eluted from patient's red cells react *in vitro* only with red cells which are preincubated with the drug.

Immune Complex or "Innocent Bystander" Mechanism

The offending drug when introduced into the body serves as a hapten and binds to a plasma protein carrier to form hapten-protein carrier complex. This elicits formation of antibodies (IgM or IgG). When re-exposure to the drug occurs, antigen-antibody immune complexes are formed. These immune complexes nonspecifically bind to the erythrocyte membranes, activate complement, and cause red cell destruction.

Patient usually experiences a severe hemolytic episode with hemoglobinemia and hemoglobinuria; renal failure may occur. Direct antiglobulin test is positive with anticomplement reagent. Indirect antiglobulin test is positive only when patient's serum is preincubated with the drug in solution (to allow formation of immune complexes) and then tested against normal red cells. Eluate from the red cells is nonreactive. The prototype drug causing hemolysis by this mechanism is quinidine; other less commonly implicated drugs include—quinine, phenacetin, hydrochlorothiazide, etc.

Production of Autoantibodies against Red Cell Antigens

α methyldopa (an antihypertensive drug) induces the formation of autoantibodies reactive against the red cell antigens (but not against the drug). Possibly, the drug in some manner alters the red cell membrane antigen so that it is recognized as foreign. Alternatively, the drug may inhibit the suppressor T lymphocytes resulting in loss of control over B-lymphocytes and production of autoantibodies. About 10 to 15% of patients who are receiving α methyldopa develop autoantibodies and 0.5 to 1% develop hemolytic anemia. Direct antiglobulin test is positive due to coating of red cells with IgG antibodies; complement is rarely demonstrated on red cells. IgG antibodies in serum react with red cells in the absence of the drug. The results of direct and indirect antiglobulin tests resemble those seen in warm antibody autoimmune hemolytic anemia.

Mild to moderate hemolytic anemia usually develops due to destruction of red cells coated with IgG in spleen. Other drugs that are implicated are L-dopa, mefenamic acid, procainamide, diclofenac, etc.

Treatment: The responsible drug should be stopped. Red cell transfusions may be required if anemia is severe.

HEMOLYTIC DISEASE OF THE FETUS AND NEWBORN

Hemolytic disease of the fetus and newborn (HDFN) is a disease in which destruction of red cells of the fetus or newborn occurs due to the passage of maternal antibodies across the placenta into the fetal circulation. The production of these maternal antibodies is stimulated due to blood group incompatibility between mother and the fetus.

This disease develops if the red cell antigens inherited by the fetus from father are foreign to the mother. Leakage of fetal red cells into the maternal circulation induces formation of antibodies; these antibodies pass across the placenta into the fetal circulation and cause hemolysis of fetal red cells. Only IgG antibodies against red cell antigens can cause HDFN since antibodies only of IgG class can traverse the placental barrier. The main red cell antigens responsible for HDFN are:
- RhD
- Rhc
- Kell
- A and B

HDFN due to anti-RhD, anti-c, and anti-Kell can cause severe fetal hemolytic anemia. HDFN due to ABO incompatibility is usually a mild disease.

Maternal and fetal blood group in compatibilities associated with HDFN are shown in Table 4.9.

Chapter 4: Anemias due to Excessive Red Cell Destruction

Table 4.9: Maternal and fetal blood group incompatibilities associated with HDFN.

Blood group system	Maternal blood group	Fetal blood group	Severity of HDFN
1. ABO	O	A	Mild
	O	B	Mild
2. Rh	C−	C+	Mild to severe
	D−	D+	Mild to severe
	E−	E+	Mild to severe
	c−	c+	Mild to severe
	e−	e+	Mild to severe
3. Kell	K−	K+	Mild to severe
4. Kidd	Jk(a−)	Jk(a+)	Mild to severe
	Jk(b−)	Jk(b+)	Mild to severe
5. Duffy	Fy(a−)	Fy(a+)	Mild to severe
6. MNS	M−	M+	Moderate to severe
	S−	S+	Moderate to severe

Note: Most cases of severe HDFN are associated with D, c, and K alloantibodies.

Rh HEMOLYTIC DISEASE OF THE FETUS AND NEWBORN

Pathogenesis

Rh HDFN develops when a Rh-negative mother who is previously sensitized to the RhD antigen carries a RhD-positive fetus. The usual causes of sensitization of Rh-negative mother to D antigen are previous pregnancy or past RhD-positive blood transfusion. During pregnancy most common cause of maternal immunization is fetomaternal hemorrhage that occurs at the time of separation of placenta during delivery. Other causes of primary immunization during pregnancy are listed in Box 4.20.

Fetomaternal hemorrhage induces primary immune response consisting of IgM antibodies. Because IgM antibodies do not cross the placenta and sensitization occurs during labor, Rh HDFN does not develop during first pregnancy. During the second and following pregnancies with Rh-positive fetus, a slight fetomaternal leak can induce a strong and rapid secondary IgG immune response. IgG anti-D antibodies cross the placenta and bind to RhD-positive red cells of the fetus. The IgG-coated red cells are destroyed by macrophages in the spleen (opsonization) (Fig. 4.54). Excessive destruction of red cells leads to anemia, compensatory erythroid hyperplasia in bone marrow, erythroblastosis in peripheral blood, and extramedullary erythropoiesis in liver and spleen. Unconjugated bilirubin in the fetal circulation crosses the placenta and is metabolized by maternal liver. After birth, unconjugated bilirubin in the neonate increases markedly due to

Box 4.20: Causes of primary immunization to blood group antigens in females of reproductive age group.

- Previous pregnancy
- Abortion
- Medical termination of pregnancy
- Amniocentesis
- Chorion villus biopsy
- Cordocentesis
- Ruptured ectopic pregnancy
- Accidental hemorrhage
- Abdominal trauma
- Lower segment caesarean section
- External cephalic version
- Previous blood transfusion

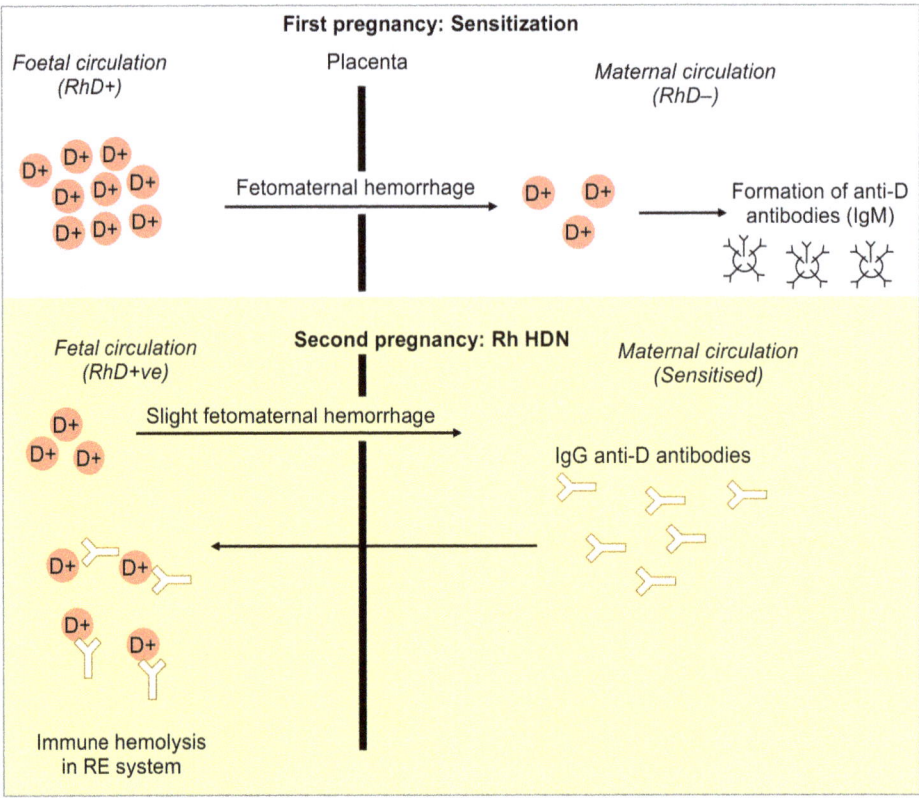

Fig. 4.54: Pathogenesis of RhD hemolytic disease of newborn.

immaturity of the glucuronyl transferase enzyme, and may cross the blood-brain barrier and damage the basal ganglia (kernicterus).

Some factors influence the production of anti-D antibodies by the RhD-negative mother. One of the major factors is **amount of fetomaternal hemorrhage**. The larger the fetomaternal bleed, the greater the risk of sensitization. For induction of secondary immune response, a very small leak may be sufficient. **ABO incompatibility** between mother and fetus reduces the risk of sensitization to RhD antigen. This is because when ABO incompatible fetal red cells enter the maternal circulation they are rapidly coated by maternal anti-A or anti-B and removed by macrophages before sensitization to RhD can occur.

Zygosity of the father decides the Rh status of the child. If father is homozygous (DD) then all his offsprings will be RhD-positive; if he is a heterozygous (Dd), then there is a 50% chance in every pregnancy of child being Rh-positive or Rh-negative.

HDFN associated with anti-Kell antibodies: The Kell antigens on erythroid cells develop early in gestation. The mechanism of fetal anemia due to anti-Kell antibodies involves destruction of sensitized red cells as well as suppression of early fetal red cell precursors by anti-Kell antibodies. There is reticulocytopenia instead of reticulocytosis. The severity is similar to that due to anti-D antibodies.

Clinical Features

Clinical presentation is variable. There may be only mild anemia and jaundice. In some cases, there is severe unconjugated hyperbilirubinemia (icterus gravis neonatorum). Jaundice is rapidly progressive and develops within 24 hours of birth. Damage to basal ganglia leads to kernicterus, which may be fatal or may cause neurological deficit. In its most severe form, Rh HDFN manifests as fresh stillbirth or as hydrops fetalis. Most of the hydropic fetuses perish in utero; if the hydropic infant has live birth, it shows severe anemia, hepatosplenomegaly, ascites, and anasarca.

The disease should be differentiated from hemolytic anemias that manifest in the newborns (Box 4.21).

> **Box 4.21:** Hemolytic anemias manifesting in the newborn period.
>
> - Hemolytic disease of fetus and newborn: Rh, ABO, minor antigens (Kell, Duffy, Kidd, MNS, Lutheran, Lewis, Kidd)
> - Infections
> - Microangiopathic hemolytic anemia in disseminated intravascular coagulation
> - Glucose-6-phosphate dehydrogenase deficiency
> - Hereditary spherocytosis
> - Hereditary elliptocytosis, pyropoikilocytosis
> - Hemoglobin H disease
> - Homozygous α thalassemia

Laboratory Features

Antenatal Investigations

Antenatal investigations are carried out to detect pregnant women with high risk of hemolytic disease developing in the fetus.

A. *Maternal investigations*
   1. Clinical history: Mothers having similar previous childbirth need careful supervision. Various possible causes of previous sensitization should be identified such as Rh-positive blood transfusion, medical termination of pregnancy, abortion, ectopic pregnancy, etc.
   2. Blood grouping: ABO and Rh typing should be done. Test for weak D antigen in the mother is not required as per current guidelines.
   3. Antibody detection: Antenatal testing for antibody detection is done to (1) identify RhD-negative women who will require Rh immune globulin, and (2) to identify women who have antibodies which can cause HDFN. Therefore antibody detection needs to be performed in all pregnant women on first antenatal check-up irrespective of their Rh status. It is done in the first trimester. Indirect Coombs' test employing two different group O screening cell panels should be used for antibody screening. If antibodies are detected, then they should be identified with the help of cells, the antigen make up of which is known. Antibody titer should be checked every month. A critical titer is defined as titer with a significant risk of fetal hydrops. Most institutes consider titer of 1:32 as critical (Box 4.22). A titer of 1:32 or more and an increasing titer on subsequent testing are reasons for fetal surveillance and/or amniocentesis.

> **Box 4.22:** Antenatal laboratory testing of women at risk of developing HDFN
>
> - First trimester: ABO grouping and RhD typing, antibody screening and identification, antibody titration to establish baseline level
> - Follow-up: Repeat antibody titration every 2–4 weeks (if antibody was identified).
>
> Note: Titer of 1:16 or 1:32 is considered as significant.

B. *Blood grouping of the father:* Father's ABO and Rh grouping should be done. ABO grouping helps in knowing the likely blood group of the fetus and also the chance of ABO incompatibility between the mother and the fetus. If the fetus is ABO-compatible then the risk of alloimmunization of the mother is more.

C. *Paternal zygosity testing:* If a significant alloantibody is detected in the mother or if there is a previous history of HDFN, fetal risk of HDFN can be initially assessed from paternal zygosity testing. If father is homozygous for the antigen in question, there is 100% risk of HDFN. If father is heterozygous, risk is 50% and further testing is required like noninvasive molecular typing of cell-free fetal DNA.

Paternal zygosity can be determined serologically for all blood groups implicated to cause HDFN except RhD; this is because there is no "d" antigen and there is no "anti-d" antibody since it represents a gene deletion. Quantitative polymerase chain reaction is available commercially to detect the number of copies of *D* gene. This technique consists of amplification of exons 5 and 7 of *RHD* gene and exon 7 of *RHCE* gene (*RHCE* gene is always present as two copies in all individuals and thus serves as an internal control). RHD-negative (d/d), homozygous RHD-positive (D/D), and heterozygous RHD-positive (D/d) can be determined from PCR products on automated sequencer.

D. *Fetal investigations:* Severity of hemolysis in the fetus is assessed by measuring the concentration of bilirubin in amniotic fluid or in fetal blood. Severity of hemolysis is also judged from previous obstetric history and maternal anti-D titer. This will help identify at risk RhD+ve fetus early in pregnancy.
   i. Amniocentesis: Amniocentesis is indicated in following situations:
      - Maternal anti-D titer of 1:32
      - Rising anti-D titer on follow-up testing
      - Bad obstetric history in Rh-negative mother (previous severely affected offspring).

   Amniotic fluid is obtained under ultrasound guidance by introducing a long needle through the abdominal wall into the uterine cavity. It is done between 28 and 32 weeks of pregnancy if there is no history of previously affected baby. If such previous history is present, then it should be done 10 weeks prior to the date of previous fetal or neonatal death. Repeat amniocentesis may be done after 2 weeks to establish whether bilirubin is rising.

   Amniotic fluid bilirubin is measured spectrophotometrically and shows peak absorbance at 450 nm. The degree of absorption at 450 nm (i.e. difference in optical density between baseline and peak of elevation) is a precise reflection of the amount of bilirubin; it is denoted as $\Delta A\ 450$.

   Level of bilirubin in amniotic fluid depends on the period of gestation. Liley's chart relates degree of absorption at 450 nm ($\Delta A\ 450$) to gestational age on a semilogarithmic graph paper. This chart is used for prediction of severity of HDFN and is divided into three zones: I (low), II (middle), and III (high). Values falling within zone III indicate severely affected fetus with imminent death. Therapy is based on gestational age or fetal maturity: intrauterine transfusion (<34 weeks) or delivery (>34 weeks). Values within zone II need observation in the form of repeated amniocentesis. Depending on the result, fetus may need intrauterine transfusion or early delivery. Before induction of early delivery, it is necessary to determine fetal lung maturity by lecithin/sphingomyelin (L/S) ratio on amniotic fluid; value > 2.0 is considered as evidence of lung maturity. The risk of respiratory distress syndrome is increased if ratio is < 2.0. Values in zone I indicate unaffected fetus and pregnancy may be continued till term.

ii. *Cordocentesis (Percutaneous umbilical blood sampling):* In this technique, under continuous ultrasound guidance, umbilical vein near the site of placental insertion is punctured and blood sample is withdrawn. Fetal blood obtained from cord blood vessel is used for assessing severity of hemolysis by estimating hemoglobin and bilirubin concentrations. Blood grouping and direct antiglobulin test can also be done. This technique is also used for direct intravascular transfusion of the fetus and for red cell genotyping by molecular methods to determine if an antigen is present on red cells. Fetal loss with this technique is reported to be 1 to 2%.
iii. Other techniques for fetal monitoring are fetal ultrasound (for determining fetal size and organomegaly) and Doppler ultrasonography of fetal middle cerebral artery peak systolic velocity or MCA-PSV (for predicting fetal hemoglobin or anemia). With increasing fetal anemia, blood flow velocity (MCV-PSV) increases due to the rise in cardiac output and vasodilatation; this measurement is specific for gestational age. This technique is replacing the amniotic fluid spectrophotometry for fetal monitoring.
iv. *Noninvasive molecular typing of fetal DNA extracted from maternal plasma:* Circulating cell-free fetal DNA or cff-DNA (from apoptotic placental trophoblast) can be identified in maternal plasma near the end of first trimester which gradually increases in amount in subsequent weeks. From this, fetal *RHD* genotype can be determined. This technique is being commonly used in developed countries. Genotyping can assist in predicting the risk of HDFN if a maternal antibody is present. Also, if the corresponding fetal antigen is absent for the maternal antibody, it can potentially avoid cordocentesis or amniocentesis.

Investigations of Newborn

Following investigations are done on the cord blood of the newborn:
1. *Blood grouping:* ABO grouping in the newborn rests solely on cell grouping since antibodies in the blood are passively acquired from the mother. Wharton's jelly of the umbilical cord may cause agglutination of red cells and therefore red cells should be washed thoroughly to avoid erroneous result. If cord blood is collected using syringe and needle, contamination with Wharton's jelly is avoided and additional washing is not needed. All infants born to D-negative mothers should be tested for D antigen and weak D antigen. This is because RhD-negative mothers with D+ or weak D+ babies should receive Rh immune globulin (RhIg). Care is needed when interpreting RhD typing on cord blood or newborn's blood sample since both false-positive and false-negative results may be obtained. If red cells of the newborn are heavily coated with anti-D antibody, false negative result may be obtained due to blocking of the D antigen sites by the antibody; red cells should be washed many times with warm saline and retested. A false-positive test may occur if weak D testing is done on red cells coated with anti-D antibodies.
2. *Blood smear:* In Rh HDFN, blood smear will show markedly increased number of nucleated red cells (erythroblastosis) and polychromasia (reticulocytosis) (Fig. 4.55).
3. *Direct antiglobulin test:* This is strongly reactive in the newborn. Positive DAT is indicative of incompatibility between red cell antigens of the fetus and antibodies in the mother. If DAT is positive, specificity of the antibody can be determined using mother's serum.
4. *Determination of hemoglobin and bilirubin concentrations:* These parameters are helpful in assessing the severity of the disease. Cord blood hemoglobin value of less than 12.0 g/dL or indirect bilirubin more than 5 mg/dL is an indication for immediate exchange transfusion.

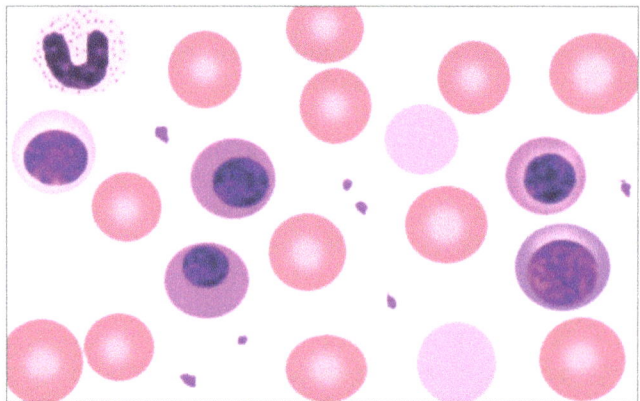

Fig. 4.55: Blood smear in Rh hemolytic disease of newborn showing many erythroblasts and polychromatic cells.

Postdelivery Maternal Investigations

After delivery, maternal investigations include repeat ABO and RhD grouping (to decide need for Rh immune globulin, or if ABO HDFN is suspected), antibody screening (by indirect antiglobulin test) and identification, rosette test, Kleihauer–Betke test (see later), and flow cytometry to assess amount of fetomaternal hemorrhage to determine dose of Rh immune globulin.

Rosette test: This is a qualitative screening test for fetomaternal hemorrhage in which maternal anticoagulated blood sample (collected within 1 hour of delivery), anti-D, and D-positive indicator cells are mixed. Anti-D gets attached to D+ve fetal red cells (if present) in the maternal sample. Indicator cells (that are D+ red cells) get attached to the free arm of the anti-D molecules that have bound to fetal red cells. The indicator cells surround antibody-coated fetal cells in the form of rosettes and indicate fetomaternal hemorrhage. This test is positive if about 10 mL of RhD+ve fetal red cells are present in the maternal circulation. If rosette test is positive, either Kleihauer–Betke test or flow cytometry analysis is done to quantify fetomaternal hemorrhage.

Flow cytometry: This is a more precise method for quantification of fetomaternal hemorrhage than Kleihauer–Betke test. Two methods are in use: anti-HbF method (detection and quantification of HbF-containing fetal red cells by anti-HbF monoclonal antibodies) and anti-D method (detection and quantification of D antigen positive fetal red cells by monoclonal antibodies).

Treatment

Fetus

If measurement of ΔA 450 indicates a severely affected fetus, then nature of treatment depends upon the maturity of the fetus. Fetal lung maturity is most commonly assessed by measuring lecithin/sphingomyelin (L/S) ratio in the amniotic fluid. L/S ratio more than 2:1 indicates fetal lung maturity. In severely affected fetus with L/S ratio > 2:1, prompt delivery is indicated; if L/S ratio indicates fetal lung immaturity, then intrauterine fetal transfusions should be given. Intrauterine fetal transfusion may be either intraperitoneal or intravascular. Packed red cells of

O Rh-negative blood group, which are compatible with mother's serum, are given. Blood to be transfused should be fresh (<5 days old). Leukocyte-poor and irradiated blood is preferred to prevent the development of alloantibodies against leukocytes and platelets in the mother, and for prevention of cytomegalovirus infection and graft-versus-host disease in the fetus. Severely affected fetuses may be transfused at 2 to 4 weeks intervals. Following this treatment, delivery is carried out at 36 weeks.

Neonate

Exchange transfusion: Rapidly rising bilirubin concentration in the neonate is associated with the danger of kernicterus. In newborns (especially in premature infants), breakdown products of hemolysis cannot be metabolized due to immaturity of the liver. Kernicterus is more likely in the presence of prematurity, septicemia, hypoxia, acidosis, hypoglycemia, and hypoproteinemia. Exchange transfusion removes antibody-coated red cells, bilirubin, and IgG anti-D antibodies from the plasma, and also corrects anemia. An exchange transfusion equal to twice the newborn's blood volume is ideal. In exchange transfusion, a small amount of patient's blood is withdrawn and replaced by equal amount of donor blood at a time (2–3 mL/kg/min). Blood for exchange transfusion should be fresh (<5 days old). Donor red cells should be cross-matched against mother's serum because any alloantibodies in the neonatal serum are derived from the mother and in the mother's serum they are more in number. If ABO blood groups of the mother and baby are identical then RhD-negative blood of the same ABO group is used. If blood groups of the mother and baby are different then O Rh-negative blood should be used.

At birth, cord blood hemoglobin concentration less than 12 g/dL and cord blood unconjugated bilirubin more than 5 mg/dL are indications for exchange transfusion. Rate of rise of unconjugated bilirubin more than 0.5 mg/dL/h is also considered by some as an indication for exchange transfusion.

Adjunctive therapy: **Phototherapy** (exposure of neonate to fluorescent blue light in the 420–475 nm range) causes unconjugated bilirubin to be converted (photoisomerization) into a soluble form that is excreted in urine and bile. **Infusion of albumin** binds free bilirubin in plasma and thus decreases the risk of kernicterus. Both phototherapy and albumin help in reducing the need for exchange transfusion.

Prevention of Rh Immunization

For prevention of immunization of Rh-negative mother against D antigen, Rh immune globulin (RhIg) is administered. It must be given before primary immunization has occurred. The mode of action of RhIg is not known. IgG anti-D in RhIg coat the D-positive fetal red cells that may have entered maternal circulation and probably blocks the antigen recognition by the immune system.

RhIg consists of IgG anti-D antibodies and is prepared from pooled plasma of donors who have high levels of anti-D antibodies. For prevention of Rh HDFN, it can be administered in different ways:
- *After delivery*: All RhD-ve women are given RhIg within 72 hours of delivery of RhD+ve infant. The usual dose is 300 mcg (1500 IU) in the USA given intramuscularly which neutralizes up to 15 mL of fetal red cells or 30 mL of whole blood (which is the usual amount of fetomaternal hemorrhage). If a larger fetomaternal leak is suspected, a maternal blood sample is taken within 1 to 2 hours of delivery to determine the amount of fetal red cells by acid elution test

of Kleihauer–Betke or flow cytometry. Principle of this test is outlined earlier in "Disorders of hemoglobin—General features and approach to diagnosis." RhD+ve red cells can also be quantitated by flow cytometry. Depending on the amount of fetomaternal hemorrhage, further RhIg can be administered.
- *During antenatal period*: All RhD-ve pregnant women are given 300 mcg of RhIg intramuscularly at 28 and 34 weeks of gestation. If infant is RhD+ve, anti-RhIg is also given following delivery.
- *Following sensitizing event during pregnancy*: RhIg is given to Rh-ve women if there is a potentially sensitizing event such as abortion, antepartum hemorrhage, abdominal trauma, external cephalic version, stillbirth, caesarean section, ectopic pregnancy, multiple pregnancy, amniocentesis, cordocentesis, and chorion villus biopsy. RhIg is given in the dose of 50 mcg intramuscularly (before 20 weeks of gestation) or 100 mcg intramuscularly (after 20 weeks).

ABO HEMOLYTIC DISEASE OF NEWBORN

Hemolytic disease of newborn due to ABO incompatibility is more common than Rh HDFN (because of low frequency of RhD-ve women in the population) and is usually a mild disease. Unlike Rh HDFN, ABO HDFN does not present *in utero* and does not cause hydrops fetalis. There is no correlation between the titer of antibodies in the mother and occurrence of HDFN. Therefore, monitoring of anti-ABO antibodies during pregnancy is not necessary. It usually develops when blood group of the mother is O and that of the fetus is A or B and when maternal high titer IgG anti-A and anti-B antibodies are present (>1:64 titer). Less commonly it results when blood group of the mother is A or B and that of the fetus is, respectively, B or A.

IgG anti-A and anti-B antibodies are naturally occurring and therefore ABO HDFN can occur in first as well as in subsequent pregnancies. The mild nature of ABO HDFN is probably related to the neutralization of anti-A and anti-B antibodies by tissue A and B antigens and also by soluble A or B substances. Incomplete expression of A and B antigens on fetal red cells also plays a role.

Differences between Rh and ABO hemolytic disease of the newborn are outlined in Table 4.10. The usual clinical manifestations are mild anemia and jaundice within 24 hours of birth. Severe anemia and kernicterus are rare.

Peripheral blood smear examination shows spherocytosis in ABO HDFN (but not in Rh HDFN) (Fig. 4.56). Blood group of the mother is O and that of the infant is A or B. Direct antiglobulin test in the infant is either negative or weakly positive. This is because of (1) weak expression of ABO antigens on red cells of newborn, and (2) neutralization of most of the IgG antibodies by tissue A and B antigens and by soluble A and B substances in the fetus so that very few antibodies remain for binding to red cells. Eluate from cord red cells will react against A or B red cells (but not against O cells) in indirect antiglobulin test.

Blood hemoglobin and bilirubin should be estimated to assess the severity of hemolysis and need for exchange transfusion.

Management usually consists of phototherapy and supportive measures. In severe hyperbilirubinemia, exchange transfusion may be necessary to prevent development of kernicterus. For exchange transfusion, group O blood with same RhD type as the neonate and which is lacking in high titer hemolytic IgG antibodies should be selected. It should be cross-matched against mother's serum.

Chapter 4: Anemias due to Excessive Red Cell Destruction

Table 4.10: Differences between Rh and ABO hemolytic disease of the newborn.

	Parameter	Rh HDFN	ABO HDFN
1.	Frequency	Less common	More common
2.	Blood group – Mother – Fetus	 Rh negative Rh positive	 O A or B
3.	Pregnancy affected	Usually second	Usually first
4.	Severity	Usually severe	Usually mild
5.	Blood smear	Erythroblastosis	Spherocytosis
6.	Direct antiglobulin test	Strongly positive	Weakly positive or negative
7.	Prevention	Rh immune globulin	Not available
8.	Stillbirth or hydrops	Common	Rare
9.	Jaundice	Marked	Mild
10.	Hepatosplenomegaly	Marked	Mild
11.	Antenatal monitoring	Required	Not required

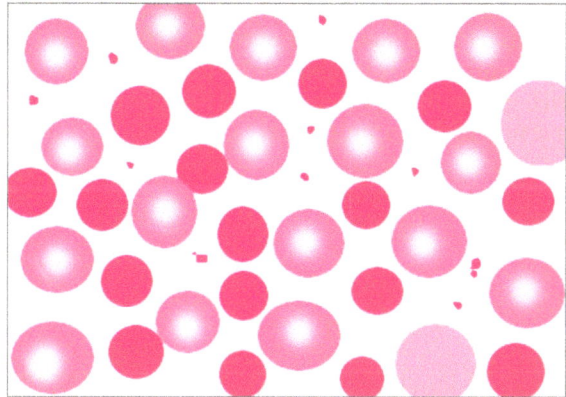

Fig. 4.56: Blood smear in ABO hemolytic disease of newborn showing numerous microspherocytes.

PAROXYSMAL NOCTURNAL HEMOGLOBINURIA

Paroxysmal nocturnal hemoglobinuria (PNH) is a rare (estimated prevalence of 2-6 per million) acquired hematopoietic stem cell disorder characterized by abnormal sensitivity of red cells to hemolytic action of complement. White cells and platelets also show similar defect. Typically, red cell destruction occurs at night so that hemoglobinuria is noticed in the first-voided urine in the morning. However, presentation is varied, e.g. iron deficiency anemia due to hemosiderinuria, pancytopenia, aplastic anemia, chronic intravascular hemolytic anemia, or repeated venous thromboses.

PATHOGENESIS

PNH is a clonal disorder characterized by expansion of defective hematopoietic stem cell. The defective stem cell in PNH gives rise to red cells, white cells, and platelets, which are abnormally sensitive to complement. The defective stem cell can arise on the background of abnormal marrow such as aplastic anemia. Both the defective and the normal clones coexist in varying proportions. Depending on the degree of sensitivity to complement, three different types of red cells are found in PNH:

- **PNH I:** Red cells with normal sensitivity to complement;
- **PNH II:** Red cells with intermediate sensitivity to complement-mediated lysis
- **PNH III:** Red cells with marked sensitivity to complement-mediated lysis.

Many patients have both PNH II and PNH III red cells. The severity of hemolysis depends on the number of PNH III red cells: mild hemolysis occurs when less than 20% PNH III red cells are present, and chronic hemolysis results when these exceed 50%.

In PNH, the abnormal sensitivity of red cells to the lytic action of complement is due to an intrinsic abnormality of red cells. In PNH, many cell membrane proteins are deficient; the most significant being (1) decay accelerating factor (DAF, CD 55) and (2) membrane inhibitor of reactive lysis (MIRL, CD 59). DAF is an inhibitor of C3 convertase, while MIRL inhibits the membrane attack complex (C5–9). Normally *in vivo*, small amount of C3b is being continuously generated via alternate complement pathway by C3 convertase (C3bBb), some of which also binds to red cell membranes. In the presence of DAF, C3bBb is inactivated and subsequent formation of membrane attack complex does not occur. The main role of MIRL is prevention of interaction between C8 and C9 thus inhibiting the formation of membrane attack complex (Fig. 4.57). Thus, in PNH, due to the deficiency of DAF and especially of MIRL, cells are more susceptible to the lytic action of the complement.

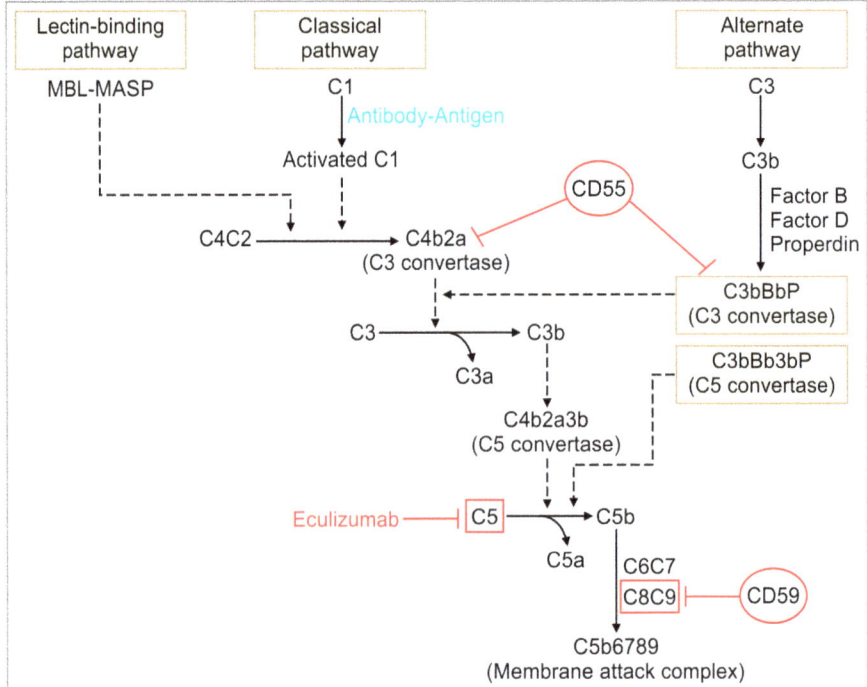

Fig. 4.57: Complement activation and roles of CD55 and CD59 in its regulation.

In addition to the deficiencies of CD 55 and CD 59, deficiencies of some other proteins also occur in PNH (Box 4.23). Normally, all these proteins are anchored to the cell membrane by a phospholipid called as glycosylphosphatidylinositol (GPI) (Figs. 4.58A and B). In PNH, GPI anchor is nonfunctional because of an acquired somatic mutation of the X-linked gene called as phosphatidylinositol glycan class A (PIG-A) in a hematopoietic stem cell. This leads to the deficiency of multiple proteins on cell membrane. About 200 different mutations of PIG-A gene have been reported.

For unknown reasons, the defective or mutated hematopoietic stem cell has proliferative advantage. The abnormal stem cell produces cells that are deficient in DAF

> **Box 4.23:** Some GPI-anchored cell surface proteins deficient in paroxysmal nocturnal hemoglobinuria
> - **All blood cells**: CD55 (Decay accelerating factor), CD59 (Membrane inhibitor of reactive lysis), CD58 (Lymphocyte function-associated antigen-3)
> - **All leukocytes**: CD48 (B-lymphocyte activation marker BLAST-1)
> - **Red blood cells**: Acetylcholinesterase
> - **Granulocytes, monocytes**: CD14 (Monocyte differentiation antigen), CD87 (Urokinase-type plasminogen activator receptor)
> - **Granulocytes, Natural killer cells:** CD16b (Low affinity Fc receptor for IgG)
> - **Granulocytes, B lymphocytes:** CD24 (Signal transducer)
> - **Granulocytes**: Neutrophil alkaline phosphatase, CD66b (Carcinoembryonic antigen-related cell adhesion molecule 8)
> - **Lymphocytes, Monocytes**: CD52 (CAMPATH-1 antigen)
> - **B and T lymphocytes**: CD73 (Ecto-5′ nucleotidase)
> - **Myeloid and erythroid cells**: Folate receptor
> - **Activated platelets and T lymphocytes**: CD109 (150 kDa TGF-beta-1-binding protein, platelet-specific Gov antigen)

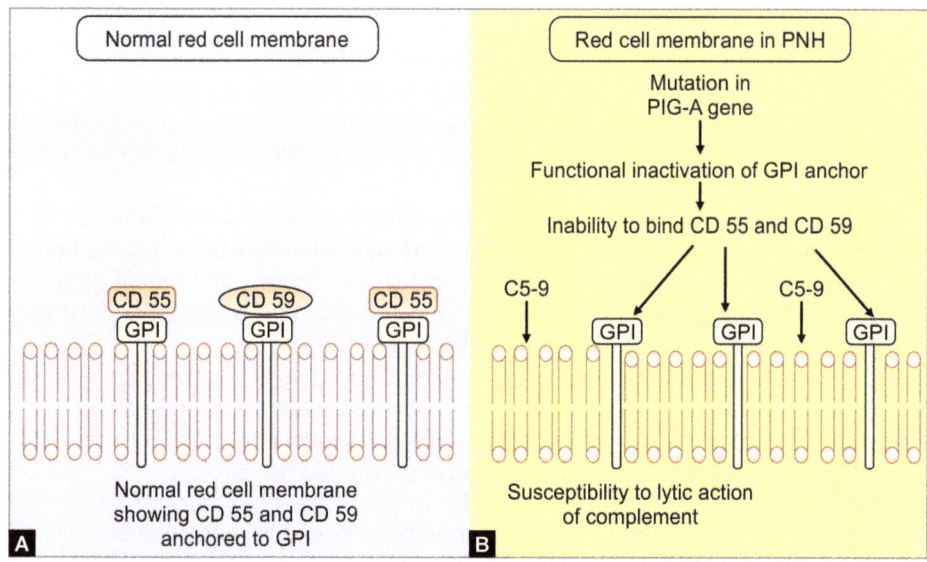

Figs. 4.58A and B: Red cell membrane in normal individuals (A) and in PNH (B).

Table 4.11: Classification of paroxysmal nocturnal hemoglobinuria (International PNH Interest Group, 2005).

Classic PNH	Severe intravascular hemolysis; cellular marrow with erythroid hyperplasia; large PNH clones
PNH in the setting of another specific bone marrow disorder	Mild to moderate intravascular hemolysis; evidence of another specific bone marrow disorder (aplastic anemia, myelodysplastic syndrome); moderate-sized PNH clones
Subclinical PNH	No evidence of intravascular hemolysis; evidence of another specific bone marrow disorder (aplastic anemia, myelodysplastic syndrome); small PNH clones detected by flow cytometry

activity, thus confirming PNH as a clonal disorder. Red cells, platelets, and neutrophils are abnormally sensitive to complement and patients have anemia, granulocytopenia, and thrombocytopenia.

Classification of PNH proposed by International PNH Interest Group is shown in Table 4.11.

CLINICAL FEATURES

The characteristic triad of PNH consists of intravascular hemolysis, pancytopenia due to bone marrow failure, and predisposition to thrombosis. Although it can occur at any age, PNH usually presents during the 3rd or 4th decade of life with features of chronic hemolytic anemia: weakness, pallor, and mild jaundice. Mild to moderate splenomegaly is present in some cases. Nocturnal hemoglobinuria (passage of reddish-brown urine after getting up in the morning) occurs in only a minority of the cases; it is due to increased hemolysis during sleep (mild respiratory acidosis during sleep due to carbon dioxide retention increases complement binding to red cells) and is not related to the time of the day. Hemosiderinuria, however, is a constant feature and leads to iron deficiency anemia.

Recurrent venous thrombosis is a common feature and probably results from activation of platelets due to complement-mediated damage with subsequent aggregation. Budd–Chiari syndrome due to hepatic vein thrombosis is a classical feature and runs a rapidly fatal course. Abdominal pain is a common complaint and may be related to thrombosis of mesenteric veins. Thrombosis of deep veins of limbs can occur.

Severe hemolysis and thrombosis typically occur in patients with large PNH clones.

Release of large amounts of free hemoglobin in circulation (due to intravascular hemolysis) results in nitric oxide scavenging (depletion). This leads to fatigue, abdominal pain, smooth muscle dystonia (esophageal spasm and dysphagia, erectile dysfunction), and thrombosis. These features are more common in patients with large PNH clones.

Bleeding (due to thrombocytopenia) and infections (due to neutropenia or impaired chemotaxis) are other common features. Thrombosis is the main cause of death.

Some cases of PNH terminate in acute myeloblastic leukemia.

Diagnosis is often delayed since presentation of PNH is heterogeneous.

Clinical features in PNH result from intravascular hemolysis, anemia, bone marrow failure, and thrombosis.

LABORATORY FEATURES

Peripheral Blood Examination

The usual manifestation of PNH is pancytopenia. Anemia is moderate to severe. If iron deficiency is present, red cells are microcytic and hypochromic. Reticulocyte count is raised.

Urine Examination

Hemoglobinuria (excretion of free hemoglobin in urine) develops when plasma haptoglobin cannot bind any more hemoglobin. Some amount of hemoglobin is reabsorbed in proximal renal tubular epithelial cells where hemoglobin iron is stored as ferritin or hemosiderin. When these cells are shed in urine, hemosiderinuria results. Hemoglobinuria is detected by benzidine or orthotoluidine test on urine sample and hemosiderinuria by Prussian blue staining of urinary sediment (Figs. 4.59A and B). Hemoglobinuria is intermittent or mild, while hemosiderinuria is a constant feature, indicating chronic intravascular hemolysis.

Complement-based Assays

These demonstrate unusual sensitivity of PNH red cells to the hemolytic action of complement. These tests are mainly of historic interest and have been replaced by flow cytometric analysis.

Sucrose Hemolysis Test (Sugar Water Test)

This is the standard screening test. In this test, red cells from the patient are added to the mixture of fresh ABO-compatible normal serum and isotonic sucrose solution. Sucrose is the low ionic strength medium and favors the attachment of IgG and complement to red cells (alternate pathway activation). After incubation at 37°C and centrifugation, amount of hemolysis is

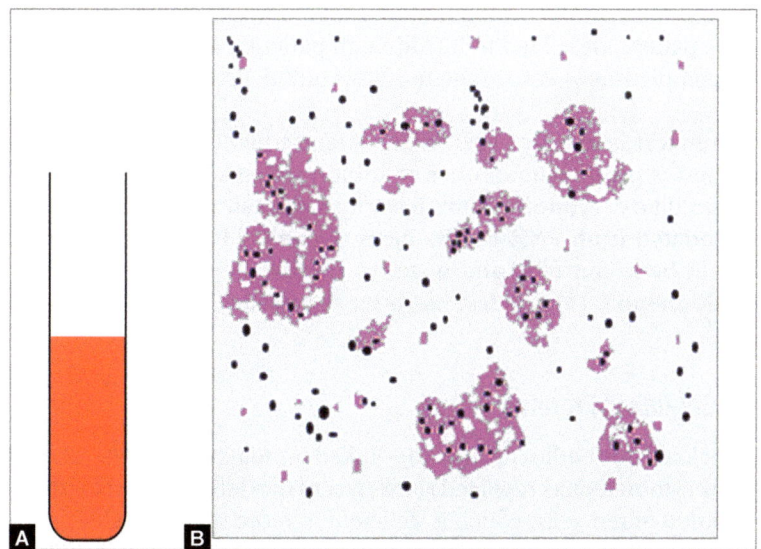

Figs. 4.59A and B: (A) Gross appearance of urine in PNH (hemoglobinuria); (B) Urine microscopy showing hemosiderinuria.

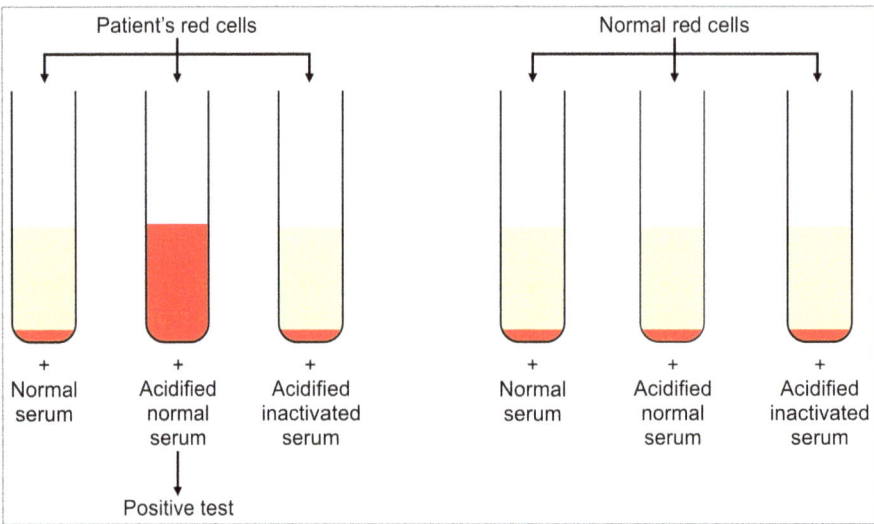

Fig. 4.60: Principle of Ham's test in PNH. Patient's red cells are hemolyzed in the presence of complement (provided by normal serum) and acid (activates complement). Inactivated serum (heated at 56°C) is devoid of complement.

quantified in a spectrophotometer. If it is more than 10%, it is indicative of PNH. This test is more sensitive but less specific than Ham test.

Acidified Serum Test (Ham Test)

Acidification of serum (to pH 6.5) activates complement via alternate pathway and causes hemolysis of red cells if they are abnormally sensitive to complement.

In this test, fresh normal ABO-compatible serum (source of complement) is acidified and red cells from the patient are added to it (Although patient's serum may also be used, it may be exhausted of complement.) Percent hemolysis is noted. PNH red cells show 10 to 50% lysis (Fig. 4.60).

Acidified serum test is usually performed if sucrose hemolysis test is positive. Although acidified serum test is positive in another condition called as congenital dyserythropoietic anemia type II (hereditary erythroid multinuclearity with positive acidified serum or HEMPAS), it can be differentiated from PNH on the basis of clinical history, abnormal morphology of erythroblasts in bone marrow, and negative sucrose hemolysis test. (See "Congenital dyserythro-poietic anemia.") Ham's test has been superseded by flowcytometric analysis for CD55 and CD59.

Assays based on GPI-linked Proteins

Analysis of monoclonal antibodies against GPI-linked proteins (like CD59, CD55, CD24, CD14, and CD16) by flow cytometry has replaced Ham's test as the definitive test for diagnosis of PNH. In PNH, a population of red cells, which is deficient in more than one GPI-anchored protein, is present. Size of the PNH clone can also be estimated by flow cytometry. This test is more sensitive and specific than complement-based assays.

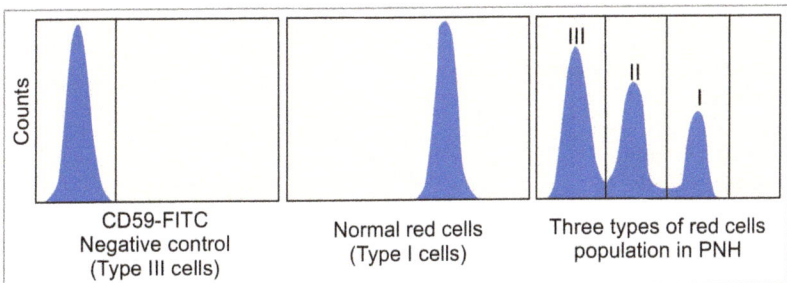

Fig. 4.61: Red cell analysis by CD59 fluorescence histogram. Figure on left shows negative control which correspond stored cells deficient in CD59 (type III red cells); figure in middle shows normal red cells which correspond to type I red cells; while figure on right shows histogram from a patient with PNH showing three distinct populations of red cells: type I (normal red cells), type II (red cells partially deficient in CD59), and type III (red cells completely deficient in CD59).

Flow cytometry can be done on red cells or granulocytes. Total size of PNH clone and relative proportions of each red cell population (type I, II, or III) can be determined. Hemolysis and thrombosis are more common in patients with large amounts of type III red cells, while patients with hypoplastic PNH are more likely to have a small type III population. As more susceptible red cells are lost through complement-mediated hemolysis, the estimated size of red cell population will be less. Many laboratories therefore prefer granulocytes for flow cytometry.

Red cell analysis by CD59 fluorescence histogram is shown in Figure 4.61.

Fluorescent Aerolysin Assay

A fluorescein-labeled proaerolysin (FLAER) is commonly being used for diagnosis of PNH by flow cytometry. It binds selectively and with high affinity to the GPI anchor on granulocytes and provides more accurate assessment of GPI anchor deficiency in PNH than traditional antibodies. FLAER is commonly used along with CD16, CD24, or CD66 when testing granulocytes (Fig. 4.62).

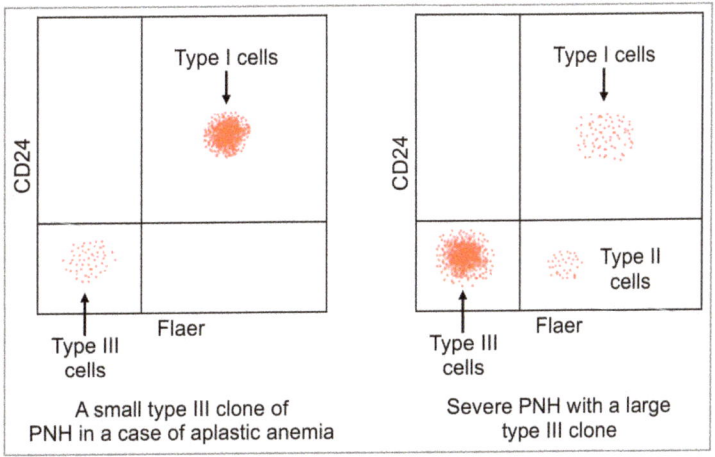

Fig. 4.62: Analysis of granulocytes for PNH by flow cytometry.

Box 4.24: Conditions requiring screening for paroxysmal nocturnal hemoglobinuria.
- Coomb's-negative intravascular hemolytic anemia
- Hemoglobinuria
- Aplastic anemia
- Myelodysplastic syndrome
- Unexplained thrombosis
- Thrombosis occurring at unusual sites (hepatic, portal, splanchnic, dermal, cerebral veins)
- Unexplained peripheral cytopenia

Conditions in which screening for paroxysmal nocturnal hemoglobinuria is recommended are listed in Box 4.24.

TREATMENT

Patients with mild disease do not require any treatment. Eculizumab is indicated in patients with severe hemolysis or thrombosis or both. Eculizumab (a humanized monoclonal antibody directed against C5 complement thus blocking terminal complement activation) is highly effective in reducing intravascular hemolysis. It is especially helpful in classic PNH. It decreases or eliminates need for blood transfusion, reduces the risk of thrombosis, and improves quality of life. However, it is very expensive and life-long treatment is required as it does not eradicate the PNH clone. It also does not have any effect on associated bone marrow failure. Since it increases the risk of infection with encapsulated organisms (due to complement inhibition), vaccination against *N. meningitidis* is necessary.

Allogeneic bone marrow transplantation is the only curative therapy but is associated with significant morbidity and mortality. It is indicated in PNH occurring in the setting of severe aplastic anemia and in myelodysplasia, or in patients not responding to eculizumab.

Supportive treatment measures include (1) blood transfusion to maintain hemoglobin level, (2) anticoagulant therapy for venous thrombosis, (3) iron supplementation, and (4) corticosteroids to reduce hemolysis.

PROGNOSIS

The median life expectancy is about 10 years. Course of PNH is variable. Patients may remain stable with chronic hemolytic anemia for many years. In some patients abnormal PNH clone may spontaneously disappear. Evolution of PNH to aplastic anemia or acute myeloblastic leukemia can occur. There is a close relationship between PNH and bone marrow failure. PNH develops in about 10% of patients with aplastic anemia and about 25% patients with PNH progress to aplastic anemia. Venous thrombosis is a major cause of morbidity and mortality.

MECHANICAL HEMOLYTIC ANEMIAS

The mechanical hemolytic anemias include:
- Microangiopathic hemolytic anemia
- March hemoglobinuria
- Cardiac hemolytic anemia.

Extra- or intravascular hemolysis and fragmented red cells or schistocytes on blood smear are the characteristic features of mechanical hemolytic anemia.

MICROANGIOPATHIC HEMOLYTIC ANEMIA

This refers to hemolytic anemia resulting from intravascular fragmentation and lysis of red cells due to alteration in small blood vessels. Usually, direct damage to red cells occurs when they pass through the fibrin strands deposited in the microcirculation.

Common causes of microangiopathic hemolytic anemia are given in Box 4.25.

Clinical features are related to the underlying disease. Severity of anemia is variable.

The characteristic feature on peripheral blood smear is fragmented red cells or schistocytes. Schistocytes include small red cell fragments with 1 to 3 sharp spicules as well as large helmet-shaped red cells from which fragments have been split off (Fig. 4.63). Evidence of intravascular hemolysis and consumptive coagulopathy is often present.

Primary treatment consists of correction of underlying cause.

> **Box 4.25:** Common causes of microangiopathic hemolytic anemia.
> 1. Thrombotic thrombocytopenic purpura
> 2. Hemolytic uremic syndrome
> 3. Disseminated intravascular coagulation
> 4. Malignant hypertension
> 5. Associated with pregnancy: Eclampsia, HELLP syndrome (**hem**olysis, **e**levated **l**iver enzymes, **l**ow **p**latelets)
> 6. Disseminated malignancy, e.g. mucin secreting adenocarcinomas
> 7. Severe infections
> 8. Generalized vasculitis due to immunologic diseases, e.g. systemic lupus erythematosus

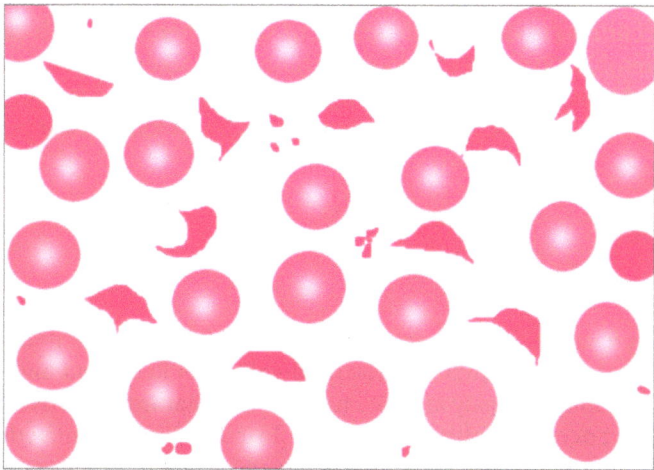

Fig. 4.63: Blood smear in microangiopathic hemolytic anemia showing many fragmented cells (schistocytes).

MARCH HEMOGLOBINURIA

Intravascular hemolysis may result following physical exercise such as marching or running on a hard surface for prolonged period (e.g. in soldiers, long-distance runners, jogging on a hard surface), conga drummers, tennis players, or in karate enthusiasts after practice. Traumatic destruction of red cells occurs within vessels of the feet. The usual complaint is of passing reddish-brown urine following physical exertion. Hemoglobinuria is transient in most cases. The degree of hemolysis is usually mild and does not cause anemia.

CARDIAC HEMOLYTIC ANEMIA

Prosthetic cardiac valves may be associated with chronic intravascular hemolysis (Waring blender syndrome). This may be related to turbulent blood flow resulting from leaking valve and presence of artificial surface in bloodstream. Degree of anemia depends upon severity of mechanical damage to red cells.

HEMOLYTIC ANEMIA DUE TO DIRECT ACTION OF PHYSICAL, CHEMICAL, OR INFECTIOUS AGENTS

PHYSICAL AGENTS

Acute intravascular hemolysis follows extensive burns and its degree depends on body surface area involved. Hemolysis usually occurs within 1 to 2 days of burn injury and is due to direct action of heat on red cells. Blood smear shows fragmented red cells, spherocytes, and erythrocyte budding.

CHEMICAL AGENTS

Hemolysis can occur due to direct toxic action of some chemicals such as lead (discussed earlier under "Sideroblastic anemia"), arsenic chloride (workers in galvanizing or soldering industries), distilled water (introduction of large quantity of distilled water in circulation may follow intravenous injection or irrigation during surgery), and some insect venoms (e.g. brown recluse spider).

INFECTIOUS AGENTS

Malaria

Malaria is caused by four species of Plasmodia: *P. vivax, P. falciparum, P. malariae,* and *P. ovale*. Infected female Anopheles mosquitoes transmit the disease. Recurrent high-grade fever with chills and rigors, and splenomegaly are the characteristic features. Icterus may be present. In *P. vivax* infection fever occurs on alternate days, while in *P. falciparum* infection it occurs daily.

In malaria, anemia is usually mild and is caused mainly by excessive destruction of parasitized red cells by spleen. Other factors in the pathogenesis of anemia are suppression of erythropoiesis by inflammatory cytokines, decreased production of erythropoietin, and shunting of iron from erythroblasts to macrophage stores.

Acute intravascular hemolysis (blackwater fever) occurs with *P. falciparum* infection and is characterized by fever, prostration, and marked hemoglobinuria. It may lead to acute renal failure. Pathogenesis is not known. It usually occurs in those patients who have had chronic malaria and were treated with quinine irregularly.

Acute intravascular hemolysis in *P. falciparum* malaria should be distinguished from drug-induced acute hemolytic episode in G6PD deficiency.

Diagnosis is based on demonstration of the parasite in blood film. Recently, immunochromatographic strip tests have been introduced that have high sensitivity and specificity.

Clostridium Perfringens

Clostridium perfringens sepsis usually follows septic abortion and frequently causes marked intravascular hemolytic anemia. Other conditions include acute cholecystitis, surgery of biliary tract, and gastrointestinal or genitourinary malignancy. *Clostridium perfringens* liberates a lecithinase that acts on red cell membranes to form lysolecithins; lysolecithins have strong hemolytic activity. Blood smear shows numerous spherocytes. Prognosis is usually serious.

HYPERSPLENISM

NORMAL STRUCTURE AND FUNCTION OF SPLEEN

The spleen is organized into two areas—white pulp and red pulp. The white pulp consists of malpighian or splenic follicles that are collections of lymphocytes around centrally located arterioles. Periarteriolar lymphocytes are mainly T lymphocytes. Adjacent to this is the area of B lymphocytes which exhibits prominent germinal centers upon antigenic stimulation. Red pulp is composed of anastomosing cords and vascular sinuses. The splenic cords are made of a meshwork of macrophages. The vascular sinuses are lined by a discontinuous layer of endothelial cells, i.e. small pores or slits occur between endothelial cells which permit blood cells to traverse between sinusoids and cords.

Most of the blood supply from the splenic artery passes from the smaller branches and arterioles into the capillaries and then into the splenic veins (closed circulation). A small proportion of the capillary blood supply passes slowly into the splenic cords; the blood from the cords then enters the sinuses through narrow slits between endothelial cells and then passes into the veins (open circulation).

Spleen plays a principle role in removal of undesirable elements from blood. As the blood passes slowly through the splenic cords, macrophages recognize and phagocytose micro-organisms, defective or damaged red cells occurring in various hemolytic anemias, senescent red cells and IgG-coated blood cells. Splenic macrophages also excise inclusions such as Howell-Jolly bodies or Heinz bodies from red cells and the remainder of the red cell is returned to the circulation.

Spleen plays a role in both B-cell mediated (humoral) and T-cell mediated (cell-mediated) immune responses.

Spleen also functions as a hematopoietic organ during fetal life. Postnatally, however, bone marrow is the sole site of blood cell production. In some disorders, such as thalassemia major and myelofibrosis, extramedullary hematopoiesis may become re-established in the spleen.

> **Box 4.26:** Common causes of splenomegaly.

Infectious diseases
- Viral: Infectious mononucleosis
- Bacterial: Typhoid fever, miliary tuberculosis, subacute bacterial endocarditis
- Protozoal: Malaria*, kala-azar*

Inflammatory diseases
- Felty's syndrome
- Systemic lupus erythematosus

Hematological disorders
- Disorders of red cells: Hereditary spherocytosis, thalassemia major*
- Disorders of white cells: Chronic myeloid leukemia*, acute leukemias, chronic lymphocytic leukemia, hairy cell leukemia*, myelofibrosis*, lymphomas

Cirrhosis of liver

Storage disorders
- Gaucher's disease*
- Niemann–Pick disease

Tropical splenomegaly syndrome (Hyperreactive malarial splenomegaly syndrome)*

* Disorders marked with asterisk can cause massive splenomegaly.

CAUSES OF SPLENOMEGALY

See Box 4.26.

DIAGNOSTIC CRITERIA

The clinical syndrome of hypersplenism occurs in only some of the cases of splenomegaly. The diagnostic criteria for hypersplenism are:
- Enlargement of spleen;
- Peripheral blood cytopenia (anemia, leukopenia, thrombocytopenia), either isolated or in combination;
- Normal or hypercellular bone marrow with normal maturation;
- Normalization of blood cell count after splenectomy.

Cytopenia in hypersplenism results from sequestration of blood cells in enlarged spleen. Normally about one-third of total platelets in the body are pooled in the spleen; enlarged spleen can sequester large number of platelets to induce thrombocytopenia. A massively enlarged spleen can also trap a considerable proportion of red cells and granulocytes to cause anemia and neutropenia, respectively.

BIBLIOGRAPHY

1. Azar S, Wong TE. Sickle cell disease. A brief update. Med Clin N Am. 2017;101:375-93.
2. Beutler E, Blume KG, Kaplan JC, et al. International Committee for Standardization in Haematology. Recommended screening test for glucose-6-phosphate dehydrogenase (G6PD) deficiency. Br J Haematol. 1979;43:465-67.
3. Brewer GJ, Tarlov AR, Alving AS. The methemoglobin reduction test for primaquine type sensitivity of erythrocytes. A simplified procedure for detecting a specific hypersusceptibility to drug hemolysis. JAMA. 1962;180:386-88.

4. Cao A, et al. Prenatal diagnosis of inherited haemoglobinopathies. Indian J Pediatr. 1989;56:707-17.
5. Cappellini MD, Porter JB, Viprakasit V, Taher AT. A paradigm shift on beta-thalassemia treatment: How will we manage this old disease with new therapies? Blood Reviews. 2018;32:300-11.
6. Chehab FF, Kan YW. Detection of sickle-cell anaemia mutation by colour DNA amplification. Lancet. 1990;335:15-17.
7. Clarke GM, Higgins TN. Laboratory investigation of hemoglobinopathies and thalassaemias:Review and update. Clin Chem. 2000;46:1284-90.
8. Fairbanks VF, Lampe LT. A tetrazolium-linked cytochemical method for estimation of glucose-6-phosphate dehydrogenase activity in individual erythrocytes:Application in the study of heterozygous for glucose-6-phosphate dehydrogenase deficiency. Blood. 1968;31:589-603.
9. Mettananda S, Higgs DR. Molecular basis and genetic modifiers of thalassemia. Hematol Oncol Clin N Am. 2018;32:177-91.
10. Mohanty D, Mukherjee MB, Colah RB. Glucose-6-phosphate dehydrogenase deficiency in India. Indian J Pediatr. 2004;71:525-9.
11. Old JM, Varawalla NY, Weatherall DJ. Rapid detection and prenatal diagnosis of β thalassaemia:Studies in Indian and Cypriot populations in the UK. Lancet. 1990;336:834-7.
12. Parker C, Omine M, Richards S, et al. Diagnosis and management of paroxysmal nocturnal hemoglobinuria. Blood. 2005;106:3699-703.
13. Parker CJ. Bone marrow failure syndromes:Paroxysmal nocturnal hemoglobinuria. Hematol Oncol Clin N Am. 2009;23:333-46.
14. Rachmilewitz EA, Giardina PJ. How I treat thalassemia. Blood. 2011;118:3479-88.
15. Richards SJ, Barnett D. The role of flowcytometry in the diagnosis of paroxysmal nocturnal hemoglobinuria in the clinical laboratory. Clin Lab Med. 2007;27:577-90.
16. Ryan K, Bain BJ, Worthington D, et al. On behalf of the British Committee for Standards in Haematology:Significant haemoglobinopathies:Guidelines for screening and diagnosis. Br J Haematol. 2010;149:35-49.
17. Taher AT, Weatherall D, Capellini MD. Thalassemia. Lancet. 2018;391:155-67.
18. Viprakasit V, Ekwattanakit S. Clinical classification, screening, and diagnosis of thalassemia. Hematol Oncol Clin N Am. 2018;32:193-211.
19. Ware RE. How I use hydroxyurea to treat young patients with sickle-cell anemia. Blood. 2010;115:5300-11.
20. Wasi P. Population screening. In Weatherall DJ (Ed):Methods in Hematology. The thalassaemias. Edinburgh. Churchill Livingstone; 1983.
21. Weatherall DJ, Provan B. Inherited anaemias. Lancet. 2000;355:1169-75.
22. Weatherall DJ, Wainscoat JS. The molecular pathology of thalassaemia. In Hoffbrand AV (Ed):Recent advances in hematology. No. 4. Edinburgh. Churchill Livingstone; 1985.
23. Weatherall DJ. Hematologic methods. In Weatherall DJ (Ed):Methods in Hematology. The thalassaemias. Edinburgh. Churchill Livingstone. 1983.
24. Weatherall DJ. The challenge of haemoglobinopathies in resource-poor countries. Br J Haematol. 2011;154:736-44.
25. Weatherall DJ. The diagnostic features of different forms of thalassaemia. In Weatherall DJ (Ed):Methods in Hematology. The thalassaemias. Edinburgh. Churchill Livingstone; 1983.
26. Working Party of the General Haematology Task Force of the British Committee for Standards in Haematology:The laboratory diagnosis of haemoglobinopathies. Br J Haematol. 1998;101:783-92.

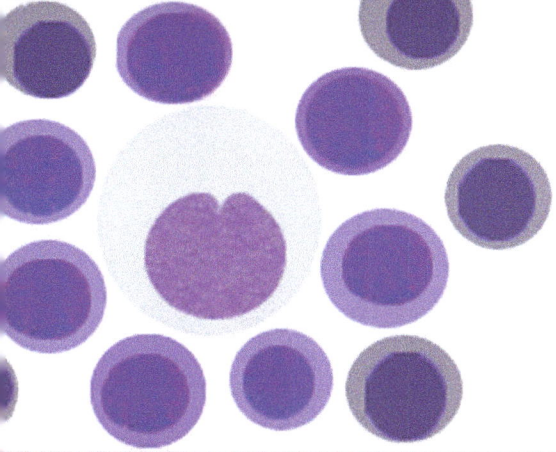

Disorders of White Blood Cells

Section Outline

5. Acute Leukemias   *235*
6. Myelodysplastic Syndromes   *287*
7. Myeloproliferative Neoplasms   *299*
8. Chronic Lymphoid Leukemias   *325*
9. Plasma Cell Dyscrasias   *341*
10. Malignant Lymphomas   *369*
11. Quantitative and Qualitative Disorders of Leukocytes   *389*
12. Hematopoietic Stem Cell Transplantation   *414*

SECTION 3

CHAPTER 5

Acute Leukemias

▍DIAGNOSIS AND CLASSIFICATION

Acute leukemias are malignant clonal disorders originating in hematopoietic stem cells characterized by the proliferation of poorly differentiated blast (immature) cells in the bone marrow and a rapidly progressive fatal course if untreated (survival <6 months without treatment).

Acute leukemias primarily originate in the bone marrow. Proliferating leukemic blasts replace normal bone marrow cells and subsequently enter into the peripheral blood. They are clonal disorders that arise from malignant transformation of a single hematopoietic progenitor cell followed by proliferation and accumulation of abnormal clone. There is an arrest in the differentiation of immature cells into functionally mature cells.

Acute leukemias comprise about 50% of all cases of leukemias. Approximate frequencies of different types of leukemias in India are shown in Box 5.1.

Box 5.1: Leukemias in India.
- Chronic myeloid leukemia: 40%
- Acute lymphoblastic leukemia: 35%
- Acute myeloid leukemia: 15%
- Chronic lymphocytic leukemia: 10%

▍PREDISPOSING FACTORS

Various factors associated with increased risk of acute leukemias are as follows:

Hereditary Factors

Some congenital disorders are associated with increased predisposition to acute leukemia, e.g. Down's syndrome (20 times increased incidence), Fanconi's anemia, Bloom's syndrome, dyskeratosis congenita, ataxia telangiectasia, Klinefelter's syndrome, Diamond-Blackfan syndrome, Wiskott-Aldrich syndrome, and Kostmann's syndrome.

Acquired Factors

Ionizing Radiation
- Nuclear fall-out: Following nuclear explosions in Hiroshima and Nagasaki, increased incidence of leukemias (particularly acute and chronic myeloid leukemias, and less commonly acute lymphoblastic leukemia) was observed in survivors.

- Therapeutic irradiation: Patients treated with irradiation for treatment of disorders such as ankylosing spondylitis, Hodgkin's lymphoma, and polycythemia vera have an increased risk of development of acute myeloid leukemia. Acute myeloid leukemia (AML) is usually preceded by myelodysplastic syndrome in these patients.
- Diagnostic X-rays: Intrauterine fetal exposure to low-dose radiation (for X-ray pelvimetry) has been found to increase the risk of subsequent occurrence of acute leukemia in childhood.

Chemical Agents

Occupational exposure to benzene is associated with increased risk of acute myeloid leukemia and aplastic anemia.

Alkylating agents used for cytotoxic chemotherapy of neoplasms may induce acute myeloid leukemia. Such secondary leukemias develop about 5 to 6 years after chemotherapy, are usually preceded by myelodysplastic syndrome, have high incidence of clonal cytogenetic abnormalities (deletions of chromosome 5 or 7), and are resistant to treatment.

Treatment with drugs that inhibit topoisomerase II (such as epipodophyllotoxins or etoposide) are implicated in causation of AML; such type of AML develops 1 to 3 years after exposure without any preceding phase of myelodysplastic syndrome and is associated with translocations of *KMT2A* (formerly *MLL*) gene located at chromosome 11q23.

Viruses: The role of oncogenic viruses in human leukemogenesis is not established, except for one virus human T lymphotropic virus type I (HTLV-I) that is associated with adult T cell leukemia/lymphoma (ATLL). Epstein-Barr virus is implicated in the causation of African Burkitt's lymphoma.

Acquired conditions: Some acquired conditions predispose to acute leukemia such as myeloproliferative neoplasms (chronic myeloid leukemia, polycythemia vera, myelofibrosis), paroxysmal nocturnal hemoglobinuria, myelodysplastic syndromes, and aplastic anemia (treated with immunosuppressive therapy).

Influence of age and sex: Most common form of leukemia in children is acute lymphoblastic leukemia (ALL), while acute myeloid leukemia is the predominant form in adults, adolescents, and infants. Males are slightly more frequently affected than females in ALL, while AML has equal sex incidence. The incidence of acute leukemia rises steeply after the age of 50 years.

MECHANISMS OF ONCOGENESIS IN ACUTE LEUKEMIAS

Leukemias are biologically a diverse group of disorders. This is evident from differences in their morphology, antigen expression, chromosomal and molecular abnormalities, response to treatment, and prognosis.

Like all other malignant tumors, leukemia is a clonal disorder (i.e. it originates from a single hematopoietic stem cell or its committed progenitor) and evolves through more than one mutation. Interactions between exogenous factors (listed under "Predisposing factors"), endogenous factors, and genetic susceptibility are involved in its pathogenesis. The mutations in progenitors (myeloid or lymphoid) confer proliferative and/or survival advantage, and also impair hematopoietic differentiation.

A 2-hit model of leukemogenesis was proposed in 2002 by Kelly and Gilliland in which it was hypothesized that the disease emerges as a result of an interaction between two classes of mutations: class I and class II (Fig. 5.1). Class I or "activating" mutations cause aberrant activation of signal transduction pathways and confer proliferative and/or survival advantage

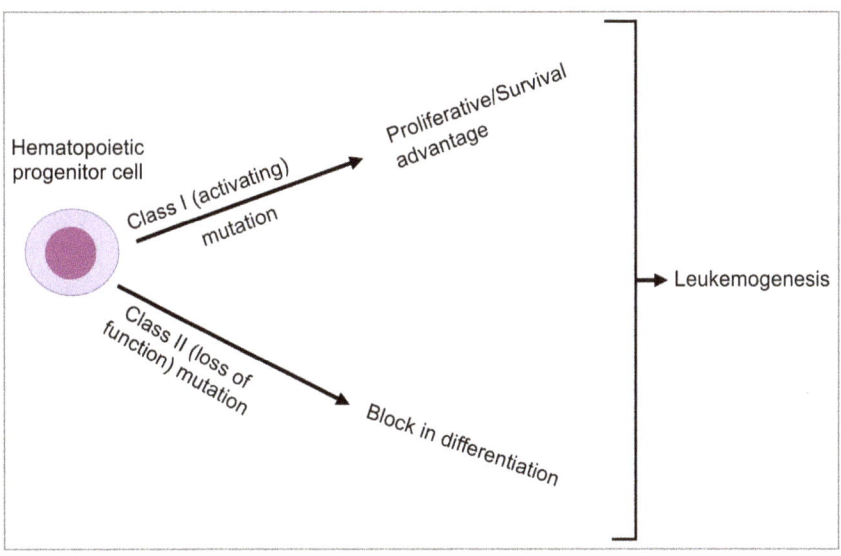

Fig. 5.1: The two-hit theory of development of leukemia.

to hematopoietic progenitor cells. These occur later in the development of leukemia and are considered as prognostic markers. Mutations in *FLT3* and *KIT* are the most common type I mutations in AML. Class II or "loss of function" mutations impair differentiation of hematopoietic progenitors and subsequent apoptosis due to mutations in transcription factors or cofactors. Type II mutations are considered as disease-defining. Type II mutations include gene fusions resulting from recurrent genetic abnormalities, and mutations of *CEBPA*, *RUNX1*, and *NPM1*.

Recent studies indicate that development of leukemia is more complex and intricate, and most AML cases have more than two mutations. Whole genome sequencing studies of AML genome have revealed numerous mutations out of which some are "driver" mutations which do not belong to either class I or class II. Also, sequence and timing of mutations during leukemogenesis appear to be important. Detection of recurrent chromosomal translocations in specific types of acute leukemia indicate that they are causal events. Identification of genes that are disrupted by chromosomal translocations and inversions has provided some insight in pathogenesis.

Current evidence indicates that the initiating event in acute leukemias is an acquired genetic abnormality in a hematopoietic progenitor cell. Chromosomal translocations occurring in specific types of leukemias play a major role in leukemogenesis. These genetic abnormalities (shown in Table 5.1) are associated with a unique disease phenotype, responsiveness to therapy, and prognosis.

Molecular pathogenesis of acute myeloid leukemia: Leukemia develops through serial acquisition of somatic mutations in progenitor cells over time. The first step in this process is establishment of preleukemic clone of cells. This preleukemic clone acquires further co-operative mutations leading to formation of subclones, which in turn acquire further mutations leading to development of frank leukemia. Studies have found that preleukemic hematopoietic stem cells survive induction chemotherapy and are a cause of relapse; therefore, identification of mutations occurring "early" in evolution of AML is of importance. AML genome was the first cancer to be sequenced, which has led to the identification of many previously unknown

Section 3: Disorders of White Blood Cells

Table 5.1: Cytogenetic and molecular abnormalities in acute leukemias.

Functional category of mutations	Gene(s) involved	Prognosis	Comment
1. Transcription factor fusions	RUNX1-RUNX1T1	Favorable	AML with t(8;21)(q22;q22.1)
2. Transcription factor fusions	PML-RARA	Favorable	AML with t(15;17); sensitive to all-transretinoic acid therapy
3. Transcription factor fusions	CBFB-MYH11	Favorable	inv(16)(p13.1q22) or t(16;16)(p13.1;q22)
4. Transcription factor fusions	BCR-ABL1	Unfavorable	AML with t(9;22)(q34.1;q11.2)
5. Nucleophosmin	NPM1	Favorable in absence of FLT3-ITD	Most common mutation in cytogenetically normal AML
6. Tumor suppressor genes	TP53	Unfavorable	Associated with complex karyotype and therapy-related AML
7. Activated signaling genes	FLT3	Unfavorable	FLT3-ITD associated with poor prognosis in cytogenetically normal AML
8. DNA methylation genes	TET2	Likely unfavorable	–
9. Myeloid transcription factors	CEBPA	Biallelic mutations associated with favorable prognosis	–
10. Chromatin modifiers	KMT2A (previously called MLL)	Unfavorable	–
11. Spliceosome complex	U2AF1	Unfavorable	Associated with multilineage dysplasia

driver mutations and improved the understanding about the pathogenesis of AML especially in cytogenetically normal AML. Many of these mutations have been shown to have prognostic significance and therefore mutational profiling of cytogenetically normal AML has assumed importance. Mutations in leukemia have been categorized into following nine functional categories (Cancer Genome Atlas Research Network) (Fig. 5.2):

1. Transcription factor fusions: *PML/RARA, MYH11/CBFB, BCR/ABL, ETV6/RUNX1*
2. Nucleophosmin: *NPM1*
3. Tumor suppressor genes: *TP53, WT1*
4. Activated signaling genes: *FLT3, KIT*
5. DNA methylation genes: *DNMT3A, TET2, IDH1*
6. Myeloid transcription factors: *RUNX1, CEBPA, Paired box protein 5 (PAX5)*
7. Chromatin modifiers: *MLL* fusions, *MLL-PTD, EZH2*
8. Cohesin complex: *STAG1/2, RAD21, SMC1A, SMC3*
9. Spliceosome complex: *SF3B1, SRSF2*

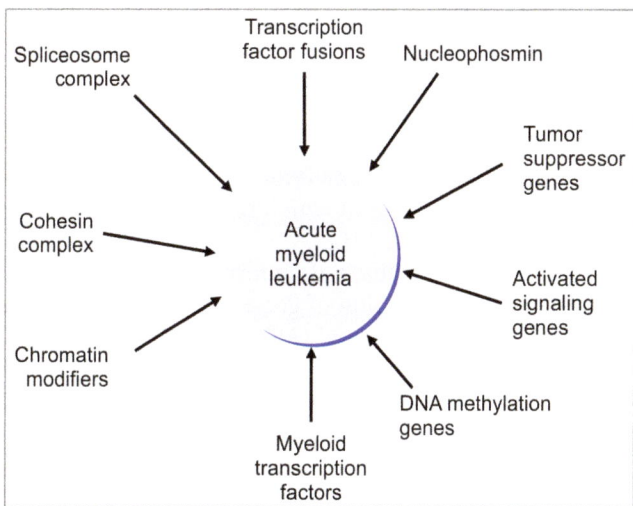

Fig. 5.2: Pathogenesis of acute myeloid leukemia (AML). Nearly all cases of AML show one of nine mutations shown above which are relevant in pathogenesis.

1. **Transcription factor fusions:** The classical example is translocation between chromosomes 15 and 17 in acute promyelocytic leukemia that leads to fusion of gene for retinoic acid receptor α *(RAR α)* on chromosome 15 with the promyelocytic leukemia *(PML)* gene on chromosome 17. Normally, RAR α can interact with both transcriptional coactivators and repressors on target gene. However, PML/RAR α fusion protein favors recruitment of transcriptional repressors. This causes block in differentiation at promyelocyte stage. Administration of all-transretinoic acid normalizes RARα signaling by releasing the transcription repressors and allowing normal maturation and differentiation of promyelocytes. However, this fusion protein is not sufficient for causation of acute promyelocytic leukemia. A second transformative event appears to be mutations in *FLT3* gene (involved in signal transduction pathway). Other examples of formation of a fusion transcription factor are (1) t(8;21)(q22;q22) generating RUNX1/CBFA2T1 fusion protein, (2) inv(16)(p13q22), which generates the CBFB/MYH11 fusion protein, and (3) t(9;22) causing formation of a fusion protein BCR/ABL that has enhanced tyrosine kinase activity.
2. **Nucleophosmin:** Mutations in *NPM1* are the most common mutations in adults with cytogenetically normal AML (30% cases). The protein encoded by *NPM1* gene is nucleophosmin that resides primarily in nucleolus and shuttles rapidly between nucleus and cytoplasm. It has multiple functions like binding to *p53* tumor suppressor gene and controlling cell proliferation and apoptosis, DNA repair, and regulation of centrosome duplication. This mutation is associated with favorable outcome in AML if not associated with *FLT3-ITD* mutations.
3. **Tumor suppressor genes:** Mutations in tumor suppressor genes *TP53* and WT1 have been found in 15% cases of AML. TP53 is called as "guardian of the genome" since it causes cell cycle arrest or apoptosis if DNA is extensively damaged.
4. **Mutations causing activation of signal transduction pathways:** These mutations provide proliferative and survival advantage to hematopoietic progenitors and include *FLT3* and *KIT* mutations. A type of *FLT3* mutation called as *FLT3-ITD* is associated with poor response to therapy and poor survival in cytogenetically normal AML. These mutations have been detected in about 60% AML cases.

5. **DNA methylation genes:** DNA methylation is an epigenetic mechanism that regulates gene transcription and genome stability. Genes involved in DNA methylation (*IDH1/2, TET2, DNMT2A*) have been consistently found to be mutated in AML (45% cases).
6. **Myeloid transcription factors:** Several transcription factors maintain renewal of hematopoietic stem cells and also regulate differentiation. In addition to fusions involving transcription factors, mutations altering their functions have also been discovered. Genes that encode transcription factors and of which mutations have been reported in acute leukemia are *CEBPA* (AML) and *PAX5* (ALL).
7. **Chromatin modifiers:** Based on epigenetic information, active chromatin remodeling is required for stimulation or repression of gene expression. The proteins involved are "writers" (KMT2A, EZH2, NSD1), "readers" (ASXL1), and "erasers" (KDM6A). Alterations in genes encoding these proteins contribute to development of AML (15%).
8. **Cohesin complex:** Cohesin complex controls cohesion of sister chromatid strands, and regulates DNA repair and transcription. Mutations in components of cohesin complex (*STAG1/2, RAD21, SMC1A, and SMC3*) are found in about 15% cases of AML.
9. **Spliceosome complex genes:** The spliceosome is a complex of multiple protein subunits that processes mRNA by removing introns. Mutations in spliceosome genes (*SF3B1, SRSF2, U2AF1*) have been found in myelodysplastic syndrome and in AML (15% cases).

Molecular pathogenesis of acute lymphoblastic leukemia: There are two main forms of ALL: B-ALL and T-ALL.
1. **B cell-acute lymphoblastic leukemia:** Evidence indicates that childhood B-ALL is initiated in utero through chromosomal translocations. Leukemia-specific fusion gene sequences *(MLL/AF4, TEL/AML1 or ETV6/RUNX1, BCR/ABL)* have been identified in archived blood spots from neonates who subsequently developed ALL after a variable latent period and their leukemic cells contained the identical fusion gene sequences. Factors associated with risk of childhood ALL have not been identified. Probably, exposure of the fetus to a mutagen induces a premalignant clone that requires subsequent additional genetic alterations ("hits") afterbirth to develop into full-blown ALL. Transplacental exposure to various compounds is implicated including some antimosquito agents, dipyrone (NSAID), and topoisomerase II inhibitors.
2. **T-cell acute lymphoblastic leukemia:** Mutations in NOTCH1 signaling pathway involving *NOTCH1* gene (activating mutation) and *FBXW7* (loss of function mutation) genes are observed in 65% cases of T-ALL and are implicated in the pathogenesis of T-ALL. NOTCH1 causes activation of MYC expression. Both NOTCH1 and MYC promote proliferation and self-renewal of leukemic cells.

CLASSIFICATION OF ACUTE LEUKEMIAS

According to current WHO classification, there are three forms of acute leukemia: Acute lymphoblastic leukemia (ALL), acute myeloid leukemia (AML), and acute leukemia of ambiguous lineage. The distinction between ALL and AML is important because of the differences in the treatment of these two types of leukemias. In 1976, hematologists from France, America, and Britain proposed a classification of acute leukemias that was designated as French-American-British (FAB) classification. In subsequent years, FAB classification was modified and newer entities were added (like M0 and M7). This classification is based on well-defined morphological criteria, cytochemical reactions, and in some cases, immunophenotyping.

Table 5.2: The French-American-British (FAB) cooperative group classification of acute leukemias.

Acute lymphoblastic leukemias (ALL)
- ALL-L1 type
- ALL-L2 type
- ALL-L3 type

Acute myeloid leukemia (AML)
- Acute myeloblastic leukemia minimally differentiated (M0)
- Acute myeloblastic leukemia without maturation (M1)
- Acute myeloblastic leukemia with maturation (M2)
- Hypergranular promyelocytic leukemia (M3)
    - Hypo- or microgranular promyelocytic leukemia (M3 variant)
- Acute myelomonocytic leukemia (M4)
    - Acute myelomonocytic leukemia with bone marrow eosinophilia (M4eo)
- Acute monocytic leukemia (M5)
    - Undifferentiated (monoblastic) (M5a)
    - Well-differentiated (promonocytic-monocytic) (M5b)
- Acute erythroleukemia (M6)
- Acute megakaryocytic leukemia (M7)

In this classification, AML is subclassified into eight categories (designated from M0 to M7) based on the lineage of leukemic cells (granulocytic, monocytic, erythroid, and megakaryocytic) and their level of differentiation. ALL is classified into three groups (designated as L1, L2, and L3) based on morphology of lymphoblasts. FAB classification is easy to use with well-defined cytological criteria, reproducible, and majority of acute leukemias can be placed in one of the categories (Table 5.2).

In recent years, several distinct categories of acute leukemias have been identified by genetic (cytogenetic and molecular genetic) studies that correlate closely with biologic behavior, treatment responsiveness, and prognosis. These features do not always correlate with FAB categories. Cytogenetic and molecular genetic studies have become vitally important in defining optimum treatment protocols.

In 2001, WHO proposed a classification of hematological malignancies based on clinical, morphologic, immunophenotypic, and genetic features which define specific entities. This classification was subsequently revised in 2008 and 2017. The 2017 classification is given in Table 5.3. This classification has clinical, therapeutic, and prognostic relevance (Tables 5.3 and 5.4).

Salient Features of WHO Classification

Acute Myeloid Leukemia

- According to WHO criteria, blast count for diagnosis of AML is ≥20% in peripheral blood or bone marrow. To obtain blast count, at least 200-cell count of all nucleated cells in peripheral blood and at least 500-cell count of all nucleated cells in bone marrow should be done. However, diagnosis of AML should be made even if blast count in peripheral blood or bone marrow is <20% in (1) AML with recurrent genetic abnormalities t(8;21), inv(16), t(16;16), and t(15;17) *PML-RARA,* and (2) myeloid sarcoma.

Table 5.3: World Health Organization (WHO) classification of acute myeloid leukemia (AML) and related precursor neoplasms, 2017.

Acute myeloid leukemia with recurrent genetic abnormalities
- AML with t(8;21)(q22;q22.1); *RUNX1-RUNX1T1*
- AML with inv(16)(p13.1q22) or t(16;16)(p13.1;q22); *CBFB-MYH11*
- Acute promyelocytic leukemia with *PML-RARA*
- AML with t(9;11)(p21.3;q23.3); *KMT2A-MLLT3*
- AML with t(6;9)(p23;q34.1); *DEK-NUP214*
- AML with inv(3)(q21.3;q26.2) or t(3;3)(q21.3;q26.2); *GATA2, MECOM*
- AML (megakaryoblastic) with t(1;22)(p13.3;q13.1); *RBM15-MKL1*
- Provisional entity: AML with *BCR/ABL1*

Acute myeloid leukemia with gene mutations
- AML with mutated *NPM1*
- AML with biallelic mutations of *CEBPA*
- Provisional entity: AML with mutated *RUNX1*

Acute myeloid leukemia with myelodysplasia-related changes

Therapy-related myeloid neoplasms

Acute myeloid leukemia, not otherwise specified
- AML with minimal differentiation
- AML without maturation
- AML with maturation
- Acute myelomonocytic leukemia
- Acute monoblastic and monocytic leukemia
- Acute erythroid leukemia
- Acute megakaryoblastic leukemia
- Acute basophilic leukemia
- Acute panmyelosis with myelofibrosis

Myeloid sarcoma

Myeloid proliferations related to Down syndrome
- Transient abnormal myelopoiesis associated with Down syndrome
- Myeloid leukemia associated with Down syndrome

Table 5.4: World Health Organization classification of precursor lymphoid neoplasms, 2017.

B lymphoblastic leukemia/lymphoma

- **B lymphoblastic leukemia/lymphoma, NOS**
- **B lymphoblastic leukemia/lymphoma with recurrent genetic abnormalities**
  - B lymphoblastic leukemia/lymphoma with(9;22)(q34.1;q11.2); *BCR-ABL1*
  - B lymphoblastic leukemia/lymphoma with t(v;11q23.3); *KMT2A* rearranged
  - B lymphoblastic leukemia/lymphoma with t(12;21)(p13.2;q22.1); *ETV6-RUNX1*
  - B lymphoblastic leukemia/lymphoma with hyperdiploidy
  - B lymphoblastic leukemia/lymphoma with hypodiploidy
  - B lymphoblastic leukemia/lymphoma with t(5;14)(q31.1;q32.1); *IGH/IL3*
  - B lymphoblastic leukemia/lymphoma with t(1;19)(q23;p13.3); *TCF3-PBX1*
  - B-lymphoblastic leukemia/lymphoma, *BCR-ABL1*–like
  - B-lymphoblastic leukemia/lymphoma with iAMP21

T lymphoblastic leukemia/lymphoma
Early T-cell precursor lymphoblastic leukemia

- AML is divided into following major categories:
  - AML with recurrent genetic abnormalities: Cytogenetic studies should be performed in all morphologically diagnosed patients of AML. Leukemias included under this category have distinctive clinical, morphological, and prognostic features in addition to specific cytogenetic and molecular genetic abnormalities.
  - AML with genetic mutations: Mutations of *NPM1*, *CEBPA*, and *RUNX1* genes are found in AML with normal karyotype as well as in association with translocations and inversions. In normal karyotype AML, mutations of *NPM1* are associated with a better prognosis if not associated with *FLT3-ITD* mutation. AML with biallelic *CEBPA* mutations are associated with a better prognosis. AML with *RUNX1* mutation have a poor outcome.
  - AML with myelodysplasia-related changes: This category comprises 25–35% of all cases of AML, mainly occurs in elderly patients, and is generally associated with a poor prognosis.
  - Therapy-related myeloid neoplasms: This category includes AML, myelodysplastic syndrome, and myelodysplastic/myeloproliferative neoplasms, which occur as a late complication of cytotoxic chemotherapy and/or radiotherapy administered for a neoplastic or non-neoplastic disorder.
  - AML, not otherwise specified: This accounts for 25–30% of all cases of AML, and includes those cases which do not fulfill the criteria for any of the previously described diagnostic categories. The subgroups under this category have no prognostic significance. Cytogenetic analysis and mutation studies are necessary before a case can be classified under this category. Morphology, cytochemistry, and immunophenotyping of leukemic cells should be done to determine the major lineage involved and their degree of maturation.
  - Myeloid sarcoma: This tumor comprises 3–7% of AML and occurs mainly in children. It is a rare extramedullary tumor of myeloid cells and is diagnostic of AML even in the absence of 20% blood or marrow blasts.
  - Myeloid proliferations related to Down syndrome: Children with Down syndrome have increased risk of AML which has unique clinical, morphologic, immunophenotypic, and molecular features. Apart from AML, transient abnormal myelopoiesis occurs in newborns with Down syndrome with clinical and morphologic features similar to AML; this disorder spontaneously resolves in majority of cases in first 3 months of life.

Acute Lymphoblastic Leukemia

Classification of ALL is presented in Table 5.4. According to WHO classification, precursor lymphoid neoplasms of either B- or T-cell type consist of ALL and lymphoblastic lymphoma. Lymphoblastic lymphoma and ALL are biologically the same disease with different clinical presentations. The distinction between lymphoblastic lymphoma and ALL is arbitrary and is based on predominant involvement of blood/bone marrow (ALL) or predominant extramedullary involvement (lymphoma). The conventional cutoff for diagnosis of ALL is 25% of lymphoblasts in blood or bone marrow. FAB categories L1, L2, and L3 do not correlate with immunophenotype, genetic abnormalities, and clinical behavior. ALL L3 is equivalent to Burkitt lymphoma/leukemia and is not considered as ALL in WHO classification.

CLINICAL FEATURES OF ACUTE LEUKEMIAS

Due to Bone Marrow Failure

Replacement of marrow and suppression of normal hemopoiesis by leukemic blasts is responsible for bone marrow failure. The main clinical features are due to lack of red cells, white cells, and platelets.
- Anemia which manifests as pallor, dyspnea, CCF
- Infections are due to neutropenia (manifests with fever)
- Bleeding due to thrombocytopenia or disseminated intravascular coagulation.

Due to Organ Infiltration

- Organomegaly (lymph nodes, spleen, liver, other); hepatosplenomegaly and lymphadenopathy are more common in ALL
- Bone pain and tenderness (common with ALL)
- Central nervous system (CNS) (meningeal) disease (common with ALL)
- Gum hypertrophy (common in monocytic leukemia)
- Testicular involvement (common in ALL)
- Mediastinal mass (T-ALL)
- Infiltration of skin (leukemia cutis) especially common with monocytic leukemia
- Chloromas (Localized proliferation of myeloblasts outside marrow producing solid tumors): Common sites are soft tissues and bones of head and neck area. Chloroma may precede or occur concurrently with overt AML.

Other

- Hyperleukocytosis (very high TLC, i.e. >1 lakh/cmm can increase blood viscosity and cause sludging of blood flow with headache, neurologic and visual changes, and respiratory distress).
- Disseminated intravascular coagulation (release of procoagulant substances from leukemic cells may induce DIC, common in acute promyelocytic leukemia).

DIAGNOSIS OF ACUTE LEUKEMIAS

The first aim of laboratory investigations is to establish the diagnosis of acute leukemia by peripheral blood and bone marrow examinations. This is followed by investigations to identify the type of acute leukemia, i.e. ALL or AML and its subtype (Box 5.2). This is essential because of differences in their management. Laboratory studies in acute leukemias (Fig. 5.3 and Box 5.3) are:
- Morphological examination of peripheral blood and bone marrow aspiration smears
- Cytochemistry
- Electron microscopy

Box 5.2: Diagnosis of acute leukemias.
- Establish the presence of acute leukemia and distinguish it from other neoplastic and reactive conditions. Acute leukemia should be differentiated from infectious mononucleosis, myelodysplastic syndrome, non-Hodgkin's lymphoma infiltrating the bone marrow, hematogones, and transient myeloproliferative disorder in Down syndrome.
- Distinguish between AML and ALL.
- Classification of AML or ALL into a specific subtype that has clinical (therapeutic and prognostic) relevance.

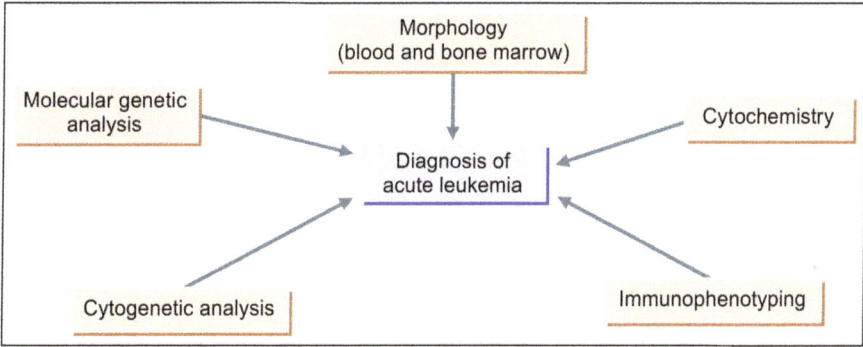

Fig. 5.3: Methods for the diagnosis of acute leukemia.

Box 5.3: Investigations for diagnosis of acute leukemias.

- Peripheral blood and bone marrow aspiration smears stained with a Romanowsky stain (e.g. Wright-Giemsa, Leishman): Determine blast percentage (count at least 200 peripheral blood leukocytes and at least 500 nucleated bone marrow cells); myeloblasts, monoblasts, promonocytes, megakaryoblasts, and lymphoblasts are counted as blasts for diagnosis of acute leukemia, proerythroblasts are counted as blasts in "pure" erythroid leukemia (must comprise ≥30% of marrow cells), while abnormal promyelocytes are counted as "blast equivalents" for diagnosis of acute promyelocytic leukemia
- Bone marrow trephine biopsy in all cases, if possible: At least 1.5 cm in length and taken at a right angle to the cortical bone surface; useful for baseline assessment, immunohistochemistry for enumeration of blasts (if aspiration is not possible)
- Cytochemistry: Myeloperoxidase, Nonspecific esterase, Periodic acid-Schiff: For assessment of blast lineage in AML, not otherwise specified
- Bone marrow aspiration sample for flow cytometry: Multiparameter flow cytometry (at least three colors) for lineage and aberrant antigen expression of neoplastic cells
- Complete cytogenetic analysis on bone marrow aspirate sample at initial diagnosis
- Bone marrow aspiration sample for mutation panels like *NPM1*, *CEBPA*, and *FLT3*

- Immunophenotyping: Flow cytometry, immunohistochemistry
- Cytogenetic analysis: Conventional, fluorescent in situ hybridization (FISH)
- Molecular genetic analysis.

Morphology

The laboratory diagnosis of acute leukemias is based mainly on morphology and cytochemistry. Morphological examination is done on both peripheral blood, and bone marrow aspiration smears or touch preparations of biopsy stained with one of the Romanowsky stains (e.g. Giemsa's, Leishman's, etc.). Bone marrow aspiration smears are necessary for confirmation of diagnosis and for morphological subclassification of acute leukemias (Fig. 5.4). Morphology of different types of blasts (myeloblast, monoblast, megakaryoblast, and lymphoblast) and blast equivalents (promyelocytes and promonocytes) is shown in Figure 5.5 and Box 5.4.

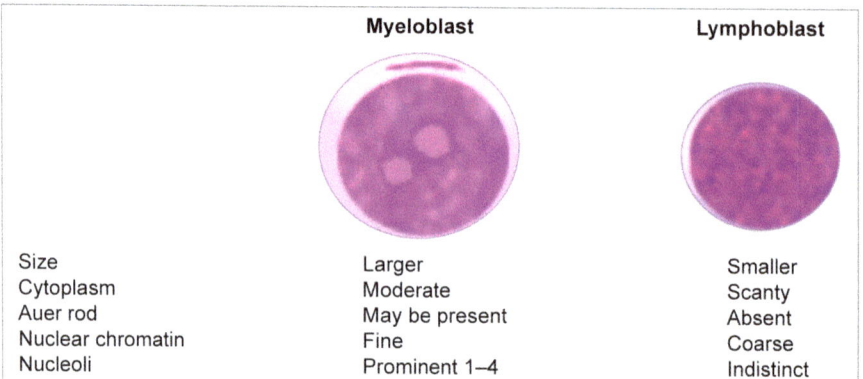

	Myeloblast	Lymphoblast
Size	Larger	Smaller
Cytoplasm	Moderate	Scanty
Auer rod	May be present	Absent
Nuclear chromatin	Fine	Coarse
Nucleoli	Prominent 1–4	Indistinct

Fig. 5.4: Morphological comparison of myeloblast and lymphoblast.

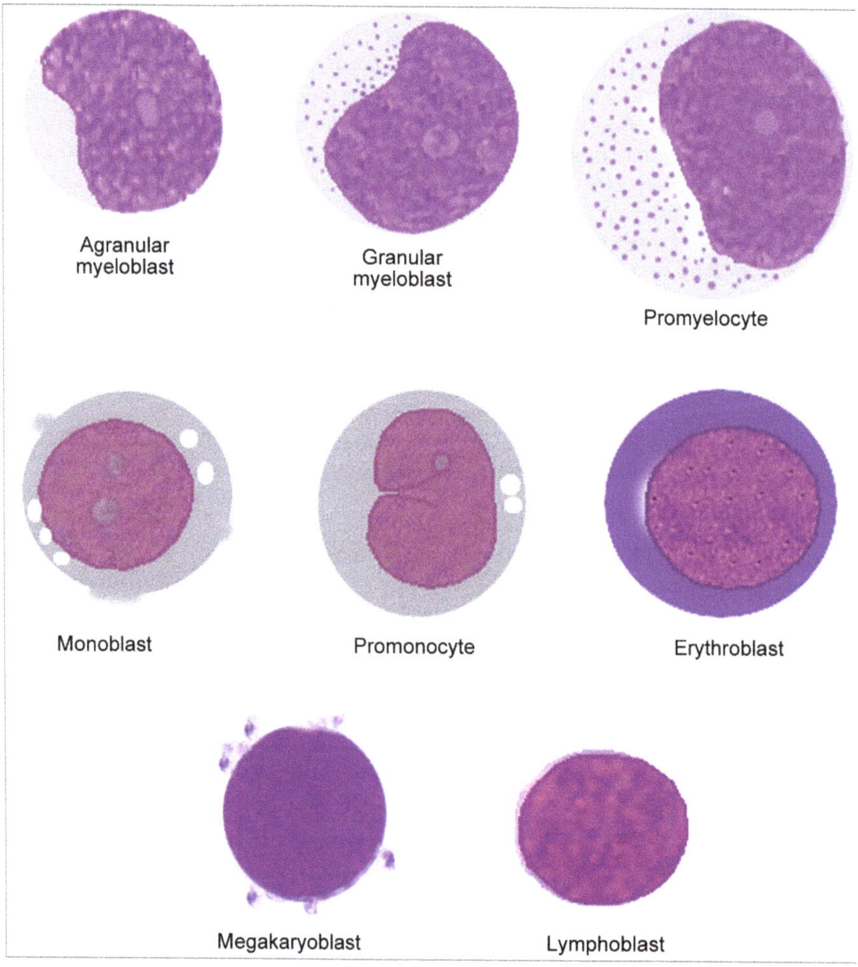

Fig. 5.5: Morphology of different types of blasts and blast equivalents in acute leukemias.

Chapter 5: Acute Leukemias

Box 5.4: Morphology of different types of blasts and blast equivalents.

- **Myeloblasts:**
  - Type 1: Agranular basophilic cytoplasm, round or invaginated nucleus, fine nuclear chromatin, 2–4 distinct nucleoli
  - Type 2: Basophilic cytoplasm with ≤20 azurophlic granules, round or invaginated nucleus, 2–4 distinct nucleoli
  - Type 3: Basophilic cytoplasm with >20 azurophilic granules, 2–4 nucleoli, round or invaginated nucleus (in contrast to promyelocyte, there is no paranuclear Golgi zone and no eccentric nuclear location)
- **Promyelocytes (in acute promyelocytic leukemia):**
  - Hypergranular: Cytoplasm with numerous dark-staining granules that often obscures the nucleus, nucleus eccentric with nucleolus, nuclear border has folded or reniform appearance, bundles of Auer rods (faggots) often present (90% cases), paranuclear Golgi zone
  - Hypogranular: Bilobate cells or cells with reniform nucleus with minimal or no granules
- **Monoblasts:** Abundant basophilic cytoplasm that may contain vacuoles or few granules, eccentric and round nucleus with delicate chromatin with prominent 1 or more nucleoli
- **Promonocytes in AML with monocytic differentiation:** Irregular or delicately convoluted nucleus, prominent nucleoli, less basophilic cytoplasm often with vacuoles, cytoplasmic azurophil granules ±
- **Erythroblasts in pure erythroid leukemia:** Deeply basophilic agranular cytoplasm often containing vacuoles (PAS+ve), round nuclei with fine to coarse chromatin, one or more nucleoli (resemble proerythroblasts or basophilic erythroblasts)
- **Megakaryoblasts:** Variable morphology from small size with dense chromatin to larger cell with fine chromatin with prominent nucleoli, cytoplasmic blebs or platelet shedding surrounding blasts may be seen
- **Lymphoblasts:** Variable morphology from small blasts with high nuclear/cytoplasmic ratio, scant cytoplasm, coarse chromatin, regular nuclear membrane, and an indistinct nucleolus to larger cells with more cytoplasm, lower nuclear/cytoplasmic ratio, irregular nuclear membrane, and one or more nucleoli.

In peripheral blood, total leukocyte count is elevated (in most cases), normal, or low. The characteristic feature is presence of blast cells. In subleukemic leukemia, total leukocyte count is normal or low but blasts are demonstrable in peripheral blood. In aleukemic leukemia, blasts are not demonstrable in peripheral smear but are present in the bone marrow; however, if buffy coat preparation is examined then some blasts will usually be seen in peripheral blood. (In buffy coat preparation, small amount of anticoagulated blood is centrifuged, smear is prepared from white cell layer, and examined).

Bone marrow aspiration smears reveal hypercellular marrow with almost complete replacement of marrow by blast cells. For diagnosis of acute leukemia, blasts should be ≥20% in blood or bone marrow. The threshold of 20% of blasts in peripheral blood or bone marrow for diagnosis of AML is not required in following cases:
- Diagnosis of AML with recurrent genetic abnormalities t(8;21), t(15;17), inv(16), and t(16;16).
- Promonocytes are considered as blast equivalents in AML with monocytic differentiation and are included along with blasts in the blast count.
- Promyelocytes are considered as blast equivalents in acute promyelocytic leukemia.
- Abnormal erythroblasts are considered as blast equivalents in pure erythroid leukemia; however, they should be more than 30%.
- Myeloid sarcoma (an extramedullary tumor of myeloid blasts) is considered as AML even if blast count is not increased in blood or marrow.

The "gold standard" for counting of myeloblasts is peripheral blood smear and/or bone marrow aspiration smears. Flow cytometry should not be used for counting of blasts. If there is "dry tap," touch smears of bone marrow biopsy are used. In rare cases in which smears are not possible, bone marrow biopsy can be used if supported by immunohistochemistry (stained with blast markers like CD34, CD117).

Normal hematopoietic cells are reduced. Morphological features of various leukemias are considered later under respective chapters. Although diagnosis of acute leukemia requires blood and bone marrow smears, bone marrow biopsy (stained with hematoxylin and eosin on paraffin-embedded tissue) is necessary in the presence of (1) "dry tap" or failure of barrow aspiration due to abundant reticulin fibrosis in acute megakaryoblastic leukemia and acute panmyelosis with myelofibrosis, and (2) hypocellular acute leukemia. Tissue biopsy is required in myeloid sarcoma.

Role of morphology in diagnosis of AML is shown in Box 5.5.

> **Box 5.5:** Role of morphology in acute myeloid leukemia.
>
> - Diagnosis of AML requires blast count ≥ 20%
> - Identification of (i) myeloblasts especially of AML M2 (blast cells with abundant, large, pink granules, and slightly basophilic cytoplasm), (ii) promyelocytes of AML M3 (folded, bilobed nuclei, abundant, small, azurophilic granules, and numerous Auer rods), (iii) abnormal eosinophils (containing basophilic granules) in AML M4 Eo, (iv) promonocytes and monocytes in AML M4 and AML M5, and (v) multilineage dysplasia
> - Provides a basis for ordering further studies, e.g. tests for disseminated intravascular coagulation in acute promyelocytic leukemia.

Cytochemistry

In many cases, it is difficult to differentiate between various types of blasts only on the basis of morphology on Romanowsky-stained smears. Various cytochemical procedures are employed to aid in this differentiation. When morphology and cytochemistry are combined together, 80 to 90% of acute leukemias can be correctly categorized. Diagnostic accuracy increases to 95 to 99% with immunophenotyping.

By cytochemical techniques, certain enzymes, fat, glycogen, or other substances are identified in blast cells. The main aim of cytochemical studies in acute leukemias is to distinguish ALL from AML. In AML, cytochemical stains allow delineation of granulocytic lineage (AML M1, M2, M3), mixed myeloid and monocytic leukemia (AML M4), and erythroid leukemia (AML M6). The cytochemical stains, which are employed in acute leukemias (Table 5.5 and 5.6), are:

- **Myeloperoxidase, Sudan black B, Chloroacetate esterase:** Positive in granulocytic lineage (AML M0, M1, M2, M3)
- **Nonspecific esterase:** Alpha naphthyl acetate esterase (ANAE), Alpha naphthyl butyrate esterase (ANBE), Naphthol AS acetate esterase (NASA), Naphthol AS-D acetate esterase (NASDA): Positive in monocyte lineage (AML M4, M5)
- **Periodic acid Schiff's (PAS) reaction:** Positive in B-ALL (block-like), and in erythroblasts in AML M6
- **Acid phosphatase:** Positive (focal) in T-ALL.

Principles and Applications of Cytochemical Reactions

Myeloperoxidase (MPO): Myeloperoxidase is an enzyme located in the azurophil (primary) granules of myeloid cells. MPO positivity appears as colored granules in the cytoplasm of cells mainly at the site of enzyme activity (Golgi zone). All the stages of neutrophil series show MPO

Table 5.5: Cytochemistry in acute leukemias.

Cytochemical stain	Reactivity	Use(s)
Myeloperoxidase (MPO)	Myeloblasts (few scattered granules ±, primary granules of promyelocytes and later cells of neutrophil series)	To distinguish AML (M1, M2, M3, M4) from ALL; to distinguish AML M3 (strong+) from AML M4 (By definition, MPO is negative in leukemic lymphoblasts*)
Chloroacetate esterase	All cells of neutrophil series	Combined with nonspecific esterase for diagnosis of AML M4
Nonspecific esterase	Granules of monocytes and precursors; megakaryocyte and platelet granules; T lymphocytes (focal)	AML M4, AML M5
Periodic acid-Schiff (PAS)	Neutrophil series, monocyte series, megakaryocytes, some lymphocytes	ALL**, erythroblasts of AML M6
Perl's Prussion blue stain for iron	Hemosiderin in erythroid cells and macrophages	Ring siderblasts in myelodysplastic syndrome
Acid phosphatase	Most bone marrow cells	T-ALL (focal)***

*MPO negative blasts: AML with minimal differentiation, lymphoblasts, megakaryoblasts, erythroblasts, some monoblasts.
**PAS: In addition to lymphoblasts in some ALL cases, block-like positivity can be seen in erythroblasts in acute erythroleukemia and in monoblasts in acute monoblastic leukemia.
***Acid phosphatase: Localized positive reaction also occurs in acute megakaryoblastic and erythroleukemia.

Table 5.6: Cytochemical reactions in acute leukemias.

Type	MPO	NSE	PAS	AP
1. AML M0	- (+ on EM)	-	-	-
2. AML M1–M3	+	-	-	-
3. AML M4	+	+	-	-
4. AML M5	±	+	-	-
5. AML M6	±	-	+	-
6. AML M7	-	-	-	-
7. B-ALL	-	-	+ (blocks)	-
8. T-ALL	-	-	-	+ (focal)

(MPO: myeloperoxidase; NSE: nonspecific esterase; PAS: periodic acid Schiff; AP: acid phosphatase; EM: electron microscopy)

positivity. In monocyte series, azurophil granules are smaller and MPO activity stains less strongly and appears late during maturation. MPO is never seen in lymphoblasts. Therefore, positive MPO stain in leukemic blasts differentiates between AML and ALL.

The main use of MPO is to distinguish AML from ALL. The blasts in AML show granular positivity while blasts in ALL are negative for MPO. MPO is positive in AML subtypes M1, M2, M3, and M4 (Figs. 5.6 and 5.7), and permits diagnosis of these leukemias. In AML M0, peroxidase activity is not visible on light microscopy, but can be demonstrated by electron microscopy. Megakaryoblasts are MPO-negative. Absence of MPO does not exclude AML since it is usually not positive in AML with minimal differentiation, acute monoblastic leukemia, and acute megakaryoblastic leukemia.

Sudan black B (SBB): Phospholipids and neutral lipids in the membrane of neutrophil granules are stained by SBB. SBB positivity parallels that of MPO in neutrophil series. SBB is reported to be less specific than MPO as positive reaction has been reported in some cases of ALL.

Chloroacetate esterase (CAE): This stain is also called as Leder stain. The reaction is present in all cells of neutrophil series (though less sensitive than MPO and SBB) and is negative in monocyte series. It is less sensitive than MPO and SBB for identification of myeloid differentiation. It is commonly used in combination with nonspecific esterase or NSE, for diagnosis of leukemia with both myeloid and monocyte components (AML M4). Both esterases (CAE for myeloid and NSE for monocytic components) can be demonstrated in the same blood film; this is called as combined or double esterase reaction. Inhibition by sodium fluoride is used for confirmation of monocytic lineage.

Nonspecific esterase (NSE) reaction (usually demonstrated by ANAE or ANBE): α-naphthyl acetate esterase is an enzyme that is present in large quantities in monocytic cells. It is present in small amounts in myeloid and lymphoid cells. The nonspecific esterase reaction is intensely and diffusely positive in monocyte series and is sensitive to sodium fluoride. In T lymphocytes it is focally positive and is resistant to sodium fluoride.

In AML M4, ANAE allows identification of blasts with monocytic differentiation (Fig. 5.7). In AML M5, reaction is strongly and diffusely positive (Fig. 5.8), while in erythroblasts in M6

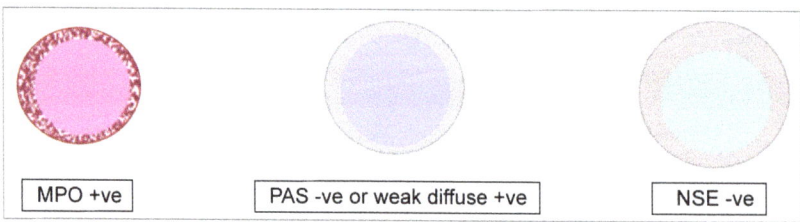

Fig. 5.6: Cytochemical reactions in AML M1, M2, and M3.

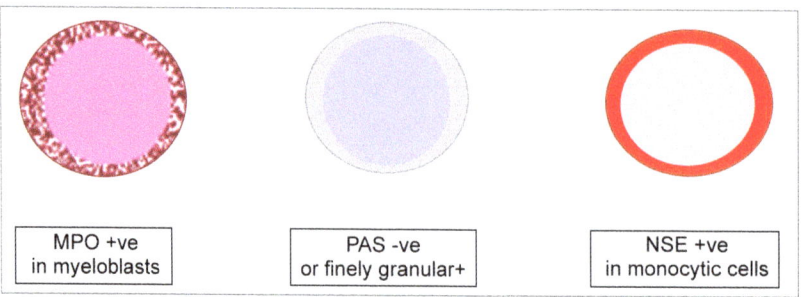

Fig. 5.7: Cytochemical reactions in AML M4. There is both granulocytic (MPO +ve blasts) and monocytic (NSE +ve cells) differentiation.

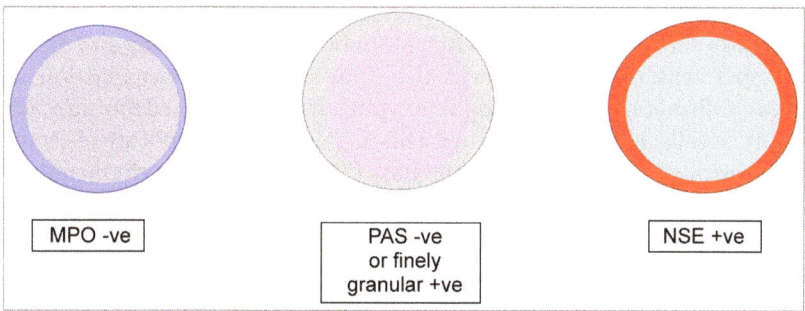

Fig. 5.8: Cytochemical reactions in AML M5.

and in megakaryoblasts in M7 it is focally positive. The reaction is strongly and focally positive also in T-ALL.

In acute leukemias, the principal role of NSE is to differentiate neutrophilic cells, i.e. myeloblasts and promyelocytes (negative reaction) from monocytic cells, i.e. monoblasts and promonocytes (positive reaction).

Periodic acid Schiff's reaction (PAS): Periodic acid is an oxidizing agent that transforms glycols and related compounds to aldehydes. The aldehyde groups then along with Schiff's reagent form an insoluble red- or magenta-colored compound. In hematopoietic cells, positive reaction is due to the abundance of glycogen in cytoplasm.

All stages in neutrophil series show a diffuse positive reaction. Monocytes show a fine, scattered, and faint staining positivity. A few small or coarse granules are present in the cytoplasm of lymphocytes. Red cell precursors do not show positive granules. Platelets are PAS-positive.

In L1 and L2 subtypes of ALL (B cell-ALL), PAS-positive "blocks" are present in lymphoblasts on a clear cytoplasmic background (Fig. 5.9). In T cell-ALL and in L3 subtype of ALL, PAS reaction is negative. PAS positivity is also seen in monoblasts (in AML M5) and in erythroblasts (in AML-M6); however, in these cells small blocks of positive material are present against a diffusely positive cytoplasmic background. Also, a fine granular positivity is seen in all AML cell types. Therefore, PAS poorly discriminates between various cell types.

When MPO, SBB, and NSE are negative and PAS shows block-like positivity in blasts, there is a strong possibility of ALL. However, such a reaction can occur in certain other cell types and therefore definitive diagnosis of ALL is made by immunophenotyping.

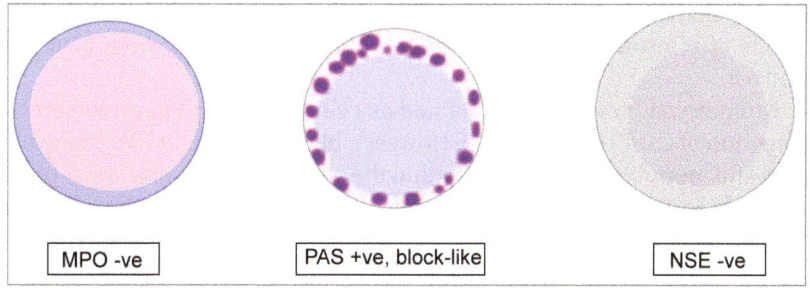

Fig. 5.9: Cytochemical reactions in ALL (70% cases).

Acid phosphatase (AP): Strong focal acid phosphatase activity is observed in T cell ALL. However, focal activity is also seen in AML M6 and M7. Monoblasts show a strong and diffuse reaction. Since aside from T cells, certain other cells also show strongly positive reaction, diagnosis of T-ALL requires confirmation by immunophenotyping. If tartrate is used during reaction, then it inhibits AP in most cells; however, abnormal cells in hairy cell leukemia are resistant to tartrate inhibition. The tartrate-resistant acid phosphatase (TRAP) activity is a characteristic feature of hairy cell leukemia.

Electron Microscopy

Electron microscopic (EM) examination is rarely used since the advent of flow cytometry on bone marrow aspirate and immunohistochemistry on paraffin-embedded sections. For ultrastructural examination, 1 mL of bone marrow aspirate sample should be immediately placed in glutaraldehyde. EM may be useful for demonstrating MPO in myeloid blasts in minimally differentiated AML (in cases with <3% MPO +ve blasts on conventional light microscopy). In acute megakaryoblastic leukemia, platelet peroxidase activity is characteristically localized on the nuclear membrane and endoplasmic reticulum and is absent from the cytoplasmic granules and Golgi complexes (in contrast to myeloblasts). Acute basophilic leukemia can be recognized by basophilic features on EM.

Immunological Cell Marker Analysis (Immunophenotyping)

The term immunophenotype refers to a combination of specific antigens identified in a cell population to determine the lineage and maturation stage of the leukemic cells. In immunophenotyping, various antigens on the surface (or in the cytoplasm or nucleus) of the leukemic cells are identified using antigen-specific antibodies. Cell surface antigens are named according to the internationally accepted CD (cluster of differentiation) system in which each cell surface antigen is ascribed a unique number (e.g. CD1, CD2, etc.). This analysis gives information about lineage and stage of development of the particular cell. Methods employed for immunophenotyping are immunofluorescence or immunoenzyme method (such as peroxidase-antiperoxidase) and flow cytometric analysis. Since blood and marrow cells are in fluid suspension, flow cytometric analysis is the method of choice. Multiple monoclonal antibodies are commercially available for this technique.

Normal hematopoietic cells have a characteristic pattern of antigen expression at different stages of maturation. A panel consisting of a combination of different antibodies is commonly employed to determine the immunophenotypic profile of a sample. The antibodies are labeled with a fluorescent marker and there activity of the cell to various antibodies can be detected.

Applications of immunophenotyping in acute leukemias are shown in Box 5.6 and in Tables 5.7 and 5.8.

On flow cytometry, a blast cells are defined as cells with low to intermediate side scatter and dim expression of CD45 ("blast gate"). However, blast equivalents like promyelocytes and promonocytes and monoblasts do not fall within the "blast gate," e.g. abnormal promyelocytes have increased side scatter and promonocytes have brighter CD45 expression. Neoplastic blasts are characterized by abnormal antigen expression that helps in distinguishing normal from neoplastic blasts. Abnormalities include expression on myeloblasts of markers not present on cells of that particular lineage, e.g. CD7 (T-lineage marker) on myeloblasts or CD13 (myeloid)

Box 5.6: Applications of immunophenotyping in acute leukemias.
- Diagnosis and classification
  - Distinction between ALL and AML
  - Diagnosis of specific types of AML: AML M0, AML M6, and AML M7
  - Distinction between B-ALL and T-ALL and further immunological subtyping of B- and T-ALL
- Assessment of prognosis
- Detection of aberrant antigen expression that corresponds with certain specific subtypes and also helps in monitoring minimal residual disease
- Monitoring of minimal residual disease (detection of the unique leukemia phenotype on a single cell amongst numerous cells allows early detection of residual disease following treatment and thus earlier institution of further treatment)
- To monitor effectiveness of monoclonal antibody therapy directed against antigens present on leukemic cells (e.g. rituximab directed against CD20 antigen in B-ALL)

Table 5.7: Monoclonal antibodies used for the diagnosis of acute leukemias by immunophenotyping.

Lineage	Primary panel*	Secondary panel**
1. Myeloid	CD13, CD33, CD117, MPO (cyt)	CD14, CD64, lysozyme, glycophorin A, CD41, CD61
2. B-lymphoid	CD19, CD79a (cyt), CD22 (cyt), CD10	Cyt IgM, surface Ig (κ/λ)
3. T-lymphoid	CD3 (cyt), CD2, CD7	CD1a, membrane CD3, CD5, CD4, CD8
4. Nonlineage restricted (primitive stem cell)	HLA DR, TdT (nuclear), CD34	

*Primary panel: To distinguish AML from ALL, and to further classify B-ALL and T-ALL.
**Secondary panel: (1) To diagnose AML of monocytic, erythroid, and megakaryocytic lines, and (2) further subtyping of B- and T-ALL.

Table 5.8: Cell antigens detected by monoclonal antibodies for characterization of acute leukemias.

- Myeloid: CD13, CD33, MPO, CD117, CD41, CD61, glycophorin A, CD14, CD15, CD36, lysozyme
- B lymphoid: CD19, CD20, CD22, CD79a, surface Ig, cytoplasmic Ig, CD38
- T lymphoid: CD2, CD3, CD5, CD7

marker in ALL. Immunophenotyping can also predict genotype and prognosis in some cases. Unique antigens or antigen patterns (called as surrogate marker profiles) are expressed in AML with t(8;21) *(RUNX1/RUNX1T1)* (immunophenotype: CD34+, CD13+, CD33+, aberrant CD19+, in some cases CD56+), and acute promyelocytic leukemia with *PML/RARA* (immunophenotype: CD34−, HLADR−, CD33+, CD13+, CD15); however, expression of such markers is only indicative and not confirmatory of genetic abnormality. Expression of CD56 in acute promyelocytic leukemia and in AML with t(8;21) is associated with worse prognosis. Determination of DNA index in ALL can provide prognostic information.

Immunophenotyping should be correlated with clinical, morphologic, and genetic features for workup of acute leukemia.

Acute myeloid leukemia: In AML, immunophenotyping is invaluable for diagnosis of certain subtypes such as AML M0, M6, and M7. The designation M0 is used for those cases of AML which have negative cytochemistry (myeloperoxidase, Sudan black B) on light microscopy, but cell surface marker studies show myeloid differentiation antigens (CD 13 or CD 33); T or B lymphoid markers are absent.

In AML M6, diagnosis is based on typical morphological features and demonstration of glycophorin A on surface.

Morphologically, megakaryoblasts (AML M7) resemble lymphoblasts. Diagnosis requires demonstration of CD41 (GPIIb) or CD61 (GPIIIa) by immunophenotyping, or platelet peroxidase by electron microscopy.

Acute lymphoblastic leukemia: Definitive identification of lymphoblasts is based on immunological cell marker studies.

Immunologically ALL is divided into B cell ALL and T cell ALL. Immunophenotyping is helpful in differentiating B cell ALL from T cell ALL and is invaluable for further subclassification of these leukemias. Immunological classification of ALL has utmost therapeutic and prognostic relevance (*see* chapter on "Acute Lymphoblastic Leukemia").

Identification of CD20 and CD22 in B-ALL has led to the development of targeted therapy in the form of rituximab (CD20 antibodies) and epratuzumab (CD22 antibodies).

In childhood ALL, flow cytometric analysis for DNA index may be of prognostic significance. Calculation of DNA index reliably detects high hyperdiploidy. DNA index >1.16 corresponds with hyperdiploidy and is associated with better survival.

Acute leukemia of ambiguous lineage: This is characterized by immunophenotypic features of both myeloid and lymphoid lineage or of neither lineage. Blasts expressing both myeloid and lymphoid markers are called as biphenotypic. In bilineage acute leukemia, there are two distinct populations of blasts.

In biphenotypic leukemia, a single abnormal blast cell population exists which demonstrates surface markers of two different lineages (e.g. blast cell exhibiting both myeloid and lymphoid antigens). Acute leukemia without any lineage-specific antigens is called as acute undifferentiated leukemia; blast cells express stem cell markers (CD34, TdT, HLA DR, CD38) but specific myeloid and/or lymphoid antigens are lacking (Fig. 5.10).

Immunohistochemistry

Immunohistochemistry (IHC) allows visualization and localization of specific lineage antigens using antibodies on paraffin-embedded tissue sections. It is especially useful if bone marrow

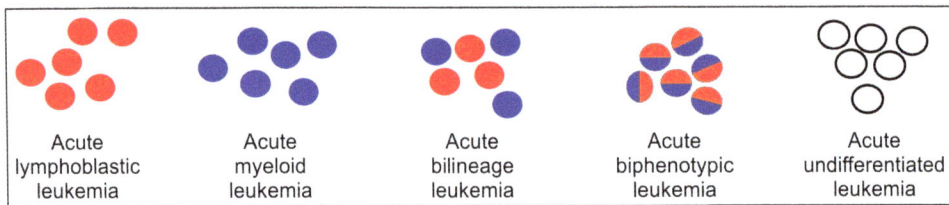

Fig. 5.10: Diagrammatic comparison based on expression or nonexpression of antigens on blasts of acute lymphoblastic, myeloid, bilineage, biphenotypic, and undifferentiated leukemias.

> **Box 5.7:** Immunohistochemical markers in acute leukemia.
> - For assessment of blast count (i.e. markers for identification of immature population): CD34 (stem cell marker expressed by both lymphoid and myeloid blasts), CD117 or C-KIT (myeloblast), TdT (lymphoblast)
> - For lineage assignment:
>   - Myeloid: Myeloperoxidase, CD33
>   - Monocytic: Lysozyme, CD11c, CD14, CD64
>   - Erythroid: CD71, glycophorin A, hemoglobin A
>   - Megakaryocyte lineage: CD42b, CD41, CD61, von Willebrand factor (F VIII-related antigen)
>   - B-lineage: CD19, CD79a, PAX-5, cytoplasmic CD22, CD10
>   - T-lineage: Cytoplasmic CD3, CD2, CD5, CD7

aspiration repeatedly yields dry tap. The immunohistochemical markers for characterization of acute leukemia are listed in Box 5.7.

Leukemia-associated immunophenotype (LAIP) and different-from-normal (DFN): Recognizing that a particular combination of antigens expressed by leukemic cells is not expressed by normal hematopoietic cells, two strategies are used for monitoring minimal residual disease (MRD) in acute leukemia after chemotherapy: LAIP and DFN. LAIP needs to be established at diagnosis before it can be used for monitoring MRD. LAIP consists of combination of antibodies, which detect expression of lineage-foreign antigens (e.g. lymphoid antigens on myeloblasts), asynchronous antigen expression, and altered density or lack of antigen expression. DFN approach does not require knowledge of immunophenotype at diagnosis and is based on recognition that antigenic expression in leukemia is different from normal cells; cells that cluster at sites where normal cells do not localize are considered as residual leukemic cells. A fixed antibody panel is used irrespective of the diagnostic baseline phenotype of leukemia. With this approach, normal cell populations like regenerating myeloid blasts or hematogones or normal precursor cells are not erroneously called as abnormal.

Cytogenetic Studies (Karyotyping) and DNA Ploidy Studies

In cancer cytogenetic studies, constitutional (or germline) chromosomal abnormalities should be differentiated from somatic or tumor-associated abnormalities. Constitutional abnormalities are detected in all cells of an individual; examples include trisomy 21 in Down syndrome, XXY karyotype in Klinefelter's syndrome, etc. Somatic or tumor-associated abnormalities are restricted to tumor cells.

Cytogenetic abnormalities in acute leukemias are of two types: numerical and structural. The term **clonal cytogenetic abnormality** refers to the same structural chromosomal abnormality or gain of the same chromosome identified in two metaphase cells, or loss of the same chromosome identified in three metaphase cells. Presence of a clonal cytogenetic abnormality usually indicates a neoplastic process. **Clonal evolution** refers to emergence of subclones containing new cytogenetic abnormalities during tumor development in a tumor cell population which is already having a chromosomal abnormality in the basic clone of tumor cells.

The sample of choice for cytogenetic analysis in acute leukemia is bone marrow aspiration since cells are spontaneously dividing. Cytogenetic analysis requires examination of 20 metaphases. Methods of chromosomal analysis include (1) conventional cytogenetic analysis (study of metaphase chromosomes obtained from viable and dividing cells stained with a

Table 5.9: Chromosomal abnormalities in AML.

Chromosomal abnormality	Type of AML	Prognosis
1. t(8;21)(q22;q22)	M2	Favorable
2. t(15;17)(q22;q12)	M3	Favorable
3. inv(16)(p13;q22) or t(16;16)(p13;q22)	M4 Eo	Favorable
4. Abnormalities of 11q23	Monocytic	Intermediate
5. –7, del(7q), –5, del(5q), +8, +9, del(11q)	AML with multilineage dysplasia, therapy-related AML	Unfavorable

Table 5.10: Chromosomal abnormalities in precursor B ALL.

Type of ALL	Chromosomal abnormality	Prognosis
Precursor B ALL	t(9;22) (q34; q11.2)	Unfavorable
	t(4;11)(q21;q23)	Unfavorable
	t(1;19)((q23;p13.3)	Unfavorable
	t(12;21)((p13;q22)	Favorable
	Hyperdiploidy > 50	Favorable
	Hypodiploidy	Unfavorable

banding technique), and (2) molecular cytogenetic analysis like FISH (study of metaphase or interphase cells with a DNA probe). FISH is more sensitive than conventional metaphase analysis for detection of chromosomal abnormalities (A molecular technique called reverse transcriptase-polymerase chain reaction is also used for identification of cryptic genetic abnormalities).

Identification of chromosomal abnormalities in acute leukemia is useful for establishing diagnosis, prognosis, selection of treatment, monitoring of disease, and assessment of response to therapy.

1. **Diagnosis:** Disease is considered as AML even if <20% blasts are present if following cytogenetic abnormalities are identified: t(8;21), inv(16)/t(16;16), and t(15;17).
2. **Prognosis:** Certain cytogenetic abnormalities are associated with favorable or unfavorable prognosis (Tables 5.9 and 5.10).
3. **Selection of treatment:** Prompt identification of acute promyelocytic leukemia with t(15;17) *PML-RARA* is important since it is treated differently from other types of AML (all-*trans* retinoic acid and chemotherapy).
4. **Monitoring of disease and response to treatment:** Cytogenetics and molecular techniques can determine response to therapy, MRD, and early or subclinical relapse.

Applications of cytogenetic analysis in acute leukemias are shown in Box 5.8.

Box 5.8: Cytogenetic analysis in acute leukemias.

- Confirmation of diagnosis of specific subtypes of leukemias (acute leukemias with recurrent genetic abnormalities)
- Assessment of prognosis
- Assessment of response to therapy
- Assessment of clonality, e.g. distinguishing hypoplastic AML from aplastic anemia
- Detection of minimal residual disease

Due to the consistent association of certain chromosomal abnormalities with particular types of leukemias, specific subtypes of AML can be diagnosed with certainty by cytogenetic studies [e.g. t(15;17) is characteristic of AML M3]. Clonal cytogenetic abnormalities are observed in about 80% cases of AML and ALL.

Cytogenetic analysis is also helpful in detection of remission and relapse.

DNA ploidy studies: In ploidy studies, number of chromosomes is determined, either by karyotyping or by measuring cellular DNA content. Cellular DNA content is measured by flow cytometry.

Ploidy studies are especially important in childhood ALL; hyperdiploid (chromosome number >50) ALL has better prognosis as compared to diploid (46 chromosomes) and hypodiploid (<46 chromosomes) ALL. DNA index >1.16 is associated with favorable prognosis and therapeutic response.

Molecular Genetic Studies

Applications of molecular genetic studies in acute leukemia are shown in Box 5.9. Methods of molecular genetic analysis are Southern blot analysis, polymerase chain reaction-based techniques, and FISH.

Principle of Southern blot analysis is given elsewhere in this book. In a clonal disorder like acute leukemia, cleaving of DNA by restriction enzyme will produce DNA fragments of same size (since all the cells of a clone will have identical gene rearrangement), which can be detected by electrophoresis of DNA. In a nonmalignant or reactive condition, due to the presence of multiple clones, fragments of DNA produced after restriction enzyme digestion are of different size.

Box 5.9: Applications of molecular genetic analysis in acute leukemias.

- Diagnosis of specific types through identification of unique fusion genes formed due to genetic rearrangements
  - Identification of mutations in a variety of genes like *FLT3*, *NPM1*, *CEBPA*, etc.
- Early detection of minimal residual disease and relapse
- Detection of clonality

Immunoglobulin and T cell receptor gene rearrangements occur during B and T lymphocyte development, respectively.

The rearrangement of immunoglobulin genes occurs in a specific sequence: μ heavy chain followed by kappa (κ) light chain that in turn is followed by lambda (λ) light chain. T gamma (Tγ) and T beta (Tβ) chain genes are rearranged earlier than T alpha (Tα) chain genes during T cell ontogeny. These rearrangements are detected by Southern blot analysis using labeled cDNA probes. The usefulness of gene rearrangement studies in acute leukemias as a lineage-specific marker is limited. This is because immunoglobulin heavy-chain gene rearrangement, which occurs during B cell ontogeny, has also been observed in some cases of T-ALL and AML. Similarly T-cell receptor gene rearrangements have been detected in some cases of B-ALL and AML. However, light chain gene rearrangements occur only in B cells and are lineage specific.

Identification of fusion genes (which are formed after translocations) such as *PML/RARA* gene in AML M3, and *BCR-ABL* and *TEL-AML1* fusion genes in ALL has prognostic and therapeutic importance.

Algorithmic approach to diagnosis of acute leukemias is shown in Figure 5.11.

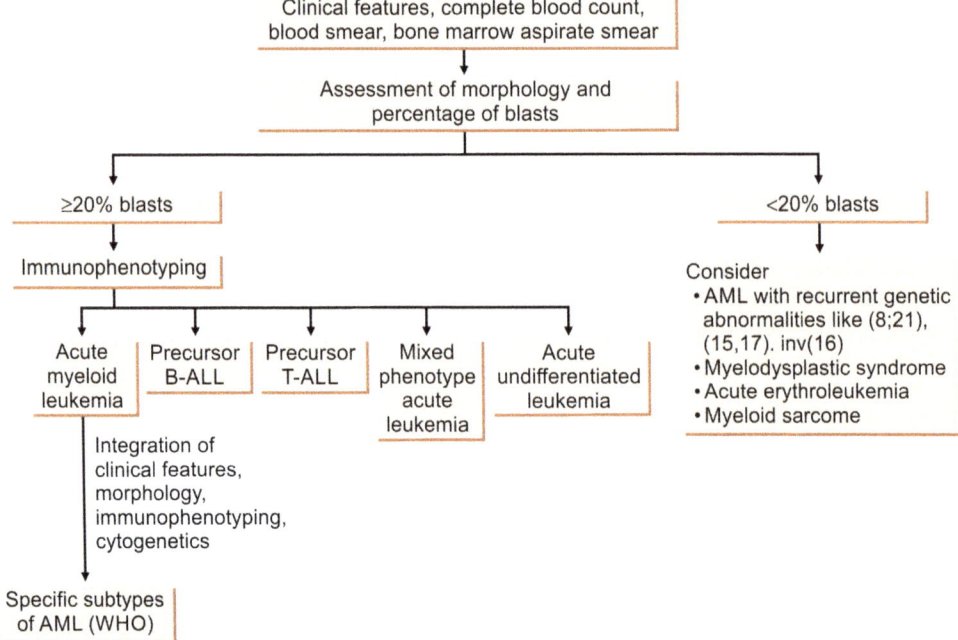

Fig. 5.11: Algorithmic approach for diagnosis of acute leukemia. Integration of clinical, morphologic, immunophenotypic, cytogenetic, and molecular genetic information is required for proper diagnosis and classification. In some cases, based on patient demographics, clinical features, and blast morphology, a specifically directed panel for immunophenotyping can be used. If blast differentiation is not apparent, then an initial full screening panel followed by specific additional markers for assignment of blast lineage need to be used. An example of screening panel is CD45 (hematopoietic), CD34 (blast), CD117 (myeloblast), CD79a or PAX-5 (B lymphoid), and CD3 (T lymphoid). Specific markers: AML-M0(CD13+,CD33+), acute promyelocytic leukemia (HLADR-), acute myelomonocytic leukemia (MPO+, CD68+), acute monoblastic leukemia (MPO-, CD68+), acute erythroleukemia (CD71+, glycophorin+, HbA+), acute megakaryoblastic leukemia (CD41+, CD61+), T-ALL (TdT, CD2, CD5, CD4, CD8), B-ALL (TdT, CD22, CD10).

ACUTE LYMPHOBLASTIC LEUKEMIA

Synonyms: Acute lymphatic leukemia

Acute lymphoblastic leukemia (ALL) is a malignant neoplasm of precursor lymphoid cells arising in the bone marrow. The clonal origin can be demonstrated by immunoglobulin or T-cell receptor gene rearrangement in most lymphoblasts. It is the commonest form of malignancy in childhood (25–30% of all childhood cancers). Malignant lymphoblasts are either B- or T-lymphoblasts. B cell-ALL (most common type) and T cell-ALL are biologically and clinically distinct.

Clinical Features

B-ALL occurs predominantly during childhood with a peak incidence at 2 to 5 years of age, while T-ALL occurs mainly in adolescents and young adults. Onset is acute with history of short duration. Children usually present with manifestations related to bone marrow and organ infiltration by leukemic cells. These include pallor, fatigue (due to anemia), bleeding in the form of bruising and petechiae (due to thrombocytopenia), and persistent fever (due to neutropenia). Enlargement of lymph nodes, spleen, and liver commonly occurs. Bone and joint pains are due to periosteal and bone involvement. Extramedullary disease can also occur in CNS, testis, eye, gastrointestinal tract, and kidneys. Anterior mediastinal mass (due to leukemic infiltration of thymus) on chest X-ray is associated with T cell-ALL; it may cause superior vena cava syndrome (obstruction of superior vena cava impairs blood drainage from head, neck, and upper limbs leading to facial and upper limb swelling, and distension of veins of neck, upper limb, and chest), tracheal obstruction, or pericardial or pleural effusions. CNS involvement is usually asymptomatic at diagnosis (diagnosed by examination of cerebrospinal fluid; Box 5.10); rarely patient may present with signs and symptoms of raised intracranial pressure (headache, vomiting, papilledema).

> **Box 5.10:** Status of central nervous system (CNS) disease at diagnosis.
>
> On cerebrospinal fluid (CSF) examination at diagnosis, CNS disease is divided into following types:
> - CNS1: No detectable blasts in CSF
> - CNS2: <5 leukocytes/μl with blast cells
> - CNS3: ≥5 leukocytes/μl with blast cells
> - TLP+: Traumatic lumbar puncture with ≥10 red cells/μl with blasts

Classification

Diagnosis of ALL requires presence of ≥25% blasts in blood or bone marrow. There are two classification schemes for ALL as follows:

Morphological Classification of ALL (FAB Cooperative Group, 1976)

According to FAB classification, there are three morphological subtypes of ALL: L1, L2, and L3 (Table 5.11). The approximate frequencies of the three subtypes in childhood ALL are: L1: 80%, L2: 15–20%, and L3: 1–2%. In adults with ALL, L2 subtype is most common. Although this classification is simple, it does not correlate adequately with immunophenotype, genetic abnormalities, clinical behavior, and response to treatment.

Although ALL-L3 is fairly easy to recognize, it was observed that morphological differentiation between L1 and L2 was not clear-cut. The FAB group, in 1981, introduced a scoring system to distinguish between L1 and L2. According to this scoring system, high nuclear/cytoplasmic ratio in >75% cells, and 0 to 1 small nucleoli in >75% of cells are each given a+ score, while low nuclear/cytoplasmic ratio in >25% of cells, one or more prominent nucleoli in >25%

Table 5.11: FAB classification of ALL.

Morphology	L1	L2	L3
1. Size of blast	Small	Large, heterogeneous	Large, homogeneous
2. Cytoplasm	Scanty	Moderate	Moderate, intensely basophilic
3. N/C ratio	High	Lower	Lower
4. Cytoplasmic vacuoles	±	±	Prominent
5. Nuclear membrane	Regular	Irregular with clefting	Regular
6. Nucleoli	Invisible or indistinct	Prominent, 1–2	Prominent, 1–2

cells, irregular nuclear membrane in >25% of cells, and large cells (double the size of small lymphocytes) in >50% of cells are each assigned a score of –. Positive score (0 to +2) is obtained in L1 while negative score (–1 to –4) is obtained in L2.

With current treatment regimens, the distinction between L1 and L2 lymphoblasts has no prognostic significance. ALL-L3 is now considered as leukemic phase or advanced stage of Burkitt lymphoma and is treated as such.

World Health Organization Classification (2017)

In WHO classification, ALL is considered as a precursor lymphoid neoplasm with following categories (*see* Table 5.4):
- B lymphoblastic leukemia/lymphoma, not otherwise specified
- B lymphoblastic leukemia/lymphoma with recurrent genetic abnormalities
- T lymphoblastic leukemia/lymphoma

Precursor B- and T-cell neoplasms are biologically and clinically distinct. In children, majority of cases are of B-cell type. Within the category of B-cell ALL, several subtypes are defined according to the genetic abnormalities. These have prognostic and therapeutic significance. There is no correlation between WHO categories and FAB subtypes L1 and L2. Leukemic phase of Burkitt's lymphoma corresponds with L3 subgroup which is now considered as a separate entity. Patients with Burkitt lymphoma who have bulky disease present with leukemic phase; pure Burkitt leukemia is rare.

The lymphoblastic lymphoma and lymphoblastic leukemia are considered as a single disease with different clinical presentations. Majority of lymphoblastic leukemias/lymphomas present as leukemia (blasts in bone marrow >25%).

Laboratory Features

Peripheral Blood Examination

Anemia, which may be severe, is present in all patients. It is normocytic and normochromic. Total leukocyte count may be raised, normal, or low. Patients with T-ALL have very high leukocyte count at presentation. Proportion of lymphoblasts is variable (Figs. 5.12A to C).

Absolute granulocytopenia and thrombocytopenia are commonly present.

Bone Marrow Examination

Bone marrow is hypercellular due to proliferation of leukemic blasts. Normal hematopoietic elements are diminished. Bone marrow aspiration smears are necessary for diagnosis and subclassification of ALL into L1, L2, and L3 subtypes. In most cases, lymphoblasts appear monotonous with small to intermediate size, scant cytoplasm, round nuclei with coarse chromatin, and indistinct nucleoli. In some cases, morphology is variable with some large cells, some cells with abundant cytoplasm, and some with prominent nucleoli. The morphologic variants of B-lymphoblasts include (a) hand-mirror variant (an asymmetric cytoplasmic projection called as uropod overlies an umbilicated nucleus; not associated with any subtype of ALL), (b) granular lymphoblasts (contain azurophil cytoplasmic granules that are MPO-negative), (c) lymphocyte-like lymphoblasts (resemble chronic lymphocyte leukemia), and (d) lymphoblasts with vacuoles (resemble Burkitt cells).

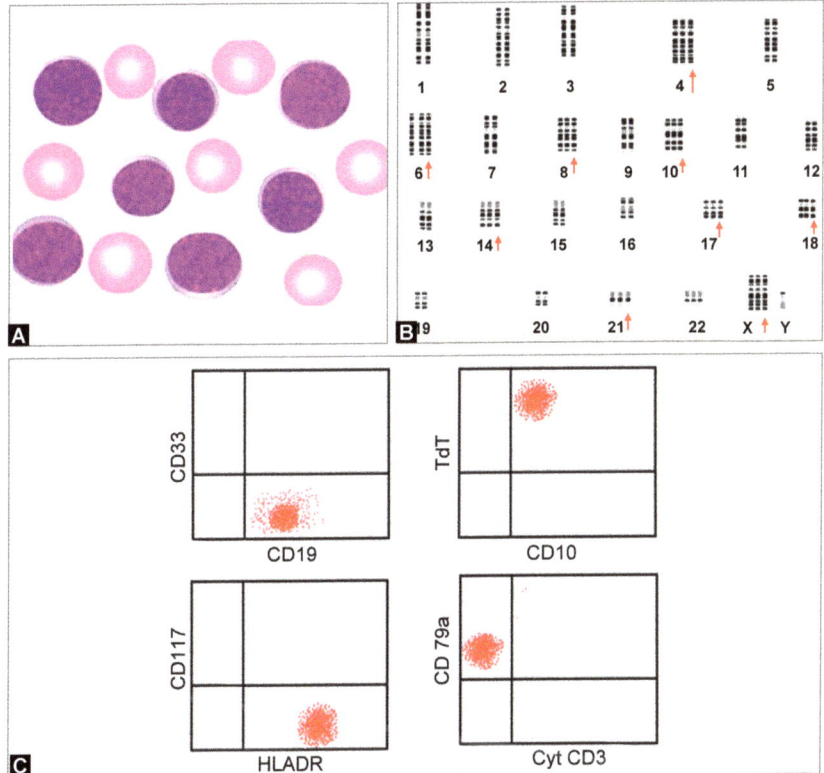

Figs. 5.12A to C: (A) Bone marrow aspiration smear in ALL; (B) Karyotyping showing hyperdiploidy; (C) Flow cytometry shows common ALL phenotype: HLADR+, TdT+, CD10+, and CD79a+ and CD33-, CD117-, and cytCD3-.

Rarely, in a distinctive variant t(5;14) of B-ALL, prominent blood and bone marrow eosinophilia is present which may obscure the lymphoblasts.

Rarely, ALL may present with hypocellular marrow (aplastic anemia) that after a few months is followed by overt manifestations of ALL.

Morphological distinction between B-lymphoblasts and T-lymphoblasts is not possible.

Cytochemistry

Cytochemical stains are an adjunct to the morphological examination of the bone marrow. By conventional definition, lymphoblasts in ALL are negative for myeloperoxidase.

Other stains which are negative in ALL are Sudan black B, chloroacetate esterase, and alpha naphthyl acetate esterase.

In leukemic lymphoblasts, PAS stain is positive in a characteristic manner and has been used for the diagnosis of ALL (Fig. 5.13). PAS-positive material (glycogen) in leukemic lymphoblasts is typically large and block-like, surrounds the nucleus, and is present against a clear cytoplasmic background. PAS stain is positive in L1 and L2 subtypes but is negative in L3 subtype. PAS stain is not specific for leukemic lymphoblasts. Also in many cases of ALL (~30% of L1 and L2), PAS stain is negative; furthermore, PAS positivity may also be observed in leukemic

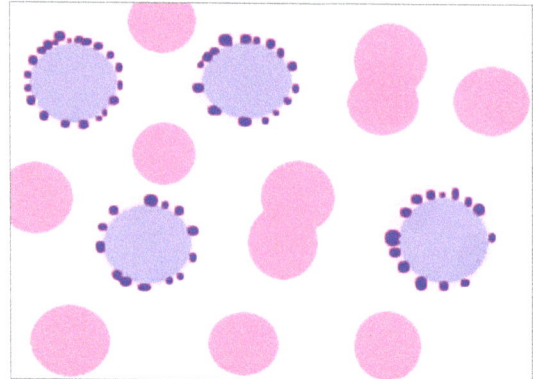

Fig. 5.13: Periodic acid Schiff stain in ALL showing block-like positivity.

myeloblasts (diffuse positivity) and in monoblasts and erythroblasts (small block-like on a diffusely positive background). No cytochemical stain is specific for lymphoblasts. Therefore, morphologic features and immunologic markers are necessary for definitive identification of lymphoblasts.

In T-ALL, acid phosphatase stain is positive in a focal paranuclear manner. In ALL L3, cytoplasmic vacuoles are positive for oil red O stain, while cytoplasm is methyl green pyronine positive.

With the wide availability of flow cytometry, cytochemical stains for the diagnosis of ALL have largely become redundant.

Immunophenotyping

By immunophenotypic analysis, ALL is divided into two main types: B-ALL and T-ALL. Each of these is further subdivided into subtypes. In addition, immunophenotyping distinguishes ALL from other acute leukemias and mature lymphoid neoplasms.

B-ALL: Accounts for 80% of all cases of childhood ALL. B lineage-specific markers are:
- Bright surface CD19 plus at least one of the following: Cytoplasmic CD79a, surface or cytoplasmic CD22, CD10, or
- Weak surface CD19 plus at least two of the following: Cytoplasmic CD79a, surface or cytoplasmic CD22, CD10

Immunological classification of ALL is as follows:
- Pro-B ALL (Early precursor B-ALL) (8–10%): TdT (terminal deoxynucleotidyl transferase) +, HLADR+, CD19+, cytoCD79a+, CD22+. This correlates with FAB subtypes L1 and L2. This type has been found to be more common in infants and children and especially in those with *KMT2A* (*MLL*) gene rearrangement.
- "Common" ALL (50%): TdT+, HLADR+, CD19+, cytoCD79a+, CD22+, CD10 (common ALL antigen or CALLA)+, CD20+. This subtype is the most common form of ALL in children, and is associated with best prognosis. It correlates with FABL1 and L2 morphological subtypes.
- Pre-B ALL (20%): TdT+, HLADR+, CD19+, cytoCD79a+, CD22+, CD10+, CD20+, Cyt μ(cytoplasmic μ chain)+.
- B-ALL (1–2%): HLADR+, CD19+, cytoCD79a+, CD22+, CD10+, CD20+, SmIg (surface membrane immunoglobulin) +. This subtype correlates with L3 morphology, is considered

as a leukemic phase of Burkitt's lymphoma, and is associated with poor prognosis. It is characterized by rearrangement of *C-MYC* caused by translocation of this gene on chromosome 8 with one of the chromosomes containing immunoglobulin gene. This is now considered as leukemic stage of Burkitt lymphoma and is not treated as childhood B-ALL.

T-ALL: Accounts for 15 to 20% cases of childhood ALL. The lineage-specific marker for T cells is cytoplasmic CD3. Immunological classification of T-ALL is as follows:
- Pro-T-ALL: CD7+, CytCD3+
- Pre-T-ALL: CD7+, CytCD3+, CD5+ and/or CD2+
- Cortical T-ALL: CD7+, CytCD3+, CD5+, CD1a+
- Mature T-ALL: CD7+, CytCD3+, CD1a+, membrane CD3+.

Recently, a distinct subtype is described called as early T-precursor ALL (ETP ALL). The immunophenotype of ETP ALL shows T-lineage markers (CD7, cytoplasmic CD3), CD1a-, CD8-, CD5- or weak+, and expression of at least one stem cell- or myeloid-associated antigen (CD34, CD117, CD33, HLA DR, CD11b, or CD64). Although there is high rate of induction failure after intensive therapy, recent studies indicate similar overall survival between ETP ALL and non-ETP ALL.

Co-expression of myeloid antigens: Some cases (20–30%) of childhood ALL co-express myeloid antigens which are often associated with genetic abnormalities like *KMT2A* rearrangement, *BCR-ABL1*, and *ETV6-RUNX1*. It has, however, no independent prognostic significance. Such cases need to be distinguished from leukemia of ambiguous lineage or mixed-phenotype acute leukemia. Lineage-specific myeloid markers (MPO) are, however, not expressed in ALL.

Cytogenetic Analysis

This is one of the most important investigations in ALL that has a great impact on selection of therapy in childhood ALL. Clonal chromosomal abnormalities occur in 80% cases of ALL (Table 5.12).

Certain chromosomal abnormalities are consistently observed in specific types of ALL. Thus, cytogenetic analysis improves the diagnostic efficiency. Secondly, chromosomal abnormalities have prognostic and therapeutic importance. Chromosomal abnormalities in ALL include both numerical and structural alterations.

Hyperdiploidy with >50 chromosomes is the most frequent abnormality in childhood CD10+ precursor or BALL. It is associated with high sensitivity to chemotherapy, complete remission rate of 100%, and long-term disease-free survival of 90%.

Patients with t(9;22)(q34;q11) and abnormalities of 11q23 have unfavorable prognosis with increased risk of relapse, lower remission rate, and poor long-term survival. In these patients, allogeneic hematopoietic stem cell transplantation should be considered in first remission.

Although multiple genetic abnormalities have been described in T-ALL, most are not clinically significant and are not used for treatment stratification.

Table 5.12: Cytogenetic abnormalities in childhood B cell ALL and their relation to prognosis with current therapy.

Chromosomal abnormality	Molecular abnormality	Prognosis
1. Hyperdiploidy (>50)	FLT3	Favorable
2. Hypodiploidy (46)	NF1, IKZF2, IKZF3, TP53, RB1	Unfavorable
3. t(12;21)(p13;q22)*	ETV6-RUNX1	Favorable
4. t(1;19)(q23;p13.3)	TCF3-PBX1	Neutral (standard risk)
5. t(9;22)(q34;q11.2)	BCR/ABL1	Unfavorable
6. t(v;11)(v;q23)	KMT2A rearrangements	Unfavorable
7. t(5;14)(q31;q32)	IL3-IGH	Standard risk
8. iAMP21	Intrachromosomal amplification of chromosome 21 (gain of at least three copies of regional chromosome 21)	Unfavorable
9. Ph-like ALL**	CRLF2, JAK2, EPOR, ABL1, ABL2, CSF1R, PDGFRB	Unfavorable

* Identified only by molecular analysis. v: variable
** High-risk ALL with gene expression profile similar to Ph+ ALL and with highly diverse range of genetic alterations that activate tyrosine kinase signaling but without *BCR-ABL1* fusion gene.

Molecular Genetic Studies

Applications of molecular genetic analysis in ALL include:
- Establishment of lineage: In those cases in which immunophenotyping fails to conclusively identify the lineage of leukemic cells, DNA analysis (Southern blot) may be carried out to detect rearrangement of heavy and light chain genes and T cell receptor genes. However, gene rearrangement studies should be interpreted carefully for reasons outlined earlier (see chapter on "Acute Leukemias"). Rearrangement of light chain genes is specific for B lineage cells.
- Establishment of clonality
- Identification of translocations that cannot be identified by cytogenetic analysis, e.g. t(12;21)(p13;q22) is identified only by molecular analysis
- Detection of MRD
- Early detection of relapse.

Other Investigations

Lumbar puncture: Not all patients with CNS involvement have clinical features of raised intracranial tension. Therefore, cerebrospinal fluid should be examined for lymphoblasts at the time of diagnosis in all patients with ALL. Lymphoblasts are detected in 15 to 20% of children at diagnosis; the incidence is higher in T-ALL. Flow cytometry is more sensitive in detection of CNS leukemia than cytology alone. CSF examination showing $\geq 5/\mu L$ of leukocytes with blast cells have higher risk of relapse. Traumatic lumbar puncture with lymphoblasts on cytologic examination is associated with adverse prognosis.

Testicular biopsy: Testis is a frequent organ of relapse in ALL. Therefore before stopping treatment, testicular biopsy may be performed to rule out residual disease.

X-ray chest: Chest X-ray examination reveals mediastinal widening especially in T-ALL.

Differential Diagnosis of ALL

Diagnosis of ALL is usually obvious in the presence of fever, anemia, thrombocytopenia, lymphadenopathy, hepatosplenomegaly, and diffuse replacement of bone marrow by lymphoblasts. However, ALL should be differentiated from following conditions:

Reactive Lymphocytosis due to Infections

Infections such as by Epstein-Barr virus or cytomegalovirus can produce fever, lymphadenopathy, splenomegaly and reactive lymphocytosis and mimick ALL. Absence of anemia and thrombocytopenia, positive serological tests (e.g. Paul-Bunnell test in infectious mononucleosis, raised IgM viral antibody titers) and morphology of reactive lymphocytes (relatively more amount of cytoplasm, coarse chromatin, scalloping and skirting of borders) are helpful in differentiating infectious lymphocytosis from ALL. Chromosomal studies and immunophenotyping can help in difficult cases.

Acute Myeloid Leukemia

Differences between ALL and AML are outlined in Table 5.13. Due to overlapping morphologic features between lymphoblasts and myeloblasts, ALL should be distinguished from AML (AML with minimal differentiation) and mixed lineage acute leukemias by immunophenotypic analysis. Lymphoblasts are negative for myeloid (MPO) and monocytic (CD11c, CD64, and CD14) markers. Acute leukemia of ambiguous lineage shows coexpression of both myeloid and lymphoid antigens.

Leukemic Phase of Non-Hodgkin's Lymphoma (Mature B- and T-cell Neoplasms)

Bone marrow and peripheral blood involvement by non-Hodgkin's lymphoma may be difficult to distinguish from acute leukemia, particularly when prior history of lymphomatous stage is absent. Small lymphocytic lymphoma/chronic lymphocytic leukemia, mantle cell lymphoma, and small cleaved cell lymphoma have a high incidence of bone marrow involvement. In these disorders, chromatin is condensed, cells express mature B cell phenotype, and immature markers like CD34 and TdT are absent.

Prolymphocytic Leukemia

Prolymphocytes have more abundant cytoplasm (low nuclear cytoplasmic ratio), a prominent nucleolus, and a mature B-cell phenotype.

Metastatic Tumors in Bone Marrow (Small Round Blue Cell Tumors)

In children, metastasis of neuroblastoma and in adolescents and adults, Ewing's sarcoma and small cell carcinoma of lung may have to be differentiated from ALL. Metastatic tumor in bone marrow occurs as clumps (or clusters) rather than as diffuse sheets. Demonstration of primary tumor and immunocytochemical studies including absence of B-cell markers, are helpful in determining the cell of origin.

Table 5.13: Differences between ALL and AML.

Parameter	ALL	AML
1. Age	More common in children	More common in infants, adolescents, and adults
2. Significant lymphadenopathy in more than one location	Common	Uncommon
3. Meningeal disease	More common	Less common
4. Mediastinal lymphadenopathy	Seen in T-ALL	Rare
5. Morphology of blasts – Size – Cytoplasm – Auer rod – Nuclear chromatin – Nucleoli	 Small to medium Scanty Absent Coarse Indistinct, 0–2	 Large Moderately abundant Pathognomonic if present Fine Prominent, 1–4
6. Myelodysplasia	Absent	May be present
7. Cytochemistry – Myeloperoxidase – PAS	 Negative Block-like positive in 70% cases	 Positive Diffuse
8. Immunophenotyping	B lineage: CD19, CD22, TdT; T lineage: CD7, cCD3, CD2, TdT	Granulocytic: CD13, CD33, CD117; Monocytic: CD14, CD64; erythroid: Glycophorin A; Megakaryocytic: CD41
8. Ig or TCR gene rearrangement	B-ALL: Clonal Ig; T-ALL: Clonal TCR	Germline configuration

Hematogones (Reactive Proliferation of Normal Precursor Cells in Bone Marrow)

Hematogones are normal B lymphocyte precursors, which increase in bone marrow in marrow regenerative states and immune cytopenias. Morphologically, they may be mistaken for lymphoblasts of ALL. Cell surface analysis of hematogones shows a spectrum of immature to mature cells (with normal antigenic evolution of B cell precursors). As they consist of different stages of maturation, they express heterogeneous pattern of CD34, TdT, CD10, and CD20. Lymphoblasts in ALL show predominance of immature cells and aberrant antigen expression. Hematogones lack chromosomal abnormalities and clonal immunoglobulin gene rearrangements.

Lymphoid Blast Crisis of Chronic Myeloid Leukemia (CML)

The distinction is based on prior history and presence of Philadelphia chromosome in CML.

Leukemic or Advanced Stage of Burkitt's Lymphoma

This was considered as ALL-L3 in FAB classification of ALL. Burkitt cells show more prominent nucleoli, deeply basophilic cytoplasm with vacuoles, mature B-cell phenotype, lack of immature markers (CD34, TdT) and characteristic t(8;14) translocation involving the *MYC* gene.

Table 5.14: Prognostic factors in ALL.

Parameter	Unfavorable	Favorable
1. Age	<1 year, >10 year	1–10 years
2. Sex	Male (testicular relapse)	Female
3. TLC	>50,000/cmm	<50,000/cmm
4. Immunophenotype	Early T-precursor ALL, pro-B ALL	'Common' ALL (CALLA+, Cμ-)
5. CNS disease	Presence of blasts in CSF	Absence of blasts in CSF
6. Cytogenetic or molecular genetic abnormalities	Hypodiploidy; t(9;22) or *BCR/ABL1* fusion; t(4;11)(q22;q23) or *KMT2A/AF4* fusion, t(17;19)	Hyperdiploidy (>50); t(12;21)(p13;q22), i.e. *TEL/AML1* fusion (*ETV6/RUNX1* fusion)
7. Remission after first induction	Time for complete remission > 4 weeks	Early achievement of remission

Prognostic Factors in ALL

At the time of diagnosis a number of factors affect prognosis (Table 5.14). These factors are used for stratification of treatment, in which more intensive and potentially more toxic treatment is reserved for patients with adverse prognostic factors.

Total Leukocyte Count

This is one of the most important prognostic variables. TLC < 50,000/cmm is associated with good prognosis while high TLC (>50,000/cmm) is associated with poor prognosis. The risk of subsequent relapse increases with increasing leukocyte count in B-ALL.

Age

Age at diagnosis is a well-recognized prognostic factor in B-ALL but not in T-ALL. Children between 1 and 10 years of age have the best prognosis with about 70% of them achieving long-term remission with current methods of treatment. These children have two favorable cytogenetic abnormalities: hyperdiploidy and *ETV6-RUNX1*. Older children and young adults with ALL have a relatively poor outcome and have unfavorable biologic factors like T-ALL, or *BCR-ABL1* fusion. Infants with ALL have the worst prognosis; majority of such infants have rearrangement of *KM2TA* gene.

Immunophenotype

Pro-B ALL and early precursor-T-cell ALL are associated with relatively poor prognosis.

Cytogenetics

Cytogenetic classification is the single most important prognostic factor in ALL. Hyperdiploidy (>50 chromosomes) has better prognosis, while prognosis is unfavorable with translocations especially Ph' chromosome.

Other Bad Prognostic Indicators

These are massive tumor burden (hepatosplenomegaly, lymphadenopathy, mediastinal mass), early CNS disease, and slow response for achieving remission.

Recently described unfavorable prognostic factors include early T-precursor phenotype, expression of CD20 antigen, and genetic mutations included under Ph-like ALL (*CRLF2, JAK2*).

The most favorable prognostic group is of children between 1 and 10 years of age who have "common" ALL (CALLA+, Cµ-) phenotype and have hyperdiploidy (>50 chromosomes). With current modes of treatment, most of these children will achieve long-term remission and many of them are probably cured.

It should be noted, however, that with successful and effective chemotherapy significance of the various prognostic factors is lost.

Risk Categorization in ALL

According to National Cancer Institute/Rome criteria, ALL is categorized into two risk categories (Table 5.15).

Infants <1 year old is a special group associated with worse prognosis. Hypodiploidy, *MLL* (*KMT2A*) rearrangement, iAMP21, Ph'+ve ALL (*BCR-ABL1*), ETP-ALL, and Ph-like ALL are also considered as high-risk in treatment protocols. Hyperdiploidy and *ETV6-RUNX1* are considered as low risk.

Table 5.15: Risk stratification in ALL.

National Cancer Institute	

• Standard risk: Both of following:
  – WBC count < 50,000/mm^3
  – Age: 1–9 years
	• High risk: Any one of following:
	  – WBC count > 50,000/mm^3
	  – Age <1 year or >9 years

Treatment

Major success has been achieved in the treatment of childhood ALL with modern chemotherapy. In Western countries, with current methods of treatment more than 90% of children with ALL achieve complete remission (CR) and majority of them are probably cured. However, in adults with ALL, complete remission is achieved only in a minority of patients.

The average duration of therapy in ALL is 2 to 2½ years.

Phases of Treatment in ALL (Box 5.11)

Remission induction: In this phase, systemic chemotherapy is given to reduce the leukemic cell load below the level of detection and to restore hematopoiesis and health. Remission induction is achieved in 90% of patients by combination of vincristine and prednisone.

Box 5.11: Phases of treatment in ALL.
- Remission induction
- CNS prophylaxis
- Consolidation (Intensification)
- Maintenance

Addition of anthracycline (daunorubicin or doxorubicin) or L-asparaginase or both can induce remission in even more number of patients. Remission is usually induced in 4 to 6 weeks.

In complete remission, there is no clinical or laboratory evidence of leukemia. Complete remission is defined as presence of less than 5% blasts in bone marrow and normalization of peripheral blood cell counts.

Central nervous system prophylaxis: After achieving CR, prophylactic therapy to CNS is necessary in ALL. Leukemic lymphoblasts infiltrate the CNS and CSF in the initial period of the disease. CNS is the sanctuary site in ALL in that the drugs used for remission induction are unable to pass through the blood-brain barrier and thus leukemic cells are protected from chemotherapeutic drugs. Subsequently, these cells may cause leukemic meningitis and relapse. If CNS prophylaxis is administered soon after completion of remission induction, risk of CNS relapse is markedly decreased.

CNS prophylaxis is achieved by combination of cranial irradiation (1800cGy for children, 2400 cGy for adults) plus intrathecal methotrexate. However, with this treatment, children often subsequently develop neuropsychological problems and CNS tumors. Therefore, many investigators omit cranial irradiation, and reserve it for high-risk cases such as T-ALL, TLC > 50,000/cmm, and translocation between chromosomes 9 and 22.

Consolidation treatment: This is the high-dose intensive chemotherapy administered immediately after remission induction to eradicate the residual blast cells and reduce the potentially resistant leukemic cell mass. In this regime, alternative drugs not used for remission induction are employed. Different protocols have been used for this purpose by different centers. The commonly used drugs are anthracycline, cytarabine, cyclophosphamide, asparagine, and thioguanine.

Recently, it has been demonstrated that addition of another block of consolidation therapy at approximately 35 weeks improves the long-term survival in high-risk patients; this is called as double-delayed intensification.

Maintenance therapy: After achieving complete remission, treatment is continued for further 2 to 2½ years. Chemotherapeutic drugs are administered for 2 to 2½ years to maintain the remission and prevent or delay the occurrence of relapse by eradicating residual leukemic cells. The usual drugs for this purpose are 6-mercaptopurine (daily) along with methotrexate (weekly). Careful monitoring is necessary for toxic side effects and compliance.

Supportive Care

- Appropriate blood product replacement therapy includes packed red cell transfusions for anemia and platelet transfusions to maintain platelet count above 20,000/cmm to reduce the risk of spontaneous hemorrhage.
- Infections: Viral infections such as measles (interstitial pneumonitis and encephalitis) and disseminated chickenpox are particularly common. Varicella-zoster immune globulin and gamma globulin for prevention of chickenpox and measles, respectively are recommended. For established chickenpox infection, acyclovir is used.
  - Cotrimoxazole is the standard form of prophylactic treatment for prevention of *Pneumocystis jiroveci (*formerly *carinii)* pneumonia.
  - Empiric antibiotic treatment is indicated in febrile neutropenic patients until definitive cause is identified.
- For prevention of uric acid nephropathy, allopurinol (or rasburicase, a recombinant urate oxidase) should be given and fluid and electrolyte balance should be maintained.
- Tumor lysis syndrome: This is a potentially life-threatening metabolic disorder resulting from destruction (spontaneous or post-treatment) of rapidly proliferating neoplastic cells. It is characterized by hyperuricemia, hyperkalemia, hyperphosphatemia, and hypocalcemia. Acute renal failure can develop. For prevention, adequate hydration should be maintained

during induction chemotherapy and patient should be closely monitored (urine output, renal function, and serum chemistry studies).

Treatment of Relapse

Despite achieving remission, relapse occurs in 25 to 30% of patients. Relapse may occur in bone marrow, central nervous system, or testis. If relapse occurs during maintenance therapy, then possibility of achieving second remission is remote as it indicates refractoriness to therapy. However, if relapse occurs sometimes after maintenance therapy is stopped, then prognosis is better and second remission can be achieved in most patients. Treatment of relapse needs to be more aggressive with induction of new drugs (podophyllins, anthracycline analogues, and fludarabine).

Long-term Side Effects of Intensive Therapy

These include:
- Deficit in intellectual and cognitive functions (in children who receive cranial irradiation at young age)
- Osteopenia, fractures, and osteonecrosis (30% survivors of childhood ALL)
- Increased risk of CNS tumors
- Therapy-related AML (with epipodophyllotoxin and alkylating drug therapy)
- Cardiac toxicity (with anthracyclines)
- Thyroid dysfunction (with cranial and neck irradiation, chemotherapy).

Hematopoietic Stem Cell Transplantation (HSCT)

Many children achieve long-term clinical remission and probably cure with modern chemotherapy. Secondly, allogeneic HSCT is associated with risk of graft-versus-host disease, opportunistic infections, and considerable morbidity and mortality. Therefore, HSCT is reserved for children with ALL in second or subsequent remission; in these cases survival with HSCT is superior as compared to chemotherapy. HSCT in first remission can be considered in those cases resistant to conventional chemotherapy and in high-risk cases such as Philadelphia chromosome-positive ALL and ALL with TLC > 50,000/cmm at diagnosis.

Risk-adapted Therapy in ALL

The aim of risk-adapted therapy in ALL is to administer therapy according to the risk category of the patient (*see* Table 5.14). The goal is to achieve cure with as little toxicity as possible (especially in low-risk patients). Low-risk patients should be treated with less intensive therapy (to limit the toxic effects of therapy), while high-risk patients are treated with more aggressive treatment (to improve survival).

Minimal Residual Disease in ALL

Although more than 95% of children achieve complete remission (i.e. presence of <5% of blast cells in marrow on microscopy) after treatment, relapse occurs in 20% of low-risk and 70% of high-risk patients. This is due to the presence of a small number of viable leukemic cells which survive the cytotoxic chemotherapy and which cannot be detected by the conventional

method. This submicroscopic persistence of disease following treatment is called as MRD. Aim of estimation of MRD following remission induction is to assess initial response to treatment, prognosis, and risk categorization so that further treatment can be individualized (less intensive, more aggressive, or stem cell transplantation) to increase the chance of cure. Currently, there are two main methods for detection of MRD:
- *Flow cytometry:* Detects aberrant antigen expression in leukemic blasts (1 leukemic cell per 10^3-10^4 normal cells)
- *Genetic analysis by quantitative polymerase chain reaction:* Detects leukemia clone-specific rearrangement of immunoglobulin heavy chain (IgH) or T-cell receptor (TCR) gene (1 leukemic cell per 10^4-10^5 normal cells)

It is necessary to establish these abnormalities at diagnosis before beginning therapy. MRD is a powerful tool to predict prognosis in childhood ALL. Outcome of poor prognostic categories like Ph-like ALL or ETP-ALL can be significantly improved if treatment is based on MRD.

Experience in India

Currently, the 5-year survival rate of ALL in children following therapy reported from major centers in India is 70%. Poor outcome in Indian children as compared to those in the Western countries appears to be due to various reasons including (1) T-ALL and molecular abnormalities associated with unfavorable prognosis (such as *BCR/ABL*, *E2A/PBX*) are more common in Indian children; (2) favorable abnormalities like hyperdiploidy and *ETV6-RUNX1* are less common, (3) noncompliance due to financial burden; and (4) poor tolerance to cytotoxic chemotherapy due to malnourishment.

ACUTE MYELOID LEUKEMIA

Synonyms: Acute myelogenous leukemia, Acute nonlymphocytic leukemia.

Acute myeloid leukemia (AML) is a malignant neoplasm of hematopoietic stem cells originating in bone marrow and characterized by proliferation of blast cells of myeloid lineage. AML is genotypically and phenotypically extremely heterogeneous. Since last 30 years, AML is being treated with the same induction regimen (cytosine arabinoside + anthracycline). With the recent identification of specific types in WHO classification (2017), individualization of treatment is possible.

Clinical Features

Acute myeloid leukemia is the most common form of acute leukemia in adults and becomes increasingly more common as age advances. Median age at diagnosis is 65 years. It is also the predominant form of leukemia before 1 year of age. It is much less frequent in children as compared to ALL.

AML can arise from pre-existing disorders such as myelodysplastic syndrome, myeloproliferative diseases (chronic myeloid leukemia, polycythemia vera, myelofibrosis), and paroxysmal nocturnal hemoglobinuria. Alkylating drugs, epipodophyllotoxins, and radiotherapy given for treatment of other neoplasms can induce AML. Genetic diseases with increased predisposition to AML include Down's syndrome, Bloom's syndrome, and Fanconi's anemia.

Clinical features are mainly due to bone marrow failure caused by infiltration by neoplastic cells, i.e. anemia (weakness, fatigue), granulocytopenia (infections), and thrombocytopenia (bleeding tendencies). Fever always indicates infection even if an identifiable focus is not found. As compared to ALL, AML is equally common between sexes and more commonly occurs in adults; bone pain, hepatomegaly, and splenomegaly are less common, and lymphadenopathy is rare (Bone pain should raise the possibility of ALL, especially in children). Skin infiltration (leukemia cutis) and gum hypertrophy occur in 50% of patients with monocytic leukemia (AML M4 and M5). About 10% of patients present with hyperleukocytosis (TLC > 100,000/cmm); these patients belong to the poor prognostic category and have increased risk of leukostasis due to intravascular clumping of blasts. Sludging of blood flow can cause pulmonary manifestations (severe dyspnea and diffuse lung shadowing), retinal hemorrhages, or neurological manifestations (altered mental status, ocular muscle palsy, etc.). CNS changes are more common in acute monocytic/monoblastic leukemia. Rarely, a patient may present with an isolated mass of leukemic cells in an extramedullary site called as chloroma or myeloid sarcoma. The common sites are soft tissues, bones (skull, sternum, ribs, vertebrae, pelvis, paranasal sinuses), skin, mucosal sites like gums, and lymph nodes. Myeloid sarcoma may precede or occur simultaneously with AML.

Disseminated intravascular coagulation (DIC) is especially likely to occur in acute promyelocytic leukemia due to release of thromboplastin-like material from primary granules of abnormal promyelocytes. DIC can also occur in monocytic leukemias (AML M4 or M5) due to the release of lysozyme.

Rapid response to chemotherapy may induce "tumor lysis syndrome" which is characterized by hyperuricemia with renal insufficiency, hyperphosphatemia, hypocalcemia, and acidosis.

History of previous cytotoxic chemotherapy and/or radiotherapy should be elicited for diagnosis of therapy-related AML. Down's syndrome and inherited bone marrow failure syndromes predispose to the development of AML and such history should be obtained.

Classification

There are two classification systems for AML
1. French-American-British Co-operative Group Classification (1976)
2. World Health Organization Classification (2017)

The French-American-British Cooperative Group Classification

The French-American-British (FAB) Co-operative Group classification is outlined in Table 5.2.

The FAB Co-operative Group has defined eight types of AML: M0 to M7. These include leukemias of granulocytic (M0, M1, M2, M3), monocytic (M4 and M5), erythroid (M6), and megakaryocytic (M7) lineages. The name "myeloid" is given because these lineages arise from the pleuripotent myeloid stem cell.

This classification is based on morphological and cytochemical features. Diagnosis of AML is made when 30% or more of nucleated cells in bone marrow are blasts (If less than 30% of all nucleated cells are blasts, then diagnosis of myelodysplastic syndrome is considered). Percentages of granulocytic and monocytic components are assessed in nonerythroid cells for classifying M1 to M5 types. Percentage of erythroblasts should be less than 50% of all nucleated cells in bone marrow. If > 50% of all nucleated cells in bone marrow are erythroblasts and >

30% of nonerythroid cells are blasts then diagnosis is AML-M6. (If erythroblasts are > 50% of all nucleated cells and < 30% of nonerythroid cells are blasts, then diagnosis is myelodysplastic syndrome.)

World Health Organization Classification

This classification is listed in Table 5.3. The new WHO classification retains the categories of FAB classification, and also creates some new categories. The blast count for diagnosis of AML is reduced to 20% from previous FAB standard of 30%. This is because studies have indicated that patients with 20 to 30% blasts (classified as "refractory anemia with excess blasts in transformation" or RAEB-T in FAB classification) have prognosis similar to patients with ≥ 30% blasts. A brief description of WHO classification (2017) follows:

AML with recurrent genetic abnormalities: This category includes specific balanced translocations, gene fusions, and gene mutations. In addition to specific genetic abnormalities, most of the diseases in this category have distinctive clinical, morphologic, and prognostic features. The abnormalities t(8;21), inv(16), t(16;16), and *PML-RARA* are diagnosed as AML even if blasts are <20%. It is necessary to perform genetic analysis in all morphologically diagnosed cases of AML.

- AML with t(8;21)(q22;q22.1) *(RUNX1-RUNX1T1):* Bone marrow shows distinctive morphologic features like abundant granules, perinuclear hofs, basophilic cytoplasm, occasional large pink or salmon-colored granules, and occasional Auer rods. Blasts express CD34, HLA-DR, myeloid antigens (MPO, CD13, CD33 weak), and aberrant lymphoid antigen (CD19). Cases with t(8;21) should be diagnosed as AML irrespective of the blast percentage in the bone marrow. The translocation disrupts function of core binding factor (which regulates normal hematopoiesis). Core binding factor is also disrupted in AML with inv(16) (p13.1q22) or t(16;16)(p13.1;q22) and these leukemias are called as core binding factor leukemias. This type of AML is associated with a favorable prognosis; however, mutations in *KIT* are associated with adverse outcome.
- AML with inv(16)(p13.1q22) or t(16;16)(p13.1;q22) *(CBFB-MYH11)*: There is evidence of both granulocytic and monocytic differentiation similar to acute myelomonocytic leukemia with abnormal eosinophils (FAB: AML M4 with Eo). Abnormal eosinophils show large basophilic granules. Immunophenotyping shows CD34, CD117, often CD2, both myeloid antigens (CD13, CD33, CD15, MPO) and monocytic differentiation antigens (CD14, CD4, CD68, lysozyme). Presence of cytogenetic abnormality is diagnostic of AML regardless of blast percentage. In the absence of *KIT* mutation, prognosis is favorable.
- Acute promyelocytic leukemia with *PML-RARA*: There is proliferation of blasts cells in bone marrow with features of promyelocytes. The abnormal promyelocytes are considered as blast equivalents for the purpose of diagnosis. Demonstration of *PML-RARA* fusion gene is diagnostic of AML regardless of blast percentage. It is of two types: hypergranular and hypogranular. In hypergranular type, there are abundant cytoplasmic granules and bundles of Auer rods (called faggots); the nuclear margin is irregular and appears folded or reniform. Myeloid antigens (MPO, CD33) are positive, HLA DR is weak or absent and CD34 is negative. In hypogranular type, cytoplasmic granules are indistinct, nuclei are folded or butterfly-shaped; immunophenotyping shows MPO+, CD33+, CD34+, and HLA-DR- or dim. DIC is common. Prognosis is good in cases with rapid diagnosis and initiation of therapy (standard induction therapy with high-dose anthracycline given with or after

all-trans retinoic acid or ATRA). *FLT3* ITD mutation occurs in a subset of patients and is associated with inferior prognosis.
- AML with t(9;11)(p21.3;q23.3) (*KMT2A-MLLT3*): This form of AML has intermediate prognosis, typically occurs in children (particularly infants) and blasts often show monocytic features.
- AML with t(6;9)(p23;q34.1); *DEK-NUP214*: There are no specific blast cell features. It is often associated with erythroid hyperplasia, multilineage dysplasia and basophilia. Occurrence of *FLT3* mutation is common and prognosis is poor.
- AML with inv(3)(q21.3q26.2) or t(3;3)(q21.3;q26.2); *GATA2, MECOM*: Myeloid blasts are associated with multilineage dysplasia and small monolobed or bilobed megakaryocytes. Prognosis is poor.
- Acute myeloid leukemia (megakaryoblastic) with t(1;22)(p13.3;q13.1) (*RBM15-MKL1*): This subtype most often occurs in infants without Down's syndrome and blasts have megakaryoblastic features like cytoplasmic blebs or budding of platelets. Micromegakaryocytes are common. There is variable marrow fibrosis. It may present as a soft tissue mass (myeloid sarcoma) resembling other small round blue cell tumors. Outcome is generally poor.
- Acute myeloid leukemia with *BCR-ABL1*: This is a de novo disease without antecedent or concurrent chronic myeloid leukemia. Prognosis is poor but may benefit from tyrosine kinase inhibitor therapy and hematopoietic stem cell transplantation.

Acute myeloid leukemia with gene mutations:
- Acute myeloid leukemia with mutated *NPM1*: Blasts often show monocytic differentiation and cup-shaped nuclei. Prognosis is favorable in the absence of *FLT3* mutation.
- Acute myeloid leukemia with biallelic mutation of *CEBPA:* This is associated with favorable prognosis in the absence of *FLT3* mutations.
- Acute myeloid leukemia with mutated *RUNX1:* This is a provisional entity in the WHO 2016 classification and is limited to de novo AML that does not meet the criteria for any other AML types especially therapy-related AML and AML with myelodysplasia-related changes. It is associated with worse overall survival and treatment resistance.

Acute myeloid leukemia with myelodysplasia-related changes: This is more common in older patients and is associated with poor prognosis. It is characterized by ≥20% blasts in blood or bone marrow and any one of following (1) previous history of myelodysplastic syndrome, (2) cytogenetic abnormality that is related to myelodysplastic syndrome, or (3) multilineage dysplasia (excluding cases with *NPM1* and biallelic mutations of *CEBPA* which also show myelodysplasia) (Multilineage dysplasia refers to dysplastic changes in ≥50% cells in at least two myeloid cell lines; this is in contrast to myelodysplastic syndrome in which a 10% threshold is used to define a dysplastic lineage). In addition, previous history of cytotoxic therapy for an unrelated disease and recurring genetic abnormalities associated with AML should be absent.

Therapy-related myeloid neoplasms: Myeloid neoplasms can develop after chemotherapy or radiation therapy administered for other malignant or chronic disorders. Latent interval can be short (2–3 years) usually after topoisomerase II inhibitor therapy, or long (5–7 years) usually after alkylating drug therapy.

Short latency type of neoplasm usually shows monoblastic or myelomonocytic features and abnormalities of *KMT2A* or *RUNX1*. Long latency type of neoplasm shows myelodysplastic features, deletions of chromosomes 5 and 7, and complex karyotypes. Prognosis is generally poor.

Acute myeloid leukemia, not otherwise specified: This category consists of those cases of AML that do not belong to any of the previous categories. Most of these subtypes are similar to FAB categories, with some modifications. The nine subtypes are defined on the basis of morphology, cytochemistry, immunophenotyping, and degree of maturation.
1. Acute myeloid leukemia with minimal differentiation: Blasts comprise ≥20% in blood or marrow without cytochemical expression of myeloperoxidase or nonspecific esterase but show evidence of myeloid nature by flow cytometry. Blasts express primitive hematopoietic cell markers (CD34, HLA-DR, CD38) and myeloid markers like myeloperoxidase, CD13, CD33, or CD117. Antigens associated with myeloid or monocytic maturation or erythroid or megakaryocytic lineage are lacking.
2. Acute myeloid leukemia without maturation: Blasts are ≥20% in blood or bone marrow which are cytochemically positive for myeloperoxidase (≥3%) and negative for nonspecific esterase (<20%). Blasts comprise ≥90% of nonerythroid marrow cells and <10% maturing myeloid elements.
3. Acute myeloid leukemia with maturation: Blasts are ≥20% in blood or bone marrow and there are >10% maturing elements (promyelocytes or later stages).
4. Acute myelomonocytic leukemia: There are ≥20% blasts (sum of myeloblasts, monoblasts, and promonocytes) with expression of myeloperoxidase by cytochemistry (≥3%) and >20% monocytic cells identified by morphology and/or cytochemical nonspecific esterase stain.
5. Acute monoblastic and monocytic leukemia: Blasts comprise ≥20% with ≥80% monocytic cells identified by morphology and/or cytochemical nonspecific esterase stain.
6. Pure erythroid leukemia: This is an extremely rare and aggressive type of AML that does not have increased myeloblasts but has > 80% marrow erythroid cells of which ≥30% are pronormoblasts.
7. Acute megakaryoblastic leukemia: Blasts comprise ≥20% out of which ≥50% express megakaryocytic markers (CD41, CD42, or CD61).
8. Acute basophilic leukemia: Blasts are ≥20% with basophilic morphology (basophilic granules) and positivity for basophilic markers on flow cytometry (expression of CD203c in the absence of CD117).
9. Acute panmyelosis with myelofibrosis: This very rare and rapidly progressive form of AML shows ≥20% blasts, diffusely fibrotic bone marrow stroma, panmyelosis (trilineage proliferation of immature granulocytes, megakaryocytes, and erythroid precursors), and markedly dysplastic megakaryocytes. Peripheral blood shows pancytopenia. Splenomegaly is lacking.

Myeloid sarcoma: Myeloid sarcoma (also called as granulocytic sarcoma, chloroma, extramedullary myeloid tumor) is an extramedullary proliferation of myeloid blasts and is diagnostic of AML even if blasts are not increased in blood or bone marrow. Myeloid sarcoma may present (1) de novo without bone marrow involvement, (2) as relapse in a treated case of myeloid neoplasm, and (3) concurrently with acute myeloid leukemia, myelodysplastic syndrome, or myeloproliferative neoplasm.

Myeloid proliferations associated with Down syndrome:
- Transient abnormal myelopoiesis (TAM) associated with Down's syndrome: This is a unique disorder occurring in 10% of newborns (typically 3–7 days of life) with Downs' syndrome in which clinical and morphologic features are indistinguishable from AML. In most cases, spontaneous remission occurs within 3 months of life. However, 20 to 30% of these infants eventually develop AML within first 4 years of life.

- Myeloid leukemia associated with Down syndrome: AML in Down's syndrome develops in the first 3 years of life and is often of megakaryoblastic type. Prognosis is better in patients younger than 4 years of age. *GATA-1* mutations are present in both TAM and AML.

Laboratory Features of AML

Peripheral Blood Examination

Anemia is common and is normocytic and normochromic with low reticulocytes. Total leukocyte count may be low or markedly raised. Blasts are usually present in peripheral blood (Figs. 5.14A and B). Cells considered as blasts in AML are myeloblasts (types 1, 2, and 3), monoblasts,

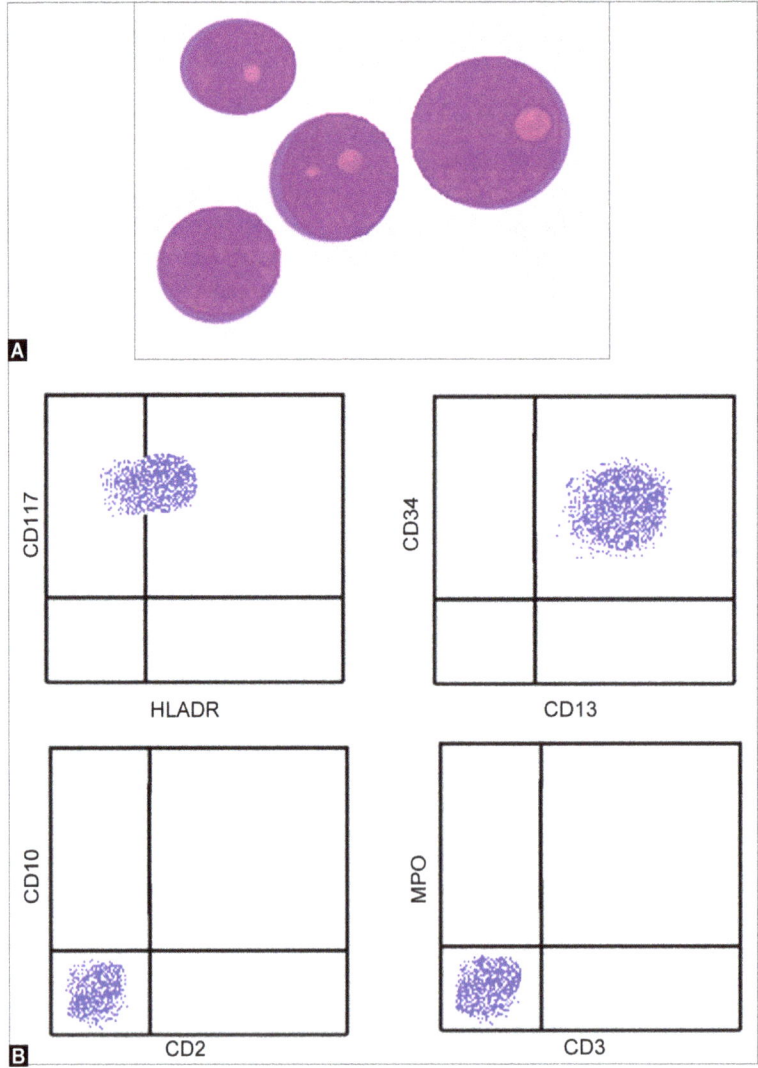

Figs. 5.14A and B: (A) Blood smear in AML M0; (B) Flow cytometry showing HLADR+, CD117+, CD13+. CD34+, CD10-, CD2-, and CD3- blasts.

and megakaryoblasts. Blast equivalents include promyelocytes (granular or hypogranular) for acute promyelocytic leukemia, promonocytes for AML with monocytic component, and pronormoblasts (atypical with cytoplasmic vacuoles) for pure erythroid leukemia. Certain AML subtypes have distinctive morphology like acute promyelocytic leukemia with *PML/RARA*, AML with t(8;21), AML with inv(16) or t(16;16), and AML with *NPM1* and/or *FLT3* mutations. Absolute granulocyte count is always low. Morphologic abnormalities of neutrophils such as Pelger-Huet cells and hypogranular forms may be seen. Thromobocytopenia is commonly present. Platelets are often large and bizarre.

Bone Marrow Examination

Bone marrow examination is necessary for diagnosis and classification of AML. The diagnosis of AML requires 20% or more blasts in all nucleated cells in bone marrow, the exceptions are given above. Bone marrow is hypercellular. However, older patients with AML may present with hypocellular marrow; in these cases interstitium of bone marrow shows blast cells. Normal hematopoietic elements are severely reduced. Morphology of non-blast myeloid population should be evaluated for dysplasia. Significant myelodysplasia is seen in AML with myelodysplasia-related changes, which is associated with poor prognosis.

The main role of morphologic examination in AML is in (1) establishing a diagnosis of AML (blast count), (2) diagnosis of AML with myelodysplasia-related changes, (3) detection of any distinctive morphology that can provide clues to certain recurrent genetic abnormalities (Box 5.12), and (4) diagnosis of subtypes under the category of AML-not otherwise specified.

Box 5.12: Association of morphologic features with genetic abnormalities.

Following genetic abnormalities have certain distinctive morphologic features that can provide clues regarding particular genetic subtype. Although they provide strong clinical suspicion, they are not always specific. If cytogenetic analysis is negative, they can guide additional genetic testing.
- AML with t(8;21);(RUNX1-RUNX1T1): Large, pink or salmon-colored granules, perinuclear hofs
- AML with inv(16)(p13.1q22) or t(16;16)(p13.1;q22); *CBFB-MYH11*: Myelomonocytic morphology, abnormal eosinophils with large, basophil granules
- Acute promyelocytic leukemia with *PML-RARA*: (1) Hypergranular: Abundant cytoplasmic granules with bundles of Auer rods, (2) Hypogranular: Folded, bilobed nuclei
- AML with mutated *NPM1*: Monocytic features with nuclear invaginations (cup-shaped nuclei)

Cytochemistry
(See also "Acute Leukemias—Diagnosis and Classification")

With careful morphological examination of blood and bone marrow aspirations smears, many cases of AML and ALL can be correctly diagnosed. Comparative morphological features of myeloblasts and lymphoblasts are shown in Figure 5.4 and Table 5.13. Additional studies (cytochemistry and immunophenotyping) are required if morphological features are equivocal.

Myeloperoxidase stain is used for identification of primary granules in myeloid precursors and is an important stain for diagnosis of AML M1, M2, M3, and M4 (*see* Fig. 5.6). In the early stage, myeloperoxidase is formed in perinuclear area which needs ultrastructural examination for its demonstration.

Section 3: Disorders of White Blood Cells

The staining reactions with Sudan black B and chloroacetate esterase are mostly similar to myeloperoxidase.

Nonspecific esterase activity (using alpha naphthyl acetate esterase) is positive in AML M4 and M5 (monocytic component) and is sensitive to sodium fluoride (see Figs. 5.7 and 5.8).

In AML M6, erythroblasts show granular positivity with PAS. Iron stain usually reveals ringed sideroblasts. Myeloperoxidase is positive in myeloblastic component.

Demonstration of platelet peroxidase in AML M7 requires electron microscopic examination.

Cytochemical reactions in different types of AML are listed in Table 5.5.

Myeloid nature of blasts can be established by (1) morphology: Auer rods, (2) cytochemistry: MPO, NSE, and (3) flow cytometry.

Immunophenotyping (Table 5.16)
(See also under "Acute Leukemias—Diagnosis and Classification")

It is recommended to perform flow cytometry in all cases of AML at diagnosis (Box 5.13). It is more sensitive than cytochemistry.

Markers of differentiation:
- Precursor cells: CD34, TdT, CD117 (CKIT)
- T lymphoid: Cytoplasmic CD3
- B lymphoid: CD19, CD22, CD79a, CD10
- Granulocytic (also called as myeloid): MPO, CD13, CD33, CD117
- Monocytic: CD11c, CD14, CD64, lysozyme
- Erythroid: Glycophorin A, hemoglobin A
- Megakaryocytic: CD41, CD42b, CD61, von Willebrand factor (F VIII-related antigen)

Box 5.13: Role of flow cytometry in AML.
- Identification of blasts: Dim expression of CD45 and low side scatter
- Differentiation of normal from abnormal (leukemic) blasts
- Lineage assignment (e.g. myeloid, monocytic, erythroid, megakaryocytic)
- Prediction of likely genetic abnormality from immunophenotype
- Detection of minimal residual disease

Table 5.16: Immunophenotypic features of AML subtypes.

AML subtype	Immunophenotyping
AML with recurrent genetic abnormalities	
AML with t(8;21)(q22;q22.1); *RUNX1-RUNX1T1*	CD34+, HLA-DR+, MPO+, CD13+, CD33 weak, aberrant expression of B antigen (like CD19, CD79a, PAX5, TdT), CD56+ in a subset of cases
AML with inv.(16) or t(16;16); *CBFB-MYH11*	Multiple populations: Immature (CD34+, CD117+), granulocytic (CD13+, CD33+, CD15+, MPO+), monocytic (CD4, CD11c, CD14, CD64, lysozyme)
Acute promyelocytic leukemia with *PML-RARA*	(1) Hypergranular: CD34-, HLA-DR-, CD33+bright, MPO+bright, CD13+/-; (2) Hypogranular: CD34dim, HLA-DRdim, CD33+bright, MPO+bright, CD13±, aberrant CD2+
AML with t(9;11)(p21.3;q23.3) *KMT2A-MLLT3*	CD34 weak to -, CD33+ CD4+, CD64+, CD65+, lysozyme+, HLA-DR+
AML with t(6;9); *DEK-NUP214*	CD34+, CD117+, MPO+, CD13+, CD33+, CD38+, CD123+, HLA-DR+, TdT+/-
inv(3)(q21.3q26.2) or t(3;3) (q21.3;q26.2); *GATA2, MECOM*	CD34+, CD13+, CD33+, CD117, HLA-DR+, aberrant CD7+/-, variable CD41 and CD61 expression

Contd...

Contd...

AML subtype	Immunophenotyping
Acute myeloid leukemia (megakaryoblastic) with t(1;22)(p13.3;q13.1); *RBM15-MKL1*	CD34-, CD13+, CD33+, HLA-DR-, megakaryocytic antigens (CD41, CD61)+, aberrant CD7+
Acute myeloid leukemia with *BCR-ABL1*	CD34+, CD13+, CD33+, aberrant expression of lymphoid antigens like CD19, CD7, and TdT common
AML with gene mutations	
Acute myeloid leukemia with mutated *NPM1*	CD34-, HLA-DR-, CD117+, CD33+ , CD11c+; monocytic differentiation may be present
Acute myeloid leukemia with biallelic mutation of *CEBPA*	HLA-DR+, CD15+, Aberrant T cell antigen (CD7)+
Acute myeloid leukemia with mutated *RUNX1*	CD34+, HLA-DR+, CD13+, variable expression of MPO, CD33, and monocytic markers
AML with myelodysplasia-related changes	
Acute myeloid leukemia with myelodysplasia-related changes	CD34+, CD117+, CD13+, CD33+, monocytic markers (CD4,CD14)+, aberrant expression of CD7, CD10, and CD56±
Therapy-related myeloid neoplasms	
Therapy-related myeloid neoplasms	CD34+, CD13+, aberrant expression of CD7 and CD56+
Acute myeloid leukemia, not otherwise specified	
Acute myeloid leukemia with minimal differentiation	CD34+, CD38+, HLA-DR+, CD13+, CD33+, CD117+, aberrant expression of TdT±, CD7 ±, TdT±
Acute myeloid leukemia without maturation	CD34±, CD117+ HLA-DR±, CD13+, CD33+ CD15−,CD14−, aberrant T cell marker CD7±
Acute myeloid leukemia with maturation	CD34+ in subset, CD117+ in subset, CD13+, CD33+, CD15-, CD14-, aberrant expression of CD7+/-
Acute myelomonocytic leukemia	Mixed population: Immature (CD34+ and/or CD117+, HLA-DR+), myeloid (CD13+, CD33+, CD15+, MPO+); monocytic (CD14+, CD4+, CD64+, lysozyme+)
Acute monoblastic and monocytic leukemia	CD34±, CD117±, HLA-DR+, MPO weak/-, CD33+bright, CD13+dim, CD15+, CD64+, lysozyme+, CD14-, aberrant expression of CD2+ and CD56+
Pure erythroid leukemia	CD34-, HLA-DR-, CD71+, glycophorin A±, hemoglobin A±
Acute megakaryoblastic leukemia	CD34-, TdT-, MPO -, CD13±, CD33±, CD41+, CD61+
Acute basophilic leukemia	CD34+, HLA-DR+, CD117-, CD13±, CD33±, CD123+, CD203c+
Acute panmyelosis with myelofibrosis	Due to dense fibrosis of marrow, aspirate is often inadequate for flow cytometry and diagnosis and immunophenotyping is based on immunohistochemistry. Precursor marker CD34+, myeloid markers CD13+ and CD33+ (MPO-), megakaryocytic markers CD41+ and CD61+, erythroid markers glycophorin+, and hemoglobin A+

Cytogenetic Analysis

Cytogenetic abnormalities are common in AML (Table 5.17). In the recent WHO classification, syndromes of AML have been characterized with recurrent genetic abnormalities that correlate with clinical features, morphology, response to therapy, and overall prognosis. Two main types of cytogenetic abnormalities are observed in AML: (1) structural rearrangements (translocations or inversions), and (2) gain or loss of whole or part of a chromosome. Genetic analysis by a sensitive method (like reverse transcriptase-polymerase chain reaction) should be carried out in all newly diagnosed cases before beginning therapy because of their prognostic and therapeutic relevance.

The genetic abnormalities play a major role in the pathogenesis of AML.

Morphology, immunophenotyping and genetic features of different types of AML are shown in Figures 5.14 to 5.17.

Table 5.17: Genetic abnormalities in acute myeloid leukemia.

Genetic abnormality	Prognosis	Comments
t(8;21)(q22;q22.1); *(RUNX1-RUNX1T1)**	Favorable	Large pink granules, perinuclear hof
inv(16)(p13q22) or t(16;16)(p13.1;q22); *(CBFB-MYH11)**	Favorable	Myelomonocytic, eosinophils increased in marrow and contain mixed eosinophilic-basophilic granules
t(15;17)(q24;q21.2); *(PML-RARA)**	Favorable	(a) Hypergranular: Numerous promyelocytes with Auer rods; (b) Hypogranular: Bilobed nuclei
t(9;11)(p21.3;q23.3); *KMT2A-MLLT3*	Intermediate	Usually monocytic
t(6;9)(p23;q34.1); *DEK-NUP214*	Unfavorable	Variable blast morphology
inv(3)(q21.3q26.2) or t(3;3)(q21.3;q26.2); *GATA2, MECOM*	Unfavorable	No specific blast morphology
t(1;22) (p13;q13.1); *RBM15-MKL1*	Unfavorable	Blasts with megakaryocytic features; more common in infants
t(9;22)(q34;q11.2); *BCR-ABL1*	Unfavorable	No evidence of previous or concurrent chronic myeloid leukemia
NPM1 mutations	Favorable	Monocytic blasts, cup-like nuclear invaginations
CEBPA mutations (biallelic)	Favorable	—
RUNX1 mutation	Unfavorable	Minimal differentiation
FLT3-ITD mutation	Unfavorable	Cup-shaped nuclear invaginations
Complex karyotype (3 or more abnormalities)	Unfavorable	Myelodysplasia

*Diagnosis can be made with <20% blasts if genetic abnormality is demonstrated.

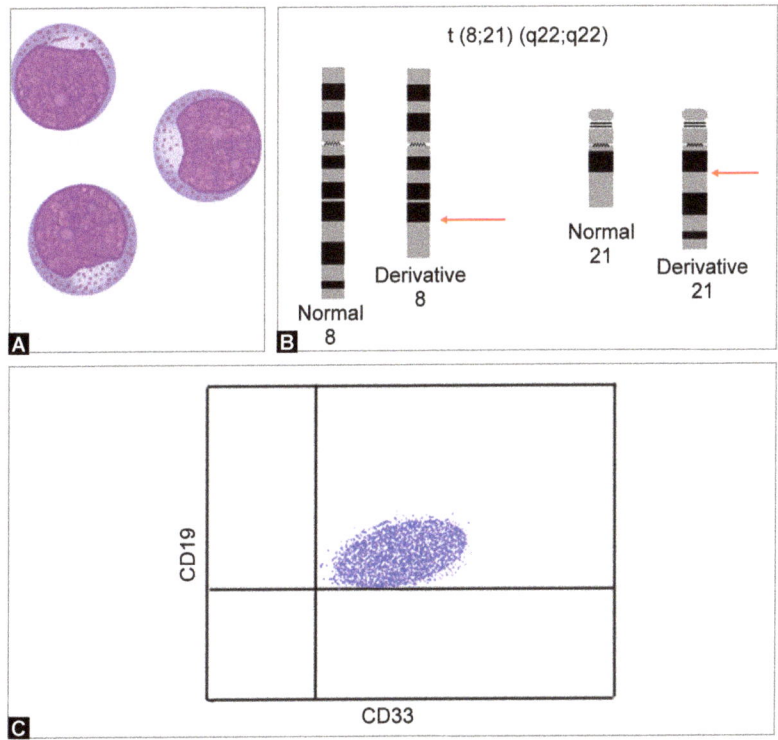

Figs. 5.15A to C: AML with t(8;21)(q22;q22). (A) Blood smear showing blasts with abundant large pink granules, basophilic cytoplasm, perinuclear hof, and thin Auer rod; (B) diagrammatic representation of t(8;21)(q22;q22); (C) flow cytometry showing expression of CD33 and aberrant expression of CD19. Other markers that are positive but not shown are CD13 and CD34.

Differential Diagnosis

Leukemoid Reaction

Presence of immature white blood cells in peripheral blood may be due to nonleukemic causes, e.g. infections, acute hemolysis, or other infiltrative diseases of the bone marrow. In leukemoid reaction, total leucocyte count is moderately increased and blast cells rarely exceed 5%. The whole range of granulocytic maturation is seen. In infections, toxic changes in neutrophils are evident. Clinical features of the causative disorder may be obvious. In difficult cases, cytogenetic analysis may be helpful.

Myelodysplastic Syndrome (MDS)

Differentiation of AML from MDS depends on proportion of myeloblasts in the bone marrow. In AML, myeloblasts are ≥20%, while in MDS they are < 20%. (*see* classification of AML).

Acute Lymphoblastic Leukemia

AML M0 and AML M7 should be differentiated from ALL (*see* Table 5.13).

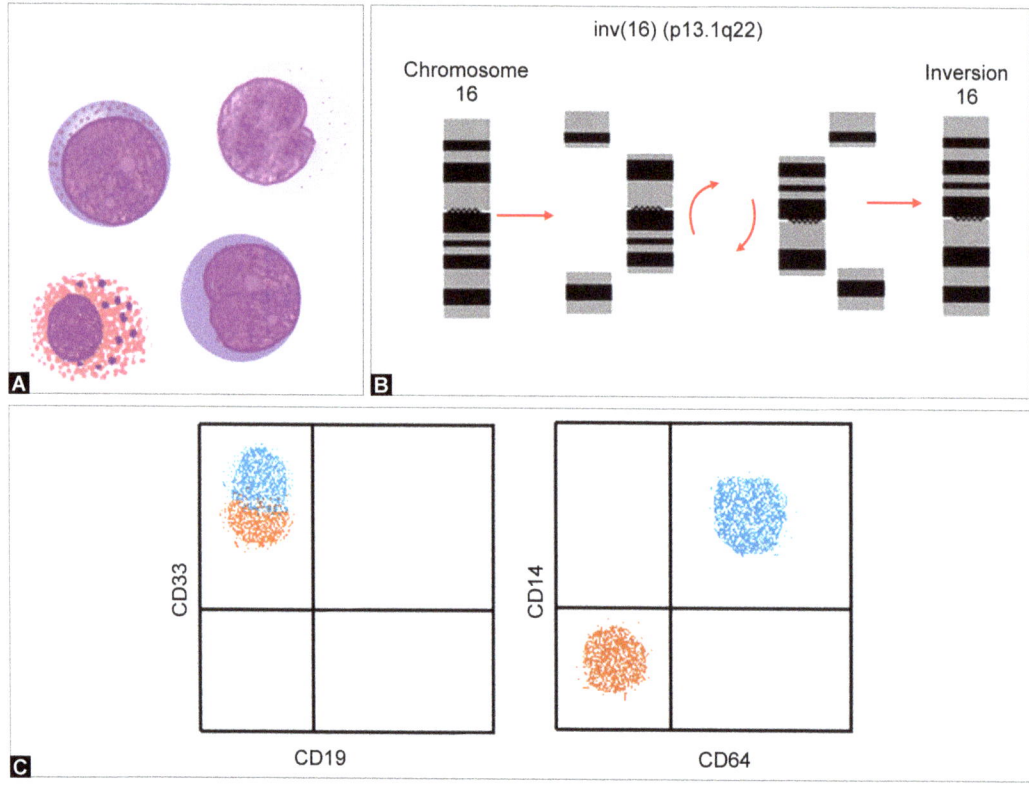

Figs. 5.16A to C: AML with inv(16)(p13.1q22). (A) Blood smear showing myelomonocytic appearance and abnormal eosinophils containing large, basophilic granules. (B) Diagrammatic representation of inv(16) (p13.1q22). (C) Representative flow cytometry graphs showing myeloblasts (orange) positive for CD33 and negative for CD19, CD14, and CD64; and monocytic cells (blue) positive for CD33, CD14, and CD64.

Blast Crisis of Chronic Myelogenous Leukemia (CML)

It may be difficult to differentiate AML from blast crisis of CML if previous history is absent. Marked splenomegaly, basophilia, and Philadelphia chromosome are suggestive of chronic myelogenous leukemia.

Prognostic Factors in AML

In AML, cytogenetic abnormalities and age are the major prognostic determinants. Depending on the risk of relapse, three prognostic categories are defined in AML as shown in Figure 5.18.

Poor prognostic factors in AML are age >60 years; chromosomal abnormalities such as monosomies of chromosome 5 or 7, deletion of long arm of chromosome 5, and complex chromosomal abnormalities; elevated lactate dehydrogenase; hyperleukocytosis (TLC > 100,000/cmm); secondary AML; and AML with myelodysplasia.

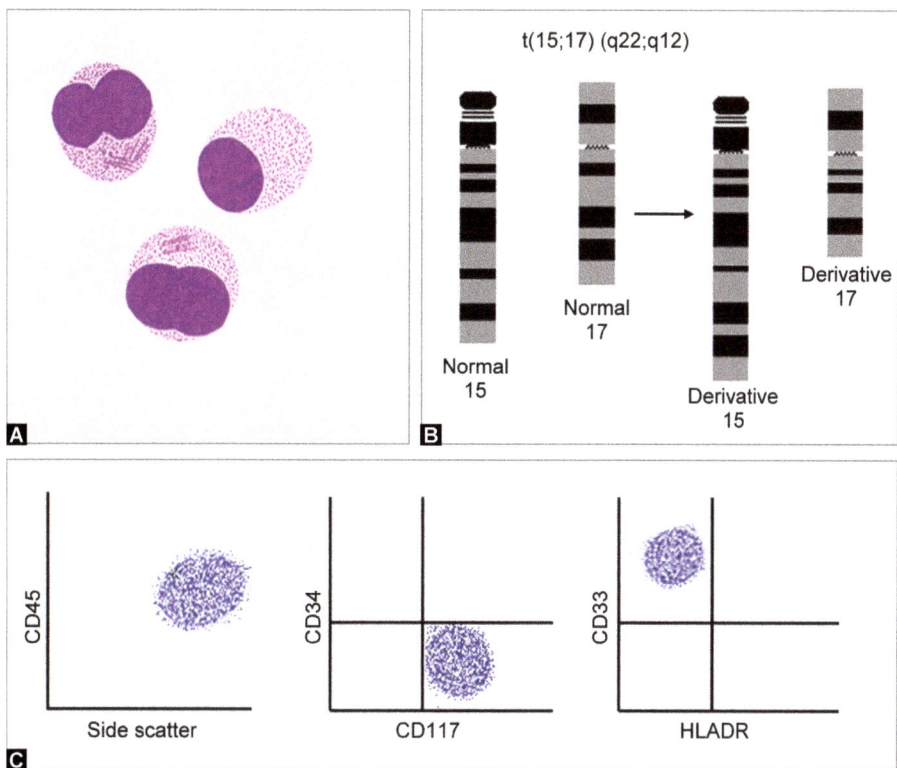

Figs. 5.17A to C: (A) Promyelocytes showing numerous azurophil granules, multiple Auer rods, and typical bilobed nucleus; (B) diagrammatic representation of t(15;17)(q22;q12); (C) dot plots of flow cytometry showing positivity for CD117, CD33 and negativity for CD34 and HLADR.

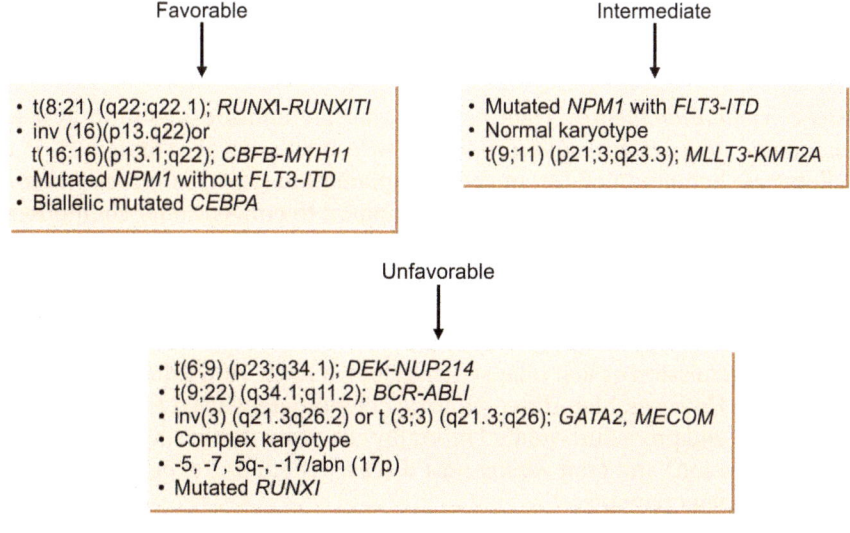

Favorable
- t(8;21) (q22;q22.1); *RUNX1-RUNX1T1*
- inv (16)(p13.q22)or t(16;16)(p13.1;q22); *CBFB-MYH11*
- Mutated *NPM1* without *FLT3-ITD*
- Biallelic mutated *CEBPA*

Intermediate
- Mutated *NPM1* with *FLT3-ITD*
- Normal karyotype
- t(9;11) (p21;3;q23.3); *MLLT3-KMT2A*

Unfavorable
- t(6;9) (p23;q34.1); *DEK-NUP214*
- t(9;22) (q34.1;q11.2); *BCR-ABL1*
- inv(3) (q21.3q26.2) or t (3;3) (q21.3;q26); *GATA2, MECOM*
- Complex karyotype
- -5, -7, 5q-, -17/abn (17p)
- Mutated *RUNX1*

Fig. 5.18: Genetic risk stratification in acute myeloid leukemia.

Treatment

Forms of therapy in AML are listed in Box 5.14.

Chemotherapy

Remission induction: The aim of therapy in AML is induction of complete remission (i.e. to eradicate the leukemic cells and restore normal hematopoiesis). Criteria for complete remission are shown in Box 5.15.

The drug combination most commonly employed for this purpose is daunorubicin (three daily infusions) and cytosine arabinoside (continuous infusion for 7 days); this regimen is commonly called as "7 and 3" regimen.

Complete remission is usually achieved in about 70% of patients who are below 60 years of age. However, significant number of leukemic cells persist (which are below the level of detection by conventional methods) that cause subsequent relapse if postremission therapy is not administered. Due to persistent toxicity of induction therapy, many patients may not be able to receive postremission therapy.

Box 5.14: Forms of therapy in AML.
• Remission induction (Daunorubicin + cytosine arabinoside)
• Postremission therapy—Options:
– Consolidation therapy (High-dose cytosine arabinoside)
– Intensive chemo- or chemoradiotherapy followed by hematopoietic stem cell transplantation (autologous or allogeneic)

Box 5.15: Criteria for complete remission (CR).
• <5% of blasts in a normocellular bone marrow
• Return of peripheral blood counts to normal
– Neutrophils > 1500/cmm
– Platelets > 100,000/cmm
– Hemoglobin > 10.0 g/dL
• Disappearance of signs and symptoms
(Note: The term "complete remission" is not synonymous with cure and blast cells may be demonstrated by a sensitive molecular technique)

In addition to "7 and 3" therapy, additional (initial) therapy in acute promyelocytic leukemia is all-transretinoic acid that induces differentiation of abnormal promyelocytes to mature cells and reduces risk of early death from bleeding. Newer agent for acute promyelocytic leukemia is arsenic trioxide.

Postremission therapy: After achieving remission, further intensive therapy is essential for eradication of residual leukemic cells and to prevent relapse. Options for postremission therapy are:

a. *Intensive consolidation therapy:* High-dose cytosine arabinoside is commonly used.
b. *Hematopoietic stem cell transplantation:* Disease-free survival of 40 to 60% is reported with allogeneic hematopoietic stem cell transplantation (HSCT) from a sibling donor in young patients during first remission. As compared to conventional chemotherapy, the risk of relapse is reduced to about 20%. High-dose marrow ablative therapy and graft-versus-leukemia effect (eradication of residual leukemic cells by donor T lymphocytes) are responsible for low risk of subsequent relapse, as compared to other forms of therapy. Long-term survival is reported in about 30% of patients with AML who are treated with HSCT during second remission or first relapse. Therefore in AML, HSCT during first remission is a better option. However, high-dose cytotoxic chemotherapy used for marrow ablation is extremely toxic, and procedure-related mortality can occur due to severe infections (due to immunosuppression) and graft versus-host disease. Therefore, allogeneic BMT is usually reserved for younger patients.

With marrow ablative therapy followed by autologous HSCT, relapse remains a major problem (due to contamination of autograft by leukemic cells and lack of graft-versus-leukemia effect).

Patients with favorable cytogenetic abnormalities are treated with intensive consolidation therapy following remission induction, while in younger patients with unfavorable cytogenetic abnormalities, more aggressive remission induction therapy followed by hematopoietic stem cell transplantation should be considered (Box 5.16).

Treatment of acute promyelocytic leukemia: All transretinoid acid (ATRA) along with concurrent anthracycline appears to be the safest treatment for acute promyelocytic leukemia.

> **Box 5.16:** Principles of therapy in AML.
> - t(8;21): Induction therapy followed by consolidation
> - t(15;17): All transretinoic acid and induction therapy, followed by consolidation
> - inv(16) or t(16;16): Induction therapy followed by consolidation
> - Unfavorable cytogenetic abnormalities: Aggressive or newer therapies; hematopoietic stem cell transplantation in first remission

Maintenance therapy is given with either ATRA or chemotherapy. Arsenic trioxide is helpful in patients who relapse or are refractory to ATRA.

The major toxic effect of ATRA is ATRA syndrome characterized by fever, fluid overload, hypoxia, and lung infiltrates. It is due to neutrophilic leukocytosis resulting from differentiation of promyelocytes followed by adhesion of differentiated cells to vascular endothelium of lung. Treatment is intravascular dexamethasone.

Supportive Therapy

Supportive therapy mainly consists of blood component replacement as required and management of infections. Platelet transfusions are indicated in treatment of hemorrhages due to thrombocytopenia and for prevention of bleeding when platelet count falls below 20,000/cmm. Packed red cell transfusion should be given for symptomatic anemia. Measures for prevention of infections include reverse isolation for neutropenic patients, oral nonabsorbable antibiotics for suppression of gastrointestinal organisms, etc. For fever in a neutropenic patient, empiric broad-spectrum antibiotic should be initiated until underlying cause is identified. In patients with hyperleukocytosis, intensive hydration and alkalinization of urine are indicated to prevent tumor lysis syndrome.

Minimal Residual Disease

Minimal residual disease (MRD) refers to disease that cannot be detected by conventional light microscopy of blood and bone marrow after administration of remission induction chemotherapy. The sensitivities of various techniques for detection of leukemic cells are one blast in 20 normal cells for morphology, one in 10^2 for cytogenetics, one in 10^4 to 10^5 for flow cytometry, and one in 10^6 for polymerase chain reaction.

There are two commonly used methods for evaluation of MRD in AML:
1. Immunophenotyping
2. Genetic tests

Immunophenotyping: For MRD detection, there are two approaches on flow cytometry which help to distinguish leukemic cells from normal precursors: (1) detection of leukemia-associated immunophenotype (LAIP), and (2) identification of different-from-normal patterns.
1. LAIP can be identified in 60–95% of patients with AML. LAIP approach detects aberrant antigen expression as follows:
    - Asynchronous antigen expression, i.e. expression of mature cell markers (CD4, CD64, CD15) by immature cells (myeloblasts)

- Lineage infidelity or cross-lineage antigen expression, e.g. expression of lymphoid antigens on myeloblasts (CD2, CD7, CD19, CD56)
- Altered level of antigen expression, e.g. decreased (CD33 or CD13) or increased (CD117)

2. In different-from-normal approach (which does not require knowledge of the presenting immunophenotype), cells that cluster at sites where normal cells do not localize are considered as residual leukemic cells. A fixed antibody panel is used irrespective of the diagnostic baseline phenotype of leukemia.

Sensitivity of flow cytometry for detection of MRD is reported to be one leukemic cell per 10^4 to 10^5 normal cells.

Genetic tests: Known disease-related genetic abnormality can be used as a marker for MRD and detected and quantified by real-time quantitative polymerase chain reaction (RQ-PCR). Sensitivity of this technique can approach one leukemic cell per 10^6 normal cells. Leukemia-specific fusion transcripts that are suitable for MRD analysis include *RUNX1-RUNX1T1*, *CBFB-MYH11*, *PML-RARA*, *KMT2A-MLLT3*, *DEK-NUP214*, and *BCR-ABL1*. In addition, gene mutations like *NPM1* are commonly used for MRD evaluation.

BIBLIOGRAPHY

1. Arya LS. Acute lymphoblastic leukaemia: current treatment concepts. Indian Pediatrics. 2000;37:397-406.
2. Bennett JM, Catovsky D, Daniel MT, et al. (FAB Cooperative Group). Proposals for the classification of the acute leukaemias. Br J Haematol. 1976;33:451-8.
3. Bennett JM, Catovsky D, Daniel MT, et al. (FAB Cooperative Group). The morphological classification of acute lymphoblastic leukaemia: concordance among observers and clinical correlations. Br J Haematol. 1981;47:553-61.
4. Bennett JM, Catovsky D, Daniel MT, et al. A variant form of hypergranular promyelocytic leukaemia. Ann Intern Med. 1980;92:261.
5. Bennett JM, Catovsky D, Daniel MT, et al. Criteria for diagnosis of acute leukaemia of megakaryocytic lineage (M7): Are port of the French-American-British Co-operative Group. Ann Intern Med. 1985;103:460-2.
6. Bennett JM, Catovsky D, Daniel MT, et al. Proposal for the recognition of minimally differentiated acute myeloid leukaemia (AML M0). The FAB Cooperative Group. Br J Haematol. 1991;789:325-9.
7. Betz BL, Hess JL. Acute myeloid leukemia diagnosis in the 21st century. Arch Pathol Lab Med. 2010;34:1427-33.
8. Cancer Genome Atlas Research Network. Genomic and epigenomic landscapes of adult de novo acute myeloid leukemia. N Engl J Med. 2013;368:2059-74.
9. Das R, Ahluwalia J, Sachdeva MUS. Hematological practice in India. Hematol Oncol Clin N Am. 2016;30:433-44.
10. Dohner H, Estey E, Grimwade D, et al. Diagnosis and management of AML in adults: 2017 ELN recommendations from an international expert panel. Blood. 2017;129(4):424-47.
11. Greaves M. Science, medicine, and the future: Childhood leukaemia. BMJ. 2002;324:283-7.
12. Schrappe M. Prognostic factors in childhood acute lymphoblastic leukaemia. Indian J Pediatr. 2003;70:817-24.
13. Swerdlow SH, Campo E, Harris NL, et al. WHO Classification of Tumours of Hematopoietic and Lymphoid Tissues. Revised 4th edition., Lyon. International Agency for Research on Cancer; 2017.
14. Swerdlow SH, Campo E, Harris NL, et al. (Eds.). WHO Classification of Tumours of Haematopoietic and Lymphoid Tissues, 4th edition. Lyon. International Agency for Research on Cancer; 2008.

CHAPTER 6

Myelodysplastic Syndromes

INTRODUCTION

Myelodysplastic syndromes (MDS) are a heterogeneous group of acquired, clonal stem cell disorders characterized by:
- Occurrence mainly in elderly individuals
- Dysplasia of one or more hematopoietic cell lines with resultant characteristic morphological abnormalities
- Ineffective erythropoiesis due to increased apoptosis causing cytopenia of one or more cell lines in peripheral blood
- Increased risk of transformation to acute myeloid leukemia

MDS was previously called as dysmyelopoietic syndrome, preleukemic syndrome, smoldering acute leukemia, and oligoblastic leukemia.

PATHOGENESIS (FIG. 6.1)

Myelodysplastic syndrome (MDS) may be primary (de novo) or secondary (e.g. following exposure to chemo- or radiotherapy) (Table 6.1). Previous exposure to chemotherapy (particularly alkylating agents and purine analogues) is associated with increased risk of development of MDS and AML. The risk is related to dose and duration of therapy and

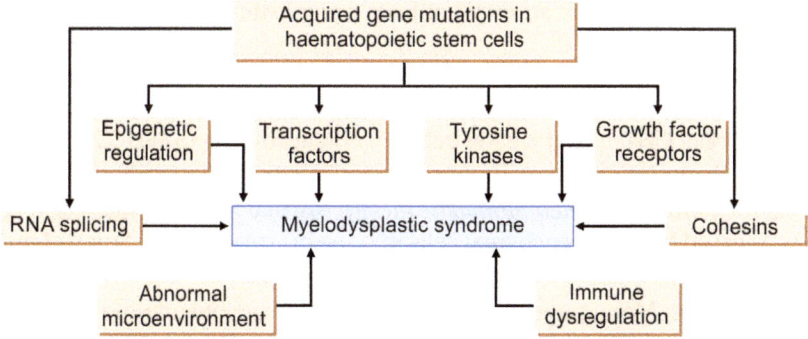

Fig. 6.1: Pathogenesis of myelodysplastic syndrome.

Table 6.1: Causes of myelodysplastic syndrome.

- Primary (Idiopathic)
- Secondary
    - Prior radiotherapy
    - Prior alkylating drug therapy
    - Exposure to chemicals, e.g. benzene, organic solvents
    - Genetic predisposition, e.g. Down's syndrome, Fanconi's anemia, neurofibromatosis type I

MDS follows about 3–7 years following exposure. The risk is increased in patients receiving combination of chemotherapy and radiotherapy. Therapy-related MDS is associated with deletions of chromosomes 5 and/or 7 and complex karyotypes, and has poor prognosis. MDS may follow environmental exposure to radiation (e.g. atomic power plant accidents) and certain toxins like benzene. However, in a majority of patients with MDS, previous exposure to chemo- or radiotherapy is lacking and the cause of MDS remains unknown (primary MDS).

MDS arises from interaction between acquired gene mutations in hematopoietic precursor cells, alteration in marrow microenvironment, and alteration in immune surveillance. A malignant clone develops from acquisition of sequential mutations in hematopoietic precursor cells, which then expands due to defective microenvironment and dysregulated immune system.

The cell of origin appears to be a hematopoietic stem cell with intrinsic self-renewal capacity. The abnormal clone expansion occurs through the acquisition of newer mutations or epigenetic alterations that increase cell proliferation and resist apoptosis. Subsequent genetic lesions cause morphologic dysplasia, ineffective hematopoiesis, or cytopenias.

Acquired gene mutations: Acquired genetic mutations in individual genes are increasingly being recognized in MDS and have been observed in majority of individuals. These include genes affecting RNA splicing (*SRSF2, SF3B1, U2AF1, ZRSR2*), chromatin remodeling and epigenetic regulation (*TET2, ASXL1, EZH2, IDH1/IDH2, DNMT3A*), transcription factors (*RUNX1, ETV6, TP53, GATA2*), tyrosine kinases and growth factor receptors (*NRAS, JAK2, CBL*), and cohesins (*RAD21, STAG2, SMC3, SMC1A*). Acquisition of genetic mutations appears to be a multistep process in MDS. It is thought that mutations occurring early (like genes affecting RNA splicing, epigenetic regulation, and transcription factors) create permissive environment for acquisition of subsequent mutations that confer proliferative advantage and induce block in differentiation (like genes affecting tyrosine kinases and growth factor receptors).

With increasing age, the number and frequency of such mutations increase.

In addition to gene mutations, various karyotypic abnormalities have been observed in MDS (like deletions and translocations) that have prognostic value and some are associated with a unique phenotype.

The term *clonal hematopoiesis of undetermined potential* (CHIP) is used when gene mutations associated with MDS are found in individuals without hematological abnormalities. The natural history of CHIP is not clearly defined, and according to WHO 2016 classification, presence of somatic mutations alone is not sufficient to make a diagnosis of MDS.

Abnormal microenvironment (Hematopoietic niche): Normal hematopoiesis is also regulated by cytokines released from mesenchymal cells in bone marrow stroma. Some of the factors in microenvironment appear to be dysregulated in MDS.

Immune dysregulation: Many aspects of immune system have been found to be abnormal in MDS and it thought that disturbance of immune regulation possibly allows persistence and propagation of abnormal clones in MDS.

Abnormal apoptosis: Abnormalities have been detected in both pathways of apoptosis (death receptor pathway and intrinsic pathway) in MDS. Enhanced apoptosis contributes to development of ineffective hematopoiesis.

Transformation to AML: It has been discovered that progression of MDS to AML results from acquisition of mutations in genes that confer constitutive proliferative advantage (like *FLT3, NRAS, KIT, CEBPA*). Development of AML in MDS tends to have poorer prognosis than de novo AML. This possibly results from older age and associated comorbidities; however, persistence of pre-existing driver mutations even after therapy is thought to play a major role.

CLASSIFICATION OF MYELODYSPLASTIC SYNDROMES

There are two classification systems for MDS:
1. French-American-British (FAB) Classification (1982)
2. World Health Organization Classification (2016)

French-American-British (FAB) Classification

In 1982, French-American-British (FAB) Cooperative Group proposed classification of MDS. The basis of this classification is type and degree of dysplasia, and percentage of ringed sideroblasts and of blast cells in bone marrow. According to FAB classification myelodysplastic syndromes are divided into five groups (Table 6.2).

World Health Organization (WHO) Classification

This classification is presented in Table 6.3. The WHO classification has set the dividing line between MDS and AML at 20% of blasts. In FAB classification, this demarcation is 30%. Also, chronic myelomonocytic leukemia (included in FAB classification) is placed under the category of "Myelodysplastic/Myeloproliferative disorders" since it shares features of both the disorders.

Table 6.2: FAB classification and laboratory features of primary myelodysplastic syndromes.

Category	Blasts (blood)	Blasts (marrow)	Ringed sideroblasts	Comments
1. Refractory anemia (RA)	<1%	<5%	<15%	Anemia with dyserythropoiesis predominant; macrocytosis
2. Refractory anemia with ringed sideroblasts (RARS)	<1%	<5%	≥15%	Dimorphic anemia
3. Refractory anemia with excess blasts (RAEB)	<5%	5–20%	Variable	Bi- or tricytopenia, trilineage dysplasia
4. Refractory anemia with excess of blasts in transformation (RAEB-T)	≥5%	21–30%	Variable	Auer rods ± (in the presence of auer rods, diagnosis is RAEB-T even if blasts are < 20%)
5. Chronic myelomonocytic leukemia	<5%	1–20%	Variable	Monocytosis >1,000/mm^3, hepatosplenomegaly

Table 6.3: World Health Organization classification of myelodysplastic syndromes, 2016.

Type	Number of Cytopenia	Blast % (Blood)	Blast % (Marrow)	Dysplasia lines	Other
1. Myelodysplastic syndrome with single lineage dysplasia (MDS-SLD)	1–2	<1	<5	1	<15% ringed sideroblasts or <5% with *SF3B1* mutation, no Auer rods
2. Myelodysplastic syndrome with multilineage dysplasia (MDS-MLD)	1–3	<1	<5	2–3	<15% ring sideroblasts or <5% with *SF3B1* mutation, no Auer rods
3. Myelodysplastic syndrome with ring sideroblasts (MDS-RS)					
– Myelodysplastic syndrome with ring sideroblasts and single lineage dysplasia (MDS-RS-SLD)	1–2	<1	<5	1	≥15% ring sideroblasts or 5–15% ring sideroblasts with *SF3B1* mutation
– Myelodysplastic syndrome with ring sideroblasts and multilineage dysplasia (MDS-RS-MLD)	1–3	<1	<5	2–3	≥15% ring sideroblasts or 5–15% ring sideroblasts in the presence of an *SF3B1* mutation
4. Myelodysplastic syndrome with excessblasts-1 (MDS-EB-1)	1–3	2–4	5–9	1–3	No Auer rods
5. Myelodysplastic syndrome with excessblasts-2 (MDS-EB-2)	1–3	5–19	10–19	1–3	Auer rods±
6. Myelodysplastic syndrome associated with isolated del(5q)	1–2	<1	<5	1–3	Hypolobated megakaryocytes
7. Refractory cytopenia of childhood (RCC) (Provisional)	1–3	<2	<5	1–3	Marrow hypocellularity common
8. Myelodysplastic syndrome-unclassifiable (MDS-U)					
– with 1% blood blasts	1–3	1 on two separate occasions	<5	1–3	No Auer rods Ring sideroblasts±
– with single lineage dysplasia and pancytopenia	Pancytopenia	<1	<5	1	No Auer rods Ring sideroblasts±
– with defining cytogenetic abnormalities	1–3	<1	<5	None	Any defining cytogenetic abnormality (table)

Note: (1) ≥10% of cells of at least one myeloid lineage (erythroid, granulocytic, megakaryocytic) should show dysplasia for diagnosis of MDS; (2) Ringed sideroblasts are defined as erythroblasts showing ≥5 iron granules encircling at least one-third diameter of nucleus (Prussian blue stain).

CLINICAL FEATURES

Myelodysplastic syndromes usually occurs in elderly persons >60 years of age (median age at diagnosis being 70 years) and is more common in males (except 5q-syndrome which has a marked female predominance). It is uncommon in children. Patients present with symptoms related to peripheral cytopenias. These are fatigue, weakness, and dyspnea due to anemia; fever and infections due to neutropenia; and easy bruising, petechiae, and other bleeding tendencies due to thrombocytopenia. Hepatosplenomegaly is usually seen in chronic myelomonocytic leukemia. A significant proportion of patients do not have clinical manifestations and are discovered incidentally on blood examination (as unexplained macrocytosis or cytopenia).

History of treatment with chemotherapy (alkylating drugs) and/or radiotherapy for malignancies is obtained in secondary MDS.

LABORATORY FEATURES

Peripheral Blood Examination

Cytopenia, such as anemia, neutropenia or thrombocytopenia, either singly or in combination, is present in majority of patients. WHO definitions for cytopenia are hemoglobin <10 g/dL, platelets <100,000/µL, and absolute neutrophil count <1800/µL.

Red Blood Cells

Anemia is present in majority (80%) of patients. Oval macrocytosis is a typical feature. Reticulocyte count is low in relation to the level of anemia. Other red cell abnormalities include basophilic stippling, hypochromia, dimorphic red cells (normocytic or microcytic and hypochromic + macrocytic), and megaloblastoid erythroblasts.

White Blood Cells

Neutropenia is seen in 60% of patients. Both immature and abnormal granulocytes are present. Neutrophils are typically hypogranular and hypolobated (pseudo-Pelger-Huét anomaly). Nuclear hypersegmentation and ring nuclei can be seen. Type I (nongranular) and type II (granular) blasts may be seen.

Platelets

Thrombocytopenia is seen in one-half of patients. Bleeding time is prolonged despite normal platelet count (due to platelet function defect). Other abnormalities include agranular, large, or vacuolated platelets, giant platelets, micromegakaryocytes, and megakaryocyte fragments. Blood smear in a case of myelodysplastic syndrome is shown in Figure 6.2.

Bone Marrow Examination

Bone Marrow Aspiration

The blast percentage is one of the most important prognostic factors in MDS. Blasts may be agranular or granular. Granular blasts should be differentiated from promyelocytes; the latter are larger in size, show clearly visible Golgi zone, and prominent azurophil granules. By

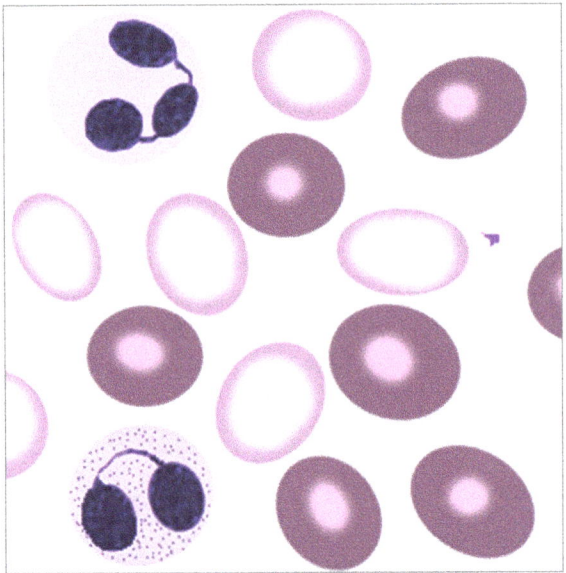

Fig. 6.2: Peripheral blood smear from a patient with myelodysplastic syndrome showing dimorphic population of red cells (one normochromic and other hypochromic), a pseudo-Pelger-Huet cell on lower left, and a hypogranulated neutrophil on upper left.

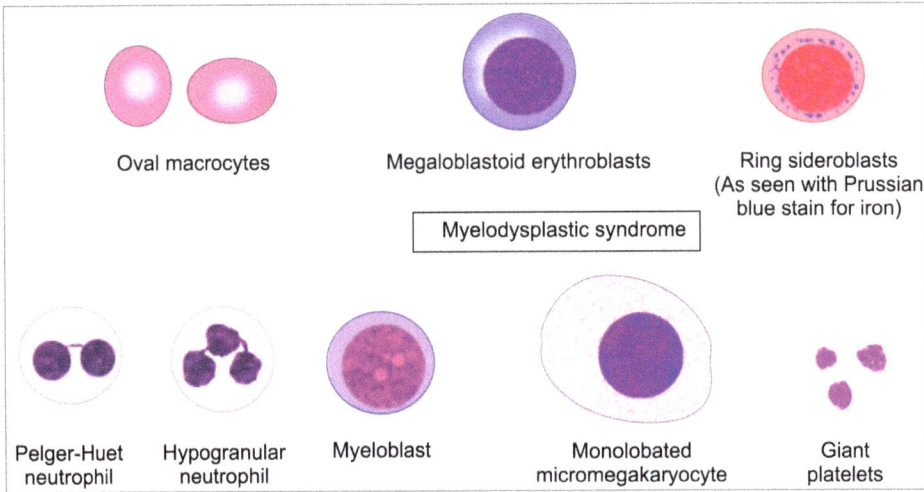

Fig. 6.3: Some characteristic morphological abnormalities in MDS.

definition, blasts are <20% in MDS, while ≥20% in AML. Blast percentage should be classified into 0–2%, 3–4%, 5–10%, and 11–19% categories for assessing prognosis according to Revised International Prognostic Scoring System, 2012. Presence of Auer rods is an independent adverse prognostic factor irrespective of blast count. Hematopoietic dysplasia is characteristic of MDS (Fig. 6.3). In MDS, ≥10% of cells of a particular lineage should be affected to term it as dysplastic. Erythroid hyperplasia with megaloblastoid maturation is a typical feature. Other dyserythropoietic features in erythroblasts include nuclear budding, multinuclearity, nuclear fragmentation, internuclear bridging, bizarre shapes, multilobation of nuclei, Howell-Jolly bodies, and cytoplasmic changes like PAS-positivity and uneven cytoplasmic staining. Iron stain (Prussian blue reaction) may reveal ringed sideroblasts (iron granules are present in mitochondria surrounding the nucleus). Ring sideroblast on iron staining is defined as having more than five granules covering at least one-third of nuclear circumference. Ring sideroblasts indicate dysplasia and their percentage has prognostic significance. In granulocytic series, myeloid precursors are increased in number. Other abnormalities include—small size, nuclear hyposegmentation (pseudo-Pelger-Huët anomaly) or hypersegmentation (ring nuclei), hypogranulation, and deficiency of myeloperoxidase. Abnormalities in megakaryocytes include micromegakaryocytes, megakaryocytes with nonlobulated nuclei, and megakaryocytes with multiple separate nuclei.

Bone Marrow Biopsy

- Bone marrow biopsy is necessary for assessment of age-adjusted cellularity (general rule: 100% cellularity at birth with its 10% deduction for every decade). Bone marrow is hypercellular or normocellular in majority of patients despite peripheral cytopenia. Some patients have hypocellular bone marrow. Hypocellularity is often seen in secondary MDS following cytotoxic chemotherapy, pediatric MDS, and MDS that follows aplastic anemia. Features favoring hypoplastic MDS over aplastic anemia are presence of dysplasia, micromegakaryocytes, increased number of myeloblasts (demonstrated with CD34 immunohistochemistry), fibrosis, and abnormal localization of immature precursors.
- Immature cells, such as myeloblasts and promyelocytes are present in the center of the marrow spaces away from the vascular structures rather than along the endosteum. This has been called as abnormal localization of immature precursors (ALIP). ALIP is positive if three or more foci of immature precursors are present. ALIP is a feature of high-grade lesion, such as RAEB. ALIP is associated with increased risk of progression to AML.
- Bone marrow fibrosis which is more common in secondary MDS (therapy-related) is assessed on bone marrow biopsy. Significant marrow fibrosis is associated with inferior prognosis.
- Immunohistochemistry (IHC): IHC on marrow biopsy is useful for (1) counting myeloblasts, (2) demonstration of ALIP, and (3) demonstration of micromegakaryocytes and dysplastic megakaryocytes (CD61).

Cytochemistry

Iron stain on bone marrow aspiration smears (with spicules) is done to identify and enumerate ring sideroblasts. Iron stain should not be done on bone marrow biopsy since iron is lost during decalcification step of tissue processing. Dysplastic vacuolated erythroblasts show globular or punctate PAS positivity.

Flow Cytometry

The immunophenotypic abnormalities detected in MDS include the following:
- Abnormal antigen expression patterns in maturing myeloid cells like CD11b, CD13, CD16; absence of CD10 expression on neutrophils
- Abnormal antigen expression patterns in CD34+ blasts like increased CD13 and CD117 and decreased expression of CD38 or HLA-DR

- Aberrant expression of antigens on myeloblasts like CD2, CD5, CD7, and CD56
- Marked reduction of CD19+, CD10+ hematogones
- Abnormal antigen expression patterns on monocytes including aberrant expression of antigens.

Cytogenetic Analysis

Conventional cytogenetic analysis is preferred over fluorescent in situ hybridization (FISH). It is necessary for diagnosis, subclassification, and prognosis. Nonrandom, clonal chromosomal abnormalities are observed in 50% of patients with primary MDS and in 80% of patients with secondary MDS, as per conventional metaphase cytogenetic analysis. Cytogenetic abnormalities in MDS are independent prognostic variables and have been incorporated into International Prognostic Scoring System. In contrast to AML, chromosomal abnormalities in MDS are numerical (i.e. loss or gain of chromosomal material) rather than structural (i.e. translocations). Common cytogenetic abnormalities in MDS include: 7q-, 20q-, +8, loss of X or Y chromosome, and 17p-. Acquisition of new chromosomal abnormalities during disease course has a poor prognosis. MDS-defining cytogenetic abnormalities are listed in Box 6.1.

Presence of a clonal chromosomal abnormality strongly favors the diagnosis of MDS over reactive conditions (Box 6.2). Patients of MDS who have complex chromosomal abnormalities (i.e. abnormality of more than three chromosomes) have poor prognosis with increased risk of progression to AML. Patients with normal or near-normal karyotype have better survival. Certain cytogenetic abnormalities are associated with distinctive clinical and hematological features. The 5q-abnormality is associated with a distinctive clinical syndrome; this entity is characterized by occurrence mainly in elderly women, presence of monolobulated megakaryocytes in bone marrow, increased platelets with giant forms, macrocytic anemia, and

---

Box 6.1: MDS-defining cytogenetic abnormalities* (WHO, 2016).

- Deletions: -7, del(7q), del(5q), -13, del(13q), del(11q), del(12p), del(9q)
- Translocations: t(5q), t(12p), t(17p), t(11;16)(q23.3;p13.3), t(3;21)(q26.2;q22.1), t(1;3)(p36.3;q21.2), t(2;11)(p21;q23.3), t(3;3;)(q21.3;q26.2), t(6;9)(p23;q34.1)
- Others: inv (3)(q21.3q26.2), idic(X)(q13), isochromosome 17q

*Cytogenetic abnormalities considered as presumptive evidence of MDS in the setting of persistent cytopenia and even in the absence of morphological abnormalities.

Box 6.2: Role of cytogenetics in myelodysplastic syndromes.

- Confirmation of clonal nature of the disorder, thus distinguishing MDS from reactive disorders
- Presumptive diagnosis of MDS in the presence of persistent unexplained cytopenia but in the absence of conclusive morphologic features if a specific cytogenetic abnormality listed below is present:
    - Unbalanced: −7 or del 7q, −5 or del 5q, i(17q) or t(17p), −13 or del 13q, del 11q, del 12p or t(12p), del 9q, idic (X)(q13)
    - Balanced: t(11;16)(q23;p13.3), t(3;21)(q26.2;q22.1), t(1;3)(p36.3;q21.2), t(2;11)(p21;q23), inv(3)(q21q26.2), t(6;9)(p23;q34)
    - Complex: ≥3 of above abnormalities
- Prognosis and selection of optimal treatment
- Documentation of additional cytogenetic abnormalities (in addition to existing) may indicate evolution to AML.

favorable prognosis. The isolated 5q-abnormality predicts favorable response to lenalidomide therapy. In addition, some cytogenetic abnormalities are more consistently observed in specific FAB subgroups. Although loss of chromosomal material is frequent, the genes affected have not been identified so far.

DIFFERENTIAL DIAGNOSIS

Typical diagnostic features of MDS are shown in Box 6.3.

In elderly subjects with RA, megaloblastic anemia due to nutritional deficiency (vitamin B_{12} or folate) should be excluded since morphological features in both the conditions are similar. A therapeutic trial should always be given even if vitamin levels are normal. Other causes of dyshematopoiesis which should be distinguished are exposure to toxic chemicals, heavy metals, or chemotherapy; inflammatory or neoplastic disease; alcohol-induced sideroblastic anemia; and HIV infection.

> **Box 6.3:** Typical diagnostic features of myelodysplastic syndromes.
>
> - Persistent unexplained cytopenia in an older adult
> - Dysplasia in ≥10% of cells in at least one myeloid lineage (erythroid, granulocytic, megakaryocytic)
> - Blasts <20% in blood or bone marrow
> - Presence of a typical cytogenetic abnormality
> - Monocyte count $<1 \times 10^9/l$ (for exclusion of chronic myelomonocytic leukemia)

Differentiation from AML has been considered earlier under AML.

MDS should also be distinguished from aplastic anemia if bone marrow is hypocellular, congenital dyserythropoietic anemia in children, and acute myelomonocytic leukemia.

PROGNOSIS

As MDS is predominantly a disease of elderly, age-related factors and associated comorbidities and therapies affect the outcome. Majority of patients die from consequences of cytopenia like infection, bleeding, anemia, and transfusion-related problems. MDS is largely an incurable disease. A minority of patients may be candidates for allogeneic hematopoietic stem cell transplantation, although only a fraction may achieve a longer disease-free survival.

- Prognostic scoring systems: Various evaluation systems have been devised to assess prognosis of MDS. The two main systems are International Prognostic Scoring System (IPSS) and WHO classification-based prognostic Scoring System (WPSS).
  1. The IPSS system should be used at diagnosis in nontherapy-related MDS (Table 6.4). This system was based on marrow blast percentage, karyotype abnormalities, and number of cytopenias. In 2012, IPSS was revised (IPSS-R) (Table 6.5) in which more strata of blast percentage, two more risk groups of cytogenetic changes and different degrees of cytopenias were added.
  2. The WPSS (Table 6.6) can be used throughout the disease course of MDS and uses karyotype risk, WHO MDS subtype, and red cell transfusion needs to identify different prognostic risk groups.
- Cytogenetics: Cytogenetic abnormalities are independent prognostic factors in MDS. Patients with clonal evolution (acquisition of new or additional cytogenetic abnormalities during disease course) have less favorable outcome.

- Bone marrow fibrosis carries less favorable prognosis.
- Therapy-related MDS: This carries adverse prognosis with high-risk of transformation to acute leukemia, and resistance to therapy.

Table 6.4: International Prognostic Scoring System for myelodysplastic syndromes (Greenberg et al, 1997).

Score	Bone marrow blasts %	Cytogenetics	Cytopenia (Hb <10 g/dL, neutrophils <1500/μL, platelets <1 lac/μL)
0	<5	Good (normal, -Y, 5q-, 20q-)	Absent or unilineage
0.5	5–10	Intermediate (other)	≥2 lineages
1.0	–	Poor (complex, chromosome 7 anomalies)	–
1.5	11–20	–	–
2.0	21–30*	–	–

Based on FAB classification of MDS; Risk groups: 0: Low; 0.5–1.0: Intermediate-1; 1.5–2.0: Intermediate-2; ≥ 2.5: High.
*Considered as AML in WHO classification

Table 6.5: Revised International Prognostic Scoring System (Greenberg et al, 2012) for myelodysplastic syndromes.

Score	Bone marrow blasts%	Cytogenetics	Hb (g/dL)	ANC (per mm^3)	Platelets (per mm^3)
0	≤2	Very good: -Y, del(11q)	≥10	≥800	≥100,000
0.5				<800	50,000–<100,000
1	>2–<5	Good: Normal, del (5q), del (12p), del (20q), double including del (5q)	8–<10		<50,000
1.5			<8		
2	5–10	Intermediate: del (7q), +8, +19, i (17q), any other single or double independent clones			
3	>10	Poor: -7, inv (3)/t (3q)/del (3q), double including -7/del (7q), complex: 3 abnormalities			
4		Very poor: Complex >3 abnormalities			

IPSS Risk group (Total score): Very low (≤1.5), Low (>1.5–3), Intermediate (>3–4.5), High (>4.5–6) , Very high (>6). These risk categories aid in estimating median overall survival and risk of progression to AML.

(ANC: absolute neutrophil count)

Table 6.6: WHO Classification-based prognostic scoring system or WPSS (Malcovati et al, 2007).

Score	WHO subtype of MDS	Chromosomal abnormalities	Need for at least one red cell transfusion every 8 weeks over a period of 4 months
0	Refractory anemia, refractory anemia with ring sideroblasts, 5q-syndrome	Good: Normal, -Y, del (5q), del (20q)	No
1	Refractory cytopenia with multilineage dysplasia (RCMD), RCMD with ring sideroblasts	Intermediate: Abnormalities other than those listed as Good or poor	
2	Refractory anemia with excess blats-1	Poor: Complex (3 or more abnormalities), abnormalities of chromosome 7	–
3	Refractory anemia with excess blats-2	–	–

Risk group (Score): Very low (0), Low (1), Intermediate (2), High (3–4), Very high (5–6)

TREATMENT

No safe and effective form of therapy is available for MDS as yet. Patients with RA and RARS have low incidence, while patients with RAEB-1 and RAEB-2 have higher incidence of transformation to AML (Table 6.7). However, even in the absence of progression to AML, patients have increased morbidity and mortality due to complications related to various cytopenias. Treatment in MDS should be individualized. Treatment options in MDS are summarized.
- Supportive therapy: This consists of red cell transfusions, platelet transfusions, and antibiotic as required. Iron chelating therapy is instituted in multiply transfused patients as ineffective erythropoiesis and frequent red cell transfusions will cause iron overload and parenchymal damage. Recently, hematopoietic growth factors (erythropoietin and G-CSF) are being tried to improve cytopenias in MDS patients. Supportive therapy is indicated as an adjunctive

Table 6.7: Median survival and risk of AML in MDS.

WHO subtype	Median survival (months)	Transformation to AML (%)
RA	69	6
RARS	69	1–2
RCMD	33	11
RCMD-RS	32	11
RAEB-1	16	25
RAEB-2	9	33
MDS-U	Unknown	Unknown
5q-	145	<10

therapy for all risk groups, elderly patients with severe comorbidities, and low-risk disease, and in patients not willing for aggressive forms of therapy.
- Hypomethylating agents (5-azacytidine, decitabine) are indicated in intermediate-1 or high-risk disease.
- Lenalidomide is useful in MDS with 5q-abnormality.
- Immuosuppressive therapy: Antilymphocyte globulin and/or cyclosporine is indicated in hypocellular MDS with normal cytogenetics and no excess blasts.
- High-dose AML-like chemotherapy: This may be tried in young patients with high-risk MDS with good performance status and nonavailability of HLA-identical sibling donor. Some of the patients treated with chemotherapy can achieve remission.
- Hematopoietic stem cell transplantation: The only curative form of therapy is hematopoietic stem cell transplantation. Transplantation may be considered in younger patients who have high-risk disease, good performance status, no comorbidities, and HLA-identical sibling donor; this form of therapy may result in long-term disease-free survival and cure.

BIBLIOGRAPHY

1. Bennett JM, Catovsky D, Daniel MT, Proposals for the classification of myelodysplastic syndromes. Br J Haematol. 1982;51:189-99.
2. Beris P. Primary clonal myelodysplastic syndromes. Semin Hematol. 1989;26:216-33.
3. Besa EG. Myelodysplastic syndromes (Refractory anemia). A perspective of the biologic, clinical, and therapeutic uses. Med Clin North Am. 1992;76:599-617.
4. British Committee for Standards in Haematology:Guidelines for the diagnosis and therapy of adult myelodysplastic syndromes. Br J Haematol. 2003;120:187-200.
5. Cheson BD. The myelodysplastic syndromes. The Oncologist. 1997;2:28-39.
6. Greenberg P, Cox C, LeBeau MM, et al. International scoring system for evaluating prognosis in myelodysplastic syndromes. Blood. 1997;89:2079-88.
7. Greenberg PL, Tuechler H, Schanz J, et al. Revised prognostic scoring system for myelodysplastic syndromes. Blood 2012;120(12):2454-65.
8. Heaney ML, Golde DW. Medical Progress. Myelodysplasia. N Engl J Med. 1999;340:1649.
9. Jaffe ES, Harris NL, Stein H, Vardiman JW (Eds.):World Health Organisation Classification of Tumours. Pathology and Genetics of Tumours of Haematopoietic and Lymphoid Tissues. Lyon. IARC Press. 2001.
10. Koeffler HP. Introduction:Myelodysplastic syndromes. Semin Hematol. 1996;33:87-94.
11. Koeffler HP. Myelodysplastic syndromes (pre-leukaemia). Semin Hematol. 1986;23:284-99.
12. Kouides PA and Bennett JM. Morphology and classification of the myelodysplastic syndromes and their pathologic variants. Semin Hematol. 1996;33:95-110.
13. Malcovati L, Germing U, Kuendgen A, et al. Time-dependent prognostic scoring system for predicting survival and leukemic evolution in myelodysplastic syndromes. J Clin Oncol. 2007;25:3503-10.
14. Nimer SD. Myelodysplastic syndromes. Blood. 2008;111:4841-51.
15. Swerdlow SH, Campo E, Harris NL, et al. WHO Classification of tumours of haematopoietic and lymphoid tissues (Revised 4th ed.). Lyon. IARC. 2017.
16. Swerdlow SH, Campo E, Harris NL, et al. WHO classification of tumours of haematopoietic and lymphoid tissues. 4th ed. Lyon. International Agency for Research on Cancer; 2008.
17. Tefferi A, Vardiman JW. Myelodysplastic syndromes. N Engl J Med. 2009;361:1872-85.
18. Tricot G, Dewolf-Peeters C, Vlietinck R, Verwilghen RL. Bone marrow histology in myelodysplastic syndromes II. Prognostic value of abnormal localization of immature precursors in MDS. Br J Haematol. 1984;58:217-25.
19. Zoumbos NC. The pathogenesis of myelodysplastic syndromes. Haema. 2001;4:151-7.

CHAPTER 7

Myeloproliferative Neoplasms

INTRODUCTION

These are clonal neoplastic disorders of pluripotent hematopoietic stem cell characterized by excessive proliferation of one or more of the myeloid cell lines like granulocytic, erythroid, and megakaryocytic. The WHO classification of myeloproliferative neoplasms is presented in Box 7.1.

The characteristic features of myeloproliferative neoplasms are:
- They are clonal hematopoietic stem cell disorders with origin from a single stem cell.
- Usually one cell line predominates in a given disorder.
- There is a close relationship between different disorders with interconversions, overlapping manifestations, and progression to myelofibrosis and acute leukemia.
- Maturation of blood cells is relatively normal, so that mature cells (red cells, granulocytes, or platelets) are increased in number.
- Enlargements of spleen and liver are common.

Myeloproliferative neoplasms should be distinguished from one another because of different treatment approaches of each.

Box 7.1: World Health Organization classification of myeloproliferative neoplasms (2016).
- Chronic myeloid leukemia, *BCR-ABL1*–positive
- Chronic neutrophilic leukemia
- Polycythemia vera
- Primary myelofibrosis
- Essential thrombocythemia
- Chronic eosinophilic leukemia, not otherwise specified
- Myeloproliferative neoplasm, unclassifiable

CLONAL ORIGIN

The myeloproliferation is the result of a genetic abnormality in a hematopoietic stem cell. Clonal nature of these disorders is established by glucose-6-phosphate dehydrogenase (G6PD) isoenzyme studies in female heterozygotes and cytogenetic analysis.

Gene for G6PD enzyme is located on X chromosome. Various isoenzymes of G6PD exist of which most common is G6PDB. G6PDA variant is more common in Africa. About one-third of black women are heterozygous for G6PDB or G6PDA. During embryogenesis there is random inactivation of one X chromosome so that heterozygous females have two populations

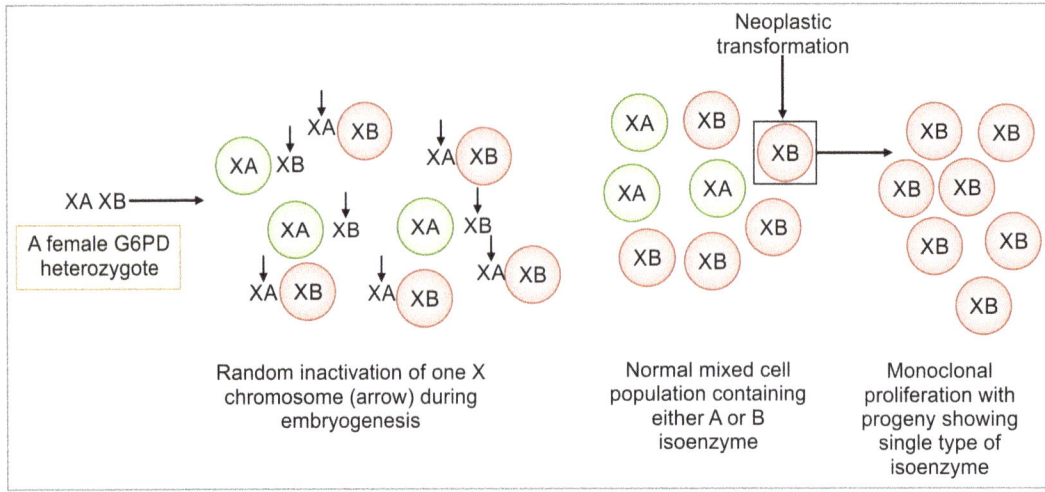

Fig. 7.1: Evidence for clonal origin of a neoplasm in a female G6PD heterozygote.

of cells—one with G6PDB and the other with G6PDA. As clonal disorders arise from a single stem cell, all the neoplastic cells contain either G6PDA or G6PDB enzyme. In myeloproliferative disorders, erythroid, myeloid, and megakaryocytic elements all contain a single G6PD enzyme (Fig. 7.1). This indicates that myeloproliferative disorders originate from a single pluripotent stem cell capable of producing erythroid, myeloid, and megakaryocytic cells. Fibroblasts are not part of the neoplastic clone in myeloproliferative disorders and their proliferation is reactive. Nonrandom chromosomal abnormalities in myeloproliferative disorders, if present, are observed in all the hematopoietic cell lines (erythroid, myeloid, megakaryocytic, and B lymphocytic) but not in fibroblasts and other nonhematopoietic tissues.

At the molecular level, neoplastic transformation results from activation of tyrosine kinase signal transduction pathway. This is exemplified in chapter on chronic myeloid leukemia.

Genetic Abnormalities in Myeloproliferative Neoplasms (Box 7.2)

Chronic myeloid leukemia is characterized by the characteristic translocation t (9;22) and formation of *BCR-ABL1* fusion gene; this gene encodes a chimeric BCR-ABL1 protein with constitutively activated tyrosine kinase. Formation of BCR-ABL1 fusion protein leads to initiation of CML. The constitutively activated tyrosine kinase causes autophosphorylation of BCR-ABL1 with subsequent activation of a network of downstream signaling pathways like JAK/STAT, PI3K/AKT, RAS/MEK, etc. This leads to growth factor independence, inhibition of cell death, and defective cell adhesion.

> **Box 7.2:** "Driver" mutations specific for myeloproliferative neoplasms.
>
> "Driver" mutations are those that confer selective growth advantage to cancer cells and are required for tumor development. (In contrast, "passenger" mutations do not impart any growth advantage and do not participate in tumorigenesis.)
> - Chronic myeloid leukemia: *BCR-ABL1* (100% cases)
> - Polycythemia vera: *JAK2* V617F (95–97% cases), *JAK2* exon 12 (2–3% cases)
> - Essential thrombocythemia: *JAK2* V617F (50–60% cases), *MPL* (3–5% cases), *CALR* (25% cases)
> - Primary myelofibrosis: *JAK2* V617F (55–60% cases), *MPL* (5–10% cases), *CALR* (25% cases)
> - Chronic neutrophilic leukemia: *CSF3R* T6181 (80% cases)

Chapter 7: Myeloproliferative Neoplasms

Polycythemia vera, essential thrombocythemia, and primary myelofibrosis have high incidence of a *V617F* point mutation in *JAK2* kinase gene. In addition, essential thrombocythemia and primary myelofibrosis both have mutations in *CALR* and *MPL*. Recently, activating mutations of colony-stimulating factor 3 receptor gene (*CSF3R*) have been identified in chronic neutrophilic leukemia.

CHRONIC MYELOID LEUKEMIA, *BCR-ABL1* POSITIVE

Chronic myeloid leukemia (CML), *BCR-ABL+* is a myeloproliferative neoplasm characterized by predominant proliferation of granulocytic cells. It is a clonal neoplastic hematopoietic stem cell disorder as evidenced by involvement of all hematopoietic cell lines. The defining characteristic of CML is presence of Philadelphia chromosome and/or *BCR/ABL1* fusion gene in all neoplastic cells. It is the most common of the myeloproliferative diseases.

Pathogenesis

CML is a clonal disorder and evidence for its origin from a single pluripotent hematopoietic stem cell is as follows:
1. A single G6PD isoenzyme is present in erythroid, granulocytic, and megakaryocytic elements, but not in fibroblasts or other somatic cells in females with CML who are heterozygous for G6PD enzyme.
2. Presence of Philadelphia chromosome in granulocytic, monocytic, erythroid, and megakaryocytic cell lines, and sometimes also in lymphoid cells.
3. Occurrence of lymphoid blast phase in CML.

The characteristic cytogenetic abnormality in CML is Philadelphia (Ph') chromosome which results from reciprocal translocation between chromosomes 9 and 22, i.e. t (9;22) (q34;q11). The Philadelphia chromosome refers to shortened chromosome 22; this was first described by investigators in Philadelphia and hence the name (Fig. 7.2). This translocation results in

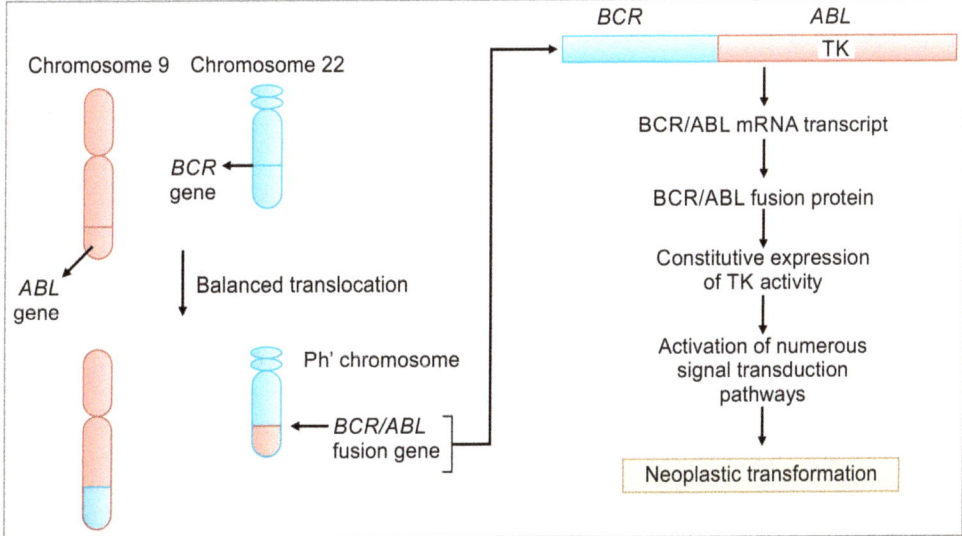

Fig. 7.2: Formation of Philadelphia chromosome and *BCR/ABL1* fusion gene product. Mechanism of leukemogenesis is shown on right side.
(TK: tyrosine kinase)

the fusion of *ABL* (Abelson leukemia virus) gene on chromosome 9 with *BCR* (breakpoint cluster region) gene on chromosome 22. Ph' chromosome is present in 95% of patients with CML. However, abnormality of chromosome 22 at the molecular level (i.e. *BCR/ABL1* gene rearrangement) is present in almost all patients with CML.

The tyrosine kinase activity resides in ABL protein; with juxtaposition of BCR sequences next to ABL, tyrosine kinase activity is constitutively activated. The site of breakpoint in *BCR* gene is variable, and therefore the size of BCR/ABL1 protein varies from 185 to 230 kDa. Most patients with typical CML have 210 kDa fusion protein. The *BCR/ABL1* fusion gene plays a central role in the pathogenesis of CML. The resultant BCR/ABL1 fusion protein is constitutively active tyrosine kinase which is confined to the cytoplasm. The BCR/ABL1 protein activates a number of cytoplasmic and nuclear signal transduction pathways affecting cell growth and differentiation. The uncontrolled activity of BCR/ABL1 tyrosine kinase ultimately results in deregulation of cellular proliferation, decreased apoptosis, and poor adherence of leukemic cells to bone marrow stroma (which causes CML cell to escape negative regulatory influences exerted by stromal cells) (Figs. 7.3A to C).

During evolution to blast phase, additional nonrandom chromosomal abnormalities occur (such as duplication of Ph' chromosome, +8, etc.) which are responsible for arrest in maturation and transformation to acute leukemia.

Pathogenesis of CML is presented in Figures 7.4 and 7.5.

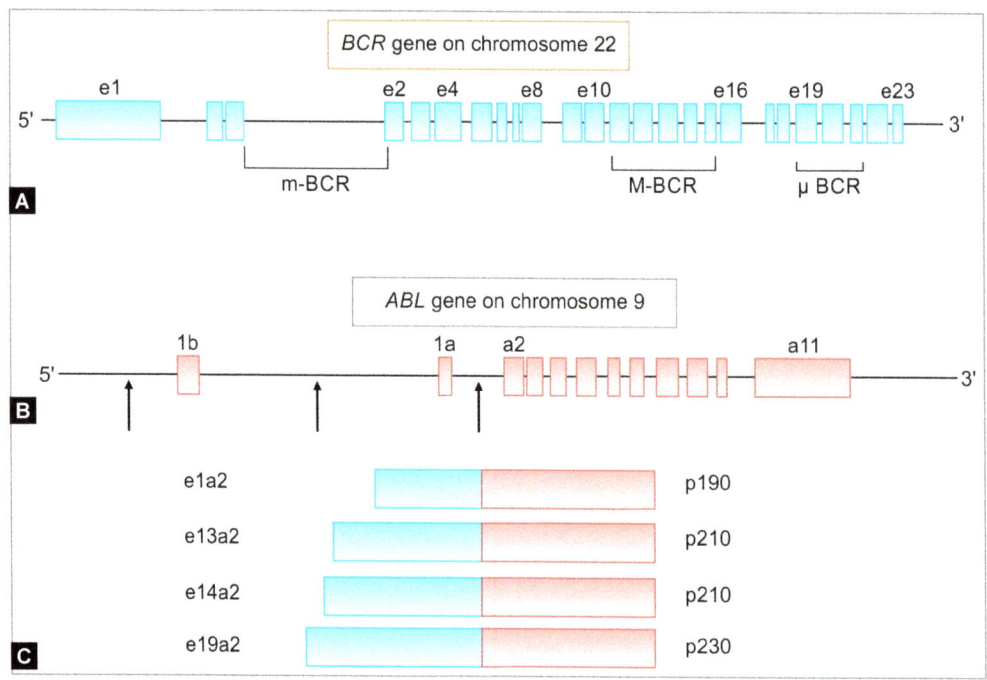

Figs. 7.3A to C: (A) *BCR* gene has 23 exons with three main breakpoint cluster regions: m-BCR, M-BCR, and μ-BCR; (B) *ABL1* gene has 11 exons with two alternative first exons (1b and 1a). Arrows show three breakpoints; (C) Structure of corresponding mRNAs according to sites of breakpoints is shown. Breakpoints in M-BCR produce p210 BCR-ABL1 fusion gene with either e13a2 or e14a2 junctions (typically seen in chronic myeloid leukemia and in some cases of acute lymphoblastic leukemia). Breakpoint in m-BCR produces p190 BCR-ABL (typically seen in acute lymphoblastic leukemia; only rarely seen in CML in which case it is associated with monocytosis). Breakpoint in micro-BCR produces p230 BCR-ABL (associated with CML with neutrophilia or thrombocytosis).

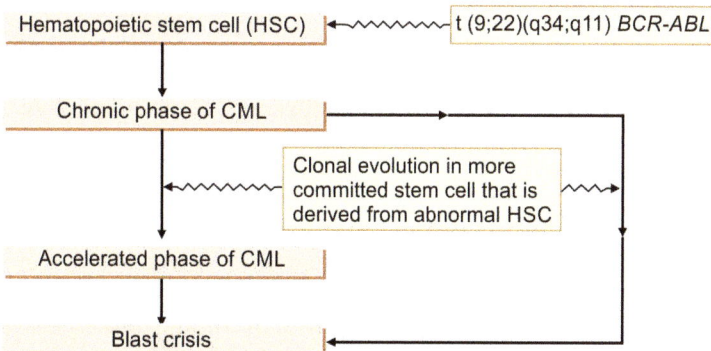

Fig. 7.4: Pathogenesis of chronic myeloid leukemia. The t(9;22)(q34;q11) *BCR-ABL* event affecting hematopoietic stem cell leads to uncontrolled expansion of a neoplastic myeloid clone that maintains differentiation. Progression to advanced phases (accelerated or blastic) results from acquisition of additional genetic abnormalities like additional Ph', +8, i (17), or +19 (termed clonal evolution). The additional genetic lesions in advanced stages cause arrest in maturation and expansion of blast population.

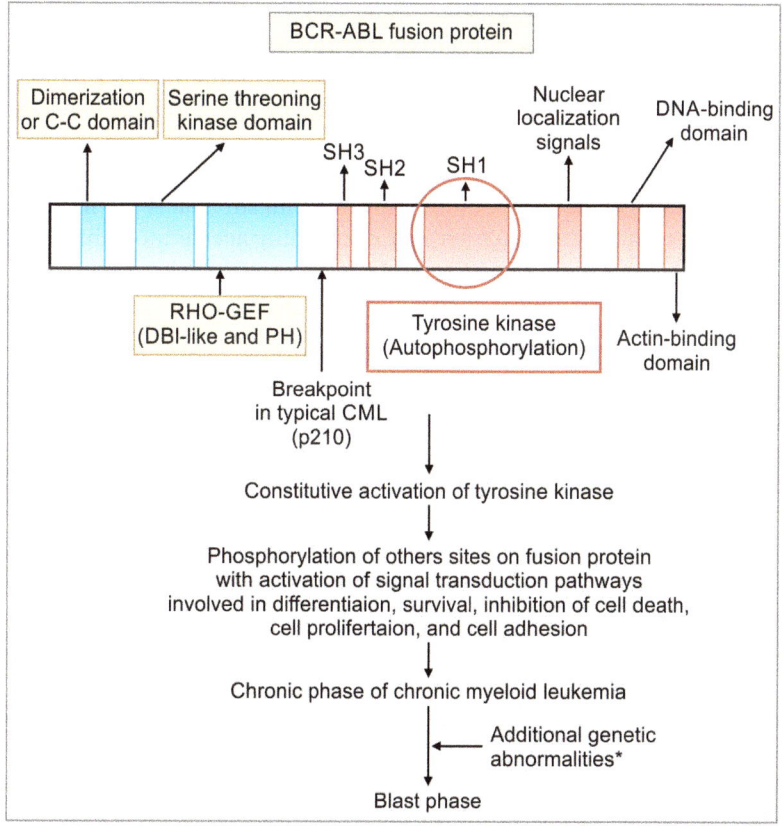

Fig. 7.5: Molecular pathogenesis of chronic myeloid leukemia. Formation of BCR-ABL1 fusion protein is central to the pathogenesis of CML. BCR proteins are colored blue and include coiled coil (C-C) domain, serine threonine kinase domain, DBL-like domain, and PH domain. ABL1 proteins are colored light brown and include SH3, SH2, SH1 (carries function of tyrosine kinase), nuclear localization signals, DNA-binding domain, and actin-binding domain.

*Additional genetic abnormalities: Double Ph chromosome, isochromosome 17, trisomy 8, trisomy 19, *TP53, CDKNA/B, EVI1/MECOM, GATA-2, RUNX1, IKZF1, ASXL1, TET2,* and *WT1*.

Incidence

CML accounts for 40% of all leukemias in the Indian population. It is slightly more common in males, with median age at diagnosis being in the fifth and sixth decades of life.

Stages of CML

There are three stages—chronic, accelerated, and acute blast phase. CML is characterized by an initial chronic stable phase which progresses to a more aggressive accelerated phase and eventually to blast phase within 3-5 years. In a proportion of patients, direct transformation from chronic phase to blastic phase occurs. In contrast to chronic phase, cells fail to mature in blast phase. In 5% of patients, presentation is in the form of accelerated phase or blast phase without preceding chronic phase.
1. *Chronic phase:* In this phase, leukemic cells retain the capacity for differentiation and maturation and are largely able to function normally. The disease is responsive to chemotherapy and remains stable for variable period. The duration of this stage is 3-5 years.
2. *Accelerated phase:* In 70% of patients, chronic phase gradually evolves into accelerated phase. In this phase, leukemic cells show increasing loss of differentiation and maturation, increased proliferation, and resistance to chemotherapy that controlled the chronic phase. Patient's disease becomes more aggressive, signs and symptoms of disease progression appear; majority of patients in this phase eventually progress to blast phase within a span of few months.
3. *Blast phase:* This occurs when there is transformation to acute leukemia and the disease becomes extremely resistant to chemotherapy. Median survival is 2-6 months. About 30% of patients progress to blastic phase without intervening accelerated phase.

Chronic Phase of CML

Clinical features: Majority (85%) of patients with CML present in chronic phase. Median age at presentation is 50 years. Patient usually presents with generalized weakness, weight loss, night sweats, and abdominal fullness (due to splenomegaly). Easy bruisability, and spontaneous bleeding, such as purpura, petechiae, and mucous membrane bleeding can occur. The principal finding on physical examination is splenomegaly which ranges in size from being just palpable to massive. Hepatomegaly is present in about half the patients. Significant lymphadenopathy is unusual and, if present, may be indicative of a localized blast phase. About 40% of patients are asymptomatic and are detected incidentally (abnormal white blood cell count).

Laboratory features:
1. *Peripheral blood examination:* Anemia is present in virtually all patients at diagnosis, and is usually mild to moderate in degree, and normocytic normochromic. There is minimal variation in size and shape of red cells. A few nucleated red cells are present in peripheral blood.
Total leukocyte count is moderately to markedly raised and is commonly more than 100,000/mm^3. Height of total leukocyte count is usually directly proportional to the size of spleen, basophil count, percentage of blast cells, and degree of anemia. All stages of maturation from myeloblast to segmented neutrophils are present with "peaks" of myelocytes and segmented neutrophils. In chronic phase, blast cells are less than 10%. Basophils and eosinophils are mildly increased. Basophilia is important for diagnosis of CML since it is rarely seen in any other disorder. Mild to moderate thrombocytosis is present in most

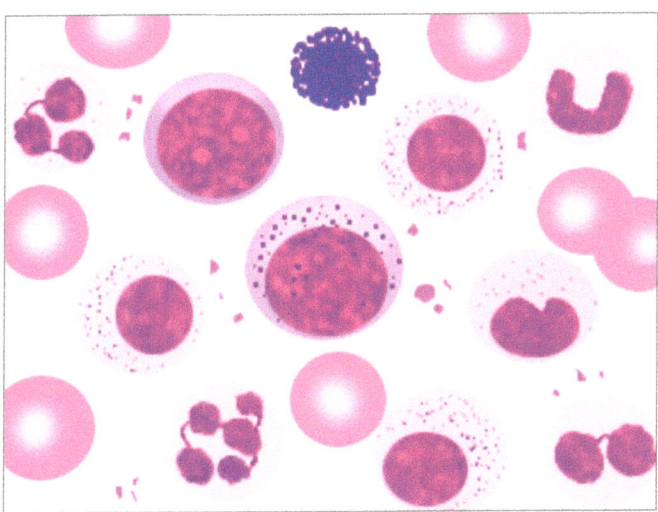

Fig. 7.6: Blood smear in chronic myeloid leukemia. All stages from myeloblast to segmented neutrophil are present. A basophil is present at the top.

patients (Fig. 7.6). Monocytes are usually <3%, although absolute monocyte count may be increased. Some patients have unusual findings like marked thrombocytosis, mature neutrophilic leukocytosis, or significant monocytosis; these may be due to variation in breakpoints in *BCR gene.*

2. *Bone marrow examination:* Bone marrow aspiration reveals hypercellular marrow with markedly increased granulopoiesis. Cells of erythroid series are usually reduced in percentage. Myeloid:erythroid ratio is 10:1 to 50:1 (normal ratio is 2:1–4:1). Myeloblasts constitute less than 10%. Basophils, eosinophils, and monocytes are increased as in peripheral blood. Megakaryocytes are frequently increased in number and are typically smaller in size with hypolobated nuclei ("dwarf"). Pseudo-Gaucher cells and sea-blue histiocytes may be observed due to increased turnover of cells.

Bone marrow aspiration is not essential for diagnosis of CML; however, it is needed to exclude accelerated or blastic phase. Also, cytogenetic analysis for Ph' chromosome is more satisfactorily done on marrow cells than on peripheral blood. In addition, bone marrow aspiration is required for fluorescent in situ hybridization (FISH) for identification of *BCR-ABL1* fusion gene and quantitative reverse transcriptase polymerase chain reaction (RT-PCR) for baseline measurement of BCR-ABL1 fusion transcripts.

Bone marrow biopsy is helpful for assessment of myelofibrosis. Previously, bone marrow fibrosis at diagnosis was associated with worse prognosis; however, with tyrosine kinase inhibitor (TKI) therapy, it has no significant effect on prognosis. Typically, bone marrow biopsy shows 5- to 10-cell-layer-thick immature granulocytes around bony trabeculae (normal thickness is two to three cell layers). "Dwarf" megakaryocytes are normally located without any cluster formation.

Role of flow cytometry in chronic phase of CML: Immunophenotyping by flow cytometry has little role in diagnosis of chronic phase of CML; however, expression of CD7 on CD34+ cells has adverse effect on prognosis.

3. *Neutrophil alkaline phosphatase (NAP) score:* Alkaline phosphatase is present in metamyelocytes, band cells, and segmented neutrophils. In this test, naphthol AS phosphate

(substrate) is converted by alkaline phosphatase in neutrophils to aryl naphthylamide which in turn combines with diazonium salt to form insoluble colored precipitate. Intensity of color reaction in neutrophils is graded 0-4+ in 100 neutrophils and values are added together to get the NAP score. Normal NAP score is 40-100. In chronic phase of CML, NAP in mature neutrophils is markedly decreased or absent. Increased NAP score is observed in leukemoid reaction due to infections, polycythemia vera, and agnogenic myeloid metaplasia with myelofibrosis. Therefore, NAP score can be used for differentiating CML from these conditions.

4. *Cytogenetic analysis:* Cytogenetic analysis in CML serves to confirm the diagnosis. It also has prognostic importance. Cytogenetic analysis of bone marrow and peripheral blood shows a characteristic abnormality, the Ph' chromosome, in more than 95% of patients with CML (Fig. 7.7). Ph' chromosome is present in all hematopoietic cell lines, i.e. erythroid,

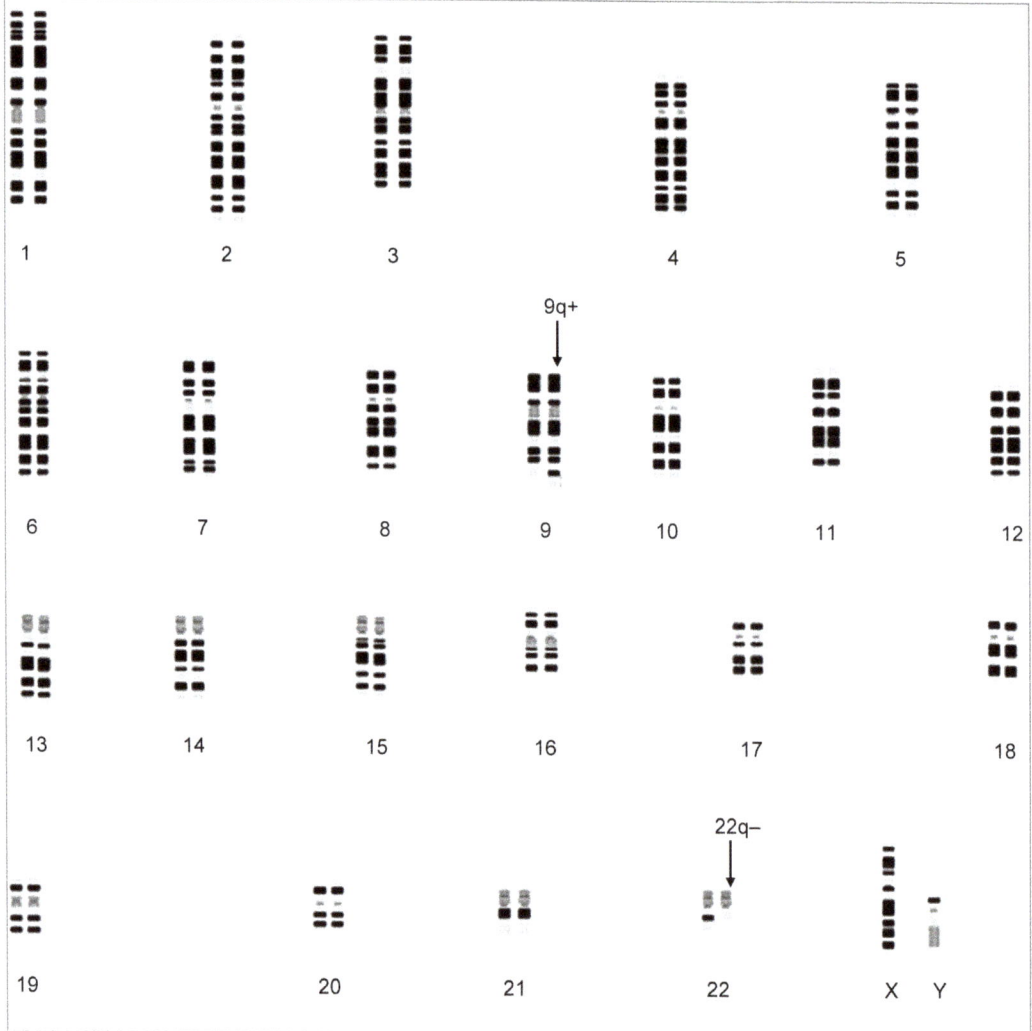

Fig. 7.7: Karyogram of a patient with chronic myeloid leukemia depicting t(9;22)(q34;q11.2). The shortened chromosome 22 (22q-) is Philadelphia chromosome.

granulocytic, monocytic, megakaryocytic, B lymphocytic, and in some cases T lymphocytic. In accelerated phase or blast phase, more chromosomal changes often develop, such as duplication of Ph' chromosome, +8, +19, and –Y.

In some cases of CML, Ph' chromosome cannot be demonstrated by cytogenetic analysis. However, in such patients rearrangement of *BCR/ABL1* can be demonstrated by fluorescent in situ hybridization (Figs. 7.8A and B), or reverse transcriptase-polymerase chain reaction.

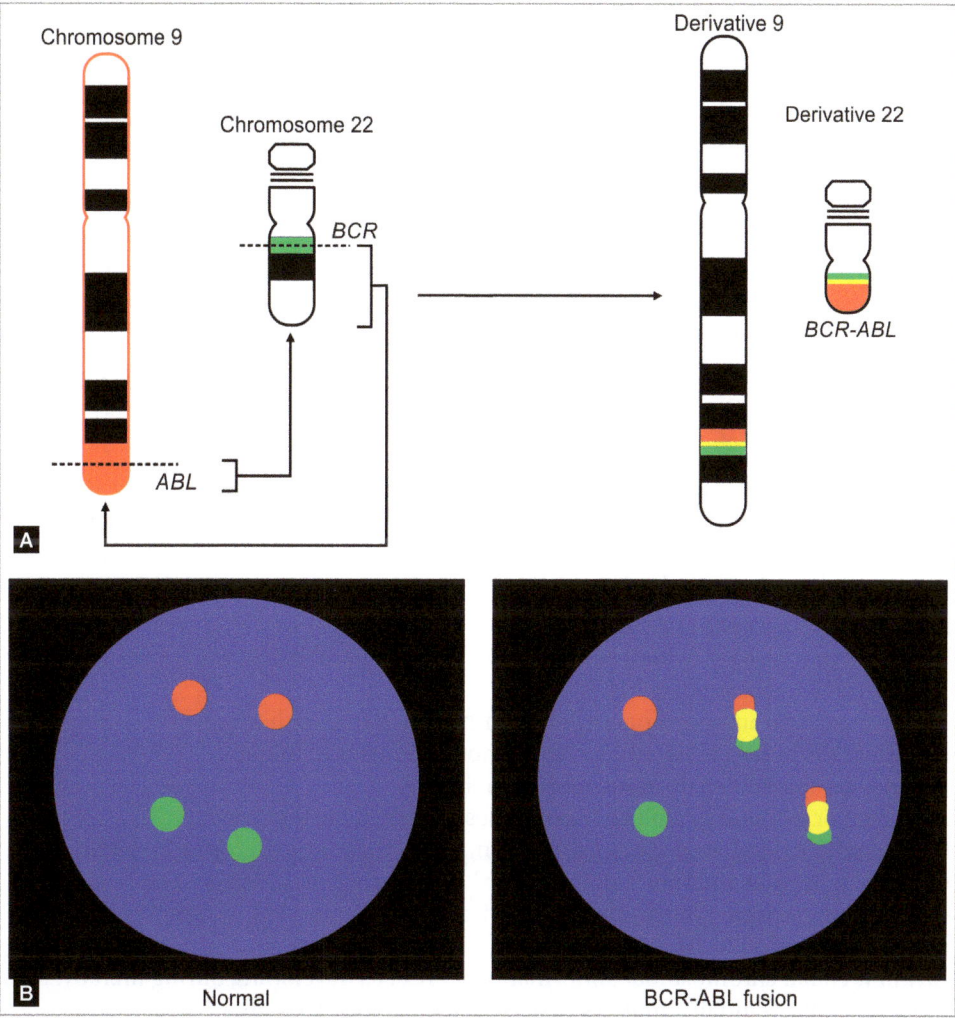

Figs. 7.8A and B: Fluorescent in situ hybridization in chronic myeloid leukemia. (A) Upper part of figure shows diagrammatic representation of t (9;22)(q34;q11) BCR-ABL. (B) Fluorescently labeled DNA probes (ABL on chromosome 9, BCR on chromosome 22) are hybridized onto interphase cells that have been attached to a glass slide. In the commonly used dual color, dual fusion method, ABL probe is labeled with a red fluorophore and BCR with a green fluorophore. In a fusion gene product, both probes overlap and produce a yellow color. The typical pattern seen in CML is 1R1G2F. 1R1G represents normal chromosomes 9 (1 red) and 22 (1 green), respectively; 2F represents reciprocal exchange of material between ABL and BCR portions of genome.

Patients without Ph' chromosome but with *BCR/ABL1* gene rearrangement have clinical and hematological features similar to Ph'-positive CML. The *BCR-ABL1* fusion gene is central to the pathogenesis of CML.

5. BCR-ABL1 analysis: Uses of BCR-ABL1 analysis in CML are listed in Box 7.3.

> **Box 7.3:** Applications of identification of BCR-ABL1 fusion gene/protein in chronic myeloid leukemia.
>
> - Diagnosis of chronic myeloid leukemia if Philadelphia chromosome is not detected on conventional karyotyping
> - Differential diagnosis of chronic phase of CML from leukemoid reaction, other myeloproliferative neoplasms, atypical CML, juvenile myelomonocytic leukemia, chronic neutrophilic leukemia, and myeloid neoplasms with prominent eosinophilia
> - Monitoring of tyrosine kinase inhibitor therapy
> - Differentiation of CML in blast phase from de novo ALL

Without any therapy, disease progression invariably occurs in CML to accelerated phase and blast phase; in such cases additional genetic abnormalities are always found. They are similar in accelerated and blast phases; these changes occur late in chronic phase or in early accelerated phase and precede clinical and morphologic evidence of disease progression. Also, about 30% of patients on tyrosine kinase inhibitor therapy develop disease progression; this is due to acquired mutations within *BCR-ABL1* that affect tyrosine kinase-binding domain rendering therapy ineffective. Other mutations like *BCR-ABL1* amplification, mutations in SH3-SH2 domain, and mutations in other signaling pathways have also been described that render tyrosine kinase inhibitor therapy ineffective.

Accelerated Phase of CML

In this phase, blood cell counts and organomegaly become increasingly resistant to chemotherapy. According to WHO classification, accelerated phase is characterized by presence of one or more of the following features (hematological/cytogenetic criteria or provisional response to tyrosine kinase inhibitor criteria).

Hematological/cytogenetic criteria:
- Increased percentages of blast cells (10–19%) in peripheral blood and/or bone marrow
- Peripheral blood basophilia ≥20%
- Persistence of thrombocytopenia (<1 lac/mm^3) unrelated to therapy
- Persistent thrombocytosis (>10 lac/mm^3) not responsive to therapy
- Progressive splenomegaly unresponsive to therapy
- Persistent or increase in leukocyte count despite adequate treatment
- Cytogenetic evidence of clonal evolution, i.e. cytogenetic changes in addition to Ph' chromosome that include "major route" abnormalities (such as duplication of Ph' chromosome, trisomy 8, trisomy 19, and isochromosome 17q), a complex karyotype, or abnormalities of 3q26.2.
- Any new clonal chromosomal abnormality in Ph' cells developing during therapy. Most of these patients eventually progress to blast phase or acute leukemia.

"Provisional" response-to-tyrosine kinase inhibitor therapy criteria:
- Hematological resistance to OR failure to achieve a complete hematologic response to the first tyrosine kinase inhibitor drug
- Any hematological, cytogenetic, or molecular indication of resistance to two sequential tyrosine kinase inhibitor drugs
- Development of two or more mutations in *BCR-ABL1 during tyrosine kinase inhibitor therapy.*

Table 7.1: Differences between chronic, accelerated, and blast phases of chronic myelogenous leukemia.

Parameter	Chronic phase	Accelerated phase	Blast phase
1. Blast%	<10%	10–19%	≥20%
2. Basophils	<20%	≥20%	Variable
3. Leukocytosis, thrombocytosis, splenomegaly	Responsive to therapy	Not responsive to therapy	–
4. LAP score	Low	Increased	Increased
5. Extramedullary blast proliferation	Absent	Absent	May be present
6. Clonal evolution	–	Yes	–
7. First-line therapy	Imatinib	Allogeneic stem cell transplantation preceded by tyrosine kinase inhibitor therapy	

Blast Phase

This represents acute leukemic transformation. According to WHO classification, blast phase is diagnosed in the presence of one or more of the following:
- Blasts in peripheral blood or bone marrow ≥20%
- Blast proliferation at a site other than bone marrow
- Focal clustering of blasts in bone marrow.

Blast phase in CML may be myeloid (70%) or lymphoid (30%); rarely it may be of mixed-lineage type. Differentiation between myeloid and lymphoid blast phase is important because of different treatment considerations.

Differences between chronic, accelerated, and blast phases of CML are shown in Table 7.1.

Differential Diagnosis of CML

Chronic Phase

Diagnosis of CML is based on presence of splenomegaly, moderate to marked granulocytosis (TLC usually >1 lac/mm^3) with presence of all stages of maturation, basophilia, decreased NAP score, and Ph' chromosome or *BCR/ABL1* gene rearrangement on chromosome 22.

Chronic phase of CML should be distinguished from following conditions:

Leukemoid reaction: Leukemoid reaction can occur in infections, inflammation, and nonmyeloid malignancy. In leukemoid reactions due to infections or hemolysis, leukocytosis is usually modest and shift to left is usually up to metamyelocyte or myelocyte stage; however, occasional blast may be seen. Underlying cause is frequently obvious. Other features favoring leukemoid reaction are absence of splenomegaly or basophilia, presence of toxic granules in neutrophils (in infections), normal or increased NAP score, and absence of Ph' chromosome and *BCR-ABL1 fusion gene* (Table 7.2). Clinical history and careful blood smear examination are the most important tools in differentiating CML from leukemoid reaction.

Table 7.2: Differences between chronic myeloid leukemia and leukemoid reaction.

Parameter	Chronic myeloid leukemia	Leukemoid reaction
1. Clinical features	Splenomegaly	As per underlying disease
2. Peripheral blood		
a. Leukocyte count	Usually >100,000/mm^3	Usually <50,000/mm^3
b. Myelocyte and neutrophil "peaks"	Present	Absent
c. Basophilia, eosinophilia, monocytosis	Present	Absent
d. "Toxic" granules, cytoplasmic vacuoles	Absent	Present
3. NAP score	Low	Normal or increased
4. Bone marrow examination	Trilineage hyperplasia, increased "dwarf" megakaryocytes, reticulin fibrosis present	Myeloid hyperplasia, no "dwarf" megakaryocytes, no reticulin fibrosis
5. Genetic analysis	Ph' chromosome or *BCR/ABL1* gene	Normal

Other myeloproliferative disorders: In polycythemia vera and myelofibrosis, in contrast to CML, leukocyte count is moderately raised, NAP score is normal or increased, and Ph' chromosome or *BCR/ABL1* gene rearrangement is absent. Packed cell volume is markedly increased in polycythemia vera, while in CML it is normal or low. In myelofibrosis, peripheral blood smear shows marked anisopoikilocytosis, numerous nucleated red cells and tear-drop red cells; bone marrow shows marked myelofibrosis at diagnosis. Comparative features of common myeloproliferative neoplasms are shown in Table 7.3.

Chronic neutrophilic leukemia (CNL): This is a very rare neoplasm characterized by persistent neutrophilia in peripheral blood without neutrophilic precursors or basophilia. Hepatosplenomegaly is common. Majority of patients with CNL show *CSF3R* gene mutation and there is absence of Ph' chromosome and *BCR-ABL1* gene fusion.

Myelodysplastic/Myeloproliferative neoplasms: Disorders that should be differentiated from CML are chronic myelomonocytic leukemia (CMML), atypical chronic myeloid leukemia (aCML), and juvenile myelomonocytic leukemia (JMML). Clinically, CMML usually presents with anemia and splenomegaly in elderly persons. There is moderate leukocytosis, neutrophils and band forms are increased, and monocyte count is in excess of 1000/mm^3 or monocytes >10%. Bone marrow typically shows dysplasia in one or more myeloid lineages, and increase in monocytic cells that can be demonstrated by nonspecific esterase reaction. Blasts are <20% in blood or bone marrow. Serum/urinary lysozyme is increased. Basophilia, Ph' chromosome, or *BCR/ABL1* gene rearrangement are absent. Atypical CML is characterized by absence of BCR-ABL1 fusion gene, presence of thrombocytopenia, dysplastic granulocytes, lack of basophilia, and multilineage dysplasia in bone marrow. JMML occurs in children (often <4 years of age) and shows leukocytosis, monocytosis >1000/mm^3, immature granulocytes, and nucleated red cells in peripheral blood. Ph' chromosome or BCR-ABL1 fusion gene are absent.

Table 7.3: Comparative features of common myeloproliferative neoplasms.

Parameter	Chronic myeloid leukemia	Polycythemia vera	Essential thrombocythemia	Primary myelofibrosis
Age	40–60 years	50–70 years	50–60 years (second peak 30 years)	60–70 years
Sex	M > F	M > F	50–60 years: M = F; 30 years: F > M	M > F
Splenomegaly	Moderate to massive	Mild to moderate	Absent or mild	Massive
Hemoglobin	Low	Raised	Normal	Low
WBC	Markedly raised	Raised	Normal	Raised/normal/low
Platelets	Normal, raised or low	Often raised	Persistently raised (>4.5 lac/μL)	Raised or low
LAP score	Low	Raised	Raised	Raised
Serum erythropoietin	Normal	Low	Normal	Normal
Blood smear	Granulocytosis with cells of all stages in chronic phase; basophilia; neutrophil and myelocyte peak	Thick smear due to erythrocytosis	Thrombocytosis with marked variation in size	Leukoerythroblastic reaction
Bone marrow examination	Trilineage hyperplasia with granulocytic predominance; small and hypolobated megakaryocytes	Trilineage hyperplasia with erythroid predominance	Numerous dispersed, large, mature hyperlobated megakaryocytes	Predominant granulocytic hyperplasia; highly bizarre megakaryocytes in tight clusters
Bone marrow fibrosis	Variable	Increased in spent phase	Minimal or absent	Marked
Predominant cell line affected	Granulocytic	Erythroid	Megakaryocytic	Granulocytic and megakaryocytic
Mutation	*BCR-ABL* fusion	*JAK2 V617F* (>95%), *JAK2* exon 12	*JAK2 V617F* (50%); *MPL*; *CALR*	*JAK2 V617F* (50%); *MPL*; *CALR*

Blast Phase

Sometimes CML may present for the first time as blast phase, in which case it may be difficult to distinguish it from Ph+ acute leukemia (ALL, AML, or mixed phenotype). Evidence favoring blast phase of CML includes large spleen (especially Ph+ ALL), basophilia, myelocyte peak, and Dwarf megakaryocytes in bone marrow. Transcript size of p190 is strongly suggestive of Ph+ ALL.

Course and Prognosis of CML

The natural history of CML is progression from chronic phase to accelerated and blastic phases and development of increasing refractoriness to previous chemotherapy. However, with the advent of tyrosine kinase inhibitor (TKI) therapy, most patients with newly diagnosed CML are expected to have a nearly normal lifespan. With TKI therapy, 5-year survival is 90% and 10-year survival is of more than 80%. Incidence of blast phase with TKI therapy is 5%; however, outlook for blast phase patients is poor.

The important prognostic factors are disease status at diagnosis and response (hematologic, cytogenetic, and molecular) to TKI therapy. However, Sokal risk assessment score based on age, spleen size, platelet count, and blast percentage in peripheral blood is also valid such that low-risk score patients respond better to TKI therapy than high-risk patients.

Treatment

Assessment of response to therapy: After initiation of therapy, response is assessed by hematologic, cytogenetic, and molecular parameters.

Complete hematologic response (CHR): CHR refers to WBC count <10,000/mm^3, platelet count <4.5 lac/mm^3, absence of immature granulocytes on differential count, and nonpalpable spleen.

Cytogenetic response (CyR):
- Complete cytogenetic response (CCyR): Absence of Ph+ metaphases in marrow cells
- Partial cytogenetic response (PCyR): Ph+ metaphases <35%.

Molecular response (MR):
- Complete molecular response (CMR): BCR-ABL transcripts nonquantifiable or nondetectable
- Major molecular response (MMR): BCR-ABL1 transcripts <0.1% (International scale).

Therapeutic agents: CML was the first malignancy to be associated with a chromosomal abnormality and the first malignancy for which targeted molecular therapy became available as the treatment of choice.

The treatment of CML was revolutionized in 1998 when imatinib mesylate, a potent and specific inhibitor of tyrosine kinase became available. It is the standard first-line treatment for newly diagnosed chronic phase CML. Eighty five percent of patients with CML present in chronic phase. The three TKI drugs approved for first-line treatment of chronic phase CML are imatinib (400 mg daily), dasatinib (100 mg daily), and nilotinib (300 mg twice a day). Patients should be monitored for response at 3, 6, and 12 months. Some patients taking imatinib may possibly be cured. The most common side effects of imatinib are nausea, periorbital swelling, edema, rash, and myalgia.

For patients showing suboptimal response, options include imatinib dose escalation or alternate tyrosine kinase inhibitors.

Second-line drugs for patients who cannot take imatinib include hydroxyurea and α-interferon.

For accelerated phase, dasatinib or nilotinib are recommended. For blast phase, tyrosine kinase inhibitor therapy either alone or in combination with chemotherapy followed by allogeneic hematopoietic transplantation is recommended.

Allogeneic hematopoietic transplantation is the only curative form of therapy. Considering the risks of significant morbidity and mortality, it is reserved for young patients with an HLA-matched sibling donor and who show inadequate response to imatinib or who show disease progression to accelerated or blast phase.

POLYCYTHEMIA VERA

Synonym: Polycythemia rubra vera

Polycythemia vera (PV) is a myeloproliferative neoplasm characterized by trilineage (granulocytic, erythroid, and megakaryocytic) hyperplasia in bone marrow with predominant involvement of erythroid series (erythrocytosis or increased red cell mass). Increased erythropoiesis in PV is independent of normal regulatory mechanisms.

The term polycythemia refers to increase in the number of red blood cells per unit volume of blood (more than two standard deviations from normal of hemoglobin, hematocrit, or red cell mass for that particular age, sex, race, and altitude). Distinction should be made between primary, secondary, and apparent polycythemias (Fig. 7.9 and Table 7.4).

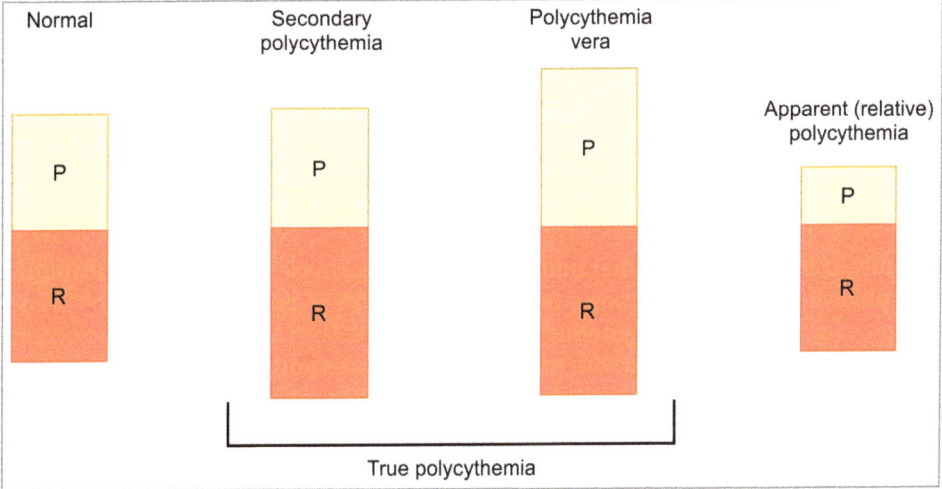

Fig. 7.9: Red cell mass and plasma volume in different types of polycythemia. P = plasma volume, R = red cell mass. In true polycythemia, red cell mass is increased and may result from PV or secondary causes. Apparent polycythemia is due to lowering of plasma volume relative to red cell mass.

Table 7.4: Causes of polycythemia.

Absolute polycythemia (Increased red cell mass)
1. Primary:
   - Congenital: Primary familial congenital erythrocytosis, truncated erythropoietin receptor due to mutation
   - Acquired: Polycythemia vera
2. Secondary:
   - Hypoxia with decreased arterial oxygen saturation (physiologically appropriate, increased erythropoietin): High altitude, chronic obstructive pulmonary disease, congenital cyanotic heart disease with right to left shunt, hemoglobins with increased oxygen affinity, heavy smoking
   - Neoplasms (physiologically inappropriate, pathologic production of erythropoietin): Renal cell carcinoma, hepatocellular carcinoma, cerebellar hemangioblastoma, uterine leiomyoma

Apparent polycythemia (Normal red cell mass)
1. Stress or spurious polycythemia
2. Dehydration

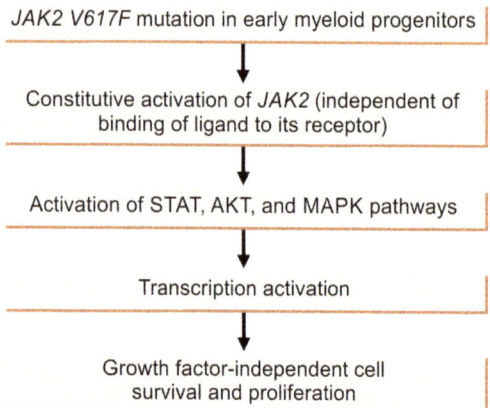

Fig. 7.10: Pathogenesis of polycythemia vera. Role of JAK2 V617F mutation in myeloproliferative neoplasms. Normally, JAK2 molecules are associated with cytoplasmic domains of cell surface receptors (e.g. erythropoietin receptors). After binding of ligand to its receptor, the receptor-associated JAKs get phosphorylated and in turn activate or phosphorylate tyrosine residues in receptor cytoplasmic tail. Activation of various pathways and signaling proteins send signals for survival, proliferation, and differentiation of erythroid progenitors.

Recently, it has been found that mutation in tyrosine kinase *JAK2 V617F* (substitution of valine to phenylalanine) on chromosome 9p24 occurs in 95% of cases and a mutation in another exon of gene (exon 12) occurs in another 4% of cases of PV. The JAK2 mutation also occurs in a significant proportion of patients with primary myelofibrosis and essential thrombocythemia. Role of this mutation in the pathogenesis of PV and other myeloproliferative neoplasms is presented in Figure 7.10.

JAK2 V617F is the most consistent molecular abnormality found in almost all patients (>95%) with PV. A guanine to cytosine substitution occurs in codon 617 of chromosome 9p24 exon 14, causing valine to phenylalanine substitution (V617F) in mRNA. This is a somatic gain of function or type I mutation ("driver" mutation) which modifies growth factor signaling. Mutation causes phosphorylation and constitutive activation of JAK2 tyrosine kinase leading to activation of signal transduction pathways and activation of transcription (*STAT5, STAT3, RAS-MAPK,* and *PI3-AKT* pathways). This leads to myeloid proliferation in the absence or reduced levels of cytokines and hypersensitivity to cytokines. Mutant allele burden is the single most important risk factor for thrombosis. Higher allele burden is also associated with more responsiveness to ruxolitinib therapy.

In about 3% of patients, *JAK2* exon 12 (9p24) mutations are found which occurs across multiple codons from 533 to 547. It is a gain of function mutation and its prognosis is similar to *JAK2* V617F mutation.

Recent studies indicate that *JAK2* mutation may be a late secondary molecular event. Although initiating molecular event is not known, evidence indicates that mutations in *TET2, ASXL1,* and *EZH2* probably precede *JAK2* V617F.

Erythropoietin (EPO) is the primary regulator of erythropoiesis. It is synthesized by peritubular cells in the kidney and its increased production occurs in response to hypoxia. Binding of EPO to EPOR receptors on erythroid progenitors leads to dimerization of EPOR and phosphorylation of associated JAK2 kinase which in turn activates downstream JAK/STAT and other pathways; this ultimately leads to proliferation and reduced apoptosis of erythroid precursors. Due to constitutive activation of JAK2, erythropoietin production is reduced in PV and abnormal erythroid stem cells require very small amounts of erythropoietin for their differentiation. The neoplastic clone suppresses normal hematopoietic stem cells as well as erythropoietin production.

There are two phases of PV:
1. Proliferative or polycythemic phase (initial phase characterized by proliferation of erythroid cells leading to increased red cell mass)
2. "Spent" or postpolycythemic phase (characterized by cytopenias, extramedullary hematopoiesis, hypersplenism, and myelofibrosis).

Progression to acute myeloid leukemia occurs in a proportion (10–15%) of patients.

Clinical Features

Polycythemia vera is an uncommon disease occurring between 50 and 70 years of age. Males are affected slightly more commonly than females.

Increased blood viscosity and volume related to erythrocytosis may lead to decreased blood flow and dilatation of blood vessels. This may cause headache, vertigo, facial plethora, blurring of vision, and congestion of conjunctiva and mucosa. Thrombosis can occur in cerebrovascular, coronary, or peripheral arteries and in deep veins of legs. Thrombosis at unusual locations such as mesenteric, portal, or hepatic veins should prompt investigations for PV. Spontaneous mucous membrane bleeding can occur such as epistaxis and gastrointestinal bleeding (due to platelet dysfunction). Incidence of peptic ulcer is higher than normal in PV. Erythromelalgia (painful and burning sensation of hands and feet associated with increased skin temperature and redness) can occur. Pruritus occurs in 30% of patients and is increased by warm bath. Moderate splenomegaly is usual and its presence virtually rules out secondary polycythemia. With progression to "spent" phase, marked enlargement of spleen occurs.

Laboratory Features

Peripheral Blood Examination

After collection, blood appears thick and viscous. The red cell count, hemoglobin concentration, and packed cell volume are raised. Initially at presentation, red cells are normocytic and normochromic; the red cells may be microcytic and hypochromic since depletion of iron stores can occur due to excess red cell production. With progression to spent phase (myelofibrosis), anisopoikilocytosis, tear drop cells, and nucleated red cells along with left-shifted myeloid cells appear (leukoerythroblastic smear).

There is usually mild to moderate leukocytosis with shift to left up to myelocyte stage. Basophils, eosinophils, and monocytes are often increased.

Platelet count is increased in 50% of patients and is usually >5 lac/mm^3. Giant platelets are often seen. Very high platelet count is associated with hemorrhage; however, there is no direct correlation between platelet count and thrombosis.

Bone Marrow Examination

In the polycythemic stage, bone marrow aspiration smears show hypercellular marrow with trilineage hyperplasia, especially involving erythroid series. Megakaryocytes are increased and show variation in size and pleomorphism.

In polycythemic phase, bone marrow biopsy shows hypercellularity (panmyelosis) and enlarged erythroblastic islands, increased megakaryocyte numbers with variability in size, and normal reticulin fiber network. Megakaryocytes do not display atypia or bizarre, dysplastic features or tight clustering. Iron stores are often absent. With progression of the disease to spent phase, myelofibrosis develops. In postpolycythemic myelofibrosis, marrow is often hypocellular and shows marked reticulin and/or collagen fibrosis (occasionally osteosclerotic bone), decreased quantity of erythropoiesis and granulopoiesis, and clusters of abnormal megakaryocytes with bizarre and dysplastic nuclei. Blasts >10% in blood or bone marrow or myelodysplastic features indicate transformation to an accelerated or myelodysplastic syndrome-like phase and if >20% indicate transformation to acute myeloid leukemia.

In myeloproliferative neoplasms, bone marrow biopsy is essential to establish the diagnosis of a particular disease, exclude other myeloproliferative neoplasms, assess the prognosis and for staging of disease.

JAK2 mutation analysis: JAK2 V617F mutation is detected in >95% of patients with polycythemia vera and is one of the diagnostic criteria for PV. It is, however, not specific for polycythemia vera since it is also observed in essential thrombocythemia and primary myelofibrosis. JAK2 exon 12 mutation is seen in 3% of patients and is specific for PV since it has not been identified in other myeloproliferative neoplasms.

Cytogenetic analysis: Demonstration of absence of Ph' chromosome or BCR-ABL1 fusion gene is essential for exclusion of CML. In addition, various cytogenetic abnormalities have been detected most frequent being +8, +9, and deletion or translocation of chromosome 20.

Serum erythropoietin (EPO) level: Low serum erythropoietin level in the presence of increased red cell mass is a key diagnostic feature that differentiates PV from other causes of polycythemia.

Other Investigations

- Neutrophil alkaline phosphatase (NAP) score is increased or normal
- Arterial oxygen saturation is normal
- Red cell mass is elevated as determined with ^{51}Cr-labeled red cells
- Spontaneous or endogenous erythroid colony formation in vitro without added erythropoietin is an important feature.
- Platelet function studies show reduced primary and secondary aggregation in response to epinephrine and ADP. Markedly increased platelet count (>1000 × 10^9/l) is associated with reduced collagen binding and ristocetin cofactor activity indicating decreased functional activity of von Willebrand factor (acquired von Willebrand syndrome). This defect is associated with hemorrhage.
- Cytochemistry and immunophenotyping: There is no role in diagnosis of polycythemia vera.

Important features necessary for diagnosis of PV are presented in Box 7.4.

Box 7.4: Diagnosis of polycythemia vera.

Diagnosis of PV should be considered in the presence of following features:
- Adult patient presenting with plethora and splenomegaly
- Raised hemoglobin and PCV above normal
- Exclusion of causes of secondary polycythemia
- Erythrocytosis, leukocytosis, and thrombocytosis in blood
- Bone marrow showing trilineage proliferation along with prominent hyperplasia of erythroid and megakaryocytic series
- Low or normal serum erythropoietin level

Chapter 7: Myeloproliferative Neoplasms

Table 7.5: Differences between polycythemia vera (PV), secondary polycythemia (SP), and relative polycythemia (RP).

	Parameter	PV	SP	RP
1.	Nature of disease	Clonal, myeloproliferative neoplasm	Hypoxia or increased erythropoietin level	Relative lowering of plasma volume
2.	Red cell mass	Increased	Increased	Normal
3.	Plasma volume	Increased	Normal	Decreased
4.	Splenomegaly	Present	Absent	Absent
5.	White blood cells	Increased, immature forms+	Normal	Normal
6.	Platelets	Increased	Normal	Normal
7.	Bone marrow	Trilineage hyperplasia	Erythroid hyperplasia	Normal
8.	Arterial O_2 saturation	Normal	Decreased or normal	Normal
9.	Erythropoietin	Decreased	Increased	Normal
10.	NAP score	Increased	Normal	Normal
11.	Cytogenetic abnormality	May be present	Absent	Absent

Differential Diagnosis

Secondary polycythemia: Various causes of polycythemia are listed in Table 7.4. Differences between them are presented in Table 7.5.

Other myeloproliferative disorders: Patients in early stage of polycythemia vera often have modestly raised hemoglobin and hematocrit values and very high platelet count; such patients may be mistakenly diagnosed as having essential thrombocythemia. In such cases, bone marrow biopsy will provide the correct diagnosis. Differentiation from other myeloproliferative disorders is considered under chronic myeloid leukemia.

Diagnosis of Polycythemia Vera

Criteria for diagnosis of polycythemia vera by World Health Organisation (2016) require either all three major criteria or the first two major criteria plus the minor criterion.

Major criteria
- Raised hemoglobin concentration (>16.5 g/dL in men; >16.0 g/dL in women) or raised hematocrit (>49% in men; >48% in women) or increased red cell mass (>25% above mean predicted value)
- Bone marrow biopsy showing trilineage (erythroid, granulocytic, megakaryocytic) hyperplasia with mature, pleomorphic megakaryocytes of varying sizes
- *JAK2 V617F* or *JAK2 exon 12* mutation.

Minor criterion: Subnormal serum erythropoietin level.

Algorithm for diagnosis of myeloproliferative neoplasms is shown in Figure 7.11. Estimation of serum erythropoietin and genetic testing for *JAK2 V617F* mutation are the frontline

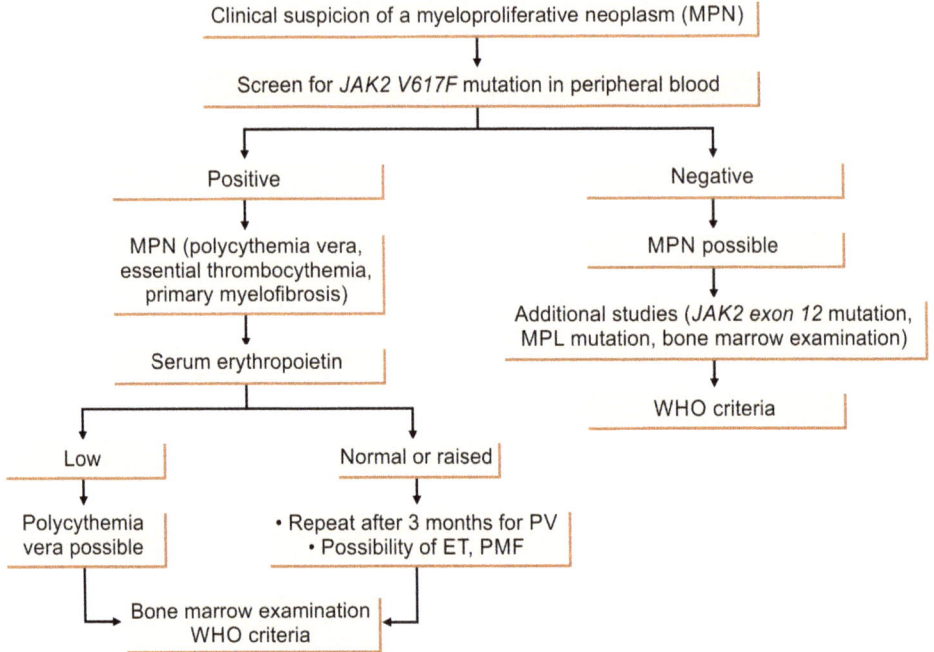

Fig. 7.11: Algorithm for diagnosis of myeloproliferative neoplasms (polycythemia vera, essential thrombocythemia, and primary myelofibrosis).

tests for diagnosis of polycythemia vera and for its differentiation from other causes of polycythemia.

Course and Prognosis

Without treatment, patients with PV have a median survival of about 18 months with death occurring most commonly from thrombotic complications (myocardial infarction, stroke, venous thromboembolism) or hemorrhage. With recent modes of therapy, survival is approximately 10–15 years. The major risk factors for thrombosis are previous history of thrombosis and older age at diagnosis. Hemorrhage is associated with extremely high platelet count ($>1000 \times 10^9$/L).

The course of PV consists of proliferative and spent phases. In the proliferative phase, trilineage proliferation with predominance of erythroid series occurs in the bone marrow. This is followed by gradual progression to a spent phase (15–20% of patients) during which clinical and hematological manifestations of myelofibrosis develop (postpolycythemic myelofibrosis).

Transformation to acute myeloid leukemia occurs in about 5% of patients of PV. Incidence of leukemia in patients treated with myelosuppression (chemo- or radiotherapy), or with radioactive phosphorous or ^{32}P (now rarely used) is higher as compared to those treated with phlebotomy alone. Transformation to AML is associated with karyotypic evolution (acquisition of chromosomal abnormalities).

Untreated patients with PV have increased risk of thrombotic complications and hemorrhage and long-term risk of myelofibrosis and acute myeloid leukemia.

Treatment

There are two modes of therapy in PV: (i) phlebotomy that aims to rapidly lower the packed cell volume or hematocrit combined with low dose aspirin, and (ii) myelosuppressive therapy to control production of blood cells in bone marrow (cytoreductive therapy).

Treatment in PV should be individualized. Patient can be treated with myelosuppressive therapy, phlebotomy plus myelosuppressive therapy, or phlebotomy combined with low-dose aspirin.

The most common form of therapy is phlebotomy combined with aspirin. All patients usually require repeated phlebotomy as an initial measure to lower the hematocrit to normal levels. This reduces the immediate risk of thrombosis. Myelosuppressive therapy (hydroxyurea), often combined with phlebotomy is indicated in patients with previous history of thrombosis, systemic symptoms, and thrombocytosis. Failure to respond to first-line therapy may warrant use of ruxolitinib, a JAK2 inhibitor; however, it does not affect the natural course of disease.

Postpolycythemic myelofibrosis and AML respond poorly to therapy.

PRIMARY MYELOFIBROSIS

Synonym: Idiopathic myelofibrosis with agnogenic myeloid metaplasia

Reticulin and collagen fibrosis are nonspecific manifestations of various diseases involving the bone marrow. Myelofibrosis is mediated by cytokines released from marrow stromal cells, megakaryocytes, T cells, monocytes and macrophages. Reticulin fibrosis (increased amount and density of network of delicate reticulin fibers) commonly occurs in response to infectious and inflammatory conditions involving the marrow, while collagen fibrosis more commonly occurs in carcinoma and lymphoma infiltrating the marrow. About 50% cases of myelofibrosis represent myeloproliferative neoplasms.

Primary myelofibrosis (PMF) is a clonal, myeloproliferative neoplasm characterized by trilineage proliferation in bone marrow (with predominance of granulocytic and megakaryocytic lines), reactive bone marrow fibrosis, and extramedullary hematopoiesis mainly in spleen. (Extramedullary hematopoiesis or "myeloid metaplasia" refers to ectopic hematopoiesis occurring in organs other than bone marrow like spleen and liver.) There is a gradual progression of disease from initial prefibrotic stage to fibrotic stage.

Studies have shown that trilineage proliferation of blood cells in bone marrow is monoclonal and arises in hematopoietic stem cell. In contrast, fibroblasts are not part of the neoplastic clone. Bone marrow fibrosis results from stimulation of fibroblastic proliferation and collagen synthesis by platelet-derived growth factor and transforming growth factor-β, which are secreted by increased numbers of abnormal megakaryocytes.

"Driver" mutations occurring in PMF include *JAK2* V617F (50% cases), *CALR* (30% cases), and *MPL* (5-10% cases). They are called "driver" mutations because they cause persistent activation of JAK/STAT signaling pathway in the absence of cytokine signaling. Cases of PMF in which any of the above three mutations are not identified are termed as triple-negative PMF.

There are two phases of PMF: Prefibrotic phase and fibrotic phase. In prefibrotic stage, marrow is hypercellular with minimal or absent fibrosis, and blood shows thrombocytosis. At fibrotic stage, bone marrow shows marked fibrosis and extramedullary hematopoiesis, and blood shows leukoerythroblastosis and tear drop red cells.

PMF, a rare disease, manifests usually in the elderly, median age at diagnosis being 65 years. Sex incidence is equal. The disease has insidious onset with fatigue and weight loss (due to production of cytokines). Splenomegaly (due to extramedullary hematopoiesis) is present in majority of patients and may be massive. Other manifestations include portal hypertension, bleeding varices, ascites, splenic pain due to infarction, and lymphadenopathy (due to extramedullary hematopoiesis). About one-third of patients are asymptomatic and detected incidentally (incidental detection of splenomegaly, or of anemia, leukocytosis, or thrombocytosis on complete blood count). Clinical features usually correlate with stage of PMF. In the prefibrotic phase, patients may present with bleeding or thrombosis. Fibrotic stage is characterized by anemia and prominent splenomegaly and often hepatomegaly.

Laboratory Evaluation

- Peripheral blood: In the prefibrotic stage, marked thrombocytosis, moderate anemia, and mild leukocytosis with shift to left are seen. Fibrotic stage is characterized by marked anisopoikilocytosis with tear drop red cells and leukoerythroblastic blood picture (presence of immature cells of erythroid and granulocytic series in peripheral blood) (Fig. 7.12). In this stage, platelet count and leukocyte count may be low due to ineffective erythropoiesis from marrow fibrosis.
- *Bone marrow examination:* In prefibrotic stage, bone marrow is hypercellular and shows granulocytic and megakaryocytic hyperplasia; megakaryocytes have pleomorphic and bizarre appearance. In fibrotic stage, bone marrow aspiration typically reveals a "dry tap," i.e. failure to obtain bone marrow with aspiration of only peripheral blood. Bone marrow trephine biopsy shows decreased cellularity, fibrosis, increase in the number of abnormal megakaryocytes that are often tightly clustered together, osteosclerosis, and dilated marrow sinuses containing intrasinusoidal hematopoiesis. Reticulin and trichrome staining can assess degree of marrow fibrosis. Myeloblasts 10–19% indicates accelerated phase, while ≥20% indicates transformation to AML.

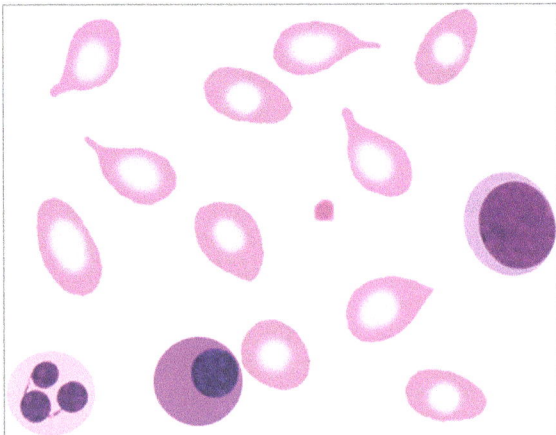

Fig. 7.12: Blood smear in primary myelofibrosis showing many tear drop cells and leukoerythroblastic reaction.

- *Cytogenetic analysis:* Chromosomal abnormalities are present in 40–50% of patients the most common of which are del (13q), del (20q), trisomy 8, trisomy 9, and abnormalities of 1q.
- *Molecular genetic analysis:* The most frequent mutation is *JAK2* V617F followed by mutations in *CALR* and *MPL*.

Highly pleomorphic and bizarre morphology of megakaryocytes is a key feature that distinguishes PMF from other myeloproliferative neoplasms. Prefibrotic stage is most likely to be confused with essential thrombocythemia from which it is distinguished by abnormal megakaryocyte morphology in the background of granulocytic hyperplasia. Differential diagnosis in fibrotic stage includes (1) other myeloproliferative diseases associated with fibrosis: CML, PV, and essential thrombocythemia; (2) myelofibrosis secondary to metastasis in marrow, lymphoma, or disseminated tuberculosis; (3) myelodysplastic syndrome with myelofibrosis; and (4) acute myelofibrosis. Causes of bone marrow fibrosis are listed in Table 7.6.

The median survival ranges from 3 to 5 years from diagnosis; however, it is highly variable. Common causes of death are infections, heart failure, hemorrhage, thrombosis, and transformation to AML (15% of patients).

Treatment is largely palliative. A trial of androgens and corticosteroids may alleviate anemia, but regular transfusions are usually required. Chemotherapy (hydroxyurea) is used for control of elevated white cell and platelet counts and to reduce the size of spleen. Splenic irradiation can result in relief of splenic pain and reduction of spleen size. Splenectomy may be considered in the presence of unacceptable transfusion needs, enlarged and painful spleen, complications of portal hypertension, and life-threatening refractory thrombocytopenia. However, splenectomy is associated with risk of considerable morbidity and mortality and should be undertaken with caution. Recently, JAK2 inhibitors like ruxolitinib have been developed which can provide palliative solutions like reducing spleen size and constitutional symptoms; however, unlike imatinib in CML, they are not curative.

Table 7.6: Causes of bone marrow fibrosis.

Hematologic disorders	Nonhematologic disorders
1. Myeloproliferative neoplasms: Chronic myelogenous leukemia, primary myelofibrosis, essential thrombocythemia, polycythemia vera, systemic mastocytosis	1. Infections: Tuberculosis, histoplasmosis, kala-azar, human immunodeficiency virus
2. Myelodysplastic syndromes	2. Metastatic carcinoma
3. Acute leukemias	3. Autoimmune disorders
4. Lymphoma	4. Hyperparathyroidism
5. Multiple myeloma	5. Renal osteodystrophy
6. Hairy cell leukemia	6. Vitamin D deficiency
7. Gray platelet syndrome	7. Paget's disease of bone

ESSENTIAL THROMBOCYTHEMIA

Synonym: Primary thrombocythemia

Essential thrombocythemia (ET) is a clonal, myeloproliferative neoplasm characterized by marked proliferation of megakaryocytes in bone marrow causing thrombocytosis in peripheral blood. It usually occurs in the elderly (50-60 years of age). Patients manifest with bleeding and/or thrombotic (digital or cerebral ischemia) manifestations. Splenomegaly is present at diagnosis in 50% of patients. Many patients are asymptomatic (50%) and are discovered incidentally on routine blood examination.

By definition, platelet count in ET is more than 4.5 lac/mm^3; in the majority of patients it exceeds 1 million/mm^3. Morphologic abnormalities of platelets, such as giant forms, marked variation in size and shape, and megakaryocyte fragments are often seen in peripheral blood. Bone marrow shows markedly increased numbers of large or giant mature megakaryocytes with hyperlobulated nuclei (staghorn appearance) which are often arranged in clusters (Figs. 7.13 and 7.14). Driver mutations in one of three genes *JAK2, CALR, or MPL* is present in 90% of patients with ET. Platelet function tests reveal defective aggregation with epinephrine.

WHO diagnostic criteria for ET (2016): Diagnosis of ET requires presence of all four major criteria or first three major and minor criterion.

Major criteria:
- Platelet count ≥ 450 × 10^9/L
- *Bone marrow biopsy:* Mainly megakaryocytic proliferation showing enlarged, mature megakaryocytes with nuclear hyperlobulation; granulocytic and erythroid series not significantly increased; if present, only minor increase in reticulin fibers (rare)
- Criteria for other myeloid neoplasms are not met
- Presence of mutation of *JAK2, CALR, or MPL*.

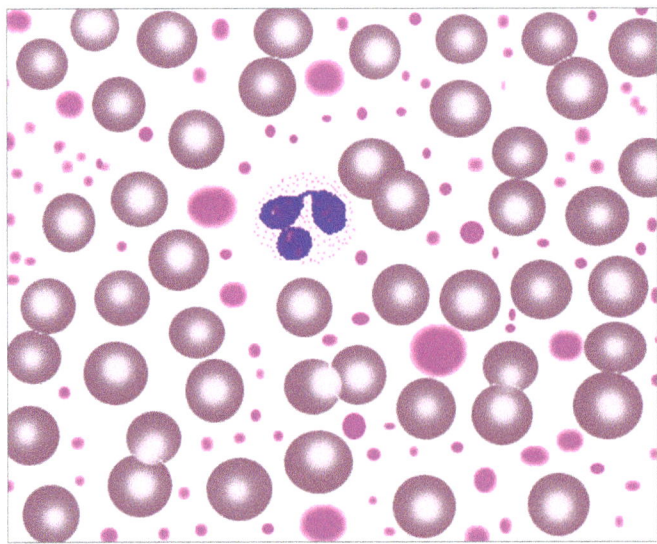

Fig. 7.13: Blood smear in essential thrombocythemia showing normal red blood cells, thrombocytosis, marked variation in size of platelets, and large and giant platelets.

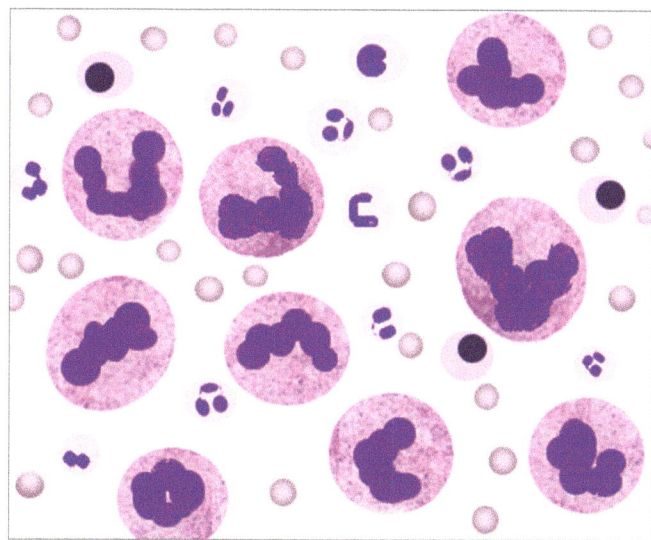

Fig. 7.14: Bone marrow aspiration smear in essential thrombocythemia showing increased number of diffusely scattered, mature, large, multilobated megakaryocytes.

Minor criterion: Presence of a clonal marker or no evidence of reactive thrombocytosis.

Differential diagnosis includes (i) other myeloproliferative disorders, and (ii) secondary (reactive) thrombocytosis which commonly occurs in infections, iron deficiency, chronic inflammatory disorders, malignant diseases, acute hemorrhage, and following splenectomy.

Amongst myeloproliferative neoplasms, ET needs to be distinguished especially from prefibrotic primary myelofibrosis, as duration of survival is longer, and progression to leukemia and to higher grade fibrosis are lower in the former. Bone marrow morphologic features favoring prefibrotic PMF over ET are marked increase in cellularity, significant granulocytic hyperplasia, reduction of erythroid cells, marked clustering of bizarre and dysplastic megakaryocytes.

Features that favor diagnosis of a clonal disorder against reactive thrombocytosis are:
- Hemorrhagic and/or thrombotic manifestations
- Splenomegaly
- Abnormal platelet function (reduced aggregation with epinephrine)
- Giant platelets on blood smear
- Abnormal megakaryocytes (e.g. giant forms) on bone marrow examination.

Features of essential thrombocythemia and reactive thrombocytosis are compared in Table 7.7.

Median survival is 10–15 years after treatment. Causes of death include thrombosis, hemorrhage, and evolution to AML (<5% of patients). Patients older than 60 years, and patients with thrombotic or hemorrhagic episodes or with very high platelet counts are treated with cytotoxic (hydroxyurea) therapy. Addition of low-dose aspirin (75 mg/day) may be helpful in the presence of thrombosis.

Table 7.7: Differences between essential thrombocythemia and reactive thrombocytosis.

Parameter	Essential thrombocythemia	Reactive thrombocytosis
1. Underlying cause for thrombocytosis	Absent	Present
2. Thrombosis	Often	No
3. Hemorrhage	Often	No
4. Splenomegaly	May be present	Absent
5. JAK2 V617F, CALR, or MPL mutation	Present (90%)	Absent
6. C-reactive protein	–	Raised
7. Giant platelets and megakaryocyte fragments on blood smear	Often present	Absent
8. Defective platelet function	Present	Absent
9. Megakaryocytes	Abnormal	Normal

BIBLIOGRAPHY

1. Baccarani M, Castagnetti F, Gugliotta G, et al. Treatment recommendations for chronic myeloid leukemia. Mediterr J Hematol Infect Dis. 2014;6:e2014005.
2. Baccarani M, Deininger MW, Rosti G, et al. European leukemiaNet recommendations for the management of chronic myeloid leukemia:2013. Blood. 2013;122(6):872–84.
3. Goldman JM, Melo JV. Chronic myeloid leukaemia—Advances in biology and new approaches to treatment. N Engl J Med.2003;349:1451-64.
4. Jaffe ES, Harris NL, Stein H, et al. World Health Organisation Classification of Tumours. Pathology and genetics of tumours of haematopoietic and lymphoid tissues. Lyon. IARC Press. 2001.
5. Sawyers CL. Chronic myeloid leukemia. N Engl J Med. 1999;340:1330-40.
6. Schafer AI. Thrombocytosis. N Engl J Med. 2004;350:1211-19.
7. Swerdlow SH, Campo E, Harris NL, et al. WHO Classification of tumours of hematopoietic and lymphoid tissues (Revised 4th Ed.). Lyon, IARC. 2017.
8. Tefferi A. Myelofibrosis with myeloid metaplasia. N Engl J Med. 2000;342:1255-65.
9. Tefferi A. Polycythemia vera: A comprehensive review and clinical recommendations. Mayo Clin Proc. 2003;78:174-94.

CHAPTER 8

Chronic Lymphoid Leukemias

These are a heterogeneous group of clonal, neoplastic disorders characterized by proliferation of mature B or T lymphoid cells (Table 8.1).

CHRONIC LYMPHOCYTIC LEUKEMIA

Chronic lymphocytic leukemia (CLL) is a neoplastic disorder characterized by monoclonal proliferation of immunologically incompetent, slowly dividing, mature B-lymphocytes. CLL is the most common form of leukemia in western countries, while it is the least common type in Asian countries including India.

Cell of Origin

CLL can be divided into two subsets based on whether CLL cells express an unmutated or mutated immunoglobulin heavy chain variable region gene (*IGVH*). Mutated *IGVH* CLL (60% cases) arises from postgerminal center B cell, while unmutated *IGVH* CLL (40% cases) originates from naïve B cells. ZAP-70 expression is used as a surrogate marker for *IGVH* mutation status since it is more highly expressed in Ig-unmutated CLL than in Ig-mutated CLL. Unmutated *IGVH* CLL is associated with inferior clinical outcome (Fig. 8.1).

Table 8.1: Chronic lymphoid leukemias.

B-cell type	T-and NK-cell type
• Chronic lymphocytic leukemia	• T-cell prolymphocytic leukemia
• B-cell prolymphocytic leukemia	• T-cell large granular lymphocytic leukemia
• Hairy cell leukemia	• Adult T cell leukemia/lymphoma
• Hairy cell leukemia variant	• Aggressive NK-cell leukemia

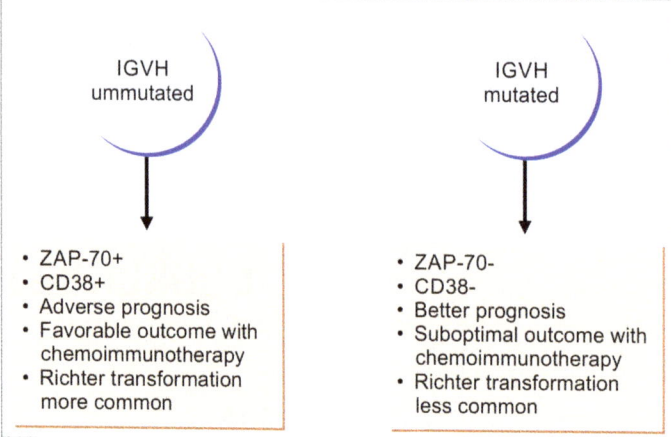

Fig. 8.1: Two types of CLL based on *IGVH* mutational status. According to some investigators, postulated cell of origin of CLL is mature, antigen-experienced postgerminal B cell. According to others, mutated *IGVH* CLL arises from mature, antigen-experienced postgerminal B cell, while unmutated *IGVH* CLL arises from pregerminal center naïve B cell.

(IGVH: immunoglobulin variable region heavy chain; ZAP-70: Zeta-chain-associated protein kinase 70)

Clinical Features

CLL occurs principally in persons over 50 years of age (median age at presentation: 65–70 years). It is twice as common in males as compared to females. First-degree relatives of the patient have significantly increased risk of developing CLL and other lymphoid malignancies. (CLL is the most common familial leukemia.) Patient may present with weakness, fatigue, and weight loss, repeated infections (due to decreased number and function of B cells and hypogammaglobulinemia) and symptoms related to anemia or thrombocytopenia. Generalized lymphadenopathy is the most common presenting feature; mild-to-moderate splenomegaly is present in two-thirds of cases. About 25% of patients are asymptomatic and are discovered incidentally on clinical or laboratory examination.

Laboratory Features

Peripheral Blood Examination

Anemia develops with progressive marrow replacement by tumor cells and is normocytic and normochromic. Other causes of anemia in CLL include hypersplenism and autoimmune hemolysis. Autoimmune hemolytic anemia occurs in about 10% of patients and is characterized by mild hyperbilirubinemia, increased reticulocytes and spherocytes, and positive Coombs' (antiglobulin) test.

Total leukocyte count is increased and is usually more than 50,000/mm^3 with >80% of cells being lymphocytes. Diagnosis of CLL requires absolute monoclonal lymphocyte count of ≥5000/mm^3.

In majority of cases, >90% of neoplastic cells are small, mature-looking lymphocytes with high N/C ratio, scanty cytoplasm and dense, clumped chromatin. Nucleoli are not seen or are inconspicuous (Fig. 8.2). In about 15% of cases, in addition to small, mature-looking lymphocytes, >10% (but <55%) cells are prolymphocytes; this category is designated as atypical CLL, mixed CLL, or CLL/PL. "Smudge" or basket cells are a characteristic feature of CLL and are produced during spreading of blood film because of fragility of lymphocytes. Although cell morphology of CLL is characteristic, flow cytometry is essential for diagnosis (WHO). Platelet count may be normal or decreased. Thrombocytopenia becomes severe with progressive replacement of

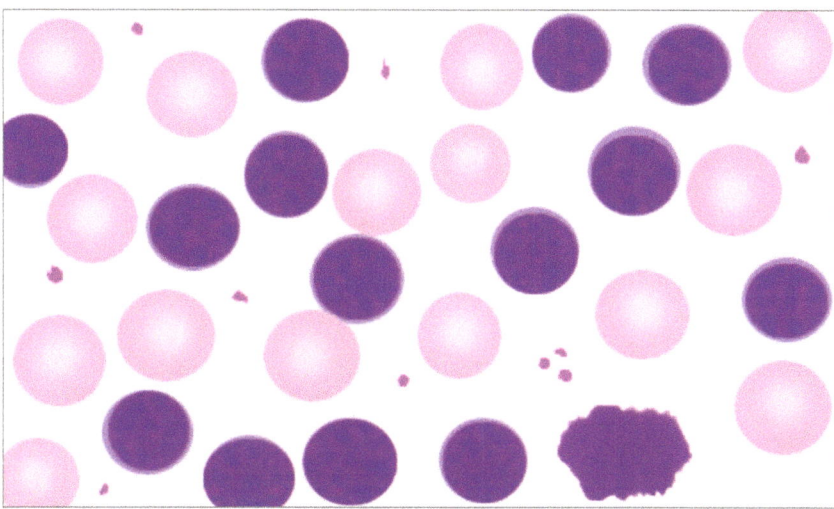

Fig. 8.2: Blood smear in chronic lymphocytic leukemia showing small, mature-looking lymphocytes with clumped chromatin. A smudge cell is seen at lower right.

bone marrow by leukemic cells. Other causes of thrombocytopenia are immune destruction of platelets and hypersplenism.

Bone Marrow Examination

Bone marrow examination is not essential for diagnosis of CLL; however, bone marrow core biopsy is useful for assessment of pattern and extent of infiltration and in assessment of residual hematopoiesis. Bone marrow lymphocytes more than 30% is a characteristic feature. Morphology of CLL cells in bone marrow is similar to that in peripheral blood.

Assessment of pattern of infiltration of neoplastic cells in bone marrow has possible prognostic importance. Four patterns of infiltration can be recognized on bone marrow trephine biopsy—interstitial, nodular, diffuse, and a combination of these. Diffuse pattern is associated with aggressive disease and worse prognosis since it is associated with cytopenias and thus higher clinical stage; diffuse pattern is also associated with ZAP-70 expression. Nodular pattern is associated with a favorable prognosis (Fig. 8.3). Pattern of marrow infiltration is also useful in differential diagnosis of CLL from other lymphoid proliferations, since paratrabecular localization is rare in CLL.

Immunophenotyping

Immunophenotyping provides definitive diagnosis and should be done in all cases before beginning therapy. It is particularly helpful in situations where lymphocytosis is less than 5000/mm^3 or when lymphocyte morphology is atypical. CLL cells usually express membrane phenotype of early B cells. Characteristically CLL cells express CD19, CD20 (weak), CD5, CD23, weak surface membrane immunoglobulin, and absent reactivity with FMC7 and with CD22. A single light chain (either κ or λ) is expressed on the surface of cells supporting the clonal origin of lymphocytes (Fig. 8.4). A newer antigen CD200 has been found to be consistently expressed on CLL cells and allows differentiation of CLL from mantle cell lymphoma and other CD5+ mature B cell neoplasms.

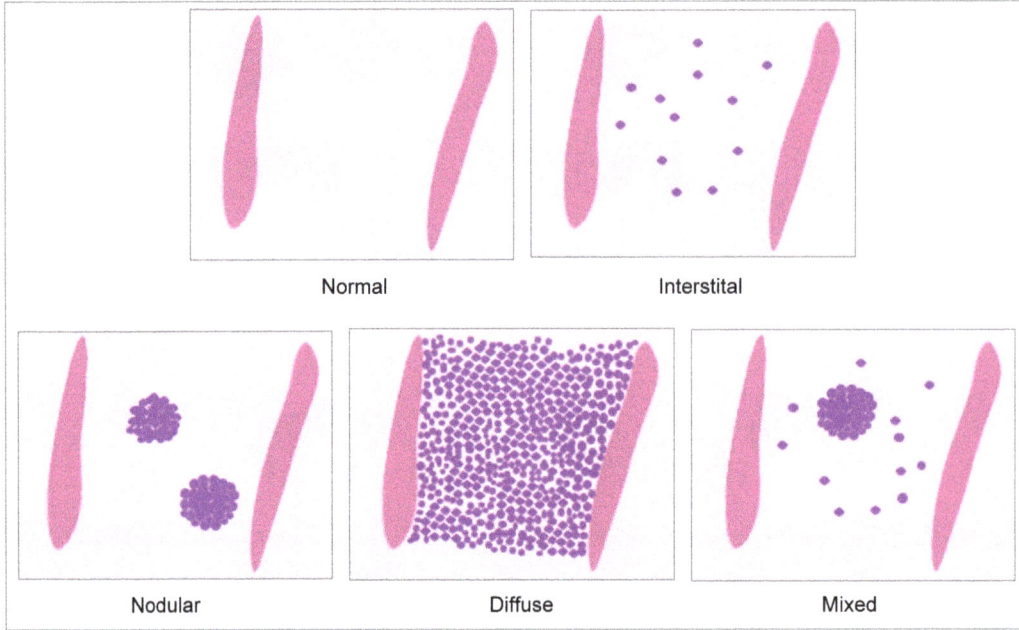

Fig. 8.3: Patterns of bone marrow infiltration in CLL. Four patterns of infiltration can be seen in CLL: (1) Interstitial: Individual neoplastic cells are interspersed between hematopoietic cells and fat cells; (2) Nodular: Well-defined round or oval aggregates of neoplastic cells that are nonparatrabecular; (3) Diffuse: Extensive replacement of both hematopoietic and fat cells so that marrow architecture is effaced and appears "packed"; (4) Mixed: Combination of nodular and interstitial pattern.

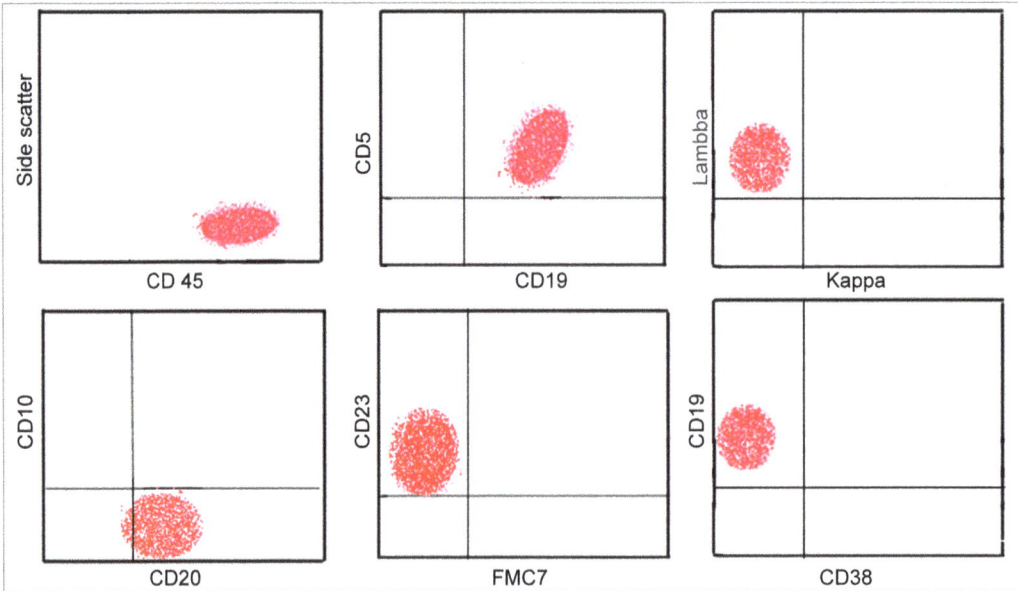

Fig. 8.4: Diagrammatic representation of immunophenotyping by flow cytometry in a case of CLL. The cells express CD19, CD5, lambda light chain (dim), CD23, CD20 (dim), and are negative for CD10, FMC7, and CD38. Absence of CD38 expression is a good prognostic indicator.

Cytogenetic Analysis

In CLL, conventional cytogenetic analysis is difficult due to low mitotic rate of CLL. Advent of fluorescent in situ hybridization (FISH) (which can detect chromosomal abnormalities in nondividing cells) has led to the identification of cytogenetic abnormalities in majority of patients with CLL. There is no single cytogenetic abnormality specific for CLL. The common abnormalities include 13q-, 11q-, trisomy 12, 17p-, and complex abnormalities. Some chromosomal abnormalities are associated with a poor outcome, such as 11q- or17p-. Clonal evolution leads to acquisition of new genetic abnormalities that may have therapeutic relevance.

Immunological Studies

Hypogammaglobulinemia is observed in two-thirds of patients and becomes severe with progression of disease; it is associated with increased risk of bacterial infections. M band (monoclonal protein) is observed in about 5% of patients.

Diagnosis

Diagnosis of CLL is based on following criteria:
- Absolute monoclonal lymphocytosis in peripheral blood ≥5 × 10^9/L in peripheral blood for a duration of at least 3 months
- Lymphocytes are small, mature-looking with high N/C ratio, round to oval nuclei and clumped chromatin (smudge or basket cells are typical)
- Characteristic immunophenotype: CD19+, weak CD20, CD23+, CD5+, and weak SmIg (kappa or lambda Ig light chains)
- Prolymphocytes ≤55%

Although ≥30% lymphocytes in bone marrow is considered characteristic, extent of bone marrow involvement is variable.

Diagnosis of small lymphocytic lymphoma is based on following features:
- Predominant extramedullary site involvement (often lymph node)
- Diffuse proliferation of small lymphocytes with scattered proliferation centers
- Monoclonal B lymphocytes in blood <5 × 10^9/L
- Immunophenotype: CD19+, coexpression of CD5 and CD23, weak CD20, weak SmIg.

Monoclonal B lymphocytosis (MBL): This refers to cases with absolute monoclonal B lymphocyte count <5000/mm^3 with immunophenotype of CLL and no symptoms or cytopenias. This is considered as precursor of CLL with rate of progression from MBL to CLL 1 to 2% per year. Cases with monlocnal B lymphocytosis <5000/mm^3 but with organomegaly or lymphadenopathy are termed as small lymphocytic lymphoma.

Atypical CLL: This refers to cases of CLL with increased numbers of cells with prominent nuclear irregularity, or with distinct nucleoli, such cases may have an aggressive course (more advanced stage, higher proliferative index, and worse prognosis). Atypical CLL is commonly associated with trisomy 12q. Some cases of atypical CLL have lymphoplasmacytic morphology.

Differential Diagnosis

Reactive Lymphocytosis

Reactive lymphocytosis occurs in infections by viruses (such as Epstein-Barr virus, cytomegalovirus, hepatitis, and influenza), postvaccination, tuberculosis, toxoplasmosis, rickettsia, and autoimmune disorders. Reactive lymphocytosis is transient and lymphocyte count is usually less than 5000/mm³. Morphology of reactive lymphocytes (large size, abundant cytoplasm, scalloping, and dark blue edges) is also helpful. In doubtful cases, surface marker analysis for monoclonality (k or λ light chain restriction) can be done.

Benign Polyclonal Lymphocytosis (Persistent Polyclonal B-Cell Lymphocytosis)

This rare condition is observed in young- to middle-aged female smokers. The lymphocytes are small with round nuclei and scant cytoplasm with some binucleate forms. Abnormalities of chromosome 3q are found in a proportion of B cells.

Other Chronic Lymphoid Leukemias

After exclusion of reactive causes, neoplastic lymphoproliferative disorders that enter into differential diagnosis. CLL in peripheral blood should be differentiated from prolymphocytic leukemia, leukemic phase of non-Hodgkin's lymphoma (especially mantle cell lymphoma and follicular lymphoma), and hairy cell leukemia (Fig. 8.5 for comparative morphological features). In addition to above, in bone marrow, CLL should be distinguished from lymphoplasmacytic lymphoma, hairy cell leukemia-variant, and splenic marginal zone lymphoma. Although flow cytometry is essential for definitive diagnosis, certain clinical and morphological features may be helpful. Prolymphocytic leukemia is characterized by massive splenomegaly, no lymphadenopathy, marked lymphocytosis, and predominance of prolymphocytes in peripheral blood (>55%). In leukemic phase of follicular small-cleaved cell lymphoma, neoplastic small lymphocytes show deep nuclear clefts and immunophenotypic analysis shows CD5-, CD19+, CD20+, BCL-2+, and strong surface membrane immunoglobulin. Paratrabecular infiltration on bone marrow biopsy is typically seen in follicular lymphoma. FISH can identify t(14;18) in 70 to 95% of cases of follicular lymphomas. In mantle cell lymphoma involving peripheral blood, neoplastic cells are small cleaved lymphocytes with a characteristic immunophenotype: CD5+, CD19+, CD20+, CD23-, and strong surface membrane immunoglobulin. In about

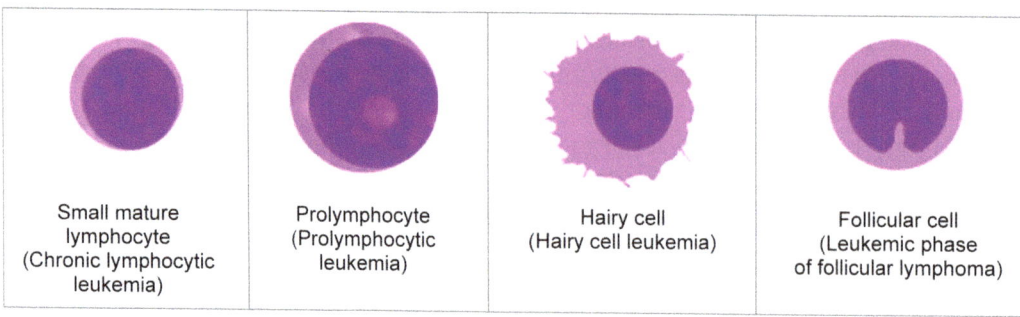

Fig. 8.5: Comparative morphological features of chronic lymphoid leukemias.

Table 8.2: Differential diagnosis of chronic lymphoid leukemias and B-cell lymphomas that can involve peripheral blood.

Parameter	CLL	MCL	SMZL/SLVL	HCL	FL	PLL
CD5	+	+	–	–	–	–
CD10	–	–/+	–	–	+	–/+
CD11c	weak	–/+	+	+	–	+
CD19	+	+	+	+	+	+
CD20	+(dim)	+(bright)	+(bright)	+(bright)	+(bright)	+(bright)
CD23	+	–/+	–/+	–	–/+	–
CD79b	–	+	+	–/+	+	+
FMC7	–	+	+	+	+	+
SmIg	+(dim)	+(bright)	+(bright)	+(bright)	+(bright)	+(bright)
CD25	–	–	–	+	–	–
CD200	+(bright)	–	+(dim)	+(bright)	+(dim)	–/+
Cyclin D1	–	+	–	+ in some cases	–	–
SOX11	–	+	–	–	–	–

(CLL: Chronic lymphocytic leukemia; MCL: Mantle cell lymphoma; SMZL/SLVL: Splenic marginal zone lymphoma/splenic lymphoma with villous lymphocytes; HCL: Hairy cell leukemia; FL: Follicular lymphoma; PLL: Prolymphocytic leukemia).

75% of patients with mantle cell lymphoma, t(11;14) chromosomal abnormality is present. Bone marrow infiltration in mantle cell lymphoma is paratrabecular or nonparatrabecular. Differentiation of CLL from hairy cell leukemia is usually not difficult. Hairy cell leukemia is characterized by massive splenomegaly, pancytopenia, lymphocytes with small, circumferential fine projections on cell surface, "fried egg" appearance on bone marrow biopsy due to abundant cytoplasm, typical immunophenotype, and tartrate-resistant acid phosphatase activity (TRAP) (Table 8.2). In lymphoplasmacytic lymphoma involving bone marrow, plasmacytoid lymphocytes, plasma cells, and mast cells are increased along with small lymphocytes. Splenic marginal zone lymphoma is characterized by peripheral blood and bone marrow involvement without significant lymphadenopathy; the neoplastic cells show polar villi and sinusoidal infiltrate in bone marrow (not seen in CLL).

Monoclonal B-cell lymphocytosis: Monoclonal B-cell lymphocytosis is defined as low level (absolute lymphocyte count <5000/mm^3) of asymptomatic proliferation of B-lymphocytes and light chain restriction on immunophenotyping by flow cytometry. There is no lymphadenopathy, organomegaly, or cytopenia and bone marrow lymphocytes are <30%. There is a small risk of progression to CLL. Recent investigations suggest that most cases of CLL are preceded by monoclonal B-lymphocytosis.

Complications of CLL

1. **Infections:** Patients with CLL have increased risk of bacterial, viral, and fungal infections, due to disease itself (from hypogammaglobulinemia) or following therapy (from neutropenia and depletion of T-lymphocytes).
2. Autoimmune hemolytic anemia and thrombocytopenic purpura.
3. **Second malignancies:** There is increased risk of second malignancies in CLL, such as skin cancer and solid tumors.
4. **Progression and transformation:** Progression to a more aggressive disorder can occur such as prolymphocytic leukemia or Richter's syndrome. Progression to prolymphocytic leukemia is characterized by ≥55% of prolymphocytes in peripheral blood; it is rare (occurring in <1% cases of CLL) and there is usually associated MYC abnormalities. Richter's syndrome is development of a diffuse large B-cell lymphoma in a patient with pre-existing CLL. It occurs in approximately 10% of cases. It should be suspected when patient develops unexplained fever, weight loss, and enlarging lymphadenopathy, particularly abdominal, and elevation of lactate dehydrogenase. It is refractory to chemotherapy and median survival is about 4 months. Other rare transformations include Hodgkin lymphoma, plasmablastic lymphoma, and B-lymphoblastic lymphoma/leukemia.

Prognosis

1. **Staging:** Prognosis depends primarily on the stage of the disease at diagnosis. There are two main staging systems for CLL: Rai (1975) and Binet (1981). These are shown in Table 8.3.
2. **Other prognostic factors:** There is a correlation between disease stage (as defined in Table 8.3) and median survival. However, the staging systems cannot accurately predict those patients in early stage who will have disease progression and those who will remain indolent. About 50% of patients in early stage will develop more advanced disease. In addition, there is marked variation in disease progression amongst patients with similar stages. Assessment of risk of progression of disease can be done from various factors as shown in Table 8.4.

Treatment

Treatment is principally symptomatic and is not curative.

Early stage disease is relatively benign and patients are often asymptomatic. Median survival of these patients is >10 years and therefore no treatment is usually indicated. Early institution of therapy does not improve survival and increases the risk of second cancers and development of resistance to treatment.

Table 8.3: Staging systems for CLL.

Binet stages	Rai stages
A: <3 lymphoid areas* enlarged	**0:** Lymphocytosis only
B: ≥3 lymphoid areas enlarged	**I:** Lymphadenopathy
C: Anemia (Hemoglobin <10 g/dL) and/or thrombocytopenia (Platelet count <1 lac/ mm^3)	**II:** Hepatomegaly and/or splenomegaly ± lymphadenopathy **III:** Hemoglobin <11 g/dL **IV:** Platelet count <100,000/mm^3

* Lymphoid areas: lymph nodes (unilateral or bilateral cervical, axillary, and inguinal), liver, and spleen

Table 8.4: Prognostic factors in CLL.

Low risk	High risk
Early stage disease (Binet: A; Rai: 0, I)	Advanced stage disease (Binet: B,C; Rai: II, III, IV)
Predominance of small mature lymphocytes	>10% prolymphocytes
Interstitial or nodular marrow infiltration	Diffuse marrow infiltration
Normal karyotype or 13q-	11q-, 12+,17p-
Antigen CD38-	Antigen CD38+
CD49d+	CD49d-
Normal β_2 microglobulin	Elevated β_2 microglobulin
Mutated *IgVH* gene	Nonmutated *IgVH* gene
LDT >12 months	LDT <12 months
Female	Male
Age <60 years	Age >60 years
ZAP-70-	ZAP-70+
Thymidine kinase low or normal	Thymidine kinase raised

(LDT: Lymphocyte doubling time or time required for lymphocyte count to double in peripheral blood)

Treatment is indicated in advanced Rai or Binet stage; and when patient develops systemic symptoms related to disease (e.g. fever, weight loss, and fatigue), evidence of disease progression (progressive worsening of anemia or thrombocytopenia, progressive enlargement of lymph nodes or spleen, lymphocyte doubling time <6 months), or presence of massively enlarged lymph nodes (>10 cm) or spleen (>6 cm) and Richter's transformation.

Treatment options for CLL have changed significantly in the last few years. The optimal first-line therapy in CLL consists of chemoimmunotherapy comprising of six cycles of fludarabine (a purine analogue), cyclophosphamide, and rituximab (anti-CD20 antibody that causes cell lysis). This is associated with a high response rate of 90 to 95% and a complete remission rate of 40 to 75%. This therapy may be curative in patients with absent nonmutated *IGVH* and deletion of 17p (or *TP53* mutation). Results of chemoimmunotherapy are not satisfactory in patients with deletion of 17p or TP53 mutation or nonmutated *IGVH* and in such cases, ibrutinib (inhibitor of Bruton tyrosine kinase) has been found to be effective. In older patients with associated comorbidities and poor performance status, frontline therapy consists of chlorambucil and rituximab. In patients with refractory disease or relapse, ibrutinib has improved the outlook. The median survival of CLL is 10 to 12 years that is likely to improve following recent introduction of novel targeted therapies.

PROLYMPHOCYTIC LEUKEMIA

Prolymphocytic leukemia (PLL) is an uncommon but a distinct form of chronic lymphoid leukemia characterized by splenomegaly, and marked lymphocytosis with predominance of prolymphocytes in the peripheral blood. PLL is of two types—B cell (75%), and T cell (25%). It is more aggressive than CLL.

Clinical Features

B-PLL is an extremely rare disease that occurs in elderly persons in the sixth or seventh decade of life. Mean age at presentation is about 10 years older than patients with typical CLL. The characteristic clinical feature is marked splenomegaly; there is minimal or no lymphadenopathy. (In typical CLL, lymph node enlargement is greater as compared to the size of the spleen). Anemia and thrombocytopenia are present in 50% of patients at diagnosis. In T-PLL, clinical features include hepatosplenomegaly, generalized lymphadenopathy, and skin involvement in the form of an erythematous, papular rash.

Laboratory Features

Total lymphocyte count is extremely high and is generally more than 1 lac/mm^3. Prolymphocytes are the most numerous cells in peripheral blood and are more than 55%. Prolymphocyte is a large lymphoid cell (more than twice the size of a small lymphocyte) with low nuclear-cytoplasmic ratio, condensed nuclear chromatin, and a prominent vesicular nucleolus (Fig. 8.6). Immunophenotypic analysis shows:
- B-PLL: CD19+, CD20+, CD22+, CD79a+, FMC7+, surface membrane immunoglobulin **(SmIg)+ (strong)**, CD23-, CD103-
- T-PLL: CD2+, CD3+, CD5+, CD7+, CD26+, CD10-, CD25-, and CD4+CD8- or CD4+CD8+ or CD4- CD8+

Genetic Analysis

In B-PLL, genetic analysis reveals del(17p) in 50% cases. Other frequent abnormalities are *TP53* mutations and del(13q). In T-PLL, inv(14) is demonstrated in 80% cases.

Differential Diagnosis

There are no specific immunophenotypic markers for B-PLL and therefore diagnosis of B-PLL depends on exclusion of other lymphoproliferative disorders like blastoid variant of mantle cell lymphoma, CLL with prolymphocytic transformation, and splenic marginal zone lymphoma.

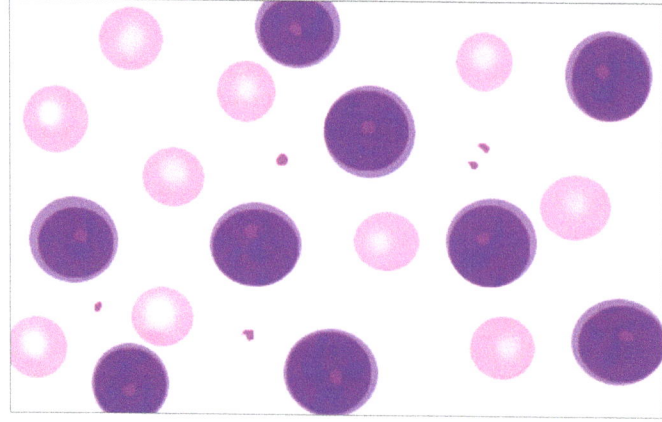

Fig. 8.6: Blood smear in prolymphocytic leukemia.

It is thought by some investigators that true B-PLL is extremely rare and many B-PLL cases diagnosed in the past actually represent leukemic mantle cell lymphomas. Assessment of t(11;14) by FISH in blood sample and/or cyclin D1 expression in tissue sections is mandatory to exclude leukemic mantle cell lymphoma before rendering a diagnosis of B-PLL.

1. **Chronic lymphocytic leukemia with prolymphocytic transformation (CLL/PLL):** CLL/PLL differs from PLL in following:
   a. Age: PLL (70 years) occurs at older age than CLL/PLL (60 years).
   b. Splenomegaly is more marked in PLL.
   c. Lymphadenopathy is moderate or marked in CLL/PLL, while it is minimal or absent in PLL.
   d. Spectrum of small lymphocytes and prolymphocytes is seen in CLL.
   e. Previous history of CLL is present in CLL/PL.
2. **CLL/PL:** Predominant cells are small; mature lymphocytes and prolymphocytes are >10% but less than 55%.
3. **Lymphosarcoma cell leukemia:** This is the leukemic phase of non-Hodgkin's lymphoma that occurs at relatively younger age. Total leukocyte count is moderately raised, and the neoplastic cells show characteristic indented or clefted nuclei.
4. **Acute lymphoblastic leukemia:** In contrast to lymphoblasts in ALL, prolymphocytes have more condensed chromatin, a conspicuous and a prominent nucleolus, and lower nuclear-cytoplasmic ratio.
5. **Pleomorphic mantle cell lymphoma:** Some cases previously diagnosed as B-PLL have now been reclassified as mantle cell lymphoma. In contrast to B-PLL, significant lymphadenopathy is present in mantle cell lymphoma. The diagnosis of mantle cell lymphoma depends on expression of cyclin D1 and demonstration of t(11;14)(q13;q32).
6. **Hairy cell leukemia variant:** These patients have prominent splenomegaly and leukocytosis, and unlike B-PLL, CD103 is positive.

Course and Prognosis

The course is aggressive with poor response to treatment; median survival is less than 3 years in B-PLL and 6 to 7 months in T-PLL.

Treatment

Patients with PLL are frequently refractory to treatment and median survival is short. Chemotherapeutic agents used include CHOP (cyclophosphamide, doxorubicin, oncovin, and prednisone), fludarabine, deoxycoformycin, and combination of chemotherapy and rituximab. Splenectomy can reduce tumor mass and cause partial improvement. In T-PLL, better responses have been reported with alemtuzumab (anti-CD52).

HAIRY CELL LEUKEMIA

Hairy cell leukemia (HCL) is a rare chronic lymphoproliferative disorder of mature B cell origin characterized by occurrence in middle-aged persons, pancytopenia, splenic enlargement, and "hairy" cells (neoplastic lymphocytes with hair-like long slender projections on cell surface) primarily in bone marrow, blood, and splenic red pulp. Most patients with HCL have a recurrent activating mutation in *BRAF* gene.

Clinical Features

The disease has male predominance and occurs mainly in middle age; it does not occur in children. The usual symptoms are tiredness, abdominal distension, easy bruisability, and repeated infections (both bacterial and opportunistic). These features result from cytopenias and splenic enlargement. The characteristic physical sign is marked splenomegaly. Mild hepatomegaly may be present. There is usually no peripheral lymphadenopathy; however, abdominal and retroperitoneal lymphadenopathy may be present. Some patients are asymptomatic and detected incidentally.

Laboratory Features

Peripheral Blood Examination

Cytopenia affecting two or more cell lines is the main laboratory feature. Anemia is mild to moderate and is normocytic and normochromic. Leukopenia is frequently present. Neutropenia and monocytopenia are usual. Monocytopenia is considered as a helpful clue for diagnosis since it is present in almost all cases. Due to low TLC, hairy cells are difficult to demonstrate. In cases with TLC greater than normal, hairy cells are increased in proportion and easily identifiable. Marked leukocytosis is unusual in HCL and, if present, should raise the possibility of hairy cell leukemia variant (a distinct disease). Hairy cells are large and are twice the size of a small lymphocyte. Their cytoplasm is clear to lightly basophilic and shows numerous fine, hair-like or broader projections on surface (best seen on thin areas of smear). Nuclear-cytoplasmic ratio is low. The nucleus is round, oval, or indented; chromatin is reticular or dispersed and nucleoli are inconspicuous (Fig. 8.7). Hairy cells are best demonstrated by phase contrast or electron microscopy. Mild-to-moderate thrombocytopenia is usual.

Bone Marrow Examination

Bone marrow is difficult to aspirate (dry tap) due to reticulin fibrosis. Bone marrow trephine biopsy is essential for definitive diagnosis. In addition, it is also helpful for assessing the extent

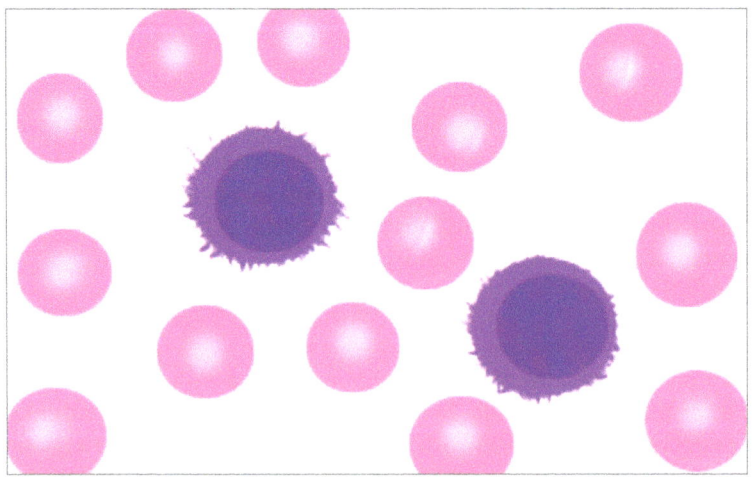

Fig. 8.7: Blood smear in hairy cell leukemia.

of disease and provides a baseline for assessment of response to therapy. It shows diffuse or interstitial infiltration by mononuclear cells, which are characteristically loosely arranged; the individual nuclei are widely spaced from each other ("fried egg appearance"). This characteristic loosely structured appearance is attributed to pericellular deposition of fibronectin. (In other leukemias and lymphomas, the nuclei of neoplastic cells are in close proximity.)

The reticulin stain demonstrates increased bone marrow fibrosis with reticulin fibers often surrounding individual cells (pericellular deposition of fibronectin). Collagen fibrosis (demonstrated by trichrome stain) is rare. Despite bone marrow fibrosis, leukoerythroblastic reaction in blood is unusual.

Cytochemistry

HCL cells show reactivity with TRAP enzyme. Alternatively, antibody to TRAP can be used in immunohistochemistry.

Immunophenotypic Analysis

On flow cytometry of peripheral blood or bone marrow aspirate, cell surface immunologic marker analysis reveals B cell nature of hairy cells (CD19+, CD20+, and CD22+). Hairy cells express SmIg (strong), CD11c, CD25, CD103, CD123, and HC2. Immunohistochemistry on bone marrow biopsy shows positivity of hairy cells for B cell markers like CD19 and CD79a; in addition, markers for HCL include TRAP, DBA.44, cyclin D1, annexin A1, and newly identified BRAF V600E monoclonal antibody.

Molecular Genetic Analysis

BRAF V600E (an oncogene *located at* chromosome 7q24) mutation occurs in majority of patients with HCL. It can be detected by allele-specific polymerase chain reaction or next generation sequencing. This mutation causes constitutive activation of mitogen-activated protein (MAP) kinase pathway. However, HCL with IGHV4-34 immunoglobulin rearrangement lacks this mutation (10% cases of HCL).

Routine cytogenetic analysis is not indicated and no prognostic cytogenetic markers have been detected.

Histology of Spleen

Spleen shows massive enlargement. Histology of spleen shows infiltration of red pulp by hairy cells, broadening of splenic cords, and formation of pseudosinuses (or blood lakes), which are lined by hairy cells (instead of endothelial cells) and filled with red cells. White pulp is atrophic.

Diagnosis and Differential Diagnosis

Diagnosis of HCL can be made when a middle-aged patient presents with marked splenomegaly, pancytopenia, hairy cells in peripheral blood which are TRAP-positive and showing activated B cell immunophenotype, and typical picture on bone marrow biopsy (Box 8.1).

Box 8.1: Diagnosis of hairy cell leukemia.

- Clinical features: Middle age, marked splenomegaly
- Blood smear: Cytopenia, hairy cells
- Bone marrow biopsy: Clear cells with "fried egg" appearance (diffuse or interstitial infiltrate), reticulin fibrosis
- Cytochemistry: Tartrate-resistant acid phosphatase (TRAP)+
- Immunophenotyping: (1) Flow cytometry: CD19+, CD20+, CD22+, CD 79A+, CD11c+, CD25+, CD103+, CD5-, CD123+; (2) Immunohistochemistry: CD20+, PAX5+, TRAP+, *DBA.44*, Cyclin D1+, Annexin A1+
- Molecular genetic analysis: *BRAF V600E* mutation

HCL should be distinguished from other low-grade lymphoid neoplasms like splenic marginal zone lymphoma, splenic diffuse red pulp small B-cell lymphoma, hairy cell leukemia-variant, B-prolymphocytic leukemia, and lymphoplasmacytic lymphoma including Waldenstrom macroglobulinemia (Table 8.5). In addition, bone marrow involvement in systemic mastocytosis can resemble infiltration by hairy cells.

Table 8.5: Differential diagnosis of hairy cell leukemia.

Neoplasm	Clinical features	CBC, morphology	Bone marrow	Immunophenotype	Genetics
Hairy cell leukemia	Splenomegaly, median age 50 years	Pancytopenia; monocytopenia; nucleus oval and indented, fine chromatin, no nucleolus, abundant cytoplasm with circumferential projections	Diffuse or interstitial infiltration; "fried egg" appearance	CD11c+, CD25+, CD103+, CD123+, CD5-, CD23-, Annexin A1+	*BRAF V600E* mutation
Splenic marginal zone lymphoma	Splenomegaly, median age 65 years	Lymphocytosis; nucleus round, clumped chromatin, small or absent nucleolus, moderately abundant cytoplasm with polar projections	Nodular and intrasinusoidal	CD11c+, CD25±, CD103-, CD123-, CD5-, CD23-, Annexin A1-	del(7q) in 40% cases, *NOTCH2* mutation in 25% cases
Splenic diffuse red pulp small B-cell lymphoma	Splenomegaly, age >40 years	Lymphocytosis, nucleus round to oval, clumped chromatin, small or absent nucleolus, abundant cytoplasm with broad polar projections	Intrasinusoidal, interstitial, nodular	CD11c±, CD25-, CD103±, CD123-, CD5±, CD23-, Annexin A1-	-

Contd...

Contd...

Neoplasm	Clinical features	CBC, morphology	Bone marrow	Immunopheno-type	Genetics
Hairy cell leukemia variant	Splenomegaly; median age 80 years	Lymphocytosis; nucleus round to oval, variable chromatin, nucleolus present, abundant cytoplasm with projections	Diffuse and interstitial	CD11c+, CD25-, CD103+, CD123-, CD5-, CD23-, Annexin A1-	MAP2K1 mutation (30-50%), 17p deletion (30%)
B-prolymphocytic leukemia	Splenomegaly; median age 69 years	Lymphocytosis; round nucleus, moderately condensed chromatin, prominent nucleolus, moderate cytoplasm	Interstitial or nodular	CD11c+, CD25±, CD103-, CD123-, CD5±, CD23+, Annexin A1-	TP53 mutation
Lymphoplasmacytic lymphoma	Hyperviscosity, median age 73 years	Lymphocytosis, round and eccentric nucleus, clumped chromatin, moderate basophilic cytoplasm (plasmacytoid morphology)	Interstitial and nodular	CD11c-, CD25±, CD103-, CD123-, CD5-, CD23-, Annexin A1-	MYD88 L265P Mutation (>90%)

Complications of HCL

1. **Infections:** These are common in HCL due to reduction in granulocytes and monocytes. Common infections are those due to Gram-negative bacteria, mycobacteria, and fungi.
2. Anemia and bleeding tendencies.
3. **Skeletal infiltration**, particularly head of femur.
4. **Vasculitis**—this occurs in small number of cases.

Course and Prognosis

Prolonged survival is possible with current modes of therapy. Death usually results from complications related to pancytopenia, particularly infections.

Treatment

In a small number of patients with HCL, manifestations of cytopenia are not present and these patients do not need treatment. Such patients are regularly observed and treatment is instituted on development of complications.

Most of the patients have cytopenia and are symptomatic at the time of diagnosis (anemia, infections, or bleeding) and require therapy. Currently available modes of therapy for HCL are purine nucleoside analogues (pentostatin or cladribine), alpha interferon (IFN-α), and splenectomy. Either pentostatin or cladribine is highly effective in inducing high rate (80%) of complete remission for prolonged duration; they have replaced alpha-interferon and splenectomy as first line therapy for HCL. Relapsed patients respond to retreatment with purine analogues. In patients resistant to purine analog therapy, monoclonal antibodies like rituximab and anti-CD22 immunotoxin have proved to be effective. An inhibitor of *BRAF*, vemurafenib, can be used in patients resistant to other forms of therapy.

BIBLIOGRAPHY

1. Bennett JM, Catovsky D, Daniel MT, Flandrin G, Galton DAG, Gralnick HR, et al. The French-American-British (FAB) Co-operative Group:Proposals for the classification of chronic (mature) B and T lymphoid leukaemias. J Clin Pathol. 1989;42:567-84.
2. Binet JL, Auquier A, Dighiero G, Chastang C, Piguer H, Goasguen J, et al. A new prognostic classification of chronic lymphocytic leukemia derived from a multivariate survival analysis. Cancer. 1981;48: 198-206.
3. Bouroncle BA. Leukemic reticuloendotheliosis (hairy cell leukemia). Blood. 1979;53:412-36.
4. British Committee for Standards in Haematology: Guidelines on the diagnosis and management of chronic lymphocytic leukaemia. Br J Haematol. 2004;125:294-17.
5. Catovsky D. Chronic lymphoid leukaemias. In Hoffbrand AV and Lewis SM (Eds.): Postgraduate Haematology. 3rd ed. London. Heinemann Professional Publishing Ltd; 1989.
6. Flinn IW, Grever MR. Chronic lymphocytic leukemia. Cancer Treat Rev. 1996;22:1-13.
7. Gale RP, Foon KA. Biology of chronic lymphocytic leukaemias. Semin Hematol. 1987;24:230-39.
8. Galton DAG, Goldman JM, Wiltshaw E, Catovsky D, Henry K, Goldenberg J. Prolymphocytic leukaemia. Br J Haematol. 1974;27:7-23.
9. International Workshop on Chronic Lymphocytic Leukemia. Chronic lymphocytic leukemia: Recommendations for diagnosis, staging and response criteria. Ann Intern Med. 1989;110:236-38.
10. Kalil N, Cheson BD. Chronic lymphocytic leukemia. The Oncologist. 1999;4:352-69.
11. Melo JV, Catovsky D, Galton DAG. The relationship between chronic lymphocytic leukaemia and prolymphocytic leukaemia. I. Clinical and laboratory features of 300 patients and characterization of an intermediate group. Br J Haematol. 1986;63:377-87.
12. Morrison VA. Chronic leukemias. CA Cancer J Clin. 1994;44:353-77.
13. Rai KR, Sawitsky A, Cronikite EP, Chanana AD, Levy RN, Pasternack BS. Clinical staging of chronic lymphocytic leukaemia. Blood. 1975;46:219-34.
14. Rozman C, Montserrat E. Chronic lymphocytic leukemia. N Engl J Med 1995;333:1052-57.
15. Rozman C, Montserrat E, Rodriguez Fernandez JM, et al. Bone marrow histologic pattern. The best single prognostic parameter in chronic lymphocytic leukemia; a multivariate survival analysis of 329 cases. Blood. 1984;64:642-8.
16. Shanafelt TD, Call TG. Current approach to diagnosis and management of chronic lymphocytic leukemia. Mayo Clin Proc. 2004;79:388-98.
17. Strati P, Jain N, O'Brien S:Chronic lymphocytic leukemia:Diagnosis and treatment. Mayo Clin Proc. 2018;93(5):651-64.
18. Swerdlow SH, Campo E, Harris NL, Jaffe ES, Pileri SA, Stein H, et al. (Eds.). WHO Classification of Tumours of Haematopoietic and Lymphoid Tissues. Revised 4th ed. Lyon. IARC. 2017.

CHAPTER 9

Plasma Cell Dyscrasias

INTRODUCTION

Plasma cell dyscrasias (also called as paraproteinemias or monoclonal gammopathies) are a group of disorders characterized by neoplastic proliferation of plasma cells and increased production of a single homogeneous immunoglobulin (paraprotein, monoclonal protein, M protein). They are listed in Box 9.1.

INVESTIGATIONS IN PLASMA CELL DYSCRASIAS (BOX. 9.2)

Peripheral Blood Examination

Rouleaux formation (refer to Fig. 9.7) and markedly raised erythrocyte sedimentation rate (ESR) are typical features and result from hyperglobulinemia. Rouleaux formation is seen when there is increased concentration of high molecular weight proteins resulting from any cause. Increased faint purple background staining of blood smear is often seen. Apart from plasma cell neoplasms (increased monoclonal immunoglobulins), rouleaux formation is also commonly seen during pregnancy (raised fibrinogen) and chronic inflammatory conditions (raised polyclonal immunoglobulins and acute phase proteins like fibrinogen). Therefore, rouleaux formation is not specific for plasma cell dyscrasias.

Plasma cell is slightly larger than a small lymphocyte, oval, with a strongly basophilic cytoplasm and having an eccentric nucleus with coarsely clumped chromatin. Plasma cells

Box 9.1: Plasma cell dyscrasias.

Plasma cell neoplasms (WHO, 2016)
- Non-IgM monoclonal gammopathy of undetermined significance
- Plasma cell myeloma (PCM)
- Plasma cell myeloma variants: Smoldering plasma cell myeloma, nonsecretory myeloma, plasma cell leukemia
- Plasmacytoma: Solitary plasmacytoma of bone, Extraosseous plasmacytoma
- Monoclonal immunoglobulin deposition diseases: Primary amyloidosis, Light chain and heavy chain deposition diseases
- Plasma cell neoplasms with associated paraneoplastic syndrome: POEMS syndrome, TEMPI syndrome

Immunoglobulin-secreting neoplasms that are composed of both plasma cells and lymphocytes
- Waldenström's macroglobulinemia (WM)
- IgM monoclonal gammopathy of undetermined significance
- Heavy chain diseases

Section 3: Disorders of White Blood Cells

> **Box 9.2:** Investigations at diagnosis in plasma cell dyscrasias.
>
> - Blood: Complete blood count including hemoglobin, blood smear, erythrocyte sedimentation rate (ESR) or plasma viscosity
> - Bone marrow: Plasma cell number and morphology, demonstration of clonality and immunophenotype
> - Serum: Albumin, immunoglobulins, protein electrophoresis, capillary electrophoresis, immunofixation electrophoresis, serum free light chain assay, calcium, β2-microglobulin, lactate dehydrogenase
> - Urine: 24-hour protein, 24-hour protein electrophoresis, 24-hour immunofixation
> - Skeletal radiological survey
> - Skeletal CT scan, skeletal MRI scan, positron emission tomography

are not seen in peripheral blood in healthy subjects; reactive plasma cells are seen in bacterial and viral infection, inflammation, postvaccination, streptokinase administration, serum sickness, dengue fever, and cirrhosis. Neoplastic plasma cells may be seen in blood in advanced plasma cell myeloma (PCM) (if >20%, diagnosis of plasma cell leukemia is suspected), rarely in Waldenström's macroglobulinemia (WM), and angioimmunoblastic T-cell lymphoma.

Bone Marrow Examination

Increased number of plasma cells in bone marrow can be reactive or neoplastic. Clonality of plasma cell population can be assessed by immunohistochemistry or flow cytometry. In plasma cell neoplasms, clonal nature is established by identification of monoclonal immunoglobulin (either kappa or lambda light chain) in the cytoplasm of plasma cells by flow cytometry or immunohistochemistry. This is crucial while evaluating plasmacytosis due to overlap of number and morphology of plasma cells in reactive plasmacytosis and plasma cell neoplasms.

In plasma cell dyscrasias, bone marrow examination (aspirate/biopsy) is necessary for:
- Differentiation of reactive from neoplastic plasmacytosis (Table 9.1)
- Assessment of morphology
- Assessing percentage of plasma cells for diagnosis and classification
- Genetic including cytogenetic and molecular studies
- Flow cytometric analysis: Diagnosis of PCM, nonsecretory myeloma, reactive plasmacytosis, detection of minimal residual disease after therapy, early detection of relapse
- Prognosis
- Immunohistochemistry
- Morphological classification and prognostic grading of PCM: According to Bartl et al, there are six morphologic types and three prognostic grades of myeloma: Low grade ("Marschalko" and "small cell" types), intermediate grade ("cleaved," "polymorphous," and "asynchronous" types), and high grade ("blastic" type).

Bone marrow aspiration is suitable for assessment of morphology, genetic and molecular studies, and flow cytometry; bone marrow biopsy is useful for accurate quantitation of disease, immunohistochemistry, and for evaluation of coexisting conditions like amyloidosis.

Table 9.1: Characteristics of reactive and neoplastic plasma cells in bone marrow.

Parameter	Reactive plasmacytosis	Neoplastic plasmacytosis
1. Localization	Perivascular or as small interstitial clusters (needs biopsy; highlighted by CD38); sometimes clustering around macrophages	Interstitial, focal, diffuse or sheet-like pattern of infiltration; lack of predilection for vascular structures
2. Marrow architecture	Preserved	Partial or complete effacement; sometimes fibrosis
3. Cytomorphology	*Small size; round, eccentric nucleus with clumped chromatin and indistinct nucleoli; basophilic cytoplasm; prominent Golgi zone; occasional binucleation; occasional cytoplasmic inclusions	**Enlarged size, immature or vesicular chromatin, distinct nucleoli, frequent binucleation or multinucleation, frequent cytoplasmic or nuclear inclusions
4. Percentage of marrow cells	<5% (normal marrow); 10–20% in reactive cases	Variable
5. Clonality	Polyclonal (κ to λ ratio 2:1)	Monoclonal (light chain restriction)
6. Causes	HIV/AIDS, Epstein–Barr virus infection, autoimmune disorders, Leishmaniasis, Castleman disease, Hodgkin lymphoma, angioimmunoblastic T-cell lymphoma	Plasma cell neoplasms

* Morphology of reactive plasma cells is also called as Marshalko or mature morphology; **Morphology of neoplastic plasma cells may sometimes be mature similar to normal plasma cells

Investigation of Protein Abnormalities

The term M (monoclonal, malignant, or myeloma) protein refers to the presence of structurally and electrophoretically homogeneous protein in serum or urine, which is synthesized by a neoplastic clone of plasma cells.

The monoclonal protein may be complete immunoglobulin molecules of the same class, or immunoglobulin light chains of the same type, or heavy chains of the same class. In contrast to monoclonal proteins, polyclonal proteins are immunoglobulins of different types. Monoclonal proteins are produced by neoplastic plasma cells that arise from a single progenitor cell, while polyclonal proteins are produced in response to the antigenic stimulation by different plasma cell clones. Disorders associated with production of monoclonal immunoglobulins are listed in Box 9.3.

Box 9.3: Disorders associated with synthesis of monoclonal immunoglobulins (M protein).

1. Plasma cell dyscrasias: Plasma cell myeloma, solitary myeloma, extramedullary plasmacytoma, Waldenström's macroglobulinemia, primary amyloidosis, heavy chain disease, monoclonal gammopathy of undetermined significance.
2. Lymphoproliferative disorders: Non-Hodgkin's lymphoma, chronic lymphocytic leukemia, Hodgkin's lymphoma.

Demonstration of monoclonal protein in serum and/or urine is an important laboratory test in plasma cell dyscrasias. It can be used as a tumor marker for diagnosing presence of a disease and also to follow the disease and assess response to therapy. Techniques employed for identification and characterizations of M proteins are shown in Box 9.4.

Currently, recommended laboratory tests for screening, identification, and quantification of abnormal or monoclonal protein in serum and/or urine include agarose gel electrophoresis, capillary zone electrophoresis, immunofixation electrophoresis, and nephelometry. International Myeloma Working Group (IMWG) recommends all the following three tests on serum for diagnosis of plasma cell dyscrasias: Agarose gel protein electrophoresis, immunofixation electrophoresis, and serum free light chain (FLC) assay as they have differing sensitivities and specificities.

Urine test for M protein is not recommended for diagnosis as 24-hour urine collection and testing are inconvenient and inaccurate, and sensitivity for M protein detection is not increased if FLC assay is done. However, for monitoring of therapy, urine protein electrophoresis is required in cases with measurable urine M protein.

Box 9.4: Laboratory characterization of monoclonal protein.

- Screening for M protein: Serum/urine protein electrophoresis by agarose gel or capillary electrophoresis method, serum free light chain assay in cases with negative SPE and free light chain production. (If quantity of M protein is very small immunofixation can confirm the presence of M protein)
- Identification of M protein: Immunofixation electrophoresis
- Quantification of M protein: Densitometer tracing of agarose gel electrophoresis, peak size of capillary electrophoresis, rate nephelometry

Serum Protein Electrophoresis

This is the initial step in the identification of abnormal proteins (Box 9.5). In this technique, separation of different proteins is achieved on the basis of their charge.

Screening for monoclonal protein in serum and urine by electrophoresis is fundamental to the diagnosis and management of plasma cell dyscrasias. Agarose gel electrophoresis is the recommended method; agarose has a relatively neutral charge and therefore decreases the electroendosmotic force in the gel when voltage is applied. (Other commonly used media for electrophoresis are polyacrylamide and cellulose acetate). Serum protein electrophoresis (SPE) is used for detection of circulating monoclonal protein, while urine protein electrophoresis (UPE) is used for detection of monoclonal protein (free immunoglobulin light chains) in urine. When SPE and UPE are combined with total protein estimation and scanning densitometry, abnormal protein can also be quantified.

Box 9.5: Serum protein electrophoresis.

- Primary screening test for detection of paraproteins
- Band patterns:
  - Polyclonal hypergammaglobulinemia—Broad band in γ region
  - M band—Dense, well-localized, narrow, band with sharp borders in γ, β, or α2 region (IgG band-γ region; IgA band-α2 region)
  - M band in serum is not detectable in nonsecretory myeloma (rare)

Serum to be tested is applied to the supporting medium that is then placed in the electrophoresis chamber containing alkaline buffer solution; electric current is applied till the desired separation is achieved. Abnormal protein is identified by visual inspection and by densitometry scanning (Fig. 9.1). Normal and abnormal patterns are shown in Figure 9.2. Normally, five zones of proteins can be distinguished from anode to cathode as shown below: *Anode (+)* Albumin- α1 globulin-α2 globulin-β globulin-γ globulin *Cathode(-)*

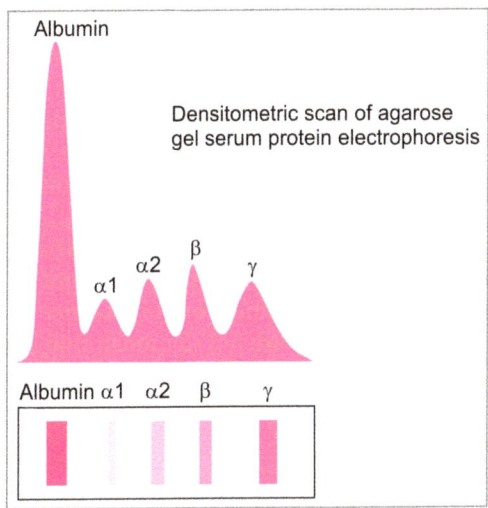

Fig. 9.1: Diagrammatic representation of densitometric scanning of serum protein electrophoresis (normal).

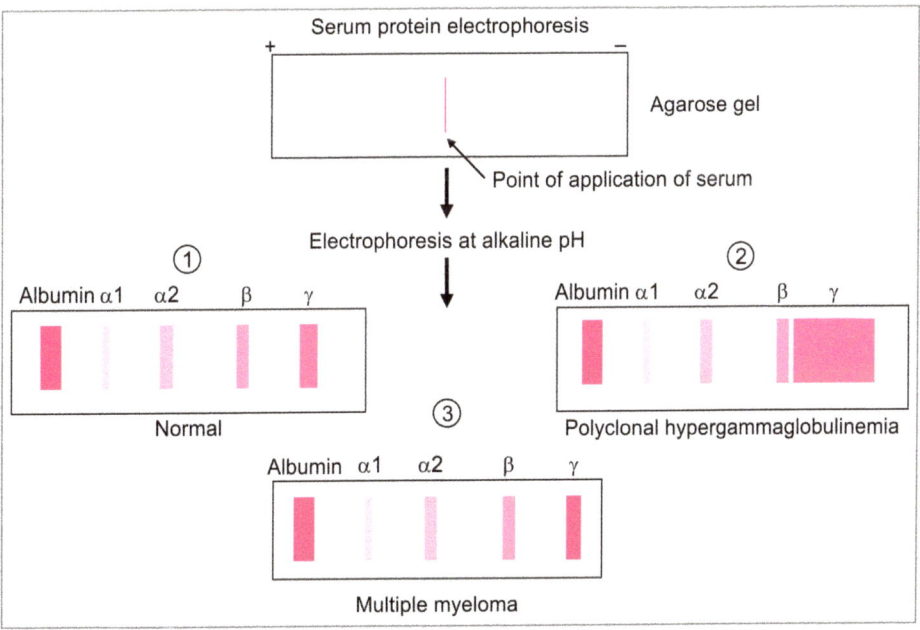

Fig. 9.2: Diagrammatic representation of serum protein electrophoresis. 1: Normal pattern; 2: Polyclonal hypergammaglobulinemia; 3: M band in myeloma.

Each zone is composed of different proteins as follows:
- Albumin
- α1 globulin—α1 antitrypsin, α1 acid glycoprotein, α1 lipoprotein, Gc-globulin
- α2 globulin—α2 macroglobulin, haptoglobin, ceruloplasmin, complement, hemopexin
- β globulin—β lipoprotein, transferrin
- γ globulin—immunoglobulins.

Immunoglobulins migrate to the γ region and may extend to the β and α2 regions. A localized dense band with sharp margins in the γ to α2 region indicates M band. On densitometer tracing, a narrow-based, tall, sharply defined spike is seen. The position of the band may suggest the type of immunoglobulin, e.g. IgG is located in γ region while IgA migrates to the β region. A wide band with indistinct borders merging into the background on electrophoresis or a broad-based peak in γ region on densitometric tracing is observed in polyclonal hypergammaglobulinemia (e.g. in chronic infections or collagen vascular diseases) (Fig. 9.2).

In about 80% of patients with monoclonal gammopathies, M band will be detected. M band or spike in serum is not observed in nonsecretory myeloma, light chain disease, and primary amyloidosis. Urine sample must also be examined for the presence of M protein because if only light chains are being produced then they are not demonstrable in serum due to their rapid excretion in urine.

Urine Protein Electrophoresis

Both serum and urine protein electrophoresis should be performed in all suspected patients of plasma cell dyscrasias. In those plasma cell dyscrasias in which only light chains are synthesized, monoclonal protein may not be detected on serum protein electrophoresis. This is because, due to their low molecular weight, light chains are excreted in urine. Bence Jones protein in urine refers to either κ or λ light chains synthesized by a neoplastic clone of plasma cells.

Reagent strip test for proteins is not sensitive for the detection of light chains in urine. However, Bence Jones proteins give a positive reaction with the sulfosalicylic acid test. One test depends upon the characteristic thermal properties of Bence Jones proteins. On heating, Bence Jones proteins precipitate at temperature between 50 and 60°C and redissolve on boiling (90–100°C). On lowering the temperature to 60°C, Bence Jones proteins reprecipitate. However, this test is not sensitive and false negative reactions occur.

Monoclonal light chains in urine (Bence Jones proteins) should be demonstrated by electrophoresis. Identification of light chain type (κ or λ) is done by immunoelectrophoresis or immunofixation.

Capillary Electrophoresis (Capillary Zone Electrophoresis)

In this technique, separation of proteins is carried out in solution (not in a gel) in a glass tube of narrow diameter with application of high voltage. Proteins are detected by a detector window near the distal end of the capillary tube by a technique like UV absorbance. Interpretation is based on derived electropherograms (and not on visualization of bands since there is no gel) that are similar to those obtained from gel electrophoresis methods. The technique is amenable to automation.

Immunofixation

This technique is the gold standard for identification of nature of M protein and is particularly helpful for the identification of a small amount of M protein. The test is more sensitive than serum protein electrophoresis. In this technique, serum proteins are separated by electrophoresis in a gel and monospecific antiserum is applied directly over the surface of the gel. Immunoprecipitation band develops in the gel between corresponding protein antigen and the monospecific antiserum. The gel is washed to remove the unbound (unprecipitated)

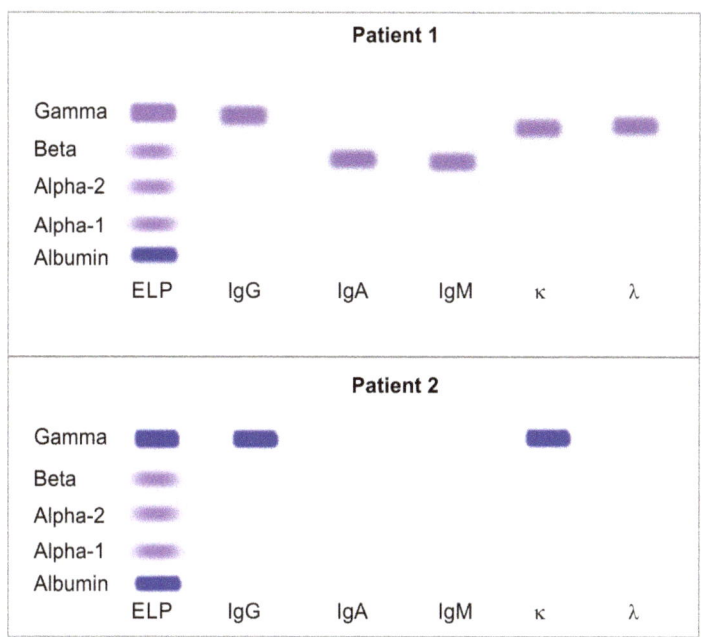

Fig. 9.3: Immunofixation. Patient 1: Normal; Patient 2: IgGκ monoclonal protein. Procedure is as follows: (1) Serum proteins are separated by agarose gel electrophoresis. (2) The M band in γ region is overlaid with monospecific antisera (IgG, IgA, IgM, and κ and λ light chains). Immunoprecipitation develops due to reaction between antigen and its corresponding antibody. Band is stained with a protein stain. The M protein (Patient 2) is IgGκ as there is development of immunoprecipitation with IgG and κ antisera; anti-λ antibody shows no immunoprecipitation band.

proteins and stained with a protein stain to demonstrate the immunoprecipitation band. The test is simple and requires shorter time than immunoelectrophoresis (Fig. 9.3).

Quantitation of Monoclonal Immunoglobulins

The quantitation of monoclonal and other immunoglobulins is necessary to assess the disease severity and follow response to treatment. The height of the peak on serum protein electrophoresis (on densitometer tracing) is directly proportional to the amount of M protein.

Previously, radial immunodiffusion (RID) was used for quantification of proteins. Nephelometry has replaced RID for measurement of immunoglobulins in most clinical laboratories because RID is labor-intensive, while nephelometry is accurate, precise, and cheaper due to automation. Nephelometry is a method that measures light scattering (when a beam of light is passed through the suspension) by small particles formed by antigen-antibody complexes in solution (Fig. 9.4). The amount of light scattered is measured as optical density in a photoelectric cell. The degree of light scattered is compared to the light scattered from standards, and the amount of the unknown is determined from a standard curve. Many automated immunology analyzers work on the principle of nephelometry. In rate or kinetic nephelometry (commonly used method), the rate of increase in light scattering is measured

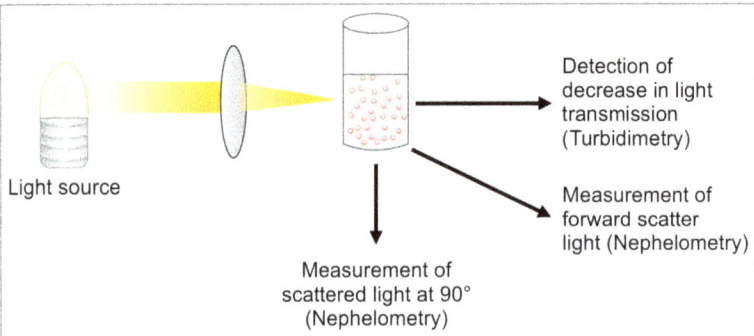

Fig. 9.4: Nephelometry versus turbidimetry. Turbidimetry measures reduction in light transmission in forward direction. Nephelometry measures light scattered in forward direction and at 90°.

immediately after addition of reagent; the rate change is directly proportional to the antigen concentration if antibody concentration is kept constant.

Other techniques for quantification are densitometer scanning of protein electrophoresis or of capillary electrophoresis.

Serum Free Light Chain Assay

Serum FLC assay is an automated assay that measures kappa (κ) and lambda (λ) FLCs that are not bound to immunoglobulins. The normal κ to λ FLC ratio is 0.26:1.65. Ratio <0.26 indicates monoclonal λ FLC and ratio >1.65 indicates monoclonal k FLC; the monoclonal light chain is called as involved FLC while the other light chain is called as uninvolved FLC. This assay can be used as a screening method for detection of M protein in place of urine protein electrophoresis and urine immunofixation electrophoresis. Serum involved/uninvolved FLC ratio of 100 or greater (provided absolute level of involved FLC is at least 100 mg/L) is considered as one of the myeloma defining events (IMWG). In addition, serum FLC assay is used to predict prognosis in monoclonal gammopathy of undetermined significance, smoldering myeloma, AL amyloidosis, and solitary plasmacytoma. It is also used to monitor disease progression in light chain only form of PCM and AL amyloidosis.

Radiological Studies

Complete skeletal survey should be obtained to detect bone lesions. The traditional skeletal survey includes plain radiographs of whole skeleton, i.e. anteroposterior and lateral views of skull, posteroanterior view of chest, anteroposterior and lateral views of the thoracic lumbar and cervical spine, humeri, and femora, and anteroposterior view of pelvis. Signs of myeloma on radiography are punched out osteolytic lesions without any reactive sclerosis, osteoporosis, and pathological fractures. However, in 15 to 20% cases X-rays are normal and are not sufficiently sensitive since osteolytic lesions are not detected by X-ray until 30% of trabecular bone is lost. Other limitations of whole body skeletal survey are difficulty to assess pelvis and spine, and difficulty to assess response to therapy since early changes of healing cannot be detected. Advanced imaging modalities include computed tomography (CT), integrated positron emission tomography/computed tomography (PET/CT) scan or a magnetic resonance imaging (MRI). They are necessary in patients with smoldering myeloma and solitary plasmacytoma of bone since they can detect additional lesions thus upstaging the disease, and alter treatment strategies.

Low-dose whole body CT scan is a better alternative to radiological survey. CT scan can detect small osteolytic lesions not detected by X-ray.

MRI is done in all patients with normal skeletal survey; its advantages are more widespread availability (as compared to PET/CT), increased sensitivity in detection of lesions in spine and pelvis, identification of extension of disease from vertebrae into soft tissue, detection of bone marrow infiltration, and detection of spinal cord compression or spinal root compression. Disadvantages of MRI as compared to PET/CT are higher cost and increased time requirement for a thorough examination, and its contraindication in patients with pacemakers, ferromagnetic aneurysm clips, or cochlear implant.

PET/CT is more helpful for determining extent of disease (including in soft tissue). As compared to MRI, PET/CT is more sensitive in assessment of active or inactive disease following therapy.

The salient features of plasma cell dyscrasias have been listed in Table 9.2.

Table 9.2: Salient features of plasma cell dyscrasias.

Plasma cell dyscrasia	Clinical features related to dyscrasia	M protein in serum by IF	Clonal plasma cells in bone marrow	Therapy
Non-IgM MGUS	Nil	<30 g/L	<10%	Observation
Plasma cell myeloma	CRAB	Any level	≥10%	Chemotherapy, HSCT, supportive therapy
Smoldering plasma cell myeloma	Nil	≥30 g/L	10–60%	Observation or clinical trial (in high-risk cases)
Nonsecretory myeloma	CRAB	Nil	≥10%	Chemotherapy, HSCT, supportive therapy
Plasma cell leukemia	CRAB	Any level	≥10% with >20% circulating plasma cells or absolute plasma cell count in blood >2 × 10^9/L	Chemotherapy, HSCT, supportive therapy
Solitary plasmacytoma	Bone lesion or depending on organ affected; absence of CRAB	Nil	Nil	Radiotherapy
Primary amyloidosis	Depending on organ affected	Present	Present	Chemotherapy, HSCT

Contd...

Contd...

Plasma cell dyscrasia	Clinical features related to dyscrasia	M protein in serum by IF	Clonal plasma cells in bone marrow	Therapy
Light chain and heavy chain deposition diseases	Depending on organ affected	±	Present	Chemotherapy, HSCT
POEMS syndrome	Polyneuropathy, organomegaly, endocrinopathy, Castleman disease, osteosclerotic bone lesions	Present	<10%	Chemotherapy, radiotherapy
TEMPI syndrome	Telangiectasias, elevated erythropoietin and erythrocytosis, monoclonal gammopathy, perinephric fluid collection, intrapulmonary shunting	Present	<10%	Bortezomib, HSCT
Waldenström's macroglobulinemia	Anemia, hyperviscosity	Present (usually IgM)	Plasma cells, plasmacytoid lymphocytes, lymphocytes	Plasma exchange, chemoimmunotherapy, HSCT
IgM-MGUS	Nil	Present (IgM)	<10%	Observation

(CRAB: hypercalcemia, renal insufficiency, anemia, bone lesions; HSCT: hematopoietic stem cell transplantation; IF: immunofixation)

PLASMA CELL MYELOMA (MULTIPLE MYELOMA)

Plasma cell myeloma (PCM) is a neoplasm of terminally differentiated B lymphocytes called plasma cells characterized by formation of multifocal tumor masses composed of plasma cells at multiple bone marrow-based locations in skeleton, and usually production of a monoclonal protein (M-protein).

Pathogenesis

The site of origin of nearly all myelomas is bone marrow. Myeloma cells originate from antigen-exposed postgerminal center B cells with somatic hypermutation, *IgH* gene rearrangement, and class switching. The progeny of this cell migrates to the bone marrow where maturation to terminally differentiated plasma cells occurs. An early event is chromosomal translocation involving 14q32 causing immortalization of plasma cell clone. Further genetic changes like del(13) lead to transformation to abnormal plasma cell clone (monoclonal gammopathy of undetermined significance or MGUS). It is now recognized that in almost all cases, PCM is preceded by asymptomatic MGUS. MGUS carries the same primary genetic abnormalities detected in PCM. Progression of MGUS to PCM is associated with acquisition of several genetic abnormalities (*RAS* mutations, p16 methylation, abnormalities of *MYC* oncogenes, secondary

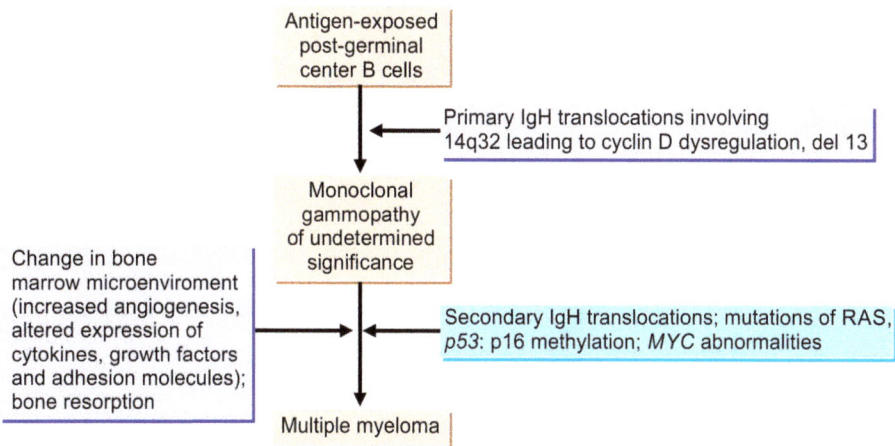

Fig. 9.5: Pathogenesis of plasma cell myeloma.

translocations, and p53 mutation) and changes in marrow microenvironment. The bone marrow microenvironment undergoes marked changes with progression like increased angiogenesis and overproduction of cytokines and growth factors by stromal cells. The cytokines and growth factors later activate multiple signaling pathways that contribute to cell growth, survival, and drug resistance of myeloma cells (Fig. 9.5). Interleukin-6 appears to promote survival and expansion of neoplastic plasma cells by stimulating their proliferation and inhibiting apoptosis.

Bone lesions in myeloma result from imbalance between activity of osteoblasts and osteoclasts. Imbalance of two molecules, receptor activator of NFκB ligand or RANKL and osteoprotegerin leads to osteoclast activation and bone resorption. In addition, macrophage inflammatory protein-1α produced by myeloma cells contributes to overactivity of osteoclasts.

Etiology

This is unknown. Risk factors include exposure to pesticides and herbicides (in farm workers), ionizing radiation, prolonged use of hair coloring agents (cosmetologists), and chronic antigenic stimulation from chronic infection or other disease.

Clinical Features

PCM occurs mainly in the older age (50–70 years) and has equal sex incidence. It does not occur in children and is rare before 35 years of age. Manifestations are as follows:

Skeletal System

Bone pain in the back and ribs, which is aggravated by movement, is the most common symptom; it is due to osteolytic lesions and osteoporosis. Bone destruction is also responsible for spontaneous fractures in weight-bearing bones, osteolytic lesions, osteoporosis, spinal cord compression, and hypercalcemia. Production of osteoclast-activating factor by myeloma cells is responsible for skeletal destruction (Fig. 9.6).

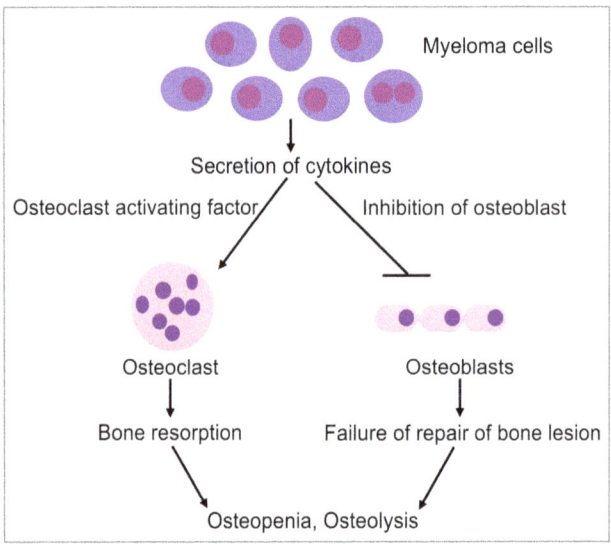

Fig. 9.6: Pathogenesis of bone lesions in myeloma.

Renal Failure

This occurs in 50% of patients. Its causes are—formation of light-chain casts in renal tubules, hypercalcemia (results from bone resorption), amyloid deposits, and pyelonephritis.

Anemia

Fatigue, weakness, and pallor result from anemia. Anemia can result from replacement of bone marrow by myeloma cells, suppression of hematopoiesis, renal failure, bleeding, infection, or hemolysis.

Infections

Patients are susceptible to bacterial infections particularity of respiratory and urinary tracts. Hypogammaglobulinemia due to suppression of normal B-lymphocytes by myeloma cells and neutropenia secondary to marrow infiltration are responsible.

Hemorrhagic Tendencies

These can occur such as purpura or mucosal bleeding. They are due to thrombocytopenia (bone marrow replacement), platelet dysfunction (due to coating of platelets by immunoglobulins which interfere with platelet aggregation), or antibodies against clotting factors.

Hyperviscosity Syndrome

A triad of visual changes, bleeding, and neurologic impairment results from increase in blood viscosity by immunoglobulins.

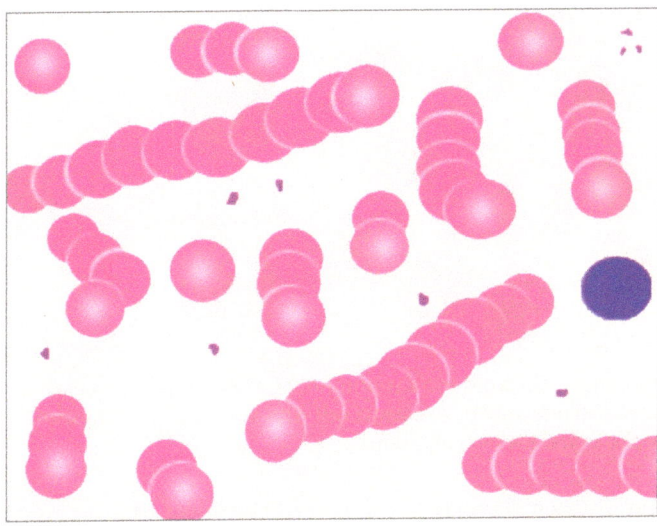

Fig. 9.7: Peripheral blood smear in plasma cell myeloma showing rouleaux formation.

Laboratory Features

Peripheral Blood Examination

Anemia develops with progression of disease in all patients and is normocytic and normochromic.

A characteristic feature on peripheral blood smear is bluish background and red cell rouleaux formation (Fig. 9.7) due to hypergammaglobulinemia.

Total leukocyte count may be normal or low. Differential count may show neutropenia with relative lymphocytic predominance and few plasma cells. Plasma cells are found in more advanced stage of disease. A leukoerythroblastic blood picture is observed in a minority of cases.

Platelet count is usually normal. Thrombocytopenia, when present, is usually mild.

A markedly increased (or rapid) ESR is a typical feature. It is due to increased immunoglobulins.

Rouleaux formation may interfere with blood grouping.

Bone Marrow Examination

Morphological examination of bone marrow in PCM is required for diagnosis, prognosis, assessment of response to therapy, and identification of recurrence. In addition, immunophenotyping, cytogenetics, and molecular analysis can be done on marrow aspiration samples. For complete evaluation, both marrow aspiration and trephine biopsy are necessary.

Bone marrow aspiration: This reveals plasmacytosis (>10%). Marrow involvement is often focal and percentage of plasma cells aspirated from different sites is variable.

The morphology of neoplastic cells varies from mature-looking plasma cells to immature cells resembling plasmablasts (Fig. 9.8). The mature cells have abundant, deeply basophilic

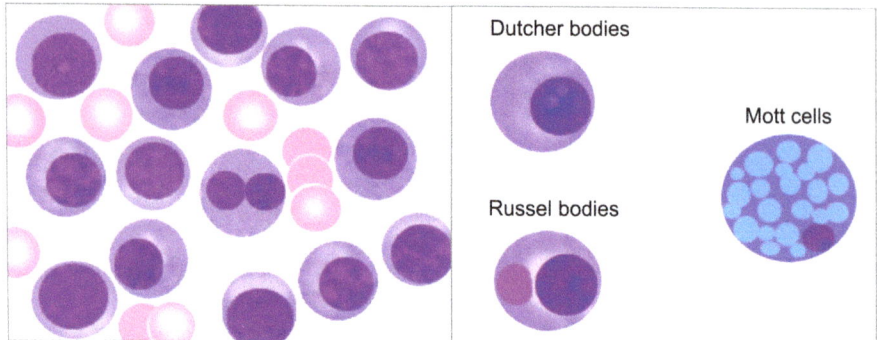

Fig. 9.8: Bone marrow smear showing increased number of plasma cells in plasma cell myeloma. One binucleated plasma cell and one immature plasma cell with nucleolus are also seen. Panel on right shows some distinctive morphological features of plasma cells.

cytoplasm with a perinuclear clear area or "hof" representing Golgi zone, and an eccentrically placed nucleus with coarse chromatin and no nucleoli; the morphology is close to that of mature plasma cells.

In intermediate type cells, features are intermediate between mature and immature myeloma cells; they have moderately dispersed chromatin and occasional small nucleoli. The immature cells are larger than typical plasma cells with larger nucleus, which may be centrally or eccentrically located, finely dispersed nuclear chromatin, one or two prominent nucleoli, and light blue cytoplasm. Bi- or multinucleated cells and pleomorphism may be seen. The nuclear-cytoplasmic dissociation, i.e. relative cytoplasmic maturity (deep basophilia) in the presence of nuclear immaturity (finely dispersed nuclear chromatin) and pleomorphism are features of neoplastic plasma cells. Plasmablastic myeloma cells show high nuclear-cytoplasmic ratio, dispersed chromatin, and small nucleoli. Plasmablastic myeloma is associated with shorter median survival.

Intracellular accumulations of immunoglobulins may produce distinctive morphological features, such as Mott cells or morula cells (numerous "grape-like" pale bluish cytoplasmic inclusions), Dutcher bodies (pale-staining, single, large intranuclear inclusions), and Russell bodies (round hyaline inclusions in cytoplasm). These features also occur in reactive plasmacytosis. Occasionally, cytoplasmic crystals and phagocytosis can be seen in plasma cells.

Certain morphological features are associated with IgA-secreting myeloma: Flaming plasma cells (cells with red cytoplasmic margin), markedly pleomorphic and multinucleated cells, and cells with frayed and fragmented cytoplasm. Otherwise, there is no morphological correlation between type of monoclonal immunoglobulin and morphology.

Bone marrow biopsy: The pattern of infiltration may be interstitial, focal, or diffuse and correlates with extent of disease. Normal hematopoiesis is mostly preserved with interstitial and focal infiltration patterns, while diffuse infiltration is associated with suppression of normal hematopoiesis and advanced stage of disease.

Protein Alterations

Zone electrophoresis of serum proteins (*see* Fig. 9.2) shows a sharply defined M band in about 80% of patients. Usually, it is located in the γ globulin region, but occasionally, it migrates to β or α2 regions.

Immunofixation using monospecific antisera reveals M protein to be IgG in 55 to 60%, light chains only in 20 to 25%, and IgA in 15 to 20% cases. Rarely, myelomas are of IgD, IgE, IgM, and biclonal (synthesis of two M proteins) type. Nonsecretory myeloma accounts for 1% myeloma cases. Approximately, 70% cases show presence of both serum and urinary monoclonal protein. Conditions associated with the production of a monoclonal protein are shown in Box 9.3.

Normal immunoglobulins in serum are markedly decreased (hypogammaglobulinemia).

Free Light Chain Assay

See earlier.

Immunophenotyping (Flow Cytometry) (Fig. 9.9)

The usual marker for identification of plasma cells on immunophenotyping is bright expression of CD38 (although not specific). CD138 appears to be specific for plasma cells amongst hematolymphoid cells. Flow cytometry appears to have a significant role in diagnosis and management of plasma cell neoplasms. Normal plasma cells express CD38 (bright), CD138

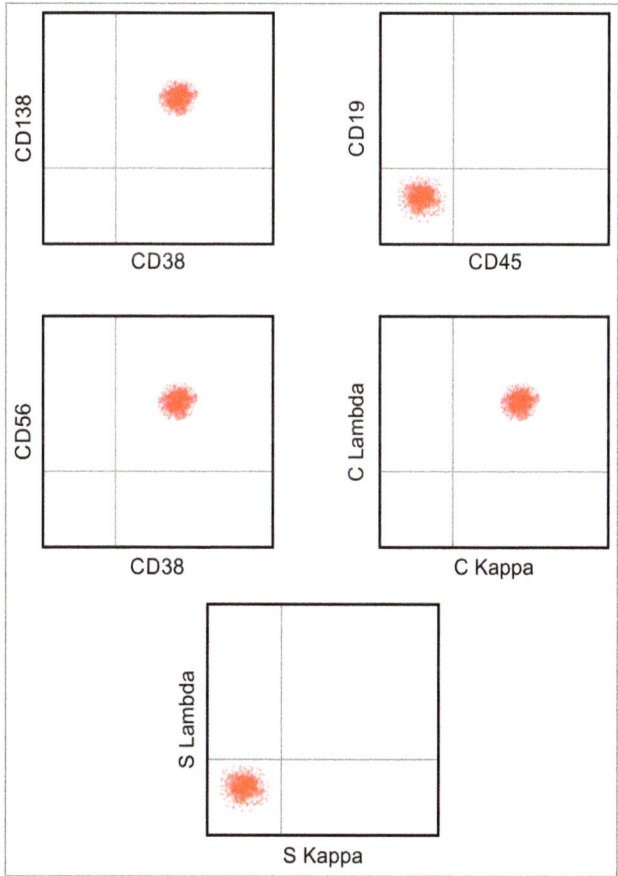

Fig. 9.9: Flow cytometry in plasma cell myeloma. Neoplastic cells are CD38+, CD138+, CD45-, CD19-, CD56+, cytoplasmic kappa+, and surface light chain negative.

(bright), CD19, CD45, and are negative for CD56, CD117, CD200, and CD20. Both kappa and lambda light chains are expressed in the ratio of 1 to 2:1. Neoplastic plasma cells express both CD38 and CD138, but are negative for CD19 and often there is acquisition of CD56, CD200, and CD117. Either kappa or lambda light chain is expressed thus confirming the clonality of a plasma cell proliferation; it also allows distinction of PCM from lymphoplasmacytic lymphoma.

Immunohistochemistry (IHC)

Applications of IHC on bone marrow biopsy are (1) accurate and easy quantification of plasma cells (after staining with plasma cell-associated antigens like CD138, CD38, kappa and lambda light chains) especially when they are distributed interstitially in marrow, (2) confirmation of plasmacytic lineage if cells are anaplastic or poorly differentiated, (3) identification of monoclonal (either kappa or lambda light chains) or polyclonal (both kappa and lambda light chains) nature of plasma cell proliferation, and (4) differentiation of poorly differentiated myeloma from other neoplasms like lymphoma or metastatic tumors.

Biochemical Abnormalities

Serum creatinine is raised in the presence of renal insufficiency and level >2 mg/dL is one of the diagnostic criteria for PCM (IMWG). *Hypercalcemia is often present and, similar to serum creatinine, is one of the diagnostic criteria for PCM; hypercalcemia is defined as serum calcium >1 mg/dL higher than upper limit of normal or >11 mg/dL (IMWG). Serum alkaline phosphatase is normal or slightly increased;* this is helpful in differentiating PCM from skeletal involvement due to hyperparathyroidism or metastatic carcinoma in which alkaline phosphatase is markedly raised. (Serum alkaline phosphatase is raised in AL amyloidosis if there is hepatic involvement.) Measurement of *serum β2-microglobulin at the time of diagnosis provides useful prognostic information.* Serum β2-microglobulin correlates with both tumor burden and renal function. β2-microglobulin level more than 5.5 mg/L is associated with high tumor mass and shorter survival as compared to patients with β2-microglobulin <5.5 mg/L. Serial estimation of β2-microglobulin is also helpful in assessing the growth rate of myeloma. Combination of serum albumin and serum β2-microglobulin provide prognostic staging of PCM.

Cytogenetic Analysis

Both structural and numerical chromosomal abnormalities have been reported in PCM including trisomies, translocations, deletions, and complex cytogenetic abnormalities. Chromosomal abnormalities in PCM are divided into two main groups: hyperdiploid (commonly trisomies) and nonhyperdiploid (structural chromosomal abnormalities most commonly involving IGH locus on 14q32). Translocations involving IGH and hyperdiploidy are probable initiating events in pathogenesis of PCM. They cause dysregulation of one of the cyclin D genes leading to overexpression of one of the cyclins.

Both conventional cytogenetic analysis and fluorescent in situ hybridization (FISH) should be done in PCM at diagnosis. Conventional analysis is performed on myeloma cells obtained by bone marrow aspirate and requires dividing or metaphase cells. At least 20 metaphase cells are analyzed; however, disadvantages include low resolution, low in vitro proliferation of myeloma cells, and common occurrence of cryptic chromosomal structural abnormalities. FISH can be performed on interphase cells and is a more sensitive technique. Certain chromosomal abnormalities like hypodiploidy, complex abnormalities, and deletion of chromosome 13 may not be completely characterized by FISH and require conventional analysis. Prognostic significance of cytogenetic abnormalities in myeloma is given under "Staging and Prognosis".

Radiological Features

Along with full skeletal X-ray survey, newer techniques like computed tomography (CT), magnetic resonance imaging (MRI), and positron emission tomography-computed tomography (PET-CT) play an important role in diagnosis and management of PCM. CT and MRI can detect smaller lesions and are more sensitive than X-ray. Bone changes in PCM include— diffuse osteoporosis, localized osteolytic lesions, and pathological fractures. The osteolytic lesions appear as multiple, rounded, punched out areas without sclerosis at the borders. Common sites for osteolytic lesions are vertebrae, ribs, skull, pelvis, and proximal areas of long bones. Rarely, the localized lesions are osteosclerotic and associated with polyneuropathy, organomegaly, endocrinopathy, monoclonal protein, and skin changes (POEMS syndrome). Diffuse osteoporosis may lead to compression fractures of thoracic or lumbar vertebrae.

Osteolytic lesions in PCM are produced by activation of osteoclasts by certain factors secreted by myeloma cells. These osteoclast-activating factors (OAF) are tumor necrosis factor α and interleukin-1β.

Diagnosis

Diagnosis of PCM requires correlation of clinical, bone marrow, immunological, and radiological findings. This is because some of the findings in PCM are also observed in other disorders (Fig. 9.10).

The parameters taken into consideration for diagnosis of PCM are shown in Box 9.6.

Criteria for diagnosis of PCM, smoldering myeloma, and monoclonal gammopathy of undetermined significance are shown in Box 9.7.

Differential Diagnosis

Reactive Bone Marrow Plasmacytosis

Marked or florid plasmacytosis in bone marrow can occur in autoimmune disorders, chronic inflammatory or infectious conditions, viral infections, Hodgkin's lymphoma, Castleman's disease, cirrhosis, carcinoma, and HIV infection. This may cause diagnostic confusion with plasma cell neoplasm. Differences between reactive plasmacytosis and PCM are shown in Table 9.3.

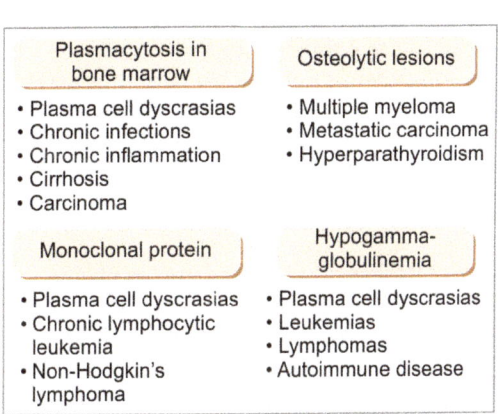

Fig. 9.10: Why multiple criteria are needed for diagnosis of myeloma. It can be seen that typical features of myeloma also occur in other acquired disorders and no single criterion is specific for myeloma.

Box 9.6: Typical features of plasma cell myeloma.

- Symptomatic patient (especially bone pain, repeated infections, fatigue) >50 years of age
- Bone marrow plasma cells increased
- Osteolytic bone lesions on skeletal X-ray survey
- Presence of M component in serum and/or urine
- Hypogammaglobulinemia (reduced levels of normal immunoglobulins)

Section 3: Disorders of White Blood Cells

> **Box 9.7:** Diagnostic criteria for Non-IgM monoclonal gammopathy of undetermined significance, smoldering myeloma, and plasma cell myeloma (International Myeloma Working Group 2014, adapted by WHO 2016 classification).

Non-IgM monoclonal gammopathy of undetermined significance (Non-IgM MGUS)
All of the following criteria should be met:
- Serum monoclonal (M) protein (IgG or IgA) <30 g/L
- Clonal plasma cells in bone marrow <10%
- Absence of features of end-organ damage i.e. CRAB (hypercalcemia, renal insufficiency, anemia, and bone lesions) that are attributed to a plasma cell disorder

Smoldering (or Asymptomatic) myeloma
Both of the following criteria should be met:
- Serum monoclonal protein (IgG or IgA) ≥30 g/L or urinary monoclonal protein ≥500 mg/24 hours and/or clonal bone marrow plasma cells—10-60%
- No evidence of myeloma-defining events or amyloidosis

Plasma cell myeloma
Both of the following criteria should be met:
- Clonal plasma cells in bone marrow ≥10% OR Biopsy proven plasmacytoma
- Any one or more of the following myeloma-defining events:
    - CRAB: End-organ damage attributed to plasma cell proliferative disorder in the form of
        - Hypercalcemia: Serum calcium >1 mg/dL higher than the upper limit of normal OR >11 mg/dL
        - Renal insufficiency: Serum creatinine >2 mg/dL
        - Anemia: Hemoglobin >2 g/dL below the lower limit of normal OR Hemoglobin <10 g/dL
        - Bone lesions: ≥1 osteolytic lesion on skeletal radiography, CT or PET-CT
    - ≥1 of the following biomarkers of malignancy:
        - Clonal plasma cells in bone marrow ≥60%
        - Involved: Uninvolved serum free light chain ratio ≥100
        - >1 focal lesion on MRI

Table 9.3: Differences between reactive plasmacytosis and plasma cell myeloma.

Parameter	Reactive plasmacytosis	Plasma cell myeloma
Bone marrow examination	Mature plasma cells; occur singly or in small groups around blood vessels	Mature plasma cells to plasmablastic cells; occur in large clusters and are not perivascular
Serum protein electrophoresis	Polyclonal hypergammaglobulinemia	Monoclonal protein
Serum free light chain ratio	Normal κ to λ ratio: 0.26 to 1.65	<0.26 or >1.65; involved/uninvolved FLC ratio ≥100
Cytogenetic analysis	No abnormality	Translocation involving 14q32 (50% cases), trisomies
Immunophenotyping of plasma cells	CD38 (bright)+, CD138 (bright)+, CD19+, CD45+, CD56-, CD117-, CD200-, CD20-, both lambda and kappa light chains+	CD38 dim+, CD138 (bright)+, CD19-, CD45-, CD56+, CD117+, CD200+, CD20+, either kappa or lambda light chain+
Associated clinical features	Abnormalities related to underlying disorder+	Abnormalities related to plasma cell proliferative disorder+, i.e. CRAB

Monoclonal Gammopathy of Undetermined Significance (MGUS)

Patients with PCM must be distinguished from those with MGUS. MGUS is considered later (refer to Table 9.8).

Systemic polyclonal immunoblastic proliferation: This rare acute immune reactive disorder is characterized by proliferation of B immunoblasts and manifests with fever, lymphadenopathy, and hepatosplenomegaly. Peripheral blood shows anemia, thrombocytopenia, and raised leukocyte count with many plasma cells, reactive lymphocytes, and immunoblasts. Bone marrow examination shows plasma cells, immunoblasts, and reactive lymphocytes. There is polyclonal hypergammaglobulinemia. Complete and rapid resolution may occur with steroids sometimes combined with chemotherapy. Mortality during acute illness is high.

Lymphomas with Plasma Cell Differentiation:

These include lymphoplasmacytic lymphoma including WM, marginal zone lymphoma, and large cell lymphoma with plasmablastic morphology (Table 9.4).

Waldenström's Macroglobulinemia

In contrast to PCM, in WM hyperviscosity syndrome, hepatosplenomegaly, and lymphadenopathy are prominent, and osteolytic lesions and hypercalcemia are rare. Bone marrow in WM shows diffuse infiltration by lymphocytes, plasmacytoid lymphocytes, and a few plasma cells; mast cells are also increased in number (refer to Table 9.6).

Metastatic Carcinoma

Carcinomas metastatic to bone can produce osteolytic lesions similar to PCM. Metastatic tumors especially from breast and prostate can morphologically resemble PCM. Diagnosis is based on identification of primary tumor and immunohistochemistry.

Table 9.4: Differentiation of PCM from lymphomas with plasma cell differentiation.

Parameter	Lymphoplasmacytic lymphoma	Marginal zone lymphoma (Nodal)	Plasmablastic lymphoma	Plasma cell myeloma
Immunophenotype	CD19+, CD20+, CD138+, CD38+, CD10-, CD5-, Cyclin D1-, CD56-, monotypic plasma cell+ (all cells)	CD19+, CD20+, CD10-, CD5-, BCL2+, monotypic plasma cells+(30%), CD38+ in plasma cell	CD38+, CD138+, CD45-, CD20-, CD3-, EBV±	CD38+, CD138+, CD45-, CD56+. CD117+, κ or λ light chain+
Clinical	Serum hyperviscosity syndrome, clinical features related to tissue infiltration	Slowly progressive lymphadenopathy	Common in HIV+ patients	CRAB
Cytogenetic and genetic features	MYD88 L265P mutations	PTPRD, NOTCH2, KLF2 mutations	MYC translocations (50% cases)	Translocations of 14q32, trisomies

Staging and Prognosis

The important prognostic factors are:
- Serum β2-microglobulin: Estimation of serum β2-microglobulin, either alone or in combination with serum albumin, is useful for predicting duration of survival and prognosis in PCM (International Staging System for Plasma Cell Myeloma).
- Genetic abnormalities: High-risk genetic abnormalities are del 17p, and *MAF* translocations t(14;16) and t(14;20). Standard or low-risk abnormalities include t(11;14), t(6;14), and hyperdiploidy. Intermediate-risk abnormalities are t(4;14), del 13, and hypodiploidy.
- High plasma cell labeling index: Proliferative activity of tumor cells measured as labeling index using [^{3}H] thymidine has prognostic importance. A low plasma cell labeling index (<1%) is indicative of low percentage of plasma cells that are actively growing and longer median survival as compared to a high index.
- Plasmablastic morphology: This is associated with adverse prognosis.
- Elevated lactate dehydrogenase level indicates high tumor burden.

There are two main staging systems of PCM: Durie and Salmon staging system and International staging system (Table 9.5). Importance of some factors affecting prognosis is as follows:

Treatment

Treatment is indicated in symptomatic patients (hypercalcemia, renal insufficiency, anemia, lytic bone lesions, hyperviscosity, repeated infections, amyloidosis). Patients with smoldering

Table 9.5: Staging systems in multiple plasma cell myeloma.

Durie and Salmon staging system	International staging system (ISS)
Stage I (all of following)	**Stage I**
• Hemoglobin >10.0 g/dL, normal serum calcium, normal immunoglobulin levels (non-M protein)	Serum β2-microglobulin <3.5 mg/L
• Low M protein: IgG <50 g/dL, IgA <30 g/dL, urine BJ protein <4 g/24 hours	Serum albumin ≥3.5 g/dL
• Normal bone X-ray or single plasmacytoma of bone	
Stage II	**Stage II**
Values between stage I and stage III	Serum β2-microglobulin <3.5 mg/L and serum albumin <3.5 g/dL or serum β2-microglobulin 3.5–5.5 mg/L irrespective of serum albumin level
Stage III (≥1 of following)	**Stage III**
• Hemoglobin <8.5 g/dL, serum calcium >12 mg/dL	Serum β2-microglobulin >5.5 mg/L
• Multiple lytic bone lesions	
• High M protein: IgG >70 g/dL, IgA >50 g/dL, urine light chains >12 g/24 hours	
Subclassification: A: Serum creatinine <2 mg/dL B: Serum creatinine ≥2 mg/dL	

myeloma are followed without therapy until symptoms develop. Although chemotherapy does not cure the disease, it relieves symptoms, controls the progression of disease, and prolongs survival. Previously, standard initial treatment for PCM was combination of alkylating agent (melphalan) and prednisone. Although objective evidence of response to therapy is observed in 50 to 60% of patients, complete remission is infrequent. However, with the introduction of proteasome inhibitor (bortezomib) and immunomodulatory drugs (thalidomide and lenalidomide), complete response and overall survival have significantly improved.

Currently, the first treatment option in symptomatic myeloma is determining whether patient is suitable for high-dose chemotherapy followed by autologous hematopoietic stem cell transplantation. This decision is based on patient's age, general health, and organ function status of kidneys, heart, liver, and lungs. If patient is eligible for transplantation, patient is given two to four cycles of three-drug induction therapy before collection of stem cells. Induction therapy usually consists of bortezomib, dexamethasone, and either thalidomide or lenalidomide or cyclophosphamide. After stem cell collection, conditioning therapy (high-dose melphalan) is given. After autologous stem cell transplantation, maintenance therapy of thalidomide or lenalidomide is given. A significant number of patients are not candidates for autologous stem cell transplantation at diagnosis.

If patient is considered to be noneligible for autologous transplantation, combination chemotherapy consisting of melphalan, prednisone, and either bortezomib or thalidomide, or lenalidomide is administered. As compared to earlier chemotherapy regimen, the newer combination therapy has led to improved response, has delayed disease progression, and improved survival.

Supportive care consists of (1) treatment of anemia: Current evidence indicates that recombinant human erythropoietin is effective in improving hemoglobin and reducing transfusion needs even in patients without renal impairment; (2) bone disease: Bisphosphonates (pamidronate, zoledronic acid) inhibit osteoclast activity and reduce skeletal pain, hypercalcemia, and other skeletal morbidity and improve quality of life; they are recommended for all patients with myeloma needing treatment for their disease; local radiotherapy is given for localized bone pain and pathological fractures; (3) renal failure is usually responsive to rehydration and chemotherapy (by reducing paraproteins and light chains); (4) hyperviscosity syndrome is treated with plasmapheresis followed by chemotherapy.

Causes of Death

With current therapy, complete remission rate and overall survival rate have improved considerably. However, myeloma is a progressive and largely incurable disease. Median survival is 5.5 years. High-risk prognostic factors are associated with survival less than 1 year. The common causes of death include (1) infection secondary to hypogammaglobulinemia, neutropenia, and immunosuppression due to chemotherapy, (2) renal failure, and (3) myelodysplastic syndrome and acute myeloid leukemia (may occur as part of the natural history of myeloma or more commonly secondary to therapy with alkylating agents).

Variant Forms of Plasma Cell Myeloma

PCM variants include smoldering (asymptomatic) myeloma, nonsecretory myeloma, and plasma cell leukemia.

Smoldering (Asymptomatic) Myeloma

These patients have 10% or more but <60% plasma cells in bone marrow and an M protein at myeloma levels but do not have evidence of myeloma-related organ damage (CRAB). These patients comprise 8 to 14% of myeloma cases. The disease remains stable for many years; treatment is initiated when evidence of disease progression develops. Both of the following criteria are required for diagnosis of smoldering PCM (IMWG 2014, WHO 2016):
- Serum M protein (IgG or IgA) ≥30 g/L or urinary M protein ≥500 mg/24 hours and/or clonal bone marrow plasma cell percentage of 10 to 60%
- Absence of myeloma—defining events or amyloidosis

Risk of progression to symptomatic PCM is higher in smoldering myeloma (10% per year for first 5 years and 75% in a lifetime) as compared to MGUS. Progression to symptomatic myeloma is more likely to occur in patients with presence of both M protein >30 g/L and >10% clonal plasma cells in bone marrow. Other risk factors for progression include bone lesions detected by MRI, high proportion of plasma cells in bone marrow with aberrant phenotype, abnormal serum FLC ratio, circulating plasma cells, and high plasma cell proliferation rate. It has been demonstrated that administration of treatment in highest risk patients slows progression to symptomatic PCM.

Nonsecretory Plasma Cell Myeloma

This accounts for 3% cases of PCM. The neoplastic plasma cells do not have the ability to secrete immunoglobulins and there is no detectable M protein in serum or urine by immunofixation electrophoresis. However, elevated serum FLC or abnormal FLC ratio is demonstrable in two-thirds of patients. Monoclonal light chains are detectable in neoplastic plasma cells in 85% cases by immunohistochemistry; in remaining cases, no such staining is observed. Morphology, immunophenotypic features, and genetic abnormalities are similar to PCM. Clinically, there is lower incidence of renal insufficiency and hypercalcemia and less suppression of normal immunoglobulins. Therapy is similar to PCM.

Plasma Cell leukemia

Plasma cell leukemia is a rare type of myeloma defined as presence of >2000/cmm or >20% of plasma cells in peripheral blood. It may be primary (de novo, i.e. present at initial diagnosis) or secondary (which occurs during late stages of 1% cases of PCM). Most cases are primary (60–70%).

The median age at diagnosis is younger, and lymphadenopathy, hepatosplenomegaly, and renal failure are more common, while lytic bone lesions are less common than myeloma.

Immunotyping is similar to PCM except for more common expression of CD20 and less common expression of CD56 (absent in 80% cases). High-risk genetic abnormalities are more frequent like hypodiploidy, del 13q, del 17p, and t(14;16).

The course is aggressive with short survival and poor response to treatment.

Solitary Plasmacytoma of Bone

This is a rare condition in which neoplastic proliferation of plasma cells is limited to a single focus in the bone. The neoplastic or clonal plasma cells are morphologically, immunophenotypically, and genetically similar to those of PCM. Patient presents with bone pain or pathological fracture at the site of the lesion. In this condition, there is only a single osteolytic bone lesion on skeletal radiological survey, MRI, or CT. MRI or CT is essential to rule out more bone lesions and thus confirming solitary nature of the lesion. Evidence of PCM (like myeloma cells in bone marrow, hypercalcemia, anemia, renal disease, and a monoclonal protein in serum and/or urine) is absent. Common sites are spine (most common site), ribs, skull, ileum, femur, clavicle, and scapula. Treatment of choice for solitary plasmacytoma of bone is local radiotherapy. Regular follow-up with serum and urine protein electrophoresis for monoclonal protein is essential after radiotherapy. About one-third of patients remain disease-free at 10 years. Most patients (two-thirds) develop additional plasmacytoma or evidence of dissemination (PCM) within 10 years.

Extramedullary (Extraosseous) Plasmacytoma

This is a rare neoplasm of plasma cells, which arises in extramedullary or extraosseous site particularly upper respiratory tract, such as oropharynx, paranasal sinuses, nasopharynx, and larynx. However, any site may be affected including gastrointestinal tract, breast, gonads, etc. Morphology, immunophenotyping, and genetics are similar to those of other plasma cell neoplasms. The condition should be differentiated from reactive plasma cell proliferations, and lymphomas with marked plasma cell differentiation like lymphoplasmacytic lymphoma and marginal zone lymphoma. PCM should be excluded by relevant investigations. Risk of progression to PCM is low. Treatment consists of surgical excision and radiotherapy.

WALDENSTRÖM'S MACROGLOBULINEMIA

Waldenström's macroglobulinemia (WM) is a lymphoplasmacytic lymphoma characterized by (1) neoplastic proliferation of small lymphocytes, plasma cells, and plasmacytoid lymphocytes involving bone marrow, and (2) production of monoclonal IgM immunoglobulin of any concentration. Macroglobulins are IgM immunoglobulins, which have high molecular weight. Recently, a recurrent somatic mutation *MYD88 L265P has been identified in more than 90% of patients with lymphoplasmacytic lymphoma/WM.*

Clinical Features

WM is a disease of the old persons with highest occurrence between 60 and 70 years. It is more common in males. Fatigue, weakness, and weight loss are common symptoms. The physical presence of macroglobulins increases blood viscosity and may produce hyperviscosity syndrome. Manifestations of hyperviscosity syndrome include visual impairment, bleeding tendencies (purpura, epistaxis), and neurological changes (headache, ataxia, vertigo, altered mental state, intracranial hemorrhage, coma). Retinal changes of hyperviscosity are distension and segmentation of retinal veins ("sausage link" pattern), hemorrhages, and exudates. Hyperviscosity syndrome usually develops when serum viscosity is more than four times normal. Sensorimotor neuropathy may develop due to binding of peripheral nerve components by monoclonal IgM. On physical examination, usual findings are lymphadenopathy and hepatosplenomegaly. Uncommon manifestations of WM are: (1) peripheral neuropathy, (2) cryoglobulinemia (patient develops Raynaud's phenomenon, urticaria, purpura on exposure to cold), (3) cold hemagglutinin disease, and (4) amyloidosis.

Bone pain and lytic bone lesions are absent in contrast to PCM. Renal involvement is also rare.

Laboratory Features

Peripheral Blood Examination

Normocytic normochromic anemia is present in majority of patients at diagnosis. Causes of anemia include expansion of plasma volume, inhibition of hematopoiesis, and sometimes hemolysis. Rouleaux formation is prominent.

Leukopenia may be present. Lymphocytes are frequently increased. Plasmacytoid lymphocytes may be present in circulation. Platelet count may be normal or low.

ESR is usually markedly raised.

Bone Marrow Examination

This reveals infiltrate of small lymphocytes, plasmacytoid lymphocytes, and plasma cells in varying proportions. Distribution may be interstitial, nodular, diffuse, or paratrabecular. Mast cells are prominent. Periodic acid Schiff-positive inclusions in nucleus and cytoplasm of some of the cells may be seen.

Immunophenotyping

This shows CD19+, CD20+, cytoplasmic IgM+, CD5-, CD10-, CD23-, CD103-, and in plasma cells CD38+ and CD138+.

Serum and Urine Protein Electrophoresis

Zone electrophoresis of serum shows a dense, well-localized band (and a narrow-based spike on densitometer tracing) in γ region. Identification of monoclonal protein is made by immunofixation using monospecific antisera. Monoclonal protein in WM shows reactivity against μ heavy chain and to one type of light chain either κ or λ. In symptomatic patients, concentration of paraprotein in serum is usually >3 g/dL. Electrophoresis of concentrated urine will reveal monoclonal light chains in majority of patients.

Genetic Analysis

Mutation in myeloid differentiation primary response gene 88 (*MYD88* L265P) *on* chromosome 3p22.2 *is detected in majority of patients with WM.*

Tests for Hemostasis

Coating of platelets by monoclonal IgM causes abnormalities in platelet function, e.g. prolongation of bleeding time, and defective platelet aggregation. Monoclonal proteins inhibit fibrin monomer polymerization, which results in prolongation of thrombin time.

Lymph Node Biopsy

It shows histologic features of lymphoplasmacytic lymphoma. In the classic pattern, there are paracortical infiltrates of lymphocytes, plasmacytoid lymphocytes, and plasma cells with dilated and open lymph sinuses. Dutcher bodies and increased numbers of mast cells may be present.

Table 9.6: Comparative features of plasma cell myeloma and Waldenström's macroglobulinemia.

Parameter	PCM	WM
1. Organomegaly, hyperviscosity syndrome	Rare	Frequent
2. Skeletal disease	Frequent	Absent
3. Renal insufficiency	Frequent	Rare
4. Bone marrow findings	Increased plasma cells	Diffuse infiltration by lymphocytes, plasmacytoid lymphocytes, and plasma cells
5. Nature of monoclonal protein	Usually IgG, IgA, or light chains only; IgM very rare	IgM
6. Drug of first choice	Melphalan + Prednisone + Bortezomib	Chlorambucil
7. Median survival	3 years	5 years

Differential Diagnosis

Plasma Cell Myeloma

Some differences between PCM and WM are outlined in Table 9.6.

IgM Monoclonal Gammopathy of Undetermined Significance

IgM monoclonal gammopathy of undermined significance (IgM MGUS) is characterized by serum IgM monoclonal protein level of <3 g/dL, clonal lymphoplasmacytic infiltrate <10% in bone marrow, and no evidence of symptoms of WM (anemia, organomegaly, hyperviscosity). MYD88 L265P mutation is observed in 50% cases. Progression to lymphoplasmacytic lymphoma/WM or primary amyloidosis can occur.

Splenic Lymphoma with Villous Lymphocytes (Splenic Marginal Zone Lymphoma)

Features favoring this disorder are marked enlargement of spleen without lymphadenopathy, moderately raised leukocyte count with villous lymphocytes, and IgM paraprotein concentration <2 g/dL (in 25% cases).

Prognosis

The disease is indolent with overall survival of 5 years. Adverse prognostic factors include advanced age (>65 years), cytopenias in peripheral blood, serum monoclonal protein >7 g/dL, and serum β2-microglobulin >3 mg/L. Transformation to a high-grade diffuse large B-cell lymphoma occurs in a minority of patients.

Treatment

Treatment is initiated when patient develops clinical manifestations or evidence of disease progression. The usual form of therapy is chlorambucil and prednisone. Other options are rituximab combined with drugs like bendamustine, or with dexamethasone and cyclophosphamide or with bortezomib. In relapsed or refractory cases, options include fludarabine-containing regimens, everolimus, or alemtuzumab. Plasmapheresis is helpful in alleviating manifestations of hyperviscosity.

MONOCLONAL GAMMOPATHY OF UNDETERMINED SIGNIFICANCE

The presence of monoclonal protein in serum without clinical or laboratory manifestations attributable to underlying plasma cell disorder or lymphoproliferative disease is referred to as monoclonal gammopathy of undetermined significance (MGUS). Previously, these disorders were called as benign monoclonal gammopathies. If such patients are followed regularly, majority remain stable over many years and consequently require no treatment. However, a small proportion will eventually develop some form of plasma cell dyscrasia such as multiple myeloma, WM, or amyloidosis. Therefore, follow-up is necessary to determine the benign or malignant nature of these disorders. Thus, the designation monoclonal gammopathy of undetermined significance appears to be more appropriate for these disorders.

MGUS is reported to occur in 3% of individuals over 50 years of age.

Two types of MGUS are distinguished: IgM MGUS (15% cases) and non-IgM MGUS (85% cases). They are biologically and clinically distinct and unified only by monoclonal protein secretion. They are compared in Table 9.7.

Criteria for diagnosis of non-IgM MGUs are as follows (IMWG 2014, adapted by WHO 2016):
1. Serum monoclonal (non-IgM) protein <3.0 g/dL
2. Bone marrow clonal plasma cells <10%
3. Absence of end-organ damage (CRAB: hypercalcemia, renal insufficiency, anemia, bone lesions) and amyloidosis due to plasma cell disorder.

There are no symptoms related to the monoclonal gammopathy. MGUS is detected in the course of evaluation of some other disorders like cardiovascular disease, liver disease, or other health problems.

Table 9.7: Comparison of IgM-MGUS and non-IgM MGUS.

Parameter	IgM MGUS	Non-IgM MGUS
Relative frequency	15%	85%
Morphology of monoclonal cells and location	Lymphoid/lymphoplasmacytic, bone marrow	Plasma cells, bone marrow
Percentage of monoclonal cells in bone marrow	<10%	<10%
Monoclonal protein	IgM	IgG, IgA, light chain only
Genetic abnormalities	MYD88 L265P mutation (50% cases)	Similar to plasma cell myeloma
Progression to plasma cell dyscrasia	Lymphoma, Waldenström's macroglobulinemia, AL amyloidosis	Plasma cell myeloma, AL amyloidosis
Risk of progression per year	1.5%	1%

Table 9.8: Comparison of plasma cell myeloma (PCM) and non-IgM MGUS.

Parameter	PCM	non-IgM MGUS
1. Clonal plasma cells in marrow	>10%	<10%
2. Anemia, hypercalcemia, lytic bone lesions, renal involvement	Frequent	Absent
3. Monoclonal protein	Variable	<3.0 g/dL
4. Normal immunoglobulins	Usually low	Usually normal
5. Plasma cell labeling index	>1%	<1%

Following features favor the diagnosis of plasma cell dyscrasia other than MGUS–bone marrow plasmacytosis greater than 10%, steadily rising M-component, significant Bence Jones proteinuria, anemia, osteolytic lesions, hypercalcemia, hepatosplenomegaly, or high plasma cell labeling index. Differences between PCM and MGUS are listed in Table 9.8.

Most cases of MGUS are benign and remain stable over many years of follow-up. In a study by Kyle, when followed for more than 10 years, malignant plasma cell dyscrasia or a lymphoproliferative disorder developed in approximately 20% of patients with MGUS.

Patients with MGUS should not be treated unless progression to a neoplastic plasma cell disorder occurs.

BIBLIOGRAPHY

1. Alexanian R, Dimopoulos MA. Management of multiple myeloma. Semin Hematol. 1975;32:20-30.
2. Alexanian R. Localized and indolent myeloma. Blood. 1980;56:521-25.
3. Barlogie B, Epstein J, Selvanayagam PI, Alexanian R. Plasma cell myeloma—New biological insights and advances in therapy. Blood. 1989;73:865-79.
4. Bartl R, Frisch B, Fateh-Moghadam A, et al. Histologic classification and staging of multiple myeloma. A retrospective and prospective study of 674 cases. Am J Clin Pathol. 1987;87:342–55.
5. Bataille R, Sany J. Solitary myeloma. Clinical and prognostic features of a review of 114 cases. Cancer. 1981;48:45-851.
6. British Committee for Standards in Haematology. Diagnosis and management of multiple myeloma. Br J Haematol. 2001;115:522-40.
7. Channing Rodgers RP. Clinical laboratory methods for detection of antigens and antibodies. In Stites DP, Terr AI, Parslow TG (Eds). Basic and Clinical Immunology. 8th Ed. Connecticut. Appleton and Lange; 1994.
8. Chesi M, Bergsagel PL. Molecular pathogenesis of multiple myeloma: Basic and clinical updates. Int J Hematol. 2013;97:313-23.
9. Dimopoulos MA and Alexanian R. Waldenstrom's macroglobulinaemia. Blood. 1994;83:1452-59.
10. Dispenzieri A, Kyle R, Merlini G, et al. International Myeloma Working Group guidelines for serum-free light chain analysis in multiple myeloma and related disorders. Leukemia. 2009;23:215–24.
11. Durie BGM, Salmon SE, Moon IE. Pretreatment tumour mass, cell kinetics, and prognosis in multiple myeloma. Blood. 1980;55:364-72.
12. Durie BGM, Salmon SE. A clinical staging system for multiple myeloma. Correlation of measured myeloma cell mass with presenting clinical features, response to treatment, and survival. Cancer. 1975;36:842-54.
13. Durie BGM, Stock-Novack D, Salmon SE, Finley P, Beckord J, Crowley J, et al. Prognostic value of pre-treatment serum β2 microglobulin in myeloma:A Southwest Oncology Group study. Blood. 1990;75:823-30.

14. Gandara DR, Mackenzie MR. Differential diagnosis of monoclonal gammopathy. Med Clin North Am. 1988;72:55-1167.
15. Gertz MA, Fonseca R, Rajkumar SV. Waldenstrom's macroglobulinaemia. The Oncologist. 2000;5:63-7.
16. Greipp P, San Miguel J, Durie B, et al. International Staging system for multiple myeloma. J Clin Oncol. 2005;23:3412.
17. Greipp PR, Kyle RA. Clinical, morphological, and cell kinetic differences among multiple myeloma, monoclonal gammopathy of undetermined significance, and smoldering multiple myeloma. Blood. 1983;62:166-71.
18. Greipp PR, Witzog TE, Gonchoroff NJ, Haberman TM, Katzman JA, O'Fallon WM, et al. Immunofluorescence labelling indices in myeloma and related monoclonal gammopathies. Mayo Clin Proc. 1987;62:969-77.
19. Joyner MV, Cassuto JP, Dujardin P, Schneider M, Ziegler G, Euller L, et al. Nonexcretory multiple myeloma. Br J Haematol. 1979;43:559-66.
20. Klein B. Cytokine, cytokine receptors, transduction signals, and oncogenes in multiple myeloma. Semin Hematol. 1995;32:4-19.
21. Kohn J. The laboratory investigation of paraproteinemia. In Dyke SC (Ed.). Recent Advances in Clinical Pathology. Series 6. Edinburgh and London. Churchill Livingstone. 1973.
22. Kosmo MA, Gale RP. Plasma cell leukemia. Semin Hematol. 1987;24:202-8.
23. Kyle RA, Greipp PR. Smoldering multiple myeloma. N Engl J Med. 1980;302:1347-9.
24. Kyle RA, Greipp PR. The laboratory investigation of monoclonal gammopathies. Mayo Clin Proc. 1978;53:719-39.
25. Kyle RA. Monoclonal gammopathy of undetermined significance. Am J Med. 1978;64:814-26.
26. Kyle RA. Multiple myeloma. Review of 869 cases. Mayo Clin Proc. 1975;50:29-40.
27. Kyle RA. Why better prognostic factors for multiple myeloma are needed? Blood. 1994;83:1713-6.
28. Kyle RA. "Benign" monoclonal gammopathy. A misnomer? JAMA. 1984;251:1849-54.
29. Latrielle J, Barlogie B, Johnston D. Ploidy and proliferative characteristics in monoclonal gammopathies. Blood. 1982;59:43-51.
30. Lin P. Plasma cell myeloma. Haematol Oncol Clin N Am. 2009;23:709-27.
31. Rajkumar SV, et al. International Myeloma Working Group updated criteria for the diagnosis of multiple myeloma. Lancet Oncol. 2014;15:e538-e548.
32. Shrikhande AV, Saoji AM, Chande CA, Thakar YS. Gel immunodiffusion and discelectrophoresis. A technical manual. Dept. of Microbiology, Govt. Medical College, Nagpur. 1994.
33. Swerdlow SH, Campo E, Harris NL, Jaffe ES, Pileri SA, Stein H, et al. (Eds). WHO classification of tumours of haematopoietic and lymphoid tissues. 4th Ed. Lyon. International Agency for Research on Cancer. 2008.
34. Swerdlow SH, Campo E, Harris NL, Jaffe ES, Pileri SA, Stein H, et al. (Eds). WHO Classification of Tumours of Haematopoietic and Lymphoid Tissues. Revised 4th Ed. Lyon. IARC. 2017
35. The International Myeloma Working Group: Criteria for the classification of monoclonal gammopathies, multiplemyeloma and related disorders: A report of the International Myeloma Working Group. Br J Haematol. 2003;121:749.

CHAPTER 10

Malignant Lymphomas

INTRODUCTION

Lymphomas are a heterogeneous group of malignant neoplasms, which originate primarily in lymph nodes or other lymphoid tissues. They are divided into two major types—Hodgkin's lymphoma (HL) and non-Hodgkin's lymphoma (NHL). Clinical and biologic differences between these two are outlined in Table 10.1.

Cell of origin: NHL arises from B or T lymphocytes; cell of origin in majority of cases of Hodgkin's lymphoma is a mature B lymphocyte at the germinal center stage of differentiation.

Table 10.1: Differences between Hodgkin's and non-Hodgkin's lymphoma.

Parameter	Hodgkin's lymphoma	Non-Hodgkin's lymphoma
1. Incidence	Stable	Steadily increasing
2. Age	Bimodal; young adults and >55 years	Incidence increases with age
3. Cell of origin	Usually B lymphocyte (germinal center B cell)	B (85–90%) or T/NK lymphocyte
4. Lymphadenopathy	Axial, especially cervical or mediastinal	Multiple, peripheral
5. Extranodal disease	Rare	More common
6. Spread	Predictable, contiguous	Noncontiguous
7. Defining morphological feature	Reed-Sternberg cell in a characteristic cellular milieu (Classical type)	—
8. Proportion of neoplastic cells of the total cell population of involved tissue	Comprises a minor component	Comprises major or total component
9. Association	Often with Epstein-Barr virus (EBV) in classical type	EBV, human immunodeficiency virus, human T-lymphotropic virus-1, autoimmune disorders, immunodeficiency disorders
10. Prognosis	Curable in majority of cases; stage is the strongest predictor of prognosis	Variable; stage and histologic type significant

Clinical features: In NHL, involvement of multiple peripheral lymph nodes, extranodal disease, noncontiguous dissemination to distant organs, and bone marrow involvement are more common. In contrast, in HL, disease is usually limited to a single axial lymph node region (usually cervical), spread is in contiguous manner, and bone marrow involvement is rare. HL occurs predominantly in young adults, while NHL shows increasing incidence with age.

Cytogenetic analysis: Clonal, nonrandom chromosomal abnormalities are frequent in NHL; specific and recurrent cytogenetic changes have not been demonstrated by conventional techniques in classical HL.

Morphology: The characteristic defining feature of HL is Reed-Sternberg cells against background of inflammatory cells; such morphology is not observed in NHL.

HODGKIN'S LYMPHOMA

Thomas Hodgkin first described this disease in 1832. It is characterized histologically by presence of Reed-Sternberg (RS) cells in a background of reactive inflammatory cells such as lymphocytes, plasma cells, eosinophils, and fibroblasts. Hodgkin's lymphoma (HL) is usually localized to a single lymph node region in the initial stage; with progression it spreads to other lymph node regions by contiguity and disseminates to other organs. Previously, the term used for HL was Hodgkin's disease due to uncertainty as to whether it represents infectious, immunologic, or neoplastic disorder; however, molecular analysis of RS cells has established the clonal nature and germinal center B-cell origin of HL.

Classification of Hodgkin's lymphoma: The classification of Hodgkin's lymphoma has largely remained constant over many years. The two main types of HL are nodular lymphocyte predominant and classical. Classical type is considered as a distinct clinicopathological entity from nodular lymphocyte predominant type. Classification of Hodgkin's lymphoma (WHO, 2016) is given in Box 10.1.

Majority (95%) of HLs are of classical type. Classical HL is divided into four subtypes based on tissue architecture, morphology of neoplastic cells, and background reactive cell population. Morphology plays a key role in the diagnosis of Hodgkin's lymphoma, especially nodular sclerosis and mixed cellularity subtypes. The lymphocyte-rich and lymphocyte-depleted subtypes always require immunohistochemistry for definitive diagnosis.

Box 10.1: WHO classification (2016) of Hodgkin's lymphoma.

1. Nodular lymphocytic predominant Hodgkin's lymphoma
2. Classical Hodgkin's lymphoma
   – Nodular sclerosis
   – Mixed cellularity
   – Lymphocyte-rich
   – Lymphocyte-depleted

Etiopathogenesis

The RS cells and their mononuclear variants are the neoplastic or malignant cells in HL. Other cells in the background such as lymphocytes, plasma cells, and eosinophils are non-neoplastic. The characteristic cell of HL was described by Sternberg (1893) and Dorothy Reed (1902). A unique feature of HL is that the malignant cells form only a minor component of the tumor, majority being composed of reactive cells. The reactive cells (granulocytes, lymphocytes, plasma cells, and fibroblasts) probably represent the immune reaction of the host against the tumor cells.

Hodgkin's lymphoma comprises of two distinct disease entities (see classification): (1) Nodular lymphocytic predominance HL, and (2) classical HL. Nature of RS cells in HL remained unknown for many years. Recent molecular studies have shown that RS cell is a B lymphocyte originating in germinal center of lymph node in majority of cases, and hence the term "Hodgkin's lymphoma" is more appropriate than the previous term "Hodgkin's disease."

Classical RS cells are hyperdiploid and extensively aneuploid. In majority of cases, immunoglobulin genes of RS cells have undergone heavy chain gene rearrangement and somatic hypermutation (indicating origin from germinal center or postgerminal center B cells). RS cells do not express immunoglobulin. NF-κB transcription factor is constitutively activated and expressed in RS cells, which promotes cell survival and proliferation, and inhibits apoptosis. Copy number gains in *c-REL* proto-oncogene on chromosome 2p are commonly found that activates NF-κB pathway. No specific "founder" mutation has been detected in RS cells.

Role of Epstein-Barr virus: Infection by Epstein-Barr virus (EBV) is thought to play a role in the causation of classical HL on the basis of identification of EBV DNA in lymph nodes and elevated antibody titers to EBV in some patients, and increased risk of HL in patients with infectious mononucleosis. EBV nucleic acids have been demonstrated by DNA *in situ* hybridization in neoplastic cells of a significant number cases. EBV latent membrane protein-1 (LMP-1) is strongly expressed in neoplastic cells in HL and has been shown to have oncogenic potential. EBV-encoded early RNAs (EBERs) are short nontranslated RNA molecules that are abundantly expressed during viral latency. Currently, the preferred methods for detection of EBV in paraffin-embedded tissue are immunohistochemistry for EBV LMP-1 and nonradioactive *in situ* hybridization for EBERs. Amongst the subtypes of HL, EBV-positivity is observed in 75% cases of mixed cellularity subtype, while 10 to 25% positivity is seen in nodular sclerosis subtype.

The risk of development of classical HL is significantly increased in patients with acquired immunodeficiency syndrome (AIDS). Such cases present with advanced stage disease, are universally associated with EBV infection, and show predominance of mixed cellularity and lymphocyte depleted subtypes of CHL. Risk of HL is also increased in recipients of organ transplantation.

Various types of cytokines have been found to be elaborated by RS cells and lymphocytes in HL. Secretion of these cytokines may be responsible for certain histologic features such as fibrosis and eosinophilia. In addition, B systemic symptoms may be related to secretion of certain cytokines.

Clinical Features

HL is a common form of lymphoid malignancy with a bimodal age distribution: higher peak in young adults (20–30 years) and a second minor peak of increased incidence is noted after 50 years of age. Males are more commonly affected. Nodular sclerosis subtype occurs mainly in young adults, while mixed cellularity subtype occurs mainly in children and older adults. Sex incidence is equal in nodular sclerosis type, while other types of classical HL have male predominance.

The usual mode of presentation is localized supradiaphragmatic lymph node enlargement, commonly in cervical region; the enlarged nodes are firm, painless, rubbery, freely mobile, and discrete. Axillary and inguinal lymph nodes are also commonly involved. Mediastinal lymphadenopathy on a routine chest radiograph is frequent, especially in asymptomatic patients. Extranodal involvement is uncommon.

About one-third of patients have systemic symptoms related to disease. These are called B symptoms and include: fever, night sweats, and weight loss > 10% in last 6 months. Presence of systemic symptoms is associated with unfavorable prognosis. Sometimes systemic symptoms are not associated with clinically evident lymphadenopathy and patient presents as a case of pyrexia of unknown origin (PUO); in these cases usually intra-abdominal disease is present. Some patients have alcohol-induced pain at the site of enlarged lymph nodes or pruritus. Splenomegaly and hepatomegaly occur in advanced stages. Bone marrow involvement is uncommon in CHL and is more likely to occur in patients with disease on both sides of diaphragm and B symptoms.

Clinical features also depend on histologic type of HL. Nodular sclerosis subtype commonly involves lower cervical, supraclavicular, and mediastinal nodes (supradiaphragmatic area); bulky mediastinal disease is also more frequent. In mixed cellularity subtype, lymphadenopathy below or on both sides of diaphragm, and presentation with stage III or IV and B symptoms are more common. Lymphocyte depletion type is more common in older adults with higher stage.

Histopathology and Classification of Hodgkin's Lymphoma

Classical Reed-Sternberg Cell and Its Variants

HL is unique amongst lymphomas in that neoplastic cells constitute only a minority of cell population in a tumor mass. The identification of classical RS cells in the characteristic cytologic environment of normal inflammatory cells is essential for diagnosis of Hodgkin's lymphoma. The classical RS cell is a giant cell (usually > 45 μ) having two nuclei or two nuclear lobes, which may appear as mirror images. Each nuclear lobe or each nucleus has an accentuated membrane, pale chromatin, and contains a prominent viral inclusion-like eosinophilic nucleolus surrounded by a clear zone ("owl-eyed" nucleoli). The cytoplasm is usually abundant and faintly eosinophilic or amphophilic. The mononuclear form has the same morphological features as the classical RS cell except a single nucleus and is called as Hodgkin's cell. In most cases, the classical RS cells comprise only a minority of the cell population. Sometimes, RS or Hodgkin's cells show degenerative changes with condensed deeply basophilic cytoplasm and condensed nuclear chromatin; such cells are called as mummified cells.

Variants of RS cells include (1) lacunar cell, and (2) lymphocyte-predominant or LP (previously called lymphocytic and histiocytic or L & H variant) or "popcorn cell. These variants are important in the histological classification of HL. The lacunar cell variant is a large cell with abundant clear to slightly eosinophilic cytoplasm, sharply defined cell borders, and a single multilobated nucleus with coarse chromatin and multiple small nucleoli (smaller than in classical RS cell). In formalin-fixed tissue, cytoplasm is condensed in perinuclear area with spider web-like extensions to the cell membrane; due to this shrinkage artifact, the cell appears to lie in a clear (lacuna-like) space. The lacunar cell variant is typically seen in nodular sclerosis HL. The LP or "popcorn" cell is particularly frequent in lymphocytic predominance type of HL and is characterized by a large, folded multilobed nucleus with multiple small nucleoli. Cells resembling RS cells are also found in other conditions (e.g. infectious mononucleosis, NHL, phenytoin-induced adenopathy, solid cancers) and therefore for diagnosis of HL, presence of RS cells in the typical background of normal inflammatory cells is essential.

World Health Organization classification of HL is presented in Box 10.1.

Chapter 10: Malignant Lymphomas

Table 10.2: Salient features of different types of Hodgkin's lymphoma.

Type	% of HL	Median age, sex	Clinical features	Microscopy	Course and prognosis
1. Nodular LPHL	5%	30–50 years; M > F	Localized peripheral lymph nodes; B symptoms rare; EBV association 3–5%	L & H variant; macronodules composed mostly of small B lymphocytes	Indolent; multiple late relapses; rarely fatal
2. Nodular sclerosis CHL	60–80% of CHL	Usually young adults; M = F	Mediastinal, supraclavicular; stage I or II; EBV association 10–40%	Lacunar variant; nodules composed of T lymphocytes, plasma cells, eosinophils, and histiocytes and surrounded by collagen bands; nodular fibrosis	Related to stage (usually low stage)
3. Mixed cellularity CHL	15–25% of CHL	Bimodal; M > F	Often high stage with B symptoms; EBV association 75%	Numerous classic RS cells and Hodgkin cells against mixed cell background of T lymphocytes, plasma cells, eosinophils, histiocytes; mild fibrosis	Related to stage (usually high stage)
4. Lymphocyte-rich CHL	5% of CHL	Older adults; M > F	Peripheral lymph node; low stage; EBV association 50%	Few classic RS or Hodgkin cells; nodular or diffuse pattern with mostly small T lymphocytes; no fibrosis	Related to stage (usually low stage)
5. Lymphocyte depleted CHL	<1% of CHL	Older age; M > F	Advanced stage, B symptoms, often in HIV +ve; EBV association 90–100% cases	Variable number of bizarre pleomorphic RS cells; depletion of small lymphocytes; disorderly diffuse fibrosis	Related to stage (usually high stage)

Note: Immunohistochemistry of RS cells and variants in all types of CHL is similar: CD30+, CD15+, CD45-, CD79a-, EMA-, CD20 weak or absent; immunohistochemistry of nodular LPHL: CD30-, CD15-, CD45+, CD79a+, EMA+, CD20+

Salient features of different types of Hodgkin's lymphoma are presented in Table 10.2. Differences between classical and nodular lymphocyte predominant Hodgkin's lymphoma are presented in Table 10.3.

Nodular lymphocyte predominant Hodgkin's lymphoma (NLPHL): There is loss of lymph node architecture by variably sized nodules composed of small lymphocytes, histiocytes, epithelioid histiocytes, and dispersed lymphocyte predominant (LP) cells (also called as popcorn cells). LP cells are large with scant cytoplasm and a single large folded or multilobed nucleus having multiple, basophilic, nucleoli that are smaller than those seen in RS cells. Eosinophils, neutrophils, and plasma cells are often not seen. Morphologically, NLPHL is most

Table 10.3: Comparison of classical and nodular lymphocyte predominance Hodgkin's lymphoma.

Parameter	Classical Hodgkin lymphoma (CHL)	Nodular lymphocyte predominance Hodgkin lymphoma (NLPHL)
1. Percent of Hodgkin lymphoma	95%	5%
2. Age	Bimodal: young adults and old age	Unimodal: Young adults
3. B symptoms	May be present	Rare
4. Association with Epstein-Barr virus	Some cases	No
5. Behavior	Aggressive; early stage can be cured with current therapy; late relapse very rare	Indolent; multiple late relapses common
6. Typical RS cells and mononuclear Hodgkin cells	+	–
7. L & H (popcorn) cells	–	+
8. Background of eosinophils, neutrophils, plasma cells	Often	Rare
9. B-cell program	Downregulated with tumor cells negative for most B-cell markers	Preserved with tumor cells positive for B-cell markers
10. Immunophenotype: – CD30 – CD15 – CD45, CD79a, EMA, J chain, BCL-6 – CD20	+ + – Weak or absent	– – + Present
11. Pathology of relapse	CHL	NLPHL or diffuse large B-cell lymphoma

likely to be confused with lymphocyte-rich classical Hodgkin's lymphoma. In some cases, growth pattern can be diffuse in NLPHL.

Nodular sclerosis classical Hodgkin's lymphoma: Lymph node shows cellular nodules surrounded by concentrically arranged bands of birefringent (in polarized light) collagen. Nodules may show areas of necrosis and microabscess (eosinophilic or neutrophilic) formation. The lacunar cells are often numerous and may occur scattered, in clusters, or in compact sheets. The classical RS cells are rare. Background reactive cells show eosinophils, neutrophils, lymphocytes (CD4+ T cells), plasma cells, macrophages, and fibroblasts. Although fibrosis is one of the diagnostic features, it may be extremely variable from minimal to completely obliterative.

Mixed cellularity classical Hodgkin's lymphoma: Lymph node architecture is diffusely obliterated (early involvement may show interfollicular growth pattern) by mixed population of small lymphocytes, eosinophils, plasma cells, and histiocytes. Classical RS cells are frequent and dispersed throughout the node. Histiocytes may show epithelioid features and may form granulomas.

Lymphocyte-rich classical Hodgkin's lymphoma: Small numbers of classical RS cells are dispersed in a nodular or rarely diffuse background of small lymphocytes (B cells); neutrophils and eosinophils are absent. Germinal centers are regressed and eccentrically placed. RS cells are present within nodules and outside of germinal centers. Some RS cells may resemble LP cells as seen in nodular lymphocyte predominant classical Hodgkin's lymphoma. Groups of epithelioid cells may be seen.

Lymphocyte-depleted classical Hodgkin's lymphoma: Two subtypes are described (Lukes and Butler): diffuse fibrosis and reticular. Diffuse fibrosis type shows diffuse reticulin fibrosis, RS cells, and a sparse heterogeneous background population. The reticular subtype shows sheets of neoplastic RS cells with anaplastic and pleomorphic features.

Staging of Hodgkin's Lymphoma

The extent of disease is determined by staging which correlates with survival and prognosis. Staging determines the prognosis and nature of treatment, and the outcome of therapy depends on accuracy of staging. The staging of Hodgkin's lymphoma is based on Ann Arbor staging system, 1971 (modified subsequently in Cotswolds meeting, 1989), which is as follows:

Stage I: Involvement of a single lymph node region or lymphoid structure (like spleen, thymus, Waldeyer's ring)

Stage II: Involvement of two or more lymph node regions on the same side of diaphragm

Stage III: Involvement of lymph node regions or structures on both sides of diaphragm

Stage IV: Involvement of extranodal site(s) (beyond that designated as E)

X: Bulky disease (>one-third mediastinal widening at T5–T6 OR > 10 cm maximum dimension of nodal mass)

E: Involvement of a single extranodal site either contiguous or proximal to a known nodal site

In **Stage I**, disease is limited to a single lymph node region (I); if the disease involves a single extralymphatic organ or site the stage is designated as IE.

In **Stage II**, two or more lymph node regions are involved but are limited to the same side of diaphragm (II); the stage is IIE if localized disease of extralymphatic organ or site is also present.

In **Stage III**, lymph node regions on both sides of diaphragm are involved (III); in addition, the disease may involve spleen (IIIS) or extralymphatic organ or site (IIIE) or both (IIISE).

Stage IV denotes disseminated or diffuse disease of one or more extralymphatic site. Involvement of liver or bone marrow indicates stage IV disease.

Staging Procedures

Once the diagnosis of HL is confirmed by histology and immunohistochemistry on biopsy, extent of disease is determined by staging procedures. Previously used staging laparotomy and lymphangiography are no longer performed due to availability of improved imaging techniques and treatment by chemotherapy (rather than radiotherapy) in many cases of early-stage disease.

History and physical examination: This includes presence or absence of B systemic symptoms, documentation of all sites of enlarged lymph nodes, presence or absence of splenomegaly or hepatomegaly.

Blood examination: Complete blood count, ESR, lactate dehydrogenase, albumin, liver and kidney function tests, serum alkaline phosphatase level, β2-microglobulin, and virological studies should be obtained.

Radiological examination: Detailed imaging studies including chest radiography and computed tomography (thoracic and abdominal) are required. X-ray-chest is obtained to detect mediastinal and hilar lymph node enlargement, pleural effusion, or pulmonary involvement. CT scan of chest, abdomen, and pelvis precisely determines the extent of disease. Newer technique of fluorodeoxyglucose positron emission tomography (FDG-PET) combined with computed tomography (PET-CT) is more specific and sensitive for staging and response to treatment.

Chest and abdominopelvic CT scan are done to detect occult nodal or extranodal disease.

Bone marrow biopsy: This is indicated in selected situations such as presence of B systemic symptoms and stage III/IV disease. Bilateral iliac crest bone marrow biopsy is performed to increase the chance of detection of bone marrow involvement. Bone marrow biopsy is generally not necessary in early stage disease and if PET-CT is negative.

Liver biopsy: Liver biopsy needs to be performed in all patients with stage III disease.

Course and Prognosis

Stage is the most important prognostic factor in classical Hodgkin's lymphoma. Stages I and II are called as early stage, while stages III and IV are called as advanced stage. Apart from staging other prognostic factors in CHL include age, bulky mediastinal disease, erythrocyte sedimentation rate, male sex, anemia, low albumin, leukocytosis, and lymphopenia. A newer prognostic factor is response to chemotherapy assessed by FDG-PET. Histological subtype of HL is not an independent prognostic factor. With current methods of treatment, 5-year survival of patients with early disease (stages IA and IIA) is about 95% with many of them possibly cured. In advanced disease (stages III and IV), 5-year survival is about 55%; however, in many patients with advanced stage disseminated disease, complete and durable remission can be achieved. However, patients with HL have increased risk of radiotherapy- or chemotherapy-induced malignancies such as cancer of lung, colon, breast, sarcomas, cancer in head or neck region, acute myeloid leukemia, and non-Hodgkin's lymphoma in 1% CHL cases (usually extranodal diffuse large B-cell lymphoma).

Treatment

Mode of therapy depends on stage of disease. Patients with early or localized HL are treated with curative intent. Patients with early-stage disease (IA or IIA) with no risk factors are treated with combined modality therapy (combined chemotherapy and radiotherapy). Four courses of chemotherapy (ABVD: adriamycin, bleomycin, vinblastine, dacarbazine) followed by involved field radiation is the standard form of treatment in these patients. In advanced stage disease (III, IV, bulky I and II), combination chemotherapy (six to eight cycles of ABVD) is the usual form of treatment. For a small group of patients who are refractory to primary therapy or who relapse later, high-dose chemotherapy and radiation followed by autologous stem cell rescue can be considered.

NON-HODGKIN'S LYMPHOMA

The non-Hodgkin's lymphomas are a heterogeneous group of neoplastic disorders of lymphoid tissue, which includes distinct categories, defined by clinical, morphological, immunological, and genetic characteristics. The incidence of non-Hodgkin's lymphomas has been rising, while that of Hodgkin's lymphomas has remained stable. The reasons for rise may be related to increasing elderly population, human immunodeficiency virus infection, increasing use of immunosuppressive therapy, and availability of better diagnostic tools.

Predisposing Factors

The exact cause of non-Hodgkin's lymphoma (NHL) is unknown; however, several disorders are associated with increased risk of development of NHL (Box 10.2).

Pathogenesis

During normal B-cell development, (antigen-independent) rearrangement of immunoglobulin (Ig) genes occurs in progenitor B cells in bone marrow. This consists of somatic recombination of V (variable), D (diversity), and J (joining) segments of Ig heavy chain genes, and of V and J

Box 10.2: Predisposing factors for non-Hodgkin's lymphoma.

Congenital disorders
- Ataxia telangiectasia
- Wiskott–Aldrich syndrome
- Severe combined immunodeficiency

Acquired disorders
- Organ transplant recipients
- Autoimmune disorders (Hashimoto's thyroiditis , Sjogren's syndrome, rheumatoid arthritis, systemic lupus erythematosus)
- Infections
  – Human immunodeficiency virus or HIV (diffuse large B-cell lymphoma, Burkitt lymphoma, central nervous system lymphoma)
  – *Helicobacter pylori* (gastric extranodal marginal zone lymphoma)
  – Epstein–Barr virus (endemic Burkitt lymphoma, classical Hodgkin's lymphoma, diffuse large B-cell lymphoma, primary central nervous system lymphoma associated with HIV)
  – Human T lymphotropic virus (adult T-cell leukemia/lymphoma)
  – Human herpes virus-8 (primary effusion lymphoma, plasmablastic lymphoma)
  – Hepatitis C virus (splenic marginal zone lymphoma)

segments of Ig light chain genes. These "naïve" B cells express both IgM and IgD on their surface and migrate to the germinal centers of lymphoid tissues. The variable region genes of these "naïve" B cells are unmutated since they have not been exposed to an antigen. After exposure to an antigen in germinal center, mutation of variable region genes occurs (so as to produce antibodies with increased affinity toward immunizing antigen). B cell with mutated variable region gene may survive as a memory B cell or may undergo class switching to IgG, IgA, or IgE. The later cells evolve into immunoglobulin-producing plasma cells. Somatically mutated variable region genes are found in majority of B-cell lymphomas (e.g. follicular lymphoma and Burkitt's lymphoma) indicating their origin from germinal center or postgerminal center B cells. Unmutated variable region genes in neoplastic cells indicate derivation from naïve B cells (e.g. mantle cell lymphoma and some cases of chronic lymphocytic leukemia/small lymphocytic lymphoma) (*see* Fig 1.20: Normal stages of B-cell development). In most cases of B-cell lymphomas, nature of inciting antigen is unknown. *Helicobacter pylori* is implicated in gastric MALT lymphoma, and hepatitis C virus in splenic marginal zone lymphomas.

Chromosomal translocations involving immunoglobulin heavy chain genes have been described in several types of B-cell lymphomas (*refer* to Tables 10.4 and 10.5). These translocations probably arise from errors of VDJ recombination, somatic hypermutation in germinal centers, or class switching. These translocations involve genes that regulate cell proliferation such as *MYC* or apoptosis such as *BCL2* and play a major role in the genesis of non-Hodgkin's lymphomas. In **Burkitt's lymphoma**, translocation between chromosomes 8 and 14 places *MYC* proto-oncogene close to transcriptionally active immunoglobulin locus. This leads to overexpression of MYC protein (Fig. 10.1). MYC is a transcription factor that controls growth-regulating genes.

Constitutive expression of MYC enhances cell proliferation. In **follicular lymphoma**, reciprocal translocation between chromosomes 14 and 18 moves *BCL-2* from chromosome 18 into transcriptionally active *IgH* gene. BCL-2 is an antiapoptotic protein. Overexpression of BCL-2 protein protects lymphocytes from cell death leading to their progressive accumulation (Fig. 10.2). In **mantle cell lymphoma**, gene for cyclin D on chromosome 11 is placed next to immunoglobulin heavy chain gene that is transcriptionally active. Cyclin D is a regulator of G1 phase of cell cycle and its overexpression leads to dysregulation of cell cycle.

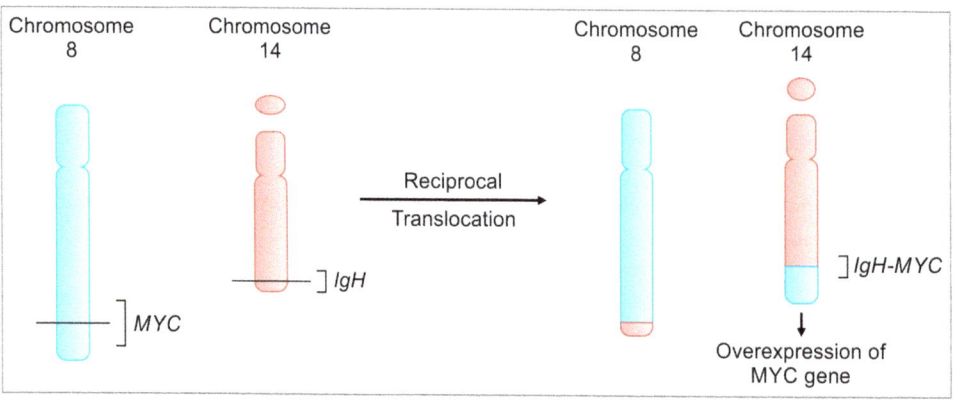

Fig. 10.1: Molecular events in pathogenesis of Burkitt lymphoma.

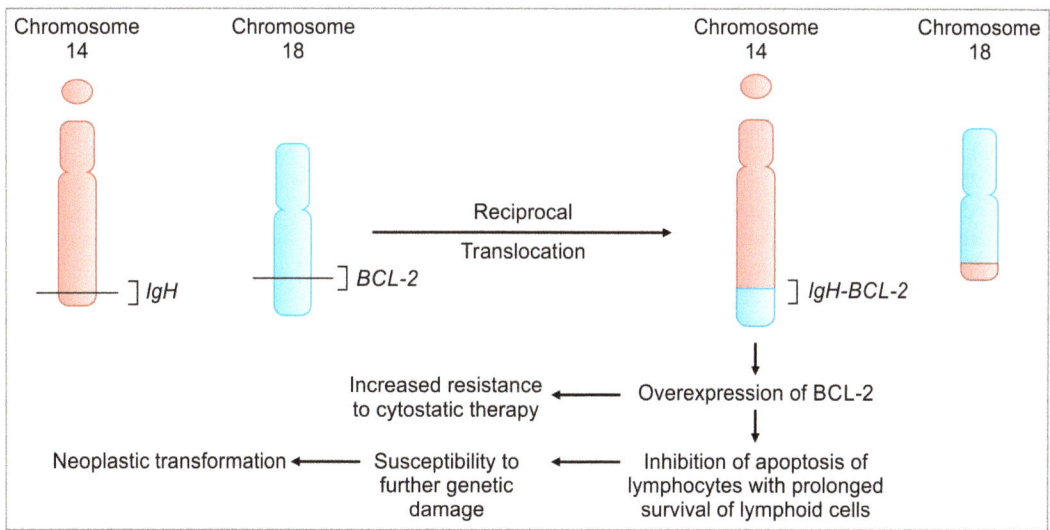

Fig. 10.2: Molecular events in pathogenesis of follicular lymphoma.

Classification of Non-Hodgkin's Lymphomas

Various classification schemes employing different terminology and criteria have been proposed for NHL, e.g. Rappaport (1956), Lukes-Collins (1974), Kiel (1975), Working formulation of non-Hodgkin's lymphomas for clinical usage (1982), Revised European-American classification of Lymphoid Neoplasms (REAL) (1994), and World Health Organization (WHO) classification (2001 and 2008).

The WHO classification (Box 10.3) is based on REAL classification, which was proposed by International Lymphoma Study Group. In this classification, distinct disease categories have been defined based on clinical, morphological, immunophenotypic, and genetic features. Each disease category has distinctive natural history and prognosis that allows planning of specific treatment.

> **Box 10.3:** WHO classification of lymphoid neoplasms (2016).
>
> **Precursor lymphoid neoplasms**
> - B-lymphoblastic leukemia/lymphoma, not otherwise specified
> - B-lymphoblastic leukemia/lymphoma with recurrent genetic abnormalities
> - T-lymphoblastic leukemia/lymphoma
> - NK-lymphoblastic leukemia/lymphoma
>
> **Mature B-cell neoplasms**
> - Chronic lymphocytic leukemia/small lymphocytic lymphoma
> - B-cell prolymphocytic leukemia
> - Splenic marginal zone lymphoma
> - Hairy cell leukemia
> - Splenic B-cell lymphoma/leukemia, unclassifiable
> - Lymphoplasmacytic lymphoma
> - IgM monoclonal gammopathy of undetermined significance
>
> *Contd...*

Contd...

- Heavy chain diseases
- Plasma cell neoplasms
- Extranodal marginal zone lymphoma of mucosa-associated lymphoid tissue (MALT lymphoma)
- Nodal marginal zone lymphoma
- Follicular lymphoma
- Pediatric-type follicular lymphoma
- Large B-cell lymphoma with *IRF4* rearrangement
- Primary cutaneous follicle center lymphoma
- Mantle cell lymphoma
- Diffuse large B-cell lymphoma (DLBCL), NOS
- T-cell/histiocyte-rich large B-cell lymphoma
- Primary diffuse large B-cell lymphoma of the CNS
- Primary cutaneous diffuse large B-cell lymphoma, leg type
- EBV-positive diffuse large B-cell lymphoma, NOS
- EBV-positive mucocutaneous ulcer
- Diffuse large B-cell lymphoma associated with chronic inflammation
- Lymphomatoid granulomatosis
- Primary mediastinal (thymic) large B-cell lymphoma
- Intravascular large B-cell lymphoma
- ALK-positive large B-cell lymphoma
- Plasmablastic lymphoma
- Primary effusion lymphoma
- HHV8-associated lymphoproliferative disorders
- Burkitt lymphoma
- Burkitt-like lymphoma with 11q aberration
- High-grade B-cell lymphoma
- B-cell lymphoma, unclassifiable, with features intermediate between DLBCL and classic Hodgkin lymphoma

Mature T- and NK-cell neoplasms

- T-cell prolymphocytic leukemia
- T-cell large granular lymphocytic leukemia
- Chronic lymphoproliferative disorder of NK cells
- Aggressive NK-cell leukemia
- EBV–positive T-cell and NK-cell lymphoproliferative diseases of childhood
- Adult T-cell leukemia/lymphoma
- Extranodal NK/T-cell lymphoma, nasal type
- Intestinal T-cell lymphoma
- Hepatosplenic T-cell lymphoma
- Subcutaneous panniculitis-like T-cell lymphoma
- Mycosis fungoides
- Sézary syndrome
- Primary cutaneous CD30-positive T-cell lymphoproliferative disorders
- Primary cutaneous peripheral T-cell lymphomas, rare subtypes
- Peripheral T-cell lymphoma, NOS
- Angioimmunoblastic T-cell lymphoma and other nodal lymphomas of T follicular helper (TFH) cell origin
- Anaplastic large cell lymphoma, ALK-positive
- Anaplastic large cell lymphoma, ALK-negative
- Breast implant–associated anaplastic large cell lymphoma

The two most common forms of NHL are follicular lymphoma and diffuse large B-cell lymphoma.

Currently, management is still based on biological behavior of the neoplasm like low-grade (indolent) or high-grade (aggressive or highly aggressive) (Box 10.4). With the introduction of WHO classification and newer therapies, it is expected that treatment will be directed against specific disease entities in future.

Salient features of some mature B- and T-cell neoplasms are given in Tables 10.4 and 10.5.

Clinical Features of NHL

The usual presentation of NHL is in the form of painless peripheral lymphadenopathy (commonly cervical or supraclavicular). Systemic symptoms

> **Box 10.4:** Categories of lymphomas/leukemias according to biological behavior.
>
> *Low-grade or indolent lymphomas/leukemias*
> - Chronic lymphocytic leukemia/Small lymphocytic lymphoma
> - Hairy cell leukemia
> - Lymphoplasmacytic lymphoma
> - Follicular lymphoma
> - Nodal marginal zone lymphoma
> - Splenic marginal zone lymphoma
> - Extranodal marginal zone B-cell lymphoma (MALT lymphoma)
>
> *Aggressive lymphomas/leukemias*
> - Precursor B- and T-cell neoplasms (B- or T-cell lymphoblastic lymphoma/leukemia)
> - Diffuse large B-cell lymphoma
> - Mantle cell lymphoma
> - Burkitt lymphoma
> - Adult T-cell lymphoma/leukemia
> - Extranodal NK/T-cell lymphoma
> - Hepatosplenic T-cell lymphoma
> - Subcutaneous panniculitis like T-cell lymphoma
> - Peripheral T-cell lymphoma, not otherwise specified
> - Anaplastic large cell lymphoma

Table 10.4: Salient features of mature B-cell neoplasms.

Disorder	Morphology of neoplastic cells	Immunophenotype	Genetic changes
Chronic lymphocytic leukemia/Small lymphocytic lymphoma	Small lymphocytes, round nuclei, dense chromatin	CD19+, CD20+(dim), surface IgM/IgD+(dim), CD79b+(dim), CD5+, CD23+, LEF1+, CD200+, CD10-, FMC7-, cyclin D1-	del(13q14), +12, del(11q22-23), del(17p13)
Splenic marginal zone lymphoma	Biphasic: small lymphocytes with round nuclei and scant cytoplasm (resembling mantle zone lymphocytes) and larger cells with irregular nuclei and moderate, pale cytoplasm (resembling marginal zone cells)	CD19+, CD20+, SIg+ (IgM±IgD), CD5-, CD10-, CD23-, CD43-, annexin A-, BCL6-, SOX11-, LEF1-, cyclin D1-	Allelic loss of 7q31-32 (40%)

Contd...

Contd...

Disorder	Morphology of neoplastic cells	Immunophenotype	Genetic changes
Hairy cell leukemia	Medium-sized cells, round/indented nuclei, hairy cytoplasmic projections	CD19+, CD22+, SIg+(bright), CD5–, CD10–, CD11c+ (bright), CD25+, CD103+, CD123+, annexin A1+	*BRAF V600E* (an oncogene located at chromosome 7q24) mutation
Lymphoplasmacytic lymphoma (Indolent)	Small lymphocytes, plasmacytoid lymphocytes, plasma cells	CD19+, CD20+, CD22+, CD79a+, PAX5+, FMC7+, Sig+; plasmacytic cells express cytoplasmic immunoglobulin, CD138, and MUM1. Unlike plasma cell myeloma, CD19 is positive and CD56 is negative	*MYD88* L265P mutation (90%)
Extranodal marginal zone lymphoma (Indolent)	Small lymphocytes, centrocyte-like cells, monocytoid cells, immunoblasts and centroblast-like cells, and sometimes plasma cells	CD19+, CD20+, sIgM+, CD43±	t(11;18)(q21;q21), t(1;14)(p22;q32), t(14;18)(q32;q21), t(3;14)(p14;q32)
Nodular marginal zone lymphoma (Indolent)	Smaller cells (monocytoid, centrocyte-like, and plasmacytoid) and larger lymphoid cells (blasts)	CD19+, CD20+, CD79a+, monotypic Ig (usually IgM without IgD), CD10-, CD5-, CD23-, BCL6-, CD43+ (50% cases), BCL2+ (weak)	+3, +8, +18
Follicular lymphoma (Indolent)	Centrocytes and centroblasts with cleaved nuclei	CD19+, CD20+ (bright), CD22+, CD79a+, PAX5+, sIg+, CD10+, BCL6+, and BCL2+, CD5-, CD43-.	t(14;18)(q32;q21) (85% cases), overexpression of cytoplasmic BCL2 protein
Mantle cell lymphoma	Monotonous small to medium-sized lymphoid cells with irregular nuclear contours	CD19+, CD20+, sIg+, CD5+, CD43+, SOX11+, Cyclin D1+, CD10-, BCL6-, CD23-	(11;14)(q13;q32) involving *CCND1* and *IGH* in virtually all cases
Diffuse large B-cell lymphoma (DLBCL), not otherwise specified	Medium to large cells with nucleus twice the size of a small lymphocyte	CD19+, CD20+, CD22+, CD79a+, PAX5+, sIg+, BCL6+ (subset), CD10+ (subset), BCL2+ (subset), MYC+ (subset)	t(14;18) (q32;q21) involving *BCL2* in 25%, t(3;14)(q27;q32) involving *BCL6* in 30%
Plasmablastic lymphoma	Plasmablasts or immunoblasts (Usually in HIV+ patients; often extranodal; often EBV+)	CD45–, CD20-, PAX5-, CD3–, CD38+, CD138+, IRF4/MUM1+, CD56-, high Ki67	*MYC* translocations (50% cases)

Contd...

Contd...

Disorder	Morphology of neoplastic cells	Immunophenotype	Genetic changes
Primary effusion lymphoma	Large cells with plasmablastic and anaplastic morphology (HHV8+)	CD45+, CD19-, CD20-, CD79a-, sIg-, CD30+, HLADR+	No recurrent abnormalities
Burkitt lymphoma	Monomorphic medium cells in diffuse pattern, basophilic cytoplasm with vacuoles	CD19+, CD20+, CD10+, BCL6+, CD5-, BCL2-, sIg+, BCL2-, Ki67+ in 100% cells	t(8;14)(q24;q32), t(8;22)(q24;q11), or t(2;8)(p12;q24) involving Ig loci and C-MYC at 8q24

Table 10.5: Salient features of mature T/NK cell neoplasms.

Disorder	Morphology of neoplastic cells	Immunophenotype	Genetic changes
T-cell large granular lymphocytic leukemia	Large granular lymphocytes with moderate to abundant cytoplasm and fine or course azurophilic granules	CD2+, CD3+, CD5+, CD7+, CD8+, CD16+, CD4-, CD56-	STAT3 mutations in 75% cases
Adult T-cell leukemia/lymphoma	Highly pleomorphic with multilobed nuclei	CD2+, CD3+, CD5+, CD7-, CD25+, FOXP3+ ; CD4+/CD8- more common than CD4-/CD8+	No specific abnormality; association with HTLV1 infection
Extranodal NK/T-cell lymphoma, nasal type	Angiocentric and angiodestructive infiltrate of atypical lymphocytes	CD45+, CD2+, cytoplasmic CD3+, CD4-, CD8-, CD5-/+, CD7+, CD56+, EBV+	No specific abnormality
Hepatosplenic T-cell lymphoma	Monotonous, medium cells with condensed chromatin	CD2+, CD3+, CD4-, CD5+, CD7±, CD8± EBV-	Isochromosome 7q
Subcutaneous panniculitis-like T-cell lymphoma	Lobular panniculitic infiltrate of pleomorphic lymphocytes of variable size	CD2+, CD3+, CD4-, CD8+, CD5+, CD7-, cytotoxic markers (perforin, granzyme, and TIA-1)	No specific abnormality
Mycosis fungoides	Small to medium lymphocytes with cerebriform nuclei	T helper phenotype is common, i.e. CD2+, CD3+,TCR beta+, CD4+, CD8-, TCR gamma-; aberrant loss of CD5 and/or CD7 often; rarely cytotoxic phenotype, i.e. CD8+ and/or TCR gamma+	Clonal rearrangement of TCR genes
Sezary syndrome	As above	As above	As above
Anaplastic large cell lymphoma (ALCL)	Large lymphoid cells with abundant cytoplasm and often horseshoe-shaped nuclei with prominent nucleoli ("hallmark" cells)	T-cell phenotype, CD30+, ALK+ (70-80%), ALK- (20–30%)	t(2;5)(p23;q35) in ALK+ ALCL(80%); DUSP22(IRF4) or TP63 rearrangement in some ALK- ALCL

are seen in advanced stage disease and indicate poor prognosis. The salient features, which distinguish NHL from Hodgkin's lymphoma, are given earlier. Involvement of multiple peripheral lymph nodes with or without hepatosplenomegaly, extranodal disease (e.g. head, neck, gastrointestinal tract, skin, testis, CNS), and dissemination to bone marrow are more commonly observed in NHL than in HL. At presentation, many patients with NHL are in stage III or IV. Mediastinal mass (lymphoblastic lymphoma), jaw tumor (African Burkitt's lymphoma), skin plaques or nodules (mycosis fungoides) are other manifestations.

Patients with low-grade NHL (Box 10.4) have gradual progression of their disease and often have a long history. Patients may present with disseminated disease, disease limited to lymph nodes, or limited to extranodal location. Low-grade lymphomas have a tendency to recur, and transformation to a high-grade lymphoma can occur after some years.

Extranodal lymphomas are lymphomas arising at sites other than lymphoid structures. Common sites are—gastrointestinal tract (most common site especially stomach followed by small intestine, colon, and esophagus), lung, thyroid, salivary glands, and skin. Some of them originate from previous non-neoplastic disorder, e.g. *Helicobacter pylori* infection of stomach, autoimmune disorders, ulcerative colitis, etc. They are slowly growing tumors and remain localized for long duration. Surgery and radiotherapy are the usual forms of treatment and often control the disease.

Patients with high-grade or aggressive lymphoma have rapid progression of their disease that is often fatal if untreated. Systemic symptoms (fever, weight loss, night sweats) are commonly present at diagnosis.

Laboratory Investigations

Lymph Node Biopsy

If lymphadenopathy is generalized, lower cervical or axillary lymph nodes are selected. Biopsy of inguinal lymph nodes is usually avoided due to frequent presence of chronic nonspecific inflammation and fibrosis. The largest lymph node in the area should be excised. Excisional biopsy should be preferred over needle or core biopsy due to difficulty in interpretation of architecture. Distortion of lymph node should be avoided during removal. Sometimes radiologically guided biopsy may be required for deep-seated abdominal or thoracic lesions. Touch imprint preparations are recommended for cytological examination which can be helpful in diagnosis of certain lymphomas, reactive conditions, and infections. Routinely, biopsied lymph node is fixed in 10% formol saline for paraffin embedding followed by hematoxylin and eosin staining.

Studies performed on biopsied lymph node are as follows:
- Morphological examination
- Immunophenotyping: For subclassification into B- or T-cell and further types.
- Cytogenetic analysis: For detection of chromosomal abnormalities
- Molecular studies: For gene rearrangement studies
- Electron microscopy: For distinction between NHL and undifferentiated tumors

Fine Needle Aspiration Cytology

FNAC of lymph node is mainly used as a screening tool for lymphomas and final diagnosis and lymphoma classification is based on biopsy. Role of cytomorphology on FNAC for diagnosis of lymphoma is limited due to inability to assess architecture. Ancillary studies like immunocytochemistry, flow cytometry, and molecular studies can be done FNAC samples and can increase diagnostic accuracy of FNAC in lymphoma cases.

Hematological Investigations

In all suspected cases of lymphoma, complete blood count and blood smear examination are initial investigations before biopsy. These are to rule out leukemia (in leukemia, lymph node biopsy is unnecessary for diagnosis) and to exclude lymphoma mimics (such as infectious mononucleosis). Bone marrow examination in NHL is mainly useful for determining the extent of disease or staging; involvement of bone marrow indicates stage IV disease.

Trephine bone marrow biopsy is preferred over marrow aspiration smears for assessment of marrow involvement. Bilateral posterior iliac crest trephine bone marrow biopsies have been advocated to increase the yield of positive bone marrow.

At presentation, marrow involvement in NHL occurs in about 50% cases. Involvement of bone marrow is common with certain types such as small lymphocytic, plasmacytoid lymphocytic, follicular small-cleaved cell, and lymphoblastic lymphomas.

Pattern of infiltration in bone marrow may be focal paratrabecular, focal nonparatrabecular (random), interstitial, or diffuse. Focal paratrabecular pattern consists of infiltration along the bony trabeculae. In focal nonparatrabecular pattern, lymphoma cells form nodules, which do not completely fill the intertrabecular space. In interstitial pattern, single or small groups of neoplastic cells infiltrate in between normal hematopoietic elements. Diffuse pattern consists of complete replacement of whole intertrabecular space by lymphoma cells.

Usually low-grade lymphomas (small lymphocytic and follicular small cleaved cell) show a focal (paratrabecular or nonparatrabecular) pattern of infiltration while high-grade (lymphoblastic and small noncleaved cell) lymphomas show a diffuse pattern.

Immunophenotyping

Identification of combination of cellular antigens (surface, cytoplasmic, or nuclear) present on a particular cell with the help of specific antibodies is called as immunophenotyping. It can be done on frozen or paraffin-embedded tissue sections or by flow cytometric analysis of cell suspensions. Applications of immunophenotyping in NHL are: (i) To differentiate neoplastic from non-neoplastic proliferation of lymphocytes, e.g. assessment of ratio of kappa to lambda light chains is helpful to demonstrate clonality in B-cell neoplasms; light chain restriction is indicative of neoplastic proliferation; (ii) to differentiate lymphoma from undifferentiated neoplasms; (iii) to identify lineage (B or T cell) and the stage of differentiation of neoplastic cells, and (iv) to assess prognosis and survival in certain lymphomas.

Cytogenetic Analysis

With recent techniques, cytogenetic abnormalities can be identified in majority of patients with NHL. Common cytogenetic abnormalities are presented (*see* Tables 10.4). Some of the cytogenetic abnormalities are consistently observed in specific morphologic subtypes of NHL and play a role in the pathogenesis of lymphomas.

Gene Rearrangement Studies

Southern blot analysis using complementary DNA probes can be used to detect rearrangement of immunoglobulin or T-cell receptor genes. Immunoglobulin gene rearrangement is indicative of B-cell nature, while TCR gene rearrangement is indicative of T-cell nature of the neoplasm. Uses of gene rearrangement studies are:

i. To differentiate neoplastic from non-neoplastic proliferation of lymphocytes. TCR gene rearrangement is the only technique available for establishing clonal nature of T-cell neoplasms;
ii. To distinguish lymphoma from undifferentiated neoplasms;
iii. To identify lineage (B or T) of lymphoid cells.

Gene rearrangement studies are especially useful in those cases in which surface antigen analysis by antibodies fails to establish the lineage or clonality of the disease.

Investigations for diagnosis of NHL are outlined in Box 10.5.

Staging of NHL

Staging is necessary to plan treatment, assign prognosis, and for post-treatment evaluation. The Ann Arbor staging system for Hodgkin's lymphoma can also be used for non-Hodgkin's lymphoma. However, as mode of spread of NHL is non-contiguous and unpredictable and as progression to distant sites occurs early, this staging system is less useful for NHL. Most patients with NHL have stage III or IV disease at presentation, and localized stage I or II disease is rare. Thus, staging is not critical for majority of cases as chemotherapy is the mainstay of treatment and radiotherapy alone is rarely indicated. Staging investigations are given in Box 10.6

An International Prognostic Index (IPI) is commonly used in aggressive NHL. This is based on age, stage (Ann Arbor), number of extranodal sites of disease, performance status, and serum

Box 10.5: Diagnosis of non-Hodgkin's lymphoma.

- Complete blood count including blood smear: This is done to rule out leukemia (e.g. CLL) and reactive conditions clinically mimicking lymphoma. Bone marrow examination may be required in some cases.
- Excisional lymph node biopsy: This is subjected to morphological examination, immunophenotypic analysis (for validation of diagnosis, determination of lineage and degree of maturation of neoplastic cells, and assessment of prognosis), and cytogenetic and molecular studies (for assessing clonality, genetic abnormalities, and prognosis).
- Integration and correlation of clinical, hematological, morphological, immunological, cytogenetic, and molecular studies to reach final diagnosis.

Box 10.6: Staging investigations in non-Hodgkin's lymphoma.

- History (B systemic symptoms), physical examination (sites of disease)
- Complete blood count, blood smear (for spillover, cytopenias, hemolysis), bilateral bone marrow aspiration and biopsy (for infiltration)
- Chest X-ray (for mediastinal adenopathy, pleural effusion, lung involvement)
- Abdominopelvic CT scan (to assess lymphadenopathy and other organs)
- Biochemical tests: liver and kidney function tests, lactate dehydrogenase
- In selected cases, CT scan of chest (for precise delineation of disease if chest X-ray is abnormal), bone scan and skeletal X-rays (if bone pain, tenderness), magnetic resonance imaging (CNS involvement), CSF examination (in high-grade lymphomas)

lactate dehydrogenase level. Four risk groups are identified using a scoring system: low, low intermediate, high intermediate, and high with predicted 5-year survival of groups being 73%, 51%, 43%, and 26%, respectively. Such a system can help in treatment planning according to the risk group, e.g. in high-risk patients, intensive or experimental form of therapy can be tried, while in low-risk patients, intensive therapy is not warranted and established form of therapy is appropriate.

Treatment of NHL

Treatment of NHL is based on histological subtype, grade of lymphoma, stage of disease, and measurable prognostic factors.

Low-Grade NHL

Those patients who have localized disease (stage I or II) are treated with involved field radiotherapy. This leads to prolonged disease-free survival in 50% of patients.

Most patients with low-grade NHL have advanced (stage III or IV) disease at presentation. In many centers, treatment is not initiated until evidence of disease progression develops (wait and watch policy). This is because low-grade NHLs are indolent neoplasms that are incurable and a period of deferral of treatment does not adversely affect the survival. Treatment options are single alkylating drug therapy.

There is increasing evidence that *Helicobacter pylori*-associated gastric MALT lymphoma can be successfully treated with antibiotics alone.

Aggressive NHL

Currently, cure can be achieved in many patients with combined chemotherapy and/or radiotherapy. Intensive combination chemotherapy is instituted immediately after diagnosis and staging. About 50 to 60% achieve complete remission and a proportion of them are probably cured. The standard regimen is CHOP (cyclophosphamide, doxorubicin, vincristine, prednisolone). Patients who relapse can be considered for high-dose chemotherapy followed by autologous bone marrow transplantation.

Intensive multiagent chemotherapy is needed for very aggressive lymphoblastic lymphoma and Burkitt's lymphoma, which often spread to CNS and bone marrow.

BIBLIOGRAPHY

1. Bennett MH, MacLennan KA, Easterling MJ, et al. The prognostic significance of cellular subtypes in nodular sclerosing Hodgkin's disease:An analysis of 271 nonlaparotomised cases (BNLI report no. 22). Clin Radiol. 1983;34:497-501.
2. Carbone PP, Kaplan HS, Musshoff K, et al. Report of the Committee on Hodgkin's lymphoma Staging Classification. Cancer Res. 1971;31:1860-61.
3. Carde P. Hodgkin's lymphoma I. Identification and classification. Br Med J. 1992;305:99.
4. Haybittle JL, Hayhoe FG, Easterling MJ, et al. Review of British National Lymphoma Investigation studies of Hodgkin's disease and development of prognostic index. Lancet. 1985;1:967-72.
5. Jaffe ES, Harris NL, Stein H, et al. (Eds). World Health Organization Classification of Tumours. Pathology and Genetics of Tumours of Haematopoietic and Lymphoid Tissues. Lyon. IARC Press. 2001.

6. Kuppers R, Klein U, Hansmann ML, et al. Cellular origin of human B-cell lymphomas. N Engl J Med. 1999;341:1520-29.
7. Lister TA, Crowther D, Sutcliffe SB, et al. Report of a committee convened to discuss the evaluation and staging of patients with Hodgkin's disease:Cotswolds meeting. J Clin Oncol. 1989;7:1630-36.
8. Lukes RJ, Butler JJ. The pathology and nomenclature of Hodgkin's disease. Cancer Res. 1966;26:1063-83.
9. Lukes RJ, Craver L, Hall T, et al. Report of the nomenclature committee. Cancer Res. 1966;26:1311.
10. Mounter PJ, Lennard AL. Management of non-Hodgkin's lymphomas. Postgrad Med J. 1999;75:2-6.
11. Skarin AT, Dorfman DM. Non-Hodgkin's lymphomas:Current classification and management. CA Cancer J Clin. 1997;47:351-72.
12. Swerdlow SH, Campo E, Harris NL, et al (Eds). WHO Classification of Tumours of Haematopoietic and Lymphoid Tissues. Revised 4th Ed. Lyon. France. IARC Press. 2017.
13. Swerdlow SH, Campo E, Harris NL, et al. (Eds). WHO classification of tumours of haematopoietic and lymphoid tissues. 4th ed. Lyon. International Agency for Research on Cancer. 2008.
14. Urba WJ, Longo DL:Hodgkin's lymphoma. N Engl J Med. 1992;326:678-87.

CHAPTER 11

Quantitative and Qualitative Disorders of Leukocytes

Disorders of leukocytes may be quantitative or qualitative. Quantitative disorders are related to the concentration of leukocytes (leukocyte counts) in peripheral blood. Qualitative disorders refer to the structural or functional abnormalities of white blood cells.

Leukocytosis is defined as an increase in the number of circulating leukocytes (total leukocyte count) above the upper level of normal. *Leukopenia* refers to total leukocyte count below the lower limit of normal. An absolute rise or fall in the count can affect any white blood cell in peripheral blood, i.e. neutrophil, eosinophil, basophil, monocyte, or lymphocyte (Box 11.1). *Leukoerythroblastic reaction* refers to the presence of immature white blood cells as well as nucleated red cells in peripheral blood. *Leukemoid reaction* refers to the presence of markedly increased leukocyte count (>50,000/mm^3) and immature white blood cells in peripheral blood resembling leukemia but occurring in nonleukemic conditions.

Box 11.1: Quantitative disorders of leukocytes.

Values in adults
- Leukocytosis: Total leukocyte count >11,000/mm^3
- Leukopenia: Total leukocyte count <4,000/mm^3
- Neutrophilia: Absolute neutrophil count >7,500/mm^3
- Neutropenia: Absolute neutrophil count <2,000/mm^3
- Lymphocytosis: Absolute lymphocyte count >4,000/mm^3
- Lymphocytopenia: Absolute lymphocyte count <1,500/mm^3
- Eosinophilia: Absolute eosinophil count >600/mm^3
- Monocytosis: Absolute monocyte count >1,000/mm^3
- Basophilia: Absolute basophil count >100/mm^3

DISORDERS OF GRANULOCYTES

NEUTROPHILIA

Neutrophilia or neutrophilic leukocytosis (Fig. 11.1) is an increase in the absolute neutrophil count above normal level (usually >7,500/mm^3). Causes of neutrophilia are listed in Box 11.2.

Section 3: Disorders of White Blood Cells

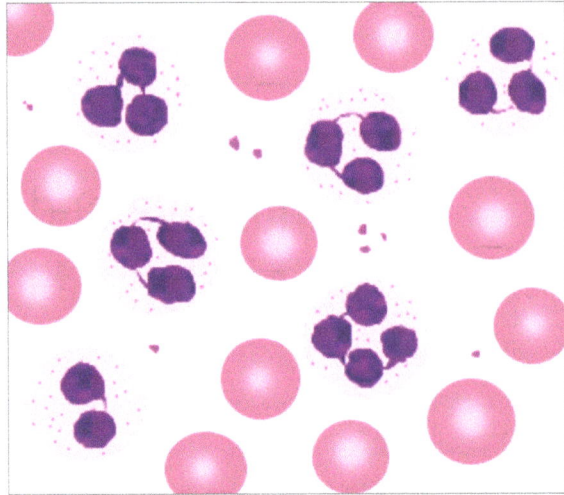

Fig. 11.1: Blood smear showing neutrophilia.

Box 11.2: Causes of neutrophilia or neutrophilic leukocytosis.

- Physiological: Newborns, pregnancy, stress, exercise
- Bacterial infections, especially pyogenic
- Tissue destruction: Surgical or other trauma, burns, myocardial infarction
- Inflammatory disorders: Vasculitis, myositis, rheumatoid arthritis
- Acute hemorrhage
- Acute hemolysis
- Metabolic disorders: Acidosis, uremia, toxins, gout
- Drugs: Corticosteroids, lithium, β-agonists, myeloid growth factors
- Solid tumors
- Hematological malignancies: Myeloproliferative neoplasms, chronic myelomonocytic leukemia, acute myeloid leukemia
- Rare inherited disorders: Down syndrome (transient myeloproliferative disorder), hereditary neutrophilia, congenital leukocyte adhesion deficiency
- Other: Cigarette smoking, asplenia

The most common cause of neutrophilic leukocytosis is bacterial infections particularly by Gram-positive cocci. Bacterial infections are frequently associated with following alterations in peripheral blood—(1) neutrophilic leukocytosis (Fig. 11.1) with shift to left (Figs. 11.2 and 11.3): Although segmented neutrophils are mainly increased some band forms and occasional metamyelocyte may be found; (2) toxic granules (*refer to* Figs. 11.4 and 11.6): These are dark blue or purple granules in the cytoplasm of segmented neutrophils, band forms, and metamyelocytes. They represent azurophil granules; toxic granules probably result from impaired cytoplasmic maturation while generating large number of neutrophils; (3) Döhle inclusion bodies: These are small, pale blue inclusion bodies in the periphery of cytoplasm of neutrophils (*see* Fig. 11.6). They represent rows of rough endoplasmic reticulum; (4) Cytoplasmic vacuoles: They are indicative of phagocytosis.

Chapter 11: Quantitative and Qualitative Disorders of Leukocytes

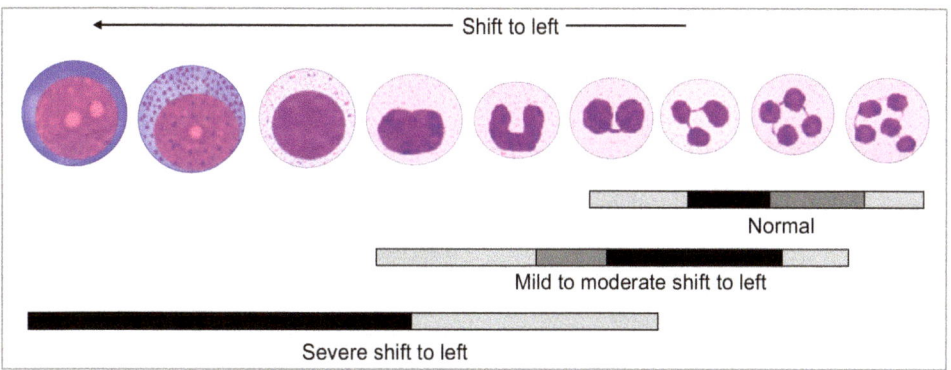

Fig. 11.2: Shift to left in neutrophil series. Normally neutrophils with three lobes predominate, while some have four lobes and only a few have two or five lobes. In mild-to-moderate left shift, immature cells are limited to band forms and metamyelocytes. In severe left shift, immature cells like myeloblast, promyelocytes, and myelocytes are also seen.

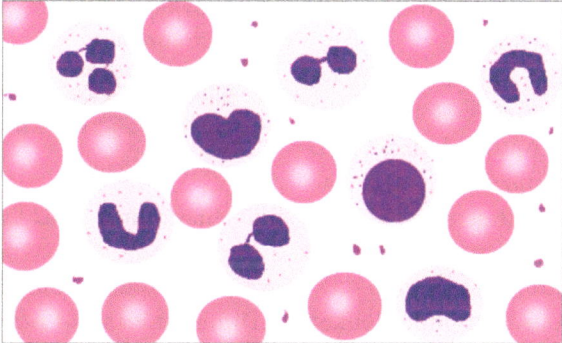

Fig. 11.3: Blood smear showing shift to left in neutrophils.

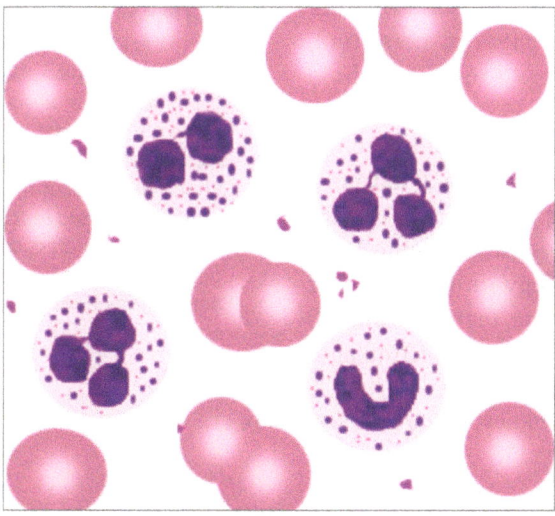

Fig. 11.4: Toxic granules in neutrophils.

In heat stroke, severe burns, and in hyperthermia (due to brain stem hemorrhage), neutrophil nuclei assume a "botryoid" morphology (nucleus resembling a bunch of grapes).

LEUKOERYTHROBLASTIC REACTION

Presence of immature cells of neutrophil series and nucleated red blood cells in peripheral blood (see Fig. 3.20) can be due to various causes (Box 11.3). Total leukocyte count may be normal or raised.

Bone marrow examination may be required to establish the underlying cause.

Box 11.3: Causes of leukoerythroblastic reaction.

Infectious diseases: Miliary tuberculosis
Cancers metastatic to bone marrow: Carcinomas of lung, breast, prostate, gastrointestinal tract, thyroid, kidney
Hematological disorders
- Myelofibrosis
- Severe hemolysis, e.g. erythroblastosis fetalis
- Lymphoma
- Myeloma
- Severe megaloblastic anemia
- Thalassemia major

Storage disorders
- Gaucher's disease
- Niemann-Pick disease

Osteopetrosis (Albers-Schönberg disease, marble bone disease)

LEUKEMOID REACTION

Definition is given earlier. It is of two types—myeloid and lymphoid (Box 11.4).

In myeloid type, blood picture resembles either acute or chronic myeloid leukemia (CML). Marked neutrophilic leukocytosis with presence of premature white cells of all stages (from myeloblasts to segmented neutrophils) may mimic CML. Differentiation of CML from leukemoid reaction is given in Table 7.2.

Lymphoid leukemoid reaction is one in which peripheral blood picture resembles that of acute or chronic lymphoid leukemia. Differentiation of reactive lymphocytosis from chronic lymphocytic leukemia may sometimes be difficult and patient may have to be followed up to decide whether lymphocytosis is transient or persistent. (See also chapter on "Chronic lymphoid leukemia.")

Differentiation of leukemoid reaction from acute (myeloid or lymphoid) leukemia is made by following features: (1) clinical presentation, (2) presence of underlying disease, (3) morphology on blood smear, (4) % of blasts in bone marrow, and (5) correction of leukemoid blood picture after treatment of underlying disease.

Box 11.4: Causes of leukemoid reaction.

Myeloid leukemoid reaction
- Severe bacterial infection (e.g. pneumonia, endocarditis, septicemia)
- Severe acute hemolysis
- Severe hemorrhage
- Cancer metastatic to bone marrow
- Other: Eclampsia, burns, mercury poisoning

Lymphoid leukemoid reaction
- Viral infections: Infectious mononucleosis, infectious lymphocytosis
- Bacterial infections: Tuberculosis, whooping cough

Terms related to leukocytosis are shown in Box 11.5.

Box 11.5: Terms related to leukocytosis.

- *Leukocytosis:* Total leukocyte count above the upper limit of normal for age
- *Shift to left:* Increased percentage of immature granulocytes in peripheral blood (usually up to bands and metamyelocytes)
- *Leukemoid reaction (myeloid type):* Marked leukocytosis (total leukocyte count >50,000/mm^3) with presence of immature granulocytes in peripheral blood (up to promyelocytes or blasts)
- *Leukoerythroblastic reaction:* Presence of immature granulocytes and nucleated red cells in peripheral blood; total leukocyte count may or may not be high
- *Hyperleukocytosis:* Total leukocyte >100,000/mm^3; it is seen almost exclusively in acute leukemia (especially AML) and myeloproliferative neoplasms; it can result in life-threatening cerebral infarcts or pulmonary insufficiency due to sludging of blood flow in small vessels
- *Pseudoneutrophilia:* Leukocytosis following vigorous exercise and acute physical or emotional stress; it results from shift of cells (neutrophils, monocytes, and lymphocytes) from the marginal to the circulating pool.

NEUTROPENIA

Neutropenia refers to reduction in the number of neutrophils in the peripheral blood below the normal level (<2,000/mm^3).

Absolute neutrophil count more than 1,000/mm^3 is usually considered as sufficient for phagocytic function of neutrophils. Neutropenia has been divided into three grades as shown in Table 11.1.

Important causes of neutropenia are given in Box 11.6.

Neutropenia due to drugs may be dose-related or idiosyncratic. Idiosyncratic neutropenia commonly occurs with following drugs—aminopyrine, phenylbutazone, chloramphenicol, sulfonamides, penicillin, antithyroid drugs, and phenothiazines. Antigens on fetal granulocytes may enter maternal circulation and induce formation of antineutrophil antibodies. Transplacental passage of these antibodies from maternal to fetal circulation can cause neonatal isoimmune neutropenia analogous to Rh hemolytic disease.

Pancytopenia is a common laboratory manifestation of megaloblastic anemia. Folic acid or vitamin B$_{12}$ deficiency causes defective maturation of hematopoietic cells, which are destroyed prematurely in bone marrow (ineffective hematopoiesis). Although bone marrow is hypercellular, there is peripheral blood cytopenia. Diagnosis is based on presence of macrocytosis and hypersegmented neutrophils in blood, megaloblastic maturation in marrow, and low levels of vitamin B$_{12}$ or folate. In megaloblastic anemia, neutropenia is usually mild.

Hematologic malignancies, myelodysplasia, and aplastic anemia require bone marrow examination for diagnosis.

Table 11.1: Grading of neutropenia.

Grade	Neutrophil count	Risk of infection
Mild	1,500–1,000/mm^3	No increased risk
Moderate	1,000–500/mm^3	Mild risk
Severe	<500/mm^3	Significant risk

> **Box 11.6:** Causes of neutropenia.
>
> 1. **Infections:** Overwhelming bacterial infections, septicemia, miliary tuberculosis, human immunodeficiency virus infection, influenza, infectious mononucleosis
> 2. **Drugs:** Antimicrobials (sulfonamides, chloramphenicol), analgesics (phenylbutazone, oxyphenbutazone), phenytoin, antithyroid drugs, cytotoxic drugs
> 3. **Immune neutropenia:** Felty's syndrome, systemic lupus erythematosus, neonatal isoimmune neutropenia, drug-induced
> 4. **Ineffective hematopoiesis:** Megaloblastic anemia
> 5. **Abnormal pooling:** Hypersplenism
> 6. **Bone marrow replacement:** Leukemia, chronic myeloproliferative disorders, myelodysplastic syndrome, myeloma, lymphoma
> 7. **Bone marrow hypoplasia:** Aplastic anemia
> 8. **Other rare conditions:** Cyclic neutropenia, Kostmann syndrome, chronic familial neutropenia, Fanconi anemia, Shwachman-Diamond syndrome, dyskeratosis congenita, myelokathexis

Kostmann syndrome is characterized by severe neutropenia at birth along with maturation arrest at promyelocyte stage. Inheritance may be autosomal recessive (mutation in *HAX1* gene) or autosomal dominant (mutation in *ELA2 or ELANE* gene). Various other mutations have also been described. Mainstay of treatment is administration of G-CSF and antibiotics; hematopoietic stem cell transplantation may be curative for those who fail to respond to G-CSF. There is a risk of transformation to myelodysplasia or AML.

Repetitive and periodic neutropenia and infections occur (usually every 3 weeks) in cyclic neutropenia. Neutrophil count returns to normal between attacks. This is a rare hereditary disease that manifests in childhood with autosomal dominant mode of inheritance. Cyclic neutropenia results from mutation in *ELA*2 gene (gene for neutrophil elastase). There is a transient arrest at promyelocyte stage before each cycle. G-CSF is the effective form of treatment.

In chronic familial neutropenia, neutrophil count is lower than "normal" in some ethnic groups but is not associated with any risk of infections.

Clinical Features

Clinical manifestations are related to the underlying disorder and neutropenia. Common sites of infection in neutropenia are skin, urinary tract, respiratory tract, and oral cavity.

Agranulocytosis is a clinical syndrome characterized by rapidly developing severe neutropenia in peripheral blood, along with fever, prostration, and painful necrotic ulcerations in oral and pharyngeal mucosa. It is of drug-induced origin.

EOSINOPHILIA

Eosinophilia refers to increase in the absolute eosinophil count in the peripheral blood above $600/mm^3$ (Fig. 11.5). Causes of eosinophilia are given in Box 11.7.

In allergic disorders, eosinophilia is transient and moderate. IgE causes release of granules from basophils and mast cells that contain chemotactic factors for eosinophils.

Eosinophilia is a regular feature of helminthic infections, particularly if the parasite invades tissues. Parasites within the lumen of the intestine or encysted parasites do not evoke significant eosinophilic response.

Loeffler's syndrome consists of transient lung infiltrates on X-ray chest, eosinophilia, and cough. It is usually caused by migration of helminth larva through the lungs.

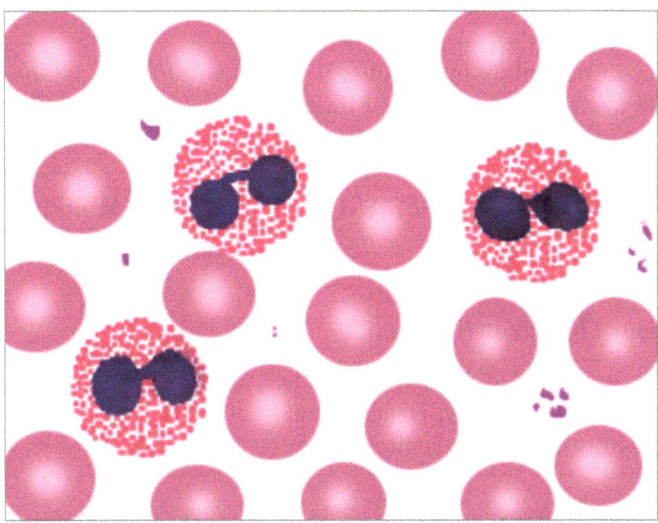

Fig. 11.5: Eosinophils in peripheral blood.

Box 11.7: Causes of eosinophilia.

1. Allergic diseases: Asthma, urticaria, rhinitis, drug reactions
2. Parasites: Filaria, trichinosis, toxocariasis, strongyloidosis, echinococcosis
3. Dermatologic disorders: Eczema, dermatitis herpetiformis, bullous pemphigoid
4. Carcinomas after radiotherapy
5. Pulmonary disorders: Loeffler's syndrome, tropical eosinophilia
6. Hematologic malignancies: Myeloproliferative disorders, Hodgkin's disease, eosinophilic leukemia, peripheral T-cell lymphoma
7. Hypereosinophilic syndrome

Tropical pulmonary eosinophilia occurs mainly in filaria-endemic regions (e.g. India, Southeast Asia) and is characterized by episodic cough with wheezing, lung infiltrates, and severe eosinophilia. High levels of antifilarial antibodies are present in the blood. Treatment is with diethylcarbamazine.

Hypereosinophilic syndrome is defined as persistent, high eosinophilia (>1,500/mm^3 for more than 6 months) without any identifiable cause and is present along with evidence of organ involvement and dysfunction. Organ damage results from tissue infiltration by eosinophils and from cytokines released from eosinophil granules. Organs commonly affected are heart, lungs, central nervous system, skin, and gastrointestinal tract. Treatment consists of corticosteroids, hydroxyurea, or α-interferon. Cardiac failure is the usual cause of death.

Both hypereosinophilic syndrome and chronic eosinophilic leukemia are associated with marked eosinophilia and organ involvement. Chronic eosinophilic leukemia is characterized by increased blasts or presence of a clonal genetic abnormality. Hypereosinophilic syndrome, on the other hand, is a diagnosis of exclusion and is not associated with increased blasts or clonal abnormality.

BASOPHILIA

Increased number of basophils in peripheral blood (>100/mm³) is observed in chronic myeloproliferative disorders especially CML, basophilic leukemia, IgE-mediated allergic disorders, ulcerative colitis, and hypothyroidism.

DISORDERS OF PHAGOCYTIC LEUKOCYTES CHARACTERIZED BY MORPHOLOGIC CHANGES

These may be acquired or hereditary.

Acquired Morphologic Changes in Neutrophils

These include toxic granules, Döhle inclusion bodies, and cytoplasmic vacuoles that are seen in bacterial infections (Fig. 11.6). Hypersegmentation of nuclei (≥5 lobes in >5% neutrophils) is a characteristic feature of megaloblastic anemia.

Inherited Morphologic Changes

Pelger-Huet Anomaly

In this autosomal dominant disorder, nuclear segmentation does not occur in granulocytes. Granulocyte nuclei may be rod-like, round, or at the most with two segments or two lobes (spectacle-like or "pince-nez" nuclei) (Fig. 11.6). Survival and function of these granulocytes is normal. The abnormality results from mutation in laminin B receptor (LBR) gene located on chromosome 1q41-q43. Such granulocytes are also seen in some acquired disorders particularly myelodysplastic syndrome, acute myeloid leukemia, and myeloproliferative disorders and are then called as pseudo-Pelger-Huet cells.

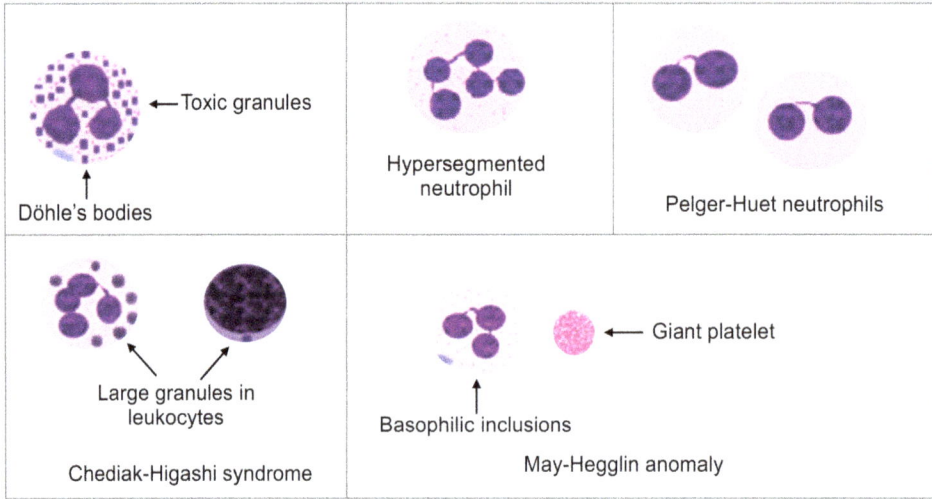

Fig. 11.6: Morphological abnormalities of neutrophils.

Alder-Reilly Anomaly

This congenital abnormality of granulocytes is characterized by the presence of abnormally large, darkly staining granules resembling toxic granules in cytoplasm. The granules are also variably present in monocytes. This abnormality is commonly seen in mucopolysaccharidoses, such as Hurler's and Hunter's syndrome.

May-Hegglin Anomaly

This uncommon condition with autosomal dominant inheritance is characterized by triad of thrombocytopenia, giant platelets, and inclusion bodies in granulocytes. The inclusions resemble Döhle bodies. Most patients are asymptomatic, although bleeding manifestations have been reported in an occasional patient. Autosomal dominant giant platelet disorders include May-Hegglin anomaly, Fechtner syndrome, Sebastian syndrome, and Epstein syndrome. All these disorders have mutations in *MYH-9* gene (that encodes nonmuscle myosin heavy chain 9) located at chromosome 22q12.3-q13.2.

Chediak-Higashi Syndrome

This rare autosomal recessive disease is characterized by immunodeficiency, poor resistance to bacterial infections (especially strepto- and staphylococcal), oculocutaneous albinism, bleeding tendency, multiple neurologic abnormalities, and giant peroxidase-positive lysosomal granules in granulocytes (Fig. 11.6). Similar lysosomal granules are also seen in other white blood cells and melanocytes. These abnormal inclusions result from the fusion of multiple cytoplasmic granules. Increased bleeding is due to defective platelet aggregation. An accelerated lymphomatous illness with lymphohistiocytic infiltrate in numerous organs develops in most patients and is characterized by fever, jaundice, hepatosplenomegaly, lymphadenopathy, pancytopenia, and bleeding. It results from mutation in the *CHS*1 gene (also called as *LYST*—lysosomal trafficking regulator gene) located on chromosome 1q42.1-1q42.2.

Myelokathexis

This is an extremely rare inherited disorder characterized by peripheral neutropenia and bone marrow hyperplasia with retention of neutrophil precursors and neutrophils in bone marrow. Neutrophils show long strands of chromatin connecting nuclear lobes, and marked abnormalities of nuclear shape and lobation. Neutrophils are also functionally defective. Recurrent bacterial and fungal infections become evident during infancy. Molecular basis of this disorder is unknown.

WHIM syndrome is a rare autosomal dominant disorder characterized by warts, hypogammaglobulinemia, infections, and myelokathexis. It is due to a mutation in *CXCR4* gene located on chromosome 2q21.

Functional Disorders of Phagocytic Leukocytes

Functional disorders of neutrophils can cause increased susceptibility to bacterial or fungal infections. Some disorders of neutrophil function are given in Box 11.8. Sites of defects in neutrophil function disorders are shown in Figure 11.7.

Section 3: Disorders of White Blood Cells

Box 11.8: Disorders characterized by neutrophil dysfunction.

1. *Impaired adhesion:*
   - Congenital leukocyte adherence deficiency (deficiency of CD11/CD18 surface glycoproteins)
   - Drugs: Corticosteroids, alcohol
2. *Impaired motility:*
   - Hyperimmunoglobulin E syndrome
   - Chediak-Higashi syndrome
   - Diabetes mellitus, Hodgkin's disease, leprosy
3. *Impaired microbicidal killing:*
   - Chronic granulomatous disease
   - Myeloperoxidase deficiency
   - Chediak-Higashi syndrome
   - Leukemias

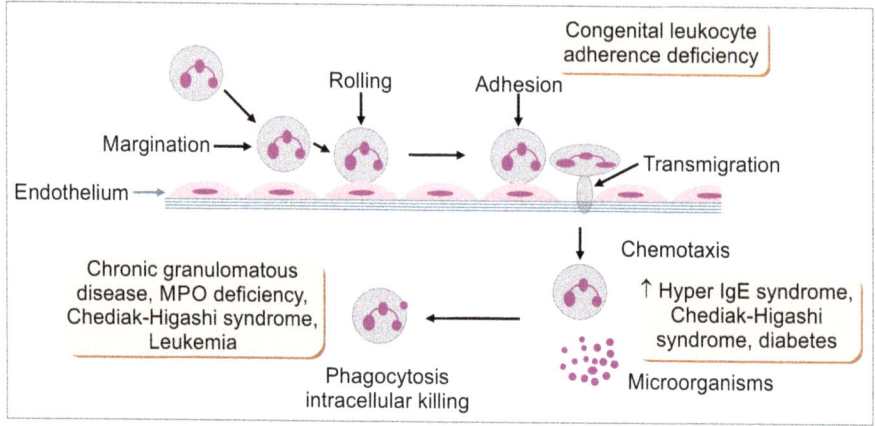

Fig. 11.7: Sites of defects in disorders of neutrophil function.

Congenital Leukocyte Adhesion Deficiency

This is a heterogeneous group of rare autosomal recessive disorders characterized by marked leukocytosis (since leukocytes are unable to leave blood vessels), defective neutrophil adhesion to endothelium, absence of extravascular neutrophils, and recurrent life-threatening bacterial infections.

Hyper IgE or Job's Syndrome

In this congenital disorder, defective neutrophil chemotaxis is present along with recurrent bacterial infections of skin and respiratory tract, recurrent cold, staphylococcal abscesses, dermatitis, eosinophilia, and markedly increased IgE.

Chronic Granulomatous Disease (CGD)

This is a group of hereditary disorders characterized by defective oxidative metabolism in phagocytic leukocytes with impaired generation of hydrogen peroxide and hydroxyl radical. There is marked chronic inflammatory reaction and granuloma formation at sites of infection.

In majority of patients, mode of inheritance is X-linked recessive while in some cases it is autosomal recessive. The disease results from mutation in one of the four genes (*CYBB*, *CYBA*, *NCF*1, *NCF*2) encoding phagocyte nicotinamide adenine dinucleotide phosphate (NADPH) oxidase subunits. As this enzyme is responsible for generation of superoxide anion, H_2O_2, and hypochlorous acid (from oxygen consumption called respiratory burst), complete absence or malfunction of NADPH oxidase leads to defective killing of bacteria by neutrophils. Patients usually present in infancy or early childhood with recurrent and severe infections by Gram +ve (*Staphylococcus aureus*) and Gram -ve (*Escherichia coli, Serratia marcescens*) microorganisms. Common sites of infection are lungs, skin, lymph nodes, gastrointestinal tract, and bones.

Diagnosis can be established by nitroblue tetrazolium (NBT) dye reduction test. NBT is a redox dye that is precipitated to blue insoluble granules of formazan by superoxide. In CGD, phagocytic cells cannot express respiratory burst and therefore do not reduce molecular oxygen to superoxide. NBT dye reduction test is thus negative in CGD.

Management consists of prompt and aggressive treatment of infections and surgical intervention when required. Long-term prophylactic antibiotics (such as cotrimoxazole) are advocated.

Myeloperoxidase Deficiency

This is the most common hereditary neutrophil function defect. In myeloperoxidase (MPO) deficient neutrophils, intracellular killing of microorganisms is slow, but is ultimately achieved. There is susceptibility to candidal and bacterial (*S. aureus*) infections. Diagnosis is established by myeloperoxidase stain of blood smear that shows lack of peroxidase activity in neutrophils.

DISORDERS OF MONOCYTE–MACROPHAGE SYSTEM

MONOCYTOSIS

Monocytosis (Fig. 11.8) refers to an increase in the monocyte count above 1,000/mm³. Causes of monocytosis are listed in Box 11.9.

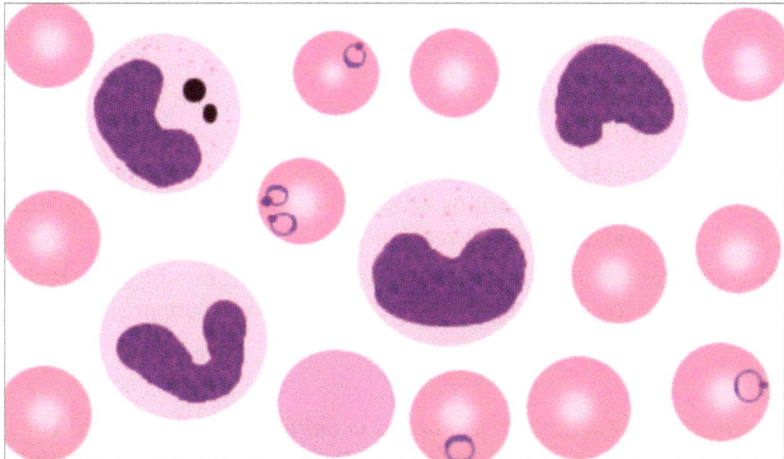

Fig. 11.8: Blood smear showing monocytosis in a case of malaria. Ring forms of *Plasmodium falciparum* are seen in some red cells. One monocyte shows brown-black malarial pigment.

> **Box 11.9:** Causes of monocytosis.
>
> **Infections:** Malaria, typhoid, tuberculosis, bacterial endocarditis, kala-azar
> **Hematological malignancies:** Acute myelomonocytic leukemia (AML M4), acute monocytic leukemia (AML M5), myeloproliferative neoplasms, chronic myelomonocytic leukemia, myelodysplastic syndrome, Hodgkin's disease
> **Others:** Sarcoidosis, ulcerative colitis, regional enteritis, carcinomas

STORAGE DISORDERS

Gaucher's Disease

Normally there is constant generation of glucocerebrosides from the breakdown of blood cell membranes. Glucocerebrosides are degraded enzymatically by lysosomal enzymes in macrophages. In Gaucher's disease, there is a hereditary deficiency of the enzyme glucocerebrosidase (acid β-glucosidase) that is required for removing glucose from ceramide. This causes accumulation of glucosylceramide (derived mainly from the phagocytosis and degradation of senescent leukocytes) within the macrophages of the reticuloendothelial system. Such enlarged macrophages are also called as Gaucher's cells. Accumulated glucosylceramide disrupts the lysosomes and damages cell structure.

Gaucher's disease is an autosomal recessive disorder. A French physician Philippe Charles Ernest Gaucher first described this disease in 1882. Many different mutations in the *glucocerebrosidase* gene (located on chromosome 1q21) can cause Gaucher's disease. There are three clinically distinct types of Gaucher's disease—type I (chronic non-neuronopathic adult type), type II (acute infantile neuronopathic type), and type III (subacute neuronopathic juvenile type).

Clinical Features

Type I: This is the most frequent type. It occurs mainly in Ashkenazi Jews. Clinical manifestations appear usually during early childhood to late adulthood and neurological involvement is absent. Splenomegaly due to accumulation of Gaucher's cells is the usual finding. Manifestations of hypersplenism may be present. Marrow expansion may lead to bone pain or fractures. The Erlenmeyer flask deformity of distal femur is a typical feature on X-ray. Progression of the disease is slow.

Type II: This is the most severe form of Gaucher's disease occurring in infants and is characterized by prominent neurologic manifestations and hepatosplenomegaly. Bone involvement is uncommon. Death often occurs before 2 years of age.

Type III: In this type, there is later onset of neurological involvement than in type II and more prolonged survival. Hepatosplenomegaly and bone involvement are present.

Diagnosis

Assay of glucocerebrosidase activity in leukocytes or cultured skin fibroblasts: The diagnosis is made by this test. This test can also be utilized for detection of heterozygotes and for prenatal diagnosis. However, as levels overlap in heterozygous and normal individuals, DNA analysis is preferred.

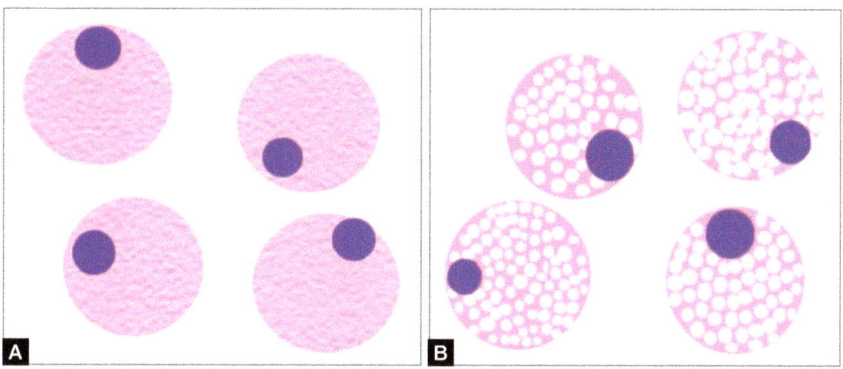

Figs. 11.9A and B: Comparative features of storage cells. Cytoplasm of Gaucher's cell (A) is fibrillary (likened to crumpled tissue paper), while that of Niemann-Pick cell (B) is vacuolated.

Demonstration of Gaucher's cells: Gaucher's cells (Fig. 11.9A) are macrophages containing large amounts of accumulated glucocerebrosides. Morphologically these are large, round to oval cells with abundant, pale, fibrillary cytoplasm (likened to a crumpled tissue paper), and have one or more dark, eccentric nuclei.

These cells are PAS-positive. Gaucher's cells can be seen in bone marrow, spleen, lymph nodes, and liver.

Ideally, diagnosis of Gaucher's disease should be established by assay of enzyme activity rather than by demonstration of Gaucher's cells in bone marrow. This is because enzymatic assay is simple and convenient. Gaucher's cells may be few in number and thus may be missed in marrow, or presence of pseudo-Gaucher's cells may lead to a mistaken diagnosis of Gaucher's disease. Pseudo-Gaucher's cells can occur in various conditions, such as chronic myeloid leukemia, lymphoproliferative disorders, Hodgkin's lymphoma, acquired immunodeficiency syndrome, and mycobacterial infections.

Treatment

Enzyme-replacement therapy with recombinant acid β-glucosidase or velaglucerase alfa has become available and can arrest and reverse the symptoms of Gaucher's disease. It is given intravenously every 2 weeks on an outpatient basis. It is now the standard form of treatment for type 1 disease. Enzyme replacement does not affect the neurologic disease progression in types 2 and 3. Splenectomy is indicated for bleeding secondary to severe thrombocytopenia or when patient develops discomfort due to massive splenomegaly. Bone marrow transplantation has been attempted in a few patients. However, due to increased morbidity and mortality associated with this procedure and good results of enzyme-replacement therapy, bone marrow transplantation is not currently advocated. Transfer of normal *glucocerebrosidase* gene into autologous stem cells is being attempted and provides the prospect of cure in Gaucher's disease.

Niemann-Pick Disease

Niemann-Pick disease is a rare, hereditary lipid-storage disorder characterized by deficiency of enzyme acid sphingomyelinase that leads to accumulation of sphingomyelin in cells of mononuclear phagocytic system. Parenchymal cells of organs are also frequently involved. Mode of inheritance is autosomal recessive.

Niemann-Pick disease is a heterogeneous disorder and different types have been described. The most common type is designated as type A (classical or infantile form) that accounts for three-fourth of the cases. It is common in Ashkenazi Jews. There is a severe deficiency of sphingomyelinase which causes widespread accumulation of sphingomyelin and other lipids in various organs. Manifestations develop early during infancy and include failure to thrive, hepatosplenomegaly, generalized lymphadenopathy, and severe neurologic symptoms. A macular cherry red spot may be present. Death usually occurs before 3–4 years of age.

Other types of Niemann-Pick disease are rare.

Diagnosis

Demonstration of Niemann-Pick cells in bone marrow: Niemann-Pick cells are mononuclear phagocytic cells containing excessive accumulations of sphingomyelin and cholesterol within lysosomes. The cells are large with multiple small vacuoles of relatively uniform size in cytoplasm and a single, small eccentric nucleus (Fig. 11.9B). Niemann-Pick cells are not pathognomonic for Niemann-Pick disease since similar cells are also found in certain other storage disorders.

Assay of sphingomyelinase: Diagnosis requires assay of acid sphingomyelinase activity in peripheral leukocytes or cultured fibroblasts. In type A Niemann-Pick disease, enzyme activity is markedly decreased (1–10%).

Treatment

Treatment is symptomatic.

Langerhans Cell Histiocytosis

Langerhans cell histiocytosis (LCH) is a group of disorders associated with clonal neoplastic proliferation of Langerhans-type cells that express CD1a, langerin, S100 protein and containing Birbeck granules. Previously these disorders were called as histiocytosis X. (Langerhans' cells are dendritic histiocytes normally residing in the epidermis. They function as antigen presenting cells). Recent evidence indicates that LCH arises from myeloid dendritic cell precursors. The *BRAF* V600E mutation has been reported to occur in 38–64% of cases of LCH in bone marrow hematopoietic precursors and circulating blood myeloid/monocytes. LCH is currently considered as an "inflammatory myeloid-derived neoplasm." The clinical spectrum of LCH varies from a single lesion to aggressive and disseminated disease. Current research indicates that mitogen-activated protein kinase (MAPK) activation in self-renewing hematopoietic progenitors causes high-risk disseminated disease, while MAPK activation in more differentiated and committed myeloid progenitors induces localized or low-risk disease.

Although LCH can occur at any age (from fetus to elderly), it is most frequent in infants and children (peak 1–5 years). Three major clinical syndromes are described:
1. *Solitary eosinophilic granuloma:* A unifocal disease usually involving the bone (especially skull, femur, pelvic bones, ribs); more frequent in older children and adults.
2. *Hand-Schuller-Christian disease:* A multifocal unisystem disease with involvement of multiple sites in one organ system, commonly bone; triad of lytic bone lesions, exophthalmos and diabetes insipidus is characteristic. It usually occurs in young children.
3. *Letterer-Siwe disease:* A multifocal multisystem progressive disease with involvement of multiple organs (skin, lymph nodes, spleen, liver, bones, and bone marrow). It occurs usually in infants.

The lesions in all the three syndromes are composed of Langerhans cells in a milieu of reactive inflammatory cells (eosinophils, histiocytes, neutrophils, and small lymphocytes). Langerhans cells are 15–25 μm in size with moderately abundant eosinophilic cytoplasm and grooved (coffee bean-like) or lobulated nucleus. The nuclear chromatin is finely dispersed and nucleoli are not prominent. On immunophenotypic analysis, Langerhans cells are positive for CD1a, langerin (CD207), and S100 protein. The ultrastructural hallmark of Langerhans cells is Birbeck granules in cytoplasm.

Unifocal bone lesions can be effectively treated with surgical curettage. As spontaneous resolution occurs in some cases, stable and asymptomatic lesions can be followed without intervention. Disseminated disease and progressive or recurrent bone lesions are treated with chemotherapy and/or steroids. Widespread organ involvement is associated with poor outcome.

LYMPHOCYTOSIS

Lymphocytosis is defined as increase in the absolute lymphocyte count above upper limit of normal for age (>4,000/mm^3 in adults). Causes of lymphocytosis are outlined in Box 11.10. Lymphocytosis in children is most often benign, while lymphocytosis in adults needs a workup to exclude a neoplastic process.

Acute infectious lymphocytosis: This is a contagious condition characterized by small mature-looking lymphocytosis occurring mainly in children; it may be related to Coxsackie virus A, Coxsackie virus B, echoviruses, and adenovirus type 12. Clinical manifestations are variable and leukocytosis varies from 20 to 50,000/mm^3 and lasts for 3 to 5 weeks.

Mononucleosis syndrome: Mononucleosis syndrome is characterized by presence of fever and reactive lymphocytes in blood (lymphocytes >50% of blood leukocytes along with >10% atypical lymphocytes). The common causes are infection by Epstein-Barr virus and cytomegalovirus. Mononucleosis-like syndrome can also be caused by *Toxoplasma gondii*, HIV-1, and several other viruses.

Monoclonal B-cell lymphocytosis: This is a monoclonal proliferation (documented by light chain restriction) of B lymphocytes (B lymphocyte count <5,000/mm^3) seen in healthy elderly individuals that is asymptomatic, and there is absence of any evidence of a lymphoproliferative, infectious, or autoimmune disorder. Monoclonal B cells may express CLL-like or non-CLL-like phenotype. Progression to CLL may occur especially in individuals with CLL immunophenotype.

Box 11.10: Causes of lymphocytosis.

1. Infections:
   Viral: Infectious mononucleosis, acute infectious lymphocytosis, cytomegalovirus, infectious hepatitis, mumps, varicella
   Bacterial: Tuberculosis, pertussis
   Protozoal: Toxoplasmosis
2. Lymphoid malignancies: Acute lymphocytic leukemia, chronic lymphocytic leukemia, prolymphocytic leukemia, leukemic phase of NHL, large granular lymphocytic leukemia
3. Monoclonal B-cell lymphocytosis
4. Persistent polyclonal B-cell lymphocytosis
5. Stress lymphocytosis: Acute cardiovascular collapse, trauma, major surgery
6. Other: Chronic infections, postvaccination, autoimmune disorders

Recent studies also indicate that nearly all cases of CLL are preceded by monoclonal B-cell lymphocytosis.

Persistent polyclonal B-cell lymphocytosis: This is a rare condition that is characterized by absolute lymphocytosis that is found to be polyclonal and B-cell in nature on immunophenotyping and is reported mainly in women who smoke and have a HLADR-7 phenotype. Small, atypical binucleated (having deep nuclear clefts) lymphocytes are characteristic. Most patients have a stable count and indolent course, but B-cell lymphomas have been reported to develop in rare patients. Patients should be followed up closely.

Stress lymphocytosis: This is a transient lymphocytosis in adults occurring immediately after acute events like trauma, surgery, acute myocardial infarction, etc. and is thus seen in emergency departments. It is usually mild and resolves shortly, and a re-evaluation after 2–4 weeks can allow distinction from a neoplastic process. It appears to be due to lymphocyte redistribution.

PLASMA CELLS IN PERIPHERAL BLOOD

Plasma cells are not seen in peripheral blood in healthy subjects. They may be seen in infection, inflammation, postvaccination, in cirrhosis, and in neoplasms of plasma cells like multiple myeloma, Waldenström macroglobulinemia, and plasma cell leukemia. A large number of reactive plasma cells are occasionally seen in Castleman disease, dengue fever, rubella, bacterial sepsis, administration of streptokinase, and angioimmunoblastic T-cell lymphoma.

INFECTIOUS MONONUCLEOSIS

Infectious mononucleosis (IM) is an acute infectious disease caused by Epstein-Barr virus (EBV) and characterized by fever, pharyngitis, lymphadenopathy, atypical lymphocytosis in peripheral blood, and heterophil and EBV-specific antibodies in serum.

Etiopathogenesis

Epstein-Barr virus is a double-stranded DNA virus of the herpes virus family. Transmission occurs chiefly by transfer of saliva from infected persons into the oropharynx of susceptible individuals usually by kissing. EBV infects B-lymphocytes of oropharyngeal tissue by binding to CD21 (which is the receptor for both C3d and EBV). EBV also spreads to other B-lymphoid sites in the body via circulation. Stimulation and proliferation of B-lymphocytes induces polyclonal hypergammaglobulinemia and formation of IgM heterophil antibodies and autoantibodies.

Binding of EBV to the B lymphocytes causes their activation with expression of activation marker CD23 on cell surface. EBV is integrated into the host genome which starts producing EBV proteins. These viral proteins are expressed on cell surface. These are recognized by T cytotoxic cells (CD8+) which undergo activation and proliferation and inhibit the activation and proliferation of EBV-infected B lymphocytes. The activated T cells represent most of the atypical or variant lymphocytes seen in peripheral blood. Multiplication of T cells also leads to enlargement of lymph nodes, spleen, and liver. Only small numbers of atypical lymphocytes are EBV-transformed B lymphocytes. EBV is characterized by its latency and EBV probably persists throughout life in the infected individual.

Clinical Features

Infectious mononucleosis is a disease of adolescents and young adults. Incubation period is 3–8 weeks. Patient usually presents with sore throat, fever, and generalized lymphadenopathy. Examination shows tonsillar enlargement, pharyngeal congestion, and transient palatal petechiae. Splenomegaly is present in 50% of patients. Less common manifestations of IM include—skin rash (resembling that occurring in typhoid fever), splenic rupture, Bell's palsy, Guillain-Barré syndrome, encephalitis, myocarditis, pericarditis, airway obstruction due to tonsillar hyperplasia, pneumonia, autoimmune hemolytic anemia, and thrombocytopenia.

X-linked lymphoproliferative disorder (Duncan's syndrome) is a rare immunodeficiency disorder in which EBV infection in childhood produces fulminant infectious mononucleosis. There is a high risk of later development of lymphoma and hypogammaglobulinemia. The disorder is due to a mutation in *SH2D1A* (also called *SAP*) gene on chromosome Xq25 that encodes SH2 domain on a signal transducing protein called SLAM-associated protein (SAP).

Laboratory Features

Peripheral blood examination: Total leukocyte count is mild to moderately raised due to absolute lymphocytosis. On differential leukocyte count, lymphocytes constitute more than 50% of cells with many (>10%) of them being atypical. Atypical or variant lymphocytes are variable in size with more abundant amount of cytoplasm that may contain vacuoles or granules. Dark basophilia of peripheral cytoplasm at points of contact with other cells ("skirting") and scalloping of cytoplasmic border around erythrocytes are characteristic (Fig. 11.10). Nucleus may be oval or irregular with coarse, clumped chromatin pattern. Sometimes one or two nucleoli may be seen.

Mild-to-moderate neutropenia and mild thrombocytopenia can occur. In a few patients, severe thrombocytopenia with purpura occurs. Mild autoimmune hemolytic anemia is observed in some cases.

Serological studies: Two types of serological tests are employed for diagnosis of IM-detection of heterophil antibodies and of EBV-specific antibodies.

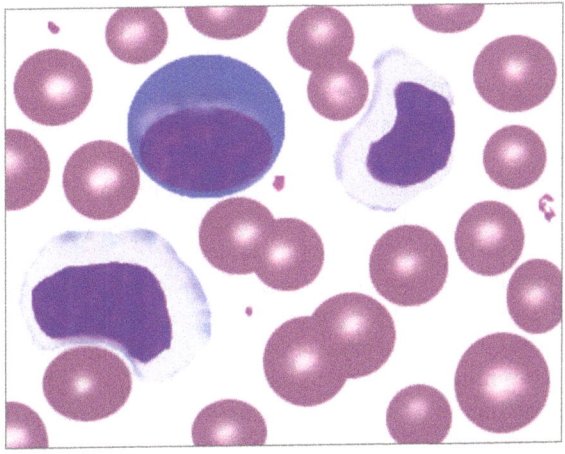

Fig. 11.10: Atypical lymphocytes in blood in infectious mononucleosis.

i. *Detection of heterophil antibodies:* An antibody which is capable of reacting with an antigen that is completely unrelated to the antigen that had originally elicited its production, is called as a heterophil antibody. Heterophil antibodies are of the IgM class. Heterophil antibodies become detectable during the second week of illness and persist for about 2 months.

Paul-Bunnell test: Paul and Bunnell in 1932 described heterophil antibodies in the sera of patients with IM that agglutinated sheep erythrocytes. The test consists of mixing sheep erythrocytes with serial dilutions of patient's serum and finding the agglutination titer (i.e. the highest dilution at which agglutination is detected). In normal individuals, agglutination titer is 1:56 or less, while in IM agglutination titers are increased (usually 1:224 or more). However, apart from IM high titers of heterophil antibodies are also found in leukemias, lymphomas, and serum sickness. Therefore, high agglutination titers (≥1:224) should be correlated with clinical and hematological findings to confirm the diagnosis of IM.

Paul-Bunnell-Davidsohn test (Differential absorption test): To distinguish heterophil antibodies in IM from those occurring in other disorders, Davidsohn in 1937 developed differential absorption test. It depends upon the finding that heterophil antibodies in IM and non-IM disorders have different antigen specificities, i.e. heterophil antibodies in IM are absorbed by beef red cells, but not completely by guinea pig kidney cells, while heterophil antibodies in other disorders are absorbed by guinea pig kidney cells, but not or only partially by beef red cells. Thus, blockage of sheep red cell agglutinating activity of patient's serum by prior absorption with beef red cells, but not by guinea pig kidney cells, indicates the presence of IM heterophil antibodies.

This test is usually employed when the agglutination titer with sheep erythrocytes is low, while clinical and hematological features are suggestive of IM.

Rapid slide tests: These are the simplest and the most widely used tests for the diagnosis of IM. Monospot test consists of mixing patients' serum with either beef red cell stromata or guinea pig kidney cell suspension on two halves of a glass slide. Horse erythrocytes are then added and presence or absence of agglutination is noted. (Substituting horse erythrocytes for sheep red cells enhances sensitivity of the test). Inhibition of agglutination by beef red cells but not by guinea pig kidney cells indicates the presence of IM heterophil antibodies.

ii. *Detection of EBV-specific antibodies:* EBV-specific serologic studies detect antibodies directed against specific EBV antigens, such as viral capsid antigen (VCA), early antigen (EA), and Epstein-Barr nuclear antigen (EBNA). Presence of IgM anti-VCA antibodies, or anti-EA-D (in D or diffuse form of EA, the whole nucleus shows antigen positivity) antibodies, and absence of anti-EBNA antibodies are diagnostic of acute infectious mononucleosis.

Lymph node biopsy: Lymph node biopsy is not performed in infectious mononucleosis as diagnosis is established on the basis of typical clinical presentation, atypical lymphocytes in blood, and serologic studies. However, if presentation is atypical, a lymph node biopsy may be done to solve the diagnostic difficulty.

Lymph node biopsy shows hyperplasia of paracortical zones due to proliferation of T lymphocytes. Lymphocytes of varying sizes ranging from small lymphocytes to immunoblasts are present in these areas. Mitotic activity is increased. Immunoblasts may show binucleation thus mimicking Reed-Sternberg cells of Hodgkin's lymphoma. Follicles often show blurring of their margins due to paracortical hyperplasia. Sinuses are filled with lymphocytes of varying sizes including immunoblasts.

Other laboratory features:
- In addition to heterophil antibodies, a variety of autoantibodies may be found in IM, such as cold-reactive autoantibodies and antinuclear antibodies. These probably result from polyclonal B cell stimulation.
- Liver function tests reveal mild elevations of liver enzymes and serum bilirubin, particularly during the second week of illness. Clinical jaundice, however, is rare.

Diagnosis and Differential Diagnosis

In majority of cases, diagnosis of IM is readily established on the basis of the following:
- Typical clinical features (adolescent or young adult patient with sore throat, fever, lymphadenopathy, and splenomegaly)
- Lymphocytosis (>50%) in peripheral blood with more than 10% atypical lymphocytes
- Positive heterophil antibody test in high titer with characteristic result on differential absorption test.

In approximately 10% cases of IM, heterophil antibody test is negative. In such cases, EBV-specific serologic tests should be done.

IM should be distinguished from CMV and toxoplasma-induced mononucleosis, human immunodeficiency virus seroconversion illness, streptococcal pharyngitis, other viral illnesses causing pharyngitis, and sometimes lymphoproliferative disorders.

Treatment

Treatment of IM is symptomatic and supportive.

IMMUNODEFICIENCY DISEASES

Immunodeficiency diseases are characterized by impairment of immune response against foreign antigens and susceptibility to infections. B and T lymphocytes, phagocytes, and complement are necessary for normal immune function and deficiency of any one of these can produce immunodeficiency.

When an immunodeficiency disorder is suspected, detailed clinical history and physical findings should be obtained. Clinical features highly suggestive of underlying immunological defect include recurrent infections, infections by unusual organisms or by organisms of low virulence, opportunistic infections, or inadequate or slow response to treatment. Causative organisms may provide clue to the type of immunodeficiency, e.g. repeated infections with encapsulated bacteria indicate defective humoral (antibody-mediated) immunity or phagocytic defense, while viral, fungal, or parasitic infections suggest impaired T-cell-mediated immune response.

Procedures for evaluation of immune function are presented in Table 11.2.

Complete blood counts and examination of peripheral blood smear are helpful for detecting neutropenia, lymphocytopenia, and morphological abnormalities of neutrophils. In assessing B lymphocyte function, hypogammaglobulinemia may be identified by serum protein electrophoresis. Quantitation of immunoglobulins can be done by single radial

Table 11.2: Laboratory tests for evaluation of immune function.

Parameter	Investigations
1. Basic blood studies	Total and absolute leukocyte counts, differential leukocyte count, blood smear for morphology of neutrophils and platelets, serum immunoglobulin levels (IgM, IgG, IgE, IgA), lymphocyte subsets by flow cytometry, complement screening tests (total hemolytic complement assay), oxidative burst test (dihydrorhodamine assay)
2. B lymphocyte function	Serum protein electrophoresis and quantification of immunoglobulins (for hypogammaglobulinemia), specific antibody titers following vaccination to diphtheria, tetanus, or pneumococci (for humoral response to antigens), quantitation of B cells by monoclonals (for deficiency of B cells)
3. T lymphocyte function	Delayed hypersensitivity skin test (for impaired cell-mediated response), absolute lymphocyte count, quantitation of T cells and T cell subsets
4. Neutrophil function	Absolute neutrophil count, Rebuck skin window test (for chemotaxis and motility), nitroblue tetrazolium dye reduction test (for phagocytic activity), cytochemical stain (myeloperoxidase)
5. Complement function	Total hemolytic complement (CH50)

immunodiffusion, nephelometry, or by ELISA. IgG, IgA, and IgM are usually moderately to markedly reduced in X-linked hypogammaglobulinemia and combined immunodeficiency. Isohemagglutinin (anti-A, anti-B) titers should be greater than 1:4 after 1 year of age and is a useful test for assessment of IgM function. B lymphocyte function can also be assessed by measuring antibody levels before and after immunization (e.g. with diphtheria or tetanus vaccines). CD19 and CD20 markers can be used for enumeration of B-lymphocytes by flow cytometry. A widely used test for evaluation of T cell function is delayed hypersensitivity skin test using purified protein derivative or candida antigen. If reaction to this test is positive, then cell-mediated immunity is largely intact.

CLASSIFICATION OF IMMUNODEFICIENCY DISEASES

Immunodeficiency diseases are classified into two major types—primary and secondary. Primary immunodeficiency diseases are genetically determined disorders which are subdivided according to the arm of the immune system that is defective. The classification of primary immunodeficiency disorders is continuously upgraded by International Union of Immunological Societies (IUIS). Primary immunodeficiencies are classified into eight categories by IUIS with numerous disorders in each category. In 2014, an additional category of "Phenocopies of primary immunodeficiency disorders" was introduced. Only a few disorders are listed in Table 11.3. Secondary immunodeficiency diseases are not intrinsic to the immune system and occur in a variety of acquired conditions, such as acquired immune deficiency syndrome (AIDS), cytotoxic chemotherapy, radiotherapy, malnutrition, etc.

Table 11.3: Classification of primary immunodeficiency disorders (International Union of Immunological Societies).

- Combined T- and B-cell immunodeficiencies
  - Severe combined immunodeficiency
- Syndromic immunodeficiencies
  - ADA deficiency
  - Omenn syndrome
  - Wiskott-Aldrich syndrome
  - Ataxia-telangiectasia
  - DiGeorge syndrome
  - Bloom syndrome
  - Chediak-Higashi syndrome
  - Leukocyte adhesion deficiency type 2
- Predominantly antibody deficiencies
  - X-linked agammaglobulinemia (*BTK* deficiency)
  - Common variable immunodeficiency
  - Selective IgA deficiency
  - Transient hypogammaglobulinemia of infancy
- Phagocytic defects
  - Chronic granulomatous disease
  - Leukocyte adhesion deficiency
  - Shwachman-Diamond syndrome
  - Severe congenital neutropenia
  - Cyclic neutropenia
  - Myeloperoxidase deficiency
- Diseases of immune dysregulation
  - Familial hemophagocytic lymphohistiocytosis
  - Autoimmune lymphoproliferative syndrome
- Defects in intrinsic and innate immunity
  - Chronic mucocutaneous candidiasis
  - WHIM syndrome
- Autoinflammatory disorders
  - Familial Mediterranean fever
- Complement deficiencies
- Phenocopies of primary immunodeficiency disorders

(ADA: adenosine deaminase deficiency)

Only lymphocytic diseases are considered below. Figure 11.11 shows sites of involvement in primary immunodeficiency disorders.

Primary Immunodeficiency

Primary immunodeficiency disorders are a group of heterogeneous genetic disorders that are associated with predisposition to recurrent infections and presentation early in life. Type of infection depends on the type of primary immunodeficiency. In addition, they are also associated with autoimmunity (e.g. autoimmune cytopenias) atopy, granulomatous disease (e.g. chronic granulomatous disease characterized by granulomas in skin, respiratory tract,

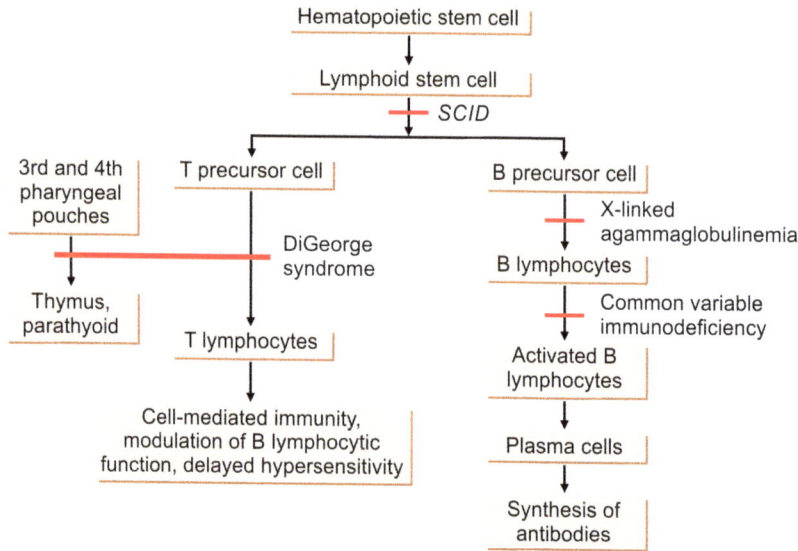

Fig. 11.11: Sites of defects in some primary immunodeficiency disorders.
(SCID: severe combined immune deficiency)

and gastrointestinal tract), lymphoproliferation (e.g. X-linked lymphoproliferative disease), and malignancies (e.g. lymphomas and leukemias). With the recent introduction of newer sophisticated genetic technique of next-generation sequencing, the number of primary immune disorders has expanded significantly.

X-Linked Agammaglobulinemia (Bruton's Disease)

This inherited immune deficiency syndrome is caused by a mutation in Bruton tyrosine kinase (BTK) gene located on chromosome Xq21.3-q22. This gene encodes a nonreceptor tyrosine kinase that is essential for B-cell development. Infants with this disorder remain normal for first few months of life due to protection by transferred maternal IgG. Afterward they start having repeated and severe bacterial infections. Although pre-B cells are identifiable in the bone marrow, they fail to differentiate into mature B cells. Lack of gammaglobulins can be detected by serum protein electrophoresis. Quantitation of immunoglobulins reveals virtual absence of IgA, IgM, IgD, and IgE (<200 mg/dL). B-lymphocytes are not detectable in the peripheral blood and plasma cells are absent in the lymphoid organs. There is inability to form antibodies after antigenic stimulation. Number and functions of T cells are adequate. Treatment consists of regular administration of intramuscular immunoglobulins. With recent availability of intravenous immunoglobulin, large doses can be given and adequate IgG levels can be achieved.

Selective Deficiency of IgA

Patients with isolated deficiency of IgA usually present with recurrent respiratory infections. IgA deficiency frequently occurs in autoimmune disorders (systemic lupus erythematosus, rheumatoid arthritis) and celiac disease. IgA-deficient patients may form anti-IgA antibodies in high titer; when such patients receive blood transfusion containing IgA, anaphylactic reaction can occur.

There appears to be an impaired release of IgA or failure of differentiation of B-lymphocytes to IgA producing plasma cells.

Quantitation of immunoglobulins shows serum IgA to be less than 5 mg/dL and normal or increased levels of other immunoglobulins. Secretory IgA is also deficient. Treatment is symptomatic. Therapeutic gammaglobulins or plasma contains small amounts of IgA. Patients requiring blood transfusion should be tested for anti-IgA antibodies and transfused washed red cells or blood from an IgA-deficient person.

Transient Hypogammaglobulinemia of Infancy

Maternally derived immunoglobulins (IgG) in infants gradually decline over the first few months of life. Immunoglobulin levels subsequently rise due to their synthesis by the infant's immune system and normal adult levels are reached by the end of 1 year. In all infants, there is a period of transient physiologic hypogammaglobulinemia around 5-6 months of age. During this period, maternally derived IgG is low, while production of immunoglobulins is yet to start in the infant. In some cases, transient hypogammaglobulinemia becomes unusually prolonged and severe due to unusual delay in beginning the synthesis of immunoglobulins, such infants may have increased susceptibility to infections. Regular follow-up is necessary to differentiate this disorder from other immunodeficiency diseases, particularly X-linked hypogammaglobulinemia. Gammaglobulin therapy is indicated when severe infections develop. Routine immunizations are deferred till the infant's immune system is established.

Common Variable Immunodeficiency

Patients with this disease usually present with history of repeated pyogenic infections. Although it can occur at any age, onset of symptoms is commonly several years after birth (often 20–30 years of age). Males and females are equally affected. Association with autoimmune disorders, such as systemic lupus erythematosus, rheumatoid arthritis, or pernicious anemia, is frequent. Other manifestations which may be present include chronic lung disease, chronic giardiasis, or malabsorption.

Common variable immunodeficiency may result from various mechanisms: Intrinsically defective B cells, circulating autoantibodies against B cells, defective B cell function due to excessive suppressor T cell activity or reduced helper T cell activity.

DiGeorge Syndrome (Thymic Hypoplasia)

In this disease, there is congenital aplasia or hypoplasia of thymus and parathyroid glands due to failure of development of 3rd and 4th pharyngeal pouches. These infants usually present with hypocalcemic tetany (due to hypoparathyroidism). There may also be congenital cardiac defects and facial abnormalities, such as low-set ears, short philtrum of upper lip, and hypertelorism. Later, defective cell-mediated immunity causes increased susceptibility to fungal, viral, bacterial, and protozoal infections. There is T-cell lymphopenia and lack of response to T cell mitogens, such as phytohemagglutinin. B cell immunity is variable.

Thymic transplantation causes correction of defective cell-mediated immunity. In some cases spontaneous improvement occurs.

Severe Combined Immunodeficiency Disease

Severe combined immunodeficiency disease (SCID) is an extremely heterogeneous group of disorders characterized by extreme form of T-cell immunodeficiency with variable amounts of B cells. Usually, there is marked deficiency of both B cell (humoral) and T cell (cell-mediated) immunity. There are two patterns of inheritance: X-linked and autosomal recessive. The basic defect may lie in the stem cell which fails to differentiate into mature B and T cells or there may be deficiency of cytokines necessary for maturation of lymphocytes. These patients usually develop symptoms of recurrent bacterial, viral, protozoal, or fungal infections during first few months of life. Candidiasis, chronic diarrhea, and pneumonia are common. Administration of live virus vaccine may cause disseminated and fatal disease. Laboratory features include marked lymphopenia, diminished T cells, lack of T lymphocyte response to phytohemagglutinin, cutaneous anergy, low or absent B lymphocytes, hypogammaglobulinemia, and lack of antibody formation after antigenic stimulation. Assay for T-cell receptor excision circles (TRECs) by polymerase chain reaction is used for screening of newborns for SCID for prompt recognition and treatment. TRECs is a biomarker for T-cell lymphopoiesis and is absent or abnormally low in SCID. Unless treated, death occurs before 1 year of age from severe infections. Bone marrow transplantation is the definitive form of treatment. Blood transfusions are contraindicated due to the risk of graft-versus-host disease.

Wiskott-Aldrich Syndrome

This is an inherited X-linked disorder characterized by severe eczema, recurrent pyogenic infections, low platelets (microthrombocytopenia), and increased risk of autoimmune disorders and hematological malignancy. It results from mutations in gene encoding *Wiskott-Aldrich syndrome protein (WASP)* which is located at Xp11.22-11.23. Usual initial presentation is bleeding secondary to thrombocytopenia in early infancy. Serum level of IgM is low, while IgA and IgE are increased. There is lack of antibody response to immunization with polysaccharide antigen. There is progressive diminution of T cell immunity. Death usually occurs in childhood from hemorrhage, severe infection, or development of a lymphoproliferative disorder. Bone marrow transplantation from HLA-identical sibling donor offers the only prospect of cure.

Ataxia-Telangiectasia

This is a rare systemic autosomal recessive disorder characterized by triad of progressive ataxia, oculocutaneous telangiectasia, and increased susceptibility to infections. There is increased risk of lymphoid malignancies. The disease is caused by mutations in ataxia-telangiectasia mutated (*ATM*) gene located on 1q22-23. There is increased susceptibility to radiation-induced damage. DNA repair is defective and spontaneous chromosomal abnormalities are frequent. Alpha-fetoprotein levels are raised. Deficiency of IgA is common; some patients may have deficiency of IgE, IgG2, or IgG4. Defect in cell-mediated immunity is variable. Therapy consists of management of infections and of other complications.

Secondary Immunodeficiency

Immunodeficiency can occur in a variety of acquired disorders, such as malnutrition, following radiotherapy or cytotoxic chemotherapy, administration of corticosteroids, hematological neoplasms, such as chronic lymphocytic leukemia, myeloma, and Hodgkin's disease, and viral infections, such as AIDS.

Immunological Abnormalities in Acquired Immunodeficiency Syndrome

AIDS is caused by a retrovirus called as human immunodeficiency virus (HIV). Individuals at high-risk of HIV infection are male homosexuals or bisexuals, intravenous drug abusers sharing needles or syringes, hemophiliacs receiving F VIII concentrate, and heterosexual contacts of above high-risk individuals.

Immunodeficient persons are susceptible to—(1) a variety of opportunistic infections especially *Pneumocystis carinii, Toxoplasma*, atypical mycobacteria, cytomegalovirus, Epstein-Barr virus, *Candida, Aspergillus,* and *Cryptococcus* and (2) neoplasms, such as Kaposi's sarcoma and non-Hodgkin's lymphomas.

Major alterations in immune system in AIDS are as follows:

T cells: HIV has tropism for CD4+ lymphocytes which causes progressive loss of CD4+ cells and reversal of CD4/CD8 ratio. Depletion of CD4+ cells profoundly affects the immune system as CD4+ cells interact with other cells of the immune system and secrete a variety of lymphokines. T lymphocytes show decreased delayed hypersensitivity response to antigens, impaired proliferative response to phytohemagglutinin, and decreased cytotoxic response.

B cells: Although polyclonal hypergammaglobulinemia is present due to stimulation of B cells, effective antibody response to new antigens is lacking.

Monocytes and macrophages: Impairment of chemotaxis and phagocytosis is present.

Other: There is decreased synthesis of interleukin-2 and gamma interferon.

BIBLIOGRAPHY

1. Al-Herz W, Bousfiha A, Casanova JL, et al. Primary immunodeficiency diseases: An update on the classification from the international union of immunological societies expert committee for primary immunodeficiency. Front Immunol. 2014;5:162.
2. Beutler E, Saven A. Misuse of marrow examination in the diagnosis of Gaucher's disease. Blood. 1990;76:646-48.
3. Beutler E. Gaucher's disease. N Engl J Med. 1991;325:1354-60.
4. Cheeseman SH. Infectious mononucleosis. Semin Hematol. 1988;25:261-68.
5. Ebeli MH. Epstein-Barr virus infectious mononucleosis. Am Fam Physician. 2004;70:1279-87.
6. Gallin JI, Buescher ES, Seligmann BE, et al. Recent advances in chronic granulomatous disease. Ann Intern Med. 1983;99:657-74.
7. McPherson RA, Pincus MR (Eds). Henry's clinical diagnosis and management by laboratory methods, 21st edition. Philadelphia: Elsevier Saunders; 2007.
8. Rosen FS, Cooper MD, Wedgwood RJ. The primary immunodeficiencies. N Engl J Med. 1995;337:431-40.
9. Stites DP. Laboratory evaluation of immune competence. In: Stites DP, Terr AI, and Parslow TG (Eds). Basic and Clinical Immunology, 8th edition. Connecticut; Appleton and Lange; 1994.
10. Stratus SE, Cohen JI, Tosato G. NIH conference. Epstein-Barr virus infections: biology, pathogenesis, and management. Ann Intern Med. 1993;118:45-58.

CHAPTER 12

Hematopoietic Stem Cell Transplantation

INTRODUCTION

This is a therapeutic procedure in which normal hematopoietic stem cells from an appropriate donor are infused intravenously to the patient having defective or diseased marrow to reconstitute normal hematopoiesis. This method is employed to treat various malignant and nonmalignant conditions. Previous term *bone marrow transplantation* is now replaced with hematopoietic stem cell transplantation since hematopoietic stem cells can be obtained from other sources like peripheral blood and umbilical cord.

TYPES OF HEMATOPOIETIC STEM CELL TRANSPLANTATION

Depending on the "relatedness" of the donor and the source of hematopoietic stem cells, three main types of hematopoietic stem cell transplantation (HSCT) are distinguished as shown in Box 12.1. Each type of HSCT has specific indications, disadvantages, and complications.

Allogeneic HSCT

In allogeneic HSCT, hematopoietic stem cells are obtained from a donor (a family member or a normal unrelated volunteer). Stem cells are best obtained from the HLA (human leukocyte antigen)-matched sibling, if available. As the genes for HLA are located on chromosome 6, and inheritance follows simple Mendelian pattern of inheritance, each sibling has 1:4 chance of finding complete HLA match. Only 30% of patients have HLA-matched sibling donor. Therefore, registries of healthy volunteer donors have been set up in some western countries from which a

---

Box 12.1: Types of hematopoietic stem cell transplantation.

- Allogeneic HSCT: Hematopoietic stem cells obtained from donor are infused into another individual.
  - Related: HLA-matched or mismatched
  - Unrelated: HLA-matched or mismatched
- Autologous: Hematopoietic stem cells are obtained from the patient's own bone marrow or peripheral blood and re-infused back after administration of conditioning regimen
- Syngeneic: Hematopoietic stem cell transplant from one individual to another who are genetically identical, i.e. identical twins (peripheral blood or bone marrow)

matched-volunteer donor may be sought. It is necessary to fully or closely match HLA antigens of the recipient and the donor to reduce the risk of life-threatening complications (graft-versus-host disease or graft rejection).

Indications for Allogeneic HSCT

- Acute myeloid leukemia in poor risk adults
- Acute lymphoblastic leukemia in poor risk adults
- Chronic myeloid leukemia
- Myelodysplasia
- Severe aplastic anemia
- Severe primary immunodeficiency
- Hemoglobinopathies (thalassemia major, sickle-cell disease)
- Inborn errors of metabolism

General Principles of Allogeneic HSCT

- *"Conditioning":* Patient is administered high-dose chemotherapy (usually cyclophosphamide) alone or in combination with total body irradiation (TBI) to eradicate malignant cells, to ablate patient's marrow and create space for marrow graft, and to cause immunosuppression to prevent graft rejection. Conditioning regimen is usually administered over 1 week.
- *Transplantation:* One day after completion of "conditioning," stem cells are harvested from the selected donor (either peripheral blood or bone marrow), and infused intravenously into the recipient. As the patient is highly susceptible to infections due to "conditioning," reverse barrier nursing in a filtered air environment is necessary and prophylactic anti-infective agents are routinely administered.
- *Engraftment:* Stem cells from the donor start producing blood cells in the bone marrow 7 to 21 days following transplantation.
- *Prevention of graft-versus-host disease (GVHD) and graft rejection:* Donor T lymphocytes recognize host tissues as foreign and cause graft-versus-host disease that is associated with high morbidity and mortality. To prevent GVHD and graft rejection, patient is routinely administered immunosuppressive therapy (methotrexate + cyclosporine) in allogeneic HSCT for 6 months.
- *Follow-up care:* Regular follow-up and care is necessary to assess and manage chronic GVHD, infections, and long-term side effects of conditioning regimen.

Graft-versus-leukemia effect: Most of the curative effect of allogeneic HSCT in patients with leukemia is due to graft-versus-leukemia effect, which is mediated by donor lymphocytes. This is evident from reduced risk of relapse in patients with acute or chronic GVHD and increased risk of relapse with lymphocyte-depleted grafts.

Complications

Complications related to "conditioning" regimen: These consist of early complications (<100 days post-transplantation) such as those associated with pancytopenia, alopecia, oropharyngeal mucositis, diarrhea, hemorrhagic cystitis, cardiomyopathy, veno-occlusive disease of liver, convulsions, and interstitial pneumonitis. Late complications (>100 days) are cataracts (due to TBI), sterility, early menopause, endocrine abnormalities, osteopenia or osteoporosis, and increased risk of secondary malignancies (especially skin).

Graft rejection: Graft rejection by recipient's surviving immunocompetent T cells is more likely in the presence of HLA incompatibility and insufficient immunosuppression. It is more likely to occur in patients of aplastic anemia. It is more common in patients who are sensitized to HLA antigens by previous blood transfusions. Transplantation of T cell-depleted graft is associated with significant reduction in its survival.

Graft-versus-host disease: In GVHD, immunocompetent T lymphocytes in the transplanted graft recognize tissues of the host (who is immunodeficient) as foreign and react against them. It is of two types—acute and chronic. Risk of acute GVHD is more in unrelated HSCT and in HLA-mismatched HSCT.

Acute GVHD: Acute GVHD develops within 100 days of marrow transplantation. It principally affects skin (maculopapular skin rash), liver (cholestatic hepatitis), and gastrointestinal tract (nausea, vomiting, diarrhea, and ileus), and the severity is variable. Acute GVHD delays recovery of the immune system thus increasing susceptibility to infections. Diagnosis can be made by biopsy of the involved organ. GVHD can be prevented or its severity reduced by immunosuppressive therapy (usually methotrexate and cyclosporine). Another form of GVHD prophylaxis consists of depleting lymphocytes from the bone marrow graft; this procedure however increases the rate of graft rejection and also of relapse due to the loss of graft versus leukemia effect. Treatment of acute GVHD is not satisfactory and involves corticosteroids, antithymocyte globulin, and monoclonal antibodies against lymphocytes.

Chronic GVHD: Chronic GVHD, developing after 100 days of transplantation, clinically resembles autoimmune disorder such as systemic lupus erythematosus, scleroderma, Sjögren's syndrome, or primary biliary cirrhosis. Treatment consists of immunosuppressive therapy.

Infections: This is one of the major complications of HSCT. An association of certain infections with particular post-transplant period exists. During the early neutropenic period, recipients are susceptible to bacterial, fungal, and herpes simplex infections. After engraftment, cytomegalovirus pneumonia is a frequent complication, which may be life-threatening. Late infections by varicella zoster virus and encapsulated bacteria occur many months after transplantations.

Recurrence of malignancy: Recurrence of leukemia, a major cause of graft failure, is less likely to occur when HSCT is done during first remission than in advanced stage of disease.

Autologous HSCT

In autologous HSCT, stem cells previously collected from the recipient are infused back, i.e. patient serves as his own source of stem cells.
- Stem cells are obtained from the patient during complete remission, processed to remove any contaminating malignant cells, and cryopreserved (frozen and stored in liquid nitrogen). Subsequent stem cell transplantation may be done within a few days or a few years of marrow harvest. In usual practice, conditioning regimen begins within a few days or weeks of marrow harvest.
- Conditioning regimen is administered (high-dose chemotherapy).
- One day after completion of conditioning, stem cell product is rapidly thawed and infused intravenously.

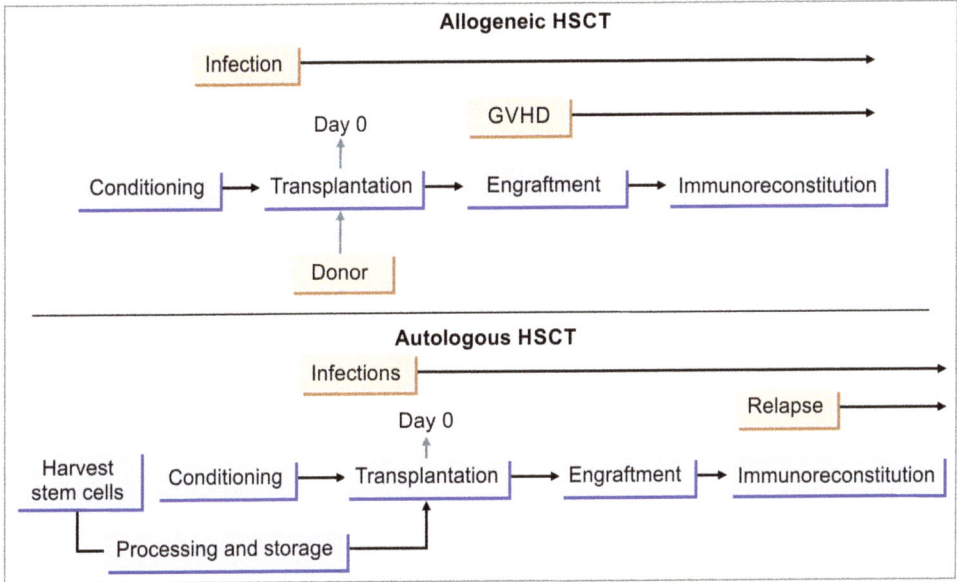

Fig. 12.1: Sequence of events (blue) in allogeneic and autologous HSCT. Main complications of each type are shown in red.
(GVHD: graft-versus-host disease; HSCT: hematopoietic stem cell transplantation)

As compared to allogeneic HSCT, intensity of conditioning regimen is less, immune restoration is quicker, and there is no potential for GVHD. This permits the procedure to be performed in older patients. Length of hospital stay and transplant-related mortality are less as compared to allogeneic HSCT. The most common complication of autologous HSCT is relapse of underlying malignant disease. Other disadvantages of autologous HSCT are failure to harvest patient's stem cells, lack of graft-versus-leukemia effect, and late development of secondary hematologic malignancies.

General principles of allogeneic and autologous HSCT are presented in Figure 12.1.

Indications for Autologous HSCT

- Relapsed aggressive non-Hodgkin's lymphoma
- Relapsed Hodgkin's lymphoma
- Plasma cell myeloma after induction chemotherapy
- Mantle cell lymphoma in first remission
- Acute myeloid leukemia in second remission if allogeneic donor is not available
- Solid tumors, for example, breast carcinoma and germ cell tumors

Complications

Complications related to conditioning regimen are similar to allogeneic HSCT, although they are less frequent and less severe. The most common late complication is relapse of the underlying malignant disease.

Allogeneic HSCT is an extremely stressful procedure associated with considerable morbidity and mortality and should be undertaken only in younger individuals (preferably less than 40 years). The major complications of allogeneic HSCT are graft-versus-host disease, graft rejection,

Table 12.1: Comparison of allogeneic and autologous hematopoietic stem cell transplantation (HSCT).

Parameter	Allogeneic HSCT	Autologous HSCT
1. Source of stem cells	Family member or unrelated donor	Stem cells previously collected from the patient
2. Age of recipient	Young, <55 years	Wide age range, can be done in older patients
3. Main indications	AML, ALL, MDS, CML, primary immunodeficiency, hemoglobinopathies	Relapsed NHL, relapsed Hodgkin's lymphoma, multiple myeloma, solid tumors
4. Risk of contamination of graft with malignant cells	Absent	Present
5. Risk of GVHD	Present	Absent
6. Graft-versus-tumor effect	Present	Absent
7. Main complication	GVHD	Relapse of malignancy
8. Overall procedure-related mortality	20–30% (if HLA-matched sibling donor), up to 45% (if unrelated donor)	5–10%
9. Treatment of inherited disease	Possible	Not possible
10. Restoration of immune function	Slower	Rapid

and infections. In contrast to allogeneic HSCT, autologous transplantation can be carried out in elderly and there is no associated problem of graft-versus-host disease. However, autologous marrow for infusion may be contaminated with tumor cells with associated increased risk of post-transplantation relapse; also, autologous HSCT cannot be used for treatment of genetic disorders. An advantage of allogeneic HSCT is graft-versus-tumor (leukemia) effect in which donor lymphocytes cause destruction of residual leukemic cells by recognizing them as nonself; this beneficial effect is lacking with autologous HSCT. Allogeneic and autologous HSCT are compared in Table 12.1.

As identical twins are rarely encountered, syngeneic HSCT is not possible in majority of cases.

SOURCES OF HEMATOPOIETIC STEM CELLS

Hematopoietic stem cells for transplantation can be obtained from peripheral blood or from bone marrow of a donor. For allogeneic HSCT, donor should be healthy, HLA-compatible, and free from infections transmissible by the procedure.

Peripheral Blood Stem Cell Mobilization and Harvesting

The current preferred method for harvesting hematopoietic stem cells or HSCs is from peripheral blood mononuclear cells. Although HSCs were known to circulate in peripheral blood, their very small number precluded their use for transplantation. Administration of recombinant hematopoietic growth factor (e.g. G-CSF ± chemotherapy) mobilizes HSCs from bone marrow and enhances their subsequent yield from peripheral blood. The method of using HSCs isolated from peripheral blood for transplantation is known as peripheral blood stem cell transplantation (PBSCT). PBSCT is associated with more rapid engraftment as compared to bone marrow transplantation.

After administration of hematopoietic growth factor (+chemotherapy in autologous transplantation), donor is connected to an apheresis machine and mononuclear cells are collected. Timing of collection following administration of HGF is such that maximum yield of stem cells is obtained. The yield can be evaluated for adequacy by mononuclear cell count, CD34+ (a marker for hematopoietic stem cells) count, or assay for colony stimulating factor-granulocyte macrophage.

Bone Marrow Harvesting

Up to 1,000 mL of marrow is aspirated from the donor from several sites in iliac crest under general anesthesia. Aspirated marrow is collected in a harvest bag containing acid citrate dextrose solution. The yield is evaluated for adequacy by total white cell count of the harvest.

RECENT ADVANCES IN HEMATOPOIETIC STEM CELLS TRANSPLANTATION

Umbilical Cord Blood Transplantation

Umbilical cord blood is an important and readily available source of hematopoietic stem cells. Due to the immaturity of immunocompetent cells in cord blood, risk of graft-versus-host disease is low. This allows for possibility of greater degree of HLA-mismatch between donor and recipient. However, number of stem cells in cord blood is limited and, therefore, most of the successful cord blood transplantations have been done in small children.

Nonmyeloablative Allogeneic HSCT

In recent years, some investigators have reported encouraging results with a procedure that uses mild conditioning regimen (rather than usual intensive high-dose chemoradiotherapy) in allogeneic HSCT for malignant disease. The aim of such mild conditioning is not to eliminate malignant cells and cause myeloablation, but to induce immunosuppression sufficient to promote engraftment and to cause slow generation of "graft-versus-leukemia" effect. It is thought that major therapeutic benefit of allogeneic HSCT results from this "graft-versus-leukemia" effect mediated by donor T lymphocytes (and not only from eradication of tumor cells by high-dose conditioning regimen). This procedure is relatively less toxic and can be performed in older patients. However, more studies are required before the role of this procedure in hematological cancers is established.

BIBLIOGRAPHY

1. Appelbaum FR. Marrow transplantation for hematologic malignancies: a brief review of current status and future prospects. Semin Hematol. 1988;25:16-22.
2. Armitage JO. Bone marrow transplantation. N Engl J Med. 1994;330:827-38.
3. Klassen LW, Armitage JO, Warkentin PI. Bone marrow transplantation. In: Koepke JA (Ed). Practical Laboratory Hematology. New York: Churchill Livingstone; 1991.
4. Leger CS, Nevill TJ. Hematopoietic stem cell transplantation: a primer for primary care physician. CMAJ. 2004;170:1569-77.
5. Soutar RL, King DJ. Bone marrow transplantation. BMJ. 1995;310:31-6.

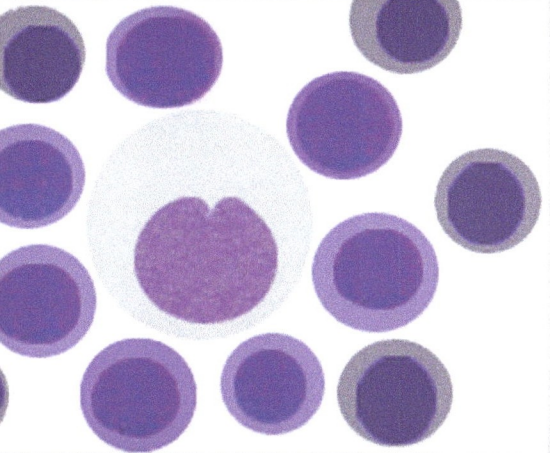

Disorders of Hemostasis

Section Outline

13. Approach to the Diagnosis of Bleeding Disorders *423*
14. Bleeding Disorders Caused by Abnormalities of Blood Vessels (The Vascular Purpuras) *442*
15. Bleeding Disorders Caused by Abnormalities of Platelets *445*
16. Disorders of Coagulation *462*

SECTION 4

CHAPTER 13

Approach to the Diagnosis of Bleeding Disorders

INTRODUCTION

Bleeding disorders result from defective hemostasis due to abnormality of vascular wall, platelets, or coagulation factors. They are one of the most commonly encountered problems in clinical hematology.

The evaluation of a patient suspected of having a bleeding disorder can be divided into two parts:
1. Clinical evaluation—history, physical examination, family history
2. Laboratory evaluation—screening tests, specific tests

CLINICAL EVALUATION

A carefully elicited history and physical examination are essential and provide clues regarding the nature of the disorder.

Clinically significant bleeding may be due to a local cause or a generalized defect in hemostasis. Features suggestive of a systemic hemostatic defect include recurrent episodes of bleeding, bleeding from more than one site, spontaneous bleeding, and severe bleeding from trivial trauma.

In mild bleeding disorders, it may be difficult to decide whether excessive bleeding is present. Such cases can be suspected by the amount of bleeding occurring following common surgical procedures such as tooth extraction, tonsillectomy, or circumcision.

Bleeding disorder may be hereditary or acquired. Hereditary nature of the disorder is suggested by presentation early in life (<5 years) and history of similar complaints in close relatives of the patient with a definite inheritance pattern. There is also past history of bleeding episodes. Not all patients, however, present in childhood (especially von Willebrand disease and mild hemophilia) and mild defect may first become manifest during later years in adults.

Family history is an essential part of the clinical evaluation as it enables to document the hereditary nature of the disorder, its pattern of inheritance, and thus limits the number of diseases to be considered, and is also helpful in genetic counseling. There are three patterns of inheritance of a hereditary disorder—X-linked recessive, autosomal recessive, and autosomal dominant (Table 13.1). History of bleeding only in males and positive family history on maternal side spanning many generations is suggestive of **X-linked disorder** (e.g. hemophilia A or B). However, in 30% of cases of hemophilia, positive family history is lacking; therefore,

Table 13.1: Inherited hemorrhagic disorders.

Deficiency (Synonym)	Mode of inheritance	Mutation (chromosome)	Incidence
Fibrinogen (afibrinogenemia, hypofibrinogenemia, dysfibrinogenemia)	AR (afibrinogenemia), AD (hypofibrinogenemia, dysfibrinogenemia)	*FGA, FGB, FGG* (4q28)	1:1 million
Prothrombin	AR	*F2* (11p11–q12)	1:2 million
FV (parahemophilia)	AR	*F5* (1q24.2)	1:1 million
FVII	AR	*F7* (13q34)	1:500000
FVIII (hemophilia A)	XR	*F8* (Xq28)	1:10,000
Combined FV and FVIII deficiency	AR	*LMAN1* (18q21.3–q22), *MCFD2* (2p21–p16.3)	1:1 million
FIX (hemophilia B)	XR	*F9* (Xq27.1)	1:60,000
FX	AR	*F10* (13q34)	1:1 million
FXI (hemophilia C)	AR	*F11* (4q35.2)	1:1 million
FXIII	AR	*F13A1* (6p24–p25) *F13B* (1q31–q32.1)	1:2 million
von Willebrand factor (von Willebrand disease)	AR ((type 3) or AD (type 1, type 2)	*VWF* (12p13.3)	1:100 (type 1), 1:1 million (type 3)

(AR: autosomal recessive; AD: Autosomal dominant; XR: X-linked recessive)
Note: Deficiencies of FXII, high molecular weight kininogen, and prekallikrein are not associated with bleeding.

negative family history does not rule out the possibility of hemophilia. In **autosomal recessive disease** (e.g. afibrinogenemia, deficiency of FV or FX, von Willebrand disease), both males and females are affected (from current generation only), and history of consanguineous marriage is common. In **autosomal dominant disorders** (e.g. some forms of von Willebrand disease, hereditary hemorrhagic telangiectasia), bleeding manifests in both sexes, in one parent, and also in older generations.

Inheritance patterns of congenital bleeding disorders are presented in Box 13.1.

Generalized bleeding is a feature of many acquired conditions such as diseases of the liver, uremia, hematological malignancies, carcinomas, sepsis, and administration of certain drugs (Box 13.2). In these cases, the underlying disease dominates the clinical picture. Important features to look for on physical examination include fever, splenomegaly, hepatomegaly, lymphadenopathy, and icterus.

Box 13.1: Inheritance patterns of congenital bleeding disorders.

- *X-linked recessive:* Hemophilia A, hemophilia B, Wiskott-Aldrich syndrome
- *Autosomal recessive:* Deficiencies of factors I, II, V, VII, X, XI, XIII; Bernard-Soulier syndrome, Glanzmann's thrombasthenia, Gray platelet syndrome, von Willebrand disease (type 3), congenital amegakaryocytic thrombocytopenia
- *Autosomal dominant:* Hereditary hemorrhagic telangiectasia, von Willebrand disease, May–Hegglin anomaly.

Box 13.2: Common drugs which can impair hemostasis and cause bleeding.

Platelet phase
Aspirin, other nonsteroidal anti-inflammatory drugs, heparin, antibacterials, thiazides, chloroquine, quinine, cytotoxic drugs, ethyl alcohol, quinidine, anticonvulsants, abciximab

Coagulation phase
Oral anticoagulants, heparin, Beta-lactam antibiotics, L-asparaginase, valproic acid

Table 13.2: Clinical differentiation between platelet/vascular and coagulation disorders.

Parameter	Platelet/vascular disorder	Coagulation disorder
1. Commonly affected sex	Female	Male
2. Family history	Often negative (as most cases are acquired)	Often positive (as most cases are hereditary)
3. Petechiae, bleeding gums, epistaxis, menorrhagia	Common	Rare
4. Deep hematoma (muscle bleeding), hemarthrosis (joint bleeding)	Not seen	Common
5. Delayed bleeding (recurrence of bleeding from the same site hours or days following injury)	Not seen	Characteristic (12–24 hours after injury)
6. Previous history of bleeding	Not present	Present since early childhood

Box 13.3: Bleeding terminology.

- Petechiae: Tiny pinpoint areas of hemorrhage (≤2 mm in diameter) due to vascular or platelet disorder. They usually occur in clusters and do not blanch on pressure.
- Purpura: Areas of hemorrhage ≥3 mm but less than 1 cm in diameter. Appearance depends on age of lesion (red → purple → brown yellow). They do not blanch on pressure. They occur in vascular or platelet disorder. Palpable purpura is indicative of vasculitis. When occurring in mucosa, it is called as wet purpura.
- Ecchymosis (Bruise): An area of extravasated blood in skin greater than 1 cm in diameter. They result from trauma or hemostatic disorder.
- Telangiectasia: These are spots or areas resulting from localized dilated blood vessels. They blanch on pressure.
- Hematoma: A swelling resulting from a large area of hemorrhage in subcutaneous tissue or muscle. It does not blanch on pressure. It results from trauma or coagulation disorder.
- Hemarthrosis: Bleeding into a joint.

In hemostatic disorders, bleeding is excessive in relation to the situation, prolonged, and recurrent.

The most common inherited bleeding disorders are von Willebrand disease, hemophilia A and hemophilia B.

Clinical history frequently indicates whether the disorder is due to abnormality of blood vessels/platelets (primary hemostasis) or coagulation factors (secondary hemostasis) (Table 13.2). Bleeding terminology is given in Box 13.3.

LABORATORY EVALUATION

This can be divided into two parts—screening tests and specific tests. Screening tests are initial tests that are simple to perform, rapid, and assess the integrity of primary or secondary hemostasis. These tests are nonspecific and do not pinpoint the nature of the defect, but assess the function of one phase of the hemostatic system. Screening tests include **tests of primary hemostasis**, such as platelet count, peripheral smear examination, bleeding time, and platelet

Table 13.3: Screening tests for hemostasis.

Test	Assessment
Tests of primary hemostasis	
Bleeding time	Platelet and vascular phases
PFA-100 system	Platelet function
Platelet count	Quantitation of platelets
Blood smear	1. Quantitative and morphological abnormalities of platelets 2. Detection of underlying hematological disorder
Tests of secondary hemostasis	
Clotting time	Crude test of coagulation phase
Prothrombin time	Extrinsic and common pathways
Activated partial thromboplastin time	Intrinsic and common pathways

function analyzer (PFA)-100 test, and **tests of secondary hemostasis** (Table 13.3), such as prothrombin time and activated partial thromboplastin time. Directed by the results of the screening tests, appropriate specific tests are performed to define the precise nature of the defect. Specific tests include platelet function studies, specific coagulation factor assays, tests for fibrinolysis, etc.

SCREENING TESTS

Screening Tests for Primary Hemostasis

Bleeding Time

The bleeding time (BT) test is an in vivo measure of primary hemostasis (vascular and platelet components). It assesses the formation of primary hemostatic plug (following a skin puncture or incision), which is dependent on adequate functioning of platelets.

In this test, time required for bleeding to cease following a skin puncture/incision is measured. Stoppage of bleeding indicates formation of a primary hemostatic plug. Three methods—Duke's, Ivy's, and template—can measure bleeding time. Duke's method, which measures bleeding time following ear lobe puncture, is not recommended since it cannot be standardized and can cause a large local hematoma. Both Ivy's and template are satisfactory methods. In Ivy's method, 2 to 3 standard punctures are made on the volar surface of the forearm with a lancet (cutting depth 2-2.5 mm) under standardized venous pressure (40 mm Hg). A stopwatch is started as soon as the punctures are made. Blood oozing from the puncture wounds is blotted with a filter paper at regular intervals. The time taken for each puncture wound to stop bleeding is noted. The average time is reported as the bleeding time. A disadvantage with this method is closure of puncture wound before stoppage of bleeding. Template method is similar to Ivy's, except that it uses a special surgical blade, which makes a larger cut (6-9 mm long and 1 mm deep).

Normal range for bleeding time is 2 to 7 minutes (Ivy's method).

Causes of prolongation of bleeding time:
- **Thrombocytopenia:** Before carrying out a bleeding time test, a platelet count should be obtained. If platelet count is less than 100,000/mm^3, bleeding time should not be carried out, as it will be prolonged.

- **Disorders of platelet function:** BT is markedly prolonged in hereditary disorders of platelet function like Glanzmann's thrombasthenia and Bernard-Soulier syndrome and mild-to-moderately prolonged in storage pool defect. Ingestion of aspirin (within last 7 days of the test) causes prolongation of BT. Uremia, myeloproliferative disorders, leukemias, myelodysplasia, and disseminated intravascular coagulation affect platelet function and prolong BT.
- **Inherited disorders of coagulation:** BT is prolonged in von Willebrand disease and afibrinogenemia.
- **Vascular disorders**.

Disadvantages of BT are operator dependency, invasive nature, low sensitivity, and poor reproducibility. It is no longer used as a routine test and has been replaced by platelet function tests like PFA-100 and whole blood aggregation in most developed countries.

Platelet Function Analyzer (PFA)-100

The conventional test for assessment of primary hemostasis has been measurement of bleeding time. However, this test is not sufficiently specific and sensitive, produces variable results, and does not correlate with significant bleeding. Recently, a new commercial automated device has been introduced, called as PFA-100 (Dade Behring) as a substitute for bleeding time. The instrument aspirates a small amount of citrated whole blood through a capillary and an aperture cut in a membrane. The membrane is coated with collagen and either epinephrine or adenosine diphosphate. Exposure of blood to these platelet agonists under high shear rates leads to binding of von Willebrand factor, platelet adhesion, activation, and aggregation. A stable platelet plug is formed which occludes the aperture. The time required for occlusion of aperture (called "closure time") is prolonged as compared to normal in most cases of von Willebrand disease and some platelet function disorders. The test can also detect aspirin-induced platelet function defect.

In severe von Willebrand disease and severe platelet function defects, closure time with both collagen/epinephrine and collagen/ADP are prolonged. Prolonged closure time result with collagen/epinephrine and normal with collagen/ADP can occur with mild platelet dysfunction, mild von Willebrand disease, and aspirin medication. The results are affected by low platelet count and low hematocrit. Interpretation requires clinical correlation along with drug history.

It should be noted that bleeding time and PFA-100 tests are not necessary in thrombocytopenia (since adequate number of platelets are required for assessment of platelet function).

If abnormal result is obtained with PFA-100, platelet aggregation studies should be performed for definitive diagnosis.

Platelet Count

For platelet count and morphological examination on blood smear, blood is collected in ethylenediaminetetraacetic (EDTA) anticoagulant. Platelet count and platelet indices (platelet distribution width and mean platelet volume) are determined on automated cell counters.

Platelets can be counted manually under a microscope or by means of an automated hematology cell analyzer.

In manual method, blood is mixed with 1% ammonium oxalate, number of platelets is counted in a counting chamber, and the result is reported as number of platelets per cubic mm. Under light microscope, platelets appear as small, roughly spherical, and refractile particles.

Differentiation of platelets from other particles is considerably aided by phase-contrast microscope. Normal range is 150,000 to 400,000/mm³.

Thrombocytopenia is defined as platelet count below 150,000/mm³. It is necessary to ascertain that platelet count is truly decreased by examination of blood smear. Thrombocytopenia is graded as mild (1,50,000 to 50,000/cmm), moderate (50,000 to 20,000/cmm), and severe (<20000/cmm). Common causes of thrombocytopenia are hematological malignancies, ingestion of certain drugs, disseminated intravascular coagulation, idiopathic thrombocytopenic purpura, connective tissue diseases, megaloblastic anemia, and aplastic anemia. Thrombocytosis (platelet count >400,000/mm³) occurs in inflammation, following hemorrhage, and in myeloproliferative disorders.

Automated hematology analyzers more precisely count platelets. However, these are expensive and have high running costs. Some electronic analyzers can also measure platelet distribution width (PDW), mean platelet volume, and reticulated platelets. **PDW** is a measure of degree of variation of platelet size present in a blood sample. High PDW is seen in myeloproliferative disorders due to the presence of marked variation in size of platelets (giant to small). In secondary or reactive thrombocytosis, PDW is normal. Thus, PDW is of some value in differentiating essential thrombocythemia from secondary or reactive thrombocytosis.

Mean platelet volume (MPV): It is increased when thrombocytopenia is due to peripheral platelet destruction (since platelet production is stimulated with release of large platelets in circulation) and is normal or low when thrombocytopenia is due to impaired platelet production. MPV is also increased in myeloproliferative disorders.

Young platelets with residual RNA are called as **reticulated platelets** (analogous to reticulocytes). They are considered as an index of platelet production. Increased values are observed in idiopathic thrombocytopenic purpura and lower values in aplastic anemia.

Complete Blood Count and Blood Smear

A complete blood count and a blood smear can provide information in the form of:
- Presence of cytopenia (anemia, leukopenia, thrombocytopenia)
- Red cell abnormalities (especially fragmented red cells, which may indicate disseminated intravascular coagulation)
- White cell abnormalities (like abnormal cells in leukemias)
- Abnormalities of platelets—thrombocytopenia (normally there is 1 platelet per 500–1000 red cells), giant platelets (seen in myeloproliferative disorders and Bernard-Soulier syndrome), and isolated discrete platelets without clumping in fingerprick smear (seen in uremia, Glanzmann's thrombasthenia).

Direct platelet count should always be accompanied by examination of a stained blood film. It is helpful in assessing the correctness of direct count, adequacy of platelets and their morphological abnormalities; in addition underlying hematological disorders can be detected, if present.

Normally, there are 8 to 20 platelets per oil immersion field or 15 to 30 platelets per high-power field (400×). A rough estimate of platelet count can be obtained from blood smear, which serves as a verification of platelet count obtained by automated analyzer. Number of platelets are counted in 8 to 10 microscopic fields under oil immersion (1000×), average is taken, which is then multiplied by 20,000 to get the platelet count per mm³ or per μL.

> **Box 13.4:** Causes of giant platelets in peripheral blood.
>
> **Inherited disorders**
> MYH-9 syndromes*: May–Hegglin anomaly, Fechtner syndrome, Sebastian syndrome, Epstein syndrome.
> Other: Bernard-Soulier syndrome, Gray platelet syndrome, velocardiofacial syndrome, hereditary macrothrombocytopenia with hearing loss, Mediterranean macrothrombocytopenia, Montreal platelet syndrome
>
> **Acquired disorders**
> Myelodysplastic syndrome, myeloproliferative neoplasms, acute megakaryoblastic leukemia, splenectomy, hyposplenism
>
> *All these disorders have mutations in *MYH-9* gene located at chromosome 22q12.3-q13.2.

Some disorders are associated with giant platelets and bleeding tendency. These are listed in Box 13.4.

Screening Tests for Secondary Hemostasis

Previously, whole blood clotting time (Lee and White) was commonly done as a screening test for hemostatic abnormality. This is the time required for whole blood to clot in a glass test tube at 37°C. This is a crude test and is affected by a number of variables. It is usually prolonged when severe deficiency of a coagulation factor in intrinsic or common pathways is present (coagulation factor level <1%) and is often normal in mild/moderate deficiency. This test has now been replaced by activated partial thromboplastin time.

The most common screening tests for assessment of coagulation phase are prothrombin time and activated partial thromboplastin time.

Collection of Blood Sample for Coagulation Studies

The prerequisites for accurate results of coagulation studies are proper collection and subsequent handling of blood sample. Certain precautions should be followed for collection, handling, and storage of specimens for coagulation studies.

Venipuncture (usually from antecubital vein) should be smooth and nontraumatic to minimize tissue thromboplastin release. As far as possible blood for coagulation studies should not be collected from an indwelling catheter as it may be contaminated with tissue fluids, intravenous fluids, or heparin which will give rise to inaccurate results. Blood should be collected with a plastic or polypropylene syringe and a large bore needle (20 G1½ or 21 G1½). Glass syringe and glass test tubes/bottles should never be used for collection of blood for coagulation studies as glass activates contact factors and initiates coagulation through intrinsic pathway. Prolonged application of tourniquet should be avoided as stasis may cause increased fibrinolysis and activation of some coagulation factors. Blood container should be made of plastic in which liquid anticoagulant has been added earlier. The anticoagulant of choice for coagulation studies is aqueous trisodium citrate (3.2%); this is because it causes rapid chelation of calcium and factors V and VIII remain relatively more stable in it. Proportion of blood to anticoagulant should be 9:1. Blood from the syringe should be allowed to flow smoothly down the side of the container. Blood and anticoagulant should be gently but thoroughly mixed.

After collection, blood sample should be transported to the laboratory without delay and kept tightly stoppered to minimize pH changes. For assay of labile coagulation factors, maintenance at 4°C is advocated.

For most coagulation studies, platelet-poor plasma (PPP) is needed. Blood sample is centrifuged at 3000 to 4000 revolutions/min for 15 to 30 minutes to obtain PPP. Platelet-rich plasma (PRP) is required for platelet function studies; it is obtained either by slow centrifugation for 5 minutes or by allowing the anticoagulated blood to settle at room temperature.

Coagulation studies need to be carried out within 2 hours of collection and centrifugation of sample.

A control (standard) sample is prepared either locally or commercially and its value is determined earlier by a reference method. A control must be run along with the patient's sample to verify the accuracy of results and to assess the reproducibility of the test system.

Prothrombin Time

Tissue thromboplastin and calcium are added to platelet-poor plasma and clotting time of the mixture is noted. This test is a measure of extrinsic and common pathways. Commercial tissue thromboplastin is prepared from rabbit brain or rabbit lung. Tissue thromboplastin serves two functions. It activates extrinsic system and provides phospholipid surface for certain coagulation reactions. Calcium ions bind vitamin K-dependent factors (II, VII, IX, and X) to phospholipid. Normal range of PT is 11 to 16 seconds. Prothrombin time measures the activity of coagulation factors VII, X, V, II (prothrombin), and I (fibrinogen) (Fig. 13.1).

Causes of prolongation of PT:
1. *Vitamin K deficiency:* PT is a useful test for detection of vitamin K deficiency as it measures three vitamin K-dependent proteins out of four, i.e. II, VII, and X.
2. *Oral anticoagulant therapy:* Oral anticoagulants interfere with the carboxylation of vitamin K-dependent factors. PT is the standard test for monitoring oral anticoagulant therapy.
3. *Disseminated intravascular coagulation*
4. *Inherited deficiency of a coagulation factor in extrinsic or common pathway,* i.e. VII, X, V, II, or I.

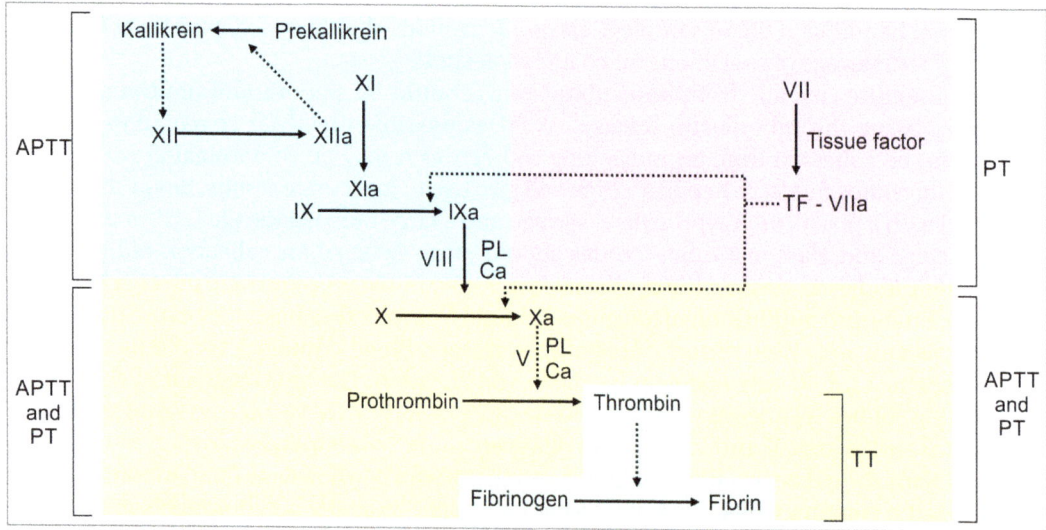

Fig. 13.1: Coagulation factors measured by three screening tests: prothrombin time (PT), activated partial thromboplastin time (APTT), and thrombin time (TT).

Activated Partial Thromboplastin Time (APTT)

In this test, platelet-poor plasma is incubated with an activator. Then phospholipid and calcium are added and clotting time is noted. An activator serves to standardize the contact activation. Commonly used activators are kaolin, celite, ellagic acid, and silica. Phospholipid is also called as partial thromboplastin; it provides surface for certain coagulation reactions. APTT measures activity of coagulation factors in intrinsic and common pathways (Fig. 13.1). Normal range of APTT is 30 to 40 seconds.

Causes of prolongation of APTT:
1. *Inherited deficiency of FVIII or FIX:* APTT is the most widely used screening test for the detection of hereditary deficiency of FVIII and FIX. APTT is also prolonged in inherited deficiencies of other coagulation factors in intrinsic and common pathways.
2. *Circulating inhibitors:* Inhibitors may be of two types—specific and nonspecific. Specific inhibitors are directed against specific coagulation factors. The most common specific inhibitor is antibody against F VIII. Nonspecific inhibitors are antibodies that are not directed against specific coagulation factors but block the interaction of clotting factors, for example, lupus inhibitor.
3. *Disseminated intravascular coagulation*
4. *Heparin:* Heparin accelerates the action of antithrombin and thus inhibits thrombin and factors Xa, XIa, and IXa. Heparin therapy is monitored by regularly performing APTT.
5. *Liver disease:* Prolongation of APTT occurs in moderate to severe liver disease due to reduced synthesis of coagulation factors.
6. *Vitamin K deficiency:* Although vitamin K deficiency prolongs APTT, the test is not affected by FVII (a vitamin-K-dependent factor with the shortest half-life). Therefore, it is not as sensitive as PT to vitamin K deficiency.

Shortening of APTT is observed in thrombosis and pregnancy. Approach to prolonged APTT is presented in Figure 13.2.

Thrombin Time

Thrombin reagent is added to platelet-poor plasma and the time required for clot formation is noted. Normal range is 8 to 12 seconds. Prolongation of thrombin time occurs in the following:
- *Disorders of fibrinogen:* These include afibrinogenemia (virtual absence of fibrinogen), hypofibrinogenemia (fibrinogen level is detectable but less than 100 mg/dL), and dysfibrinogenemia (qualitative defect of fibrinogen).
- *Presence of heparin in plasma*
- *Chronic liver disease*
- *Fibrinogen/Fibrin degradation products*

In most patients suspected of having a bleeding disorder, it is possible to arrive at a presumptive diagnosis by performing a small battery of screening tests (Fig. 13.3 and Table 13.4). Depending upon the results of the screening tests, appropriate specific studies can be performed to arrive at the final diagnosis.

In some bleeding disorders, hemostatic screening tests may be normal (Box 13.5).

Section 4: Disorders of Hemostasis

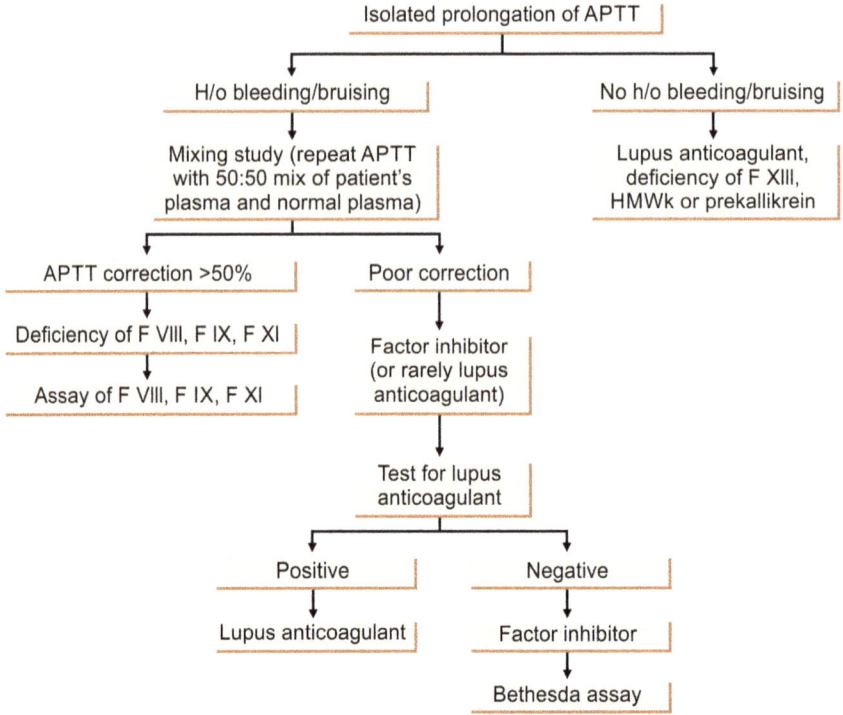

Fig. 13.2: Approach to evaluation of isolated prolongation of activated partial thromboplastin time (APTT).

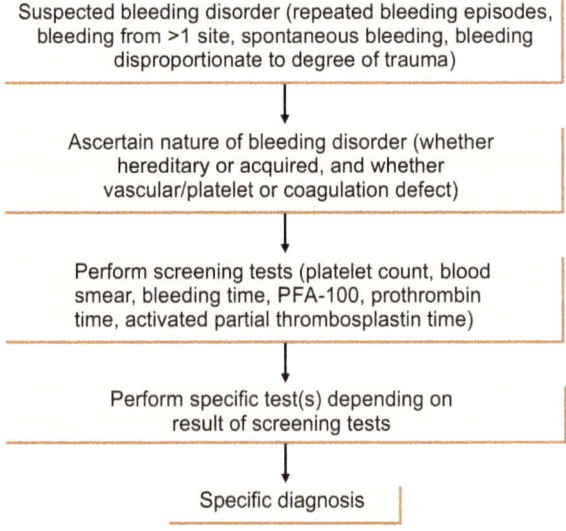

Fig. 13.3: General approach for investigation of a bleeding disorder.

Table 13.4: Interpretation of screening tests of hemostasis in a bleeding disorder.

BT	PC	PT	APTT	Hemostatic defect	Common causes
I	N	N	N	Platelet function, vascular disorder	vWD, aspirin, uremia, storage pool defect
I	D	N	N	Thrombocytopenia	Secondary causes, drugs, ITP
N	N	I	N	Extrinsic pathway	Oral anticoagulants, vitamin K deficiency, deficiency of F VII
N	N	N	I	Intrinsic pathway	Heparin, hemophilia A or B, vWD, inhibitors
N	N	I	I	Common pathway	Heparin, liver disease, vitamin K deficiency, oral anticoagulants, deficiency of V, X, II, I
I	D	I	I	Multiple pathways	Disseminated intravascular coagulation, liver disease
N	N	N	N	-	Mild vWD, vascular disorder, platelet function defect, F XIII deficiency

(N: Normal; I: increased; D: decreased; vWD: von Willebrand disease)

> **Box 13.5:** Bleeding disorders that may present with normal screening tests for hemostasis.
> - Coagulation disorders: Mild hemophilia A or B, mild von Willebrand disease, F XIII deficiency
> - Platelet disorders: Glanzmann's thrombasthenia, platelet storage pool defect
> - Vascular defects: Hereditary hemorrhagic telangiectasia, osteogenesis imperfecta, scurvy, Ehlers–Danlos syndrome
> - Defects in fibrinolysis: $\alpha 2$-antiplasmin deficiency

SPECIFIC TESTS

Specific Tests for Primary Hemostatic Disorders

Bleeding due to a defect in primary hemostasis results from following disorders:
- von Willebrand disease
- Thrombocytopenia
- Vascular disorder
- Platelet function defect

Tests for Specific Platelet Functions

Tests are available to define specific platelet functional abnormalities in adhesion, aggregation, release reaction, and platelet procoagulant activity. Commonly used platelet function tests are outlined in Table 13.5.

Platelet aggregation studies: For platelet aggregation studies, a special instrument called as aggregometer is used. This instrument has a continuous stirring device to keep the platelets in platelet-rich plasma in an even suspension; when a platelet-aggregating agent or agonist is added to platelet-rich plasma, change in light transmission occurs due to platelet aggregation, which is recorded by a photometer.

Table 13.5: Salient features of platelet function tests.

Name	Principle	Clinical applications	Comment
Bleeding time	Time needed for bleeding to cease following incision	In vivo screening test of platelet function	Invasive, low reproducibility, low sensitivity
Platelet aggregometry (light transmission)	Change in light transmission after addition of a panel of agonists	Diagnosis of inherited and acquired platelet function defects, Monitoring of antiplatelet therapy	Gold standard test; time-consuming; needs experience in performance and interpretation
PFA-100/200	High shear platelet adhesion and aggregation in whole blood	Detection of various platelet function defects and von Willebrand disease, monitoring of antiplatelet drugs like aspirin	Choice of agonists is fixed; affected by platelet count and hematocrit
Multiplate analyzer	Platelet aggregation assessed by change in impedance in whole blood	Detection of platelet function defects and monitoring antiplatelet therapy	Variety of agonists can be used; affected by platelet count and hematocrit
VerifyNow	Platelet aggregation in whole blood (light transmission)	Monitoring of antiplatelet drugs	Point of care test
Flow cytometry	Measurement of platelet glycoproteins and activation markers	Diagnosis of platelet glycoprotein defects, monitoring of antiplatelet drugs	Expensive; needs expertise
Thromboelastography (TEG/ROTEM)	Assessment of rate and quality of clot formation	Test of global hemostasis; guiding blood product replacement in major trauma or major surgery	Point of care in surgical setting
Clot retraction test	Clot retraction after recalcification of citrated plasma	Absent in Glanzmann's thrombasthenia (type 1)	Crude test

When an aggregating agent is added to platelet-rich plasma, initially there is platelet shape change from discoid to spherical. This causes a small decrease in transmission of light. As aggregates of platelets form, light transmission increases, which is recorded on the strip chart.

Commonly employed aggregating agents are ADP, epinephrine, collagen, arachidonic acid, and ristocetin. ADP and epinephrine induce primary and secondary waves of aggregation (biphasic curve). Primary wave is due to the direct action of aggregating agent on platelets with formation of small aggregates. Secondary wave is associated with thromboxane A2 synthesis and secretion from platelet granules. Collagen, arachidonic acid, and ristocetin induce a single wave of aggregation (monophasic curve).

Aggregation response is deficient or absent with ADP, epinephrine, collagen, and arachidonic acid in Glanzmann's thrombasthenia. In this disorder, there is congenital absence of platelet receptors GpIIb-IIIa necessary for fibrinogen binding during aggregation; platelet aggregation, however, is normal with ristocetin.

Table 13.6: Platelet aggregation studies in disorders of platelet function.

Disorder	Aggregating agents			
	ADP/Epinephrine		Collagen	Ristocetin
	Primary wave	Secondary wave		
1. Bernard-Soulier syndrome (BSS)*	Normal	Normal	Normal	Deficient
2. von Willebrand disease (vWD)*	Normal	Normal	Normal	Deficient
3. Glanzmann's thrombasthenia	Deficient	Deficient	Deficient	Normal
4. Storage pool deficiency**	Normal	Deficient	Deficient	Normal
5. Aspirin-like defect**	Normal	Deficient	Deficient	Normal

*Cryoprecipitate corrects abnormality in vWD but not in BSS.
** Aggregation is defective with arachidonic acid in aspirin-like defect, but not in storage pool deficiency.

Defective aggregation with ristocetin but not with other agonists is a feature of von Willebrand disease and Bernard-Soulier syndrome. Addition of normal plasma (source of von Willebrand factor) corrects the abnormality in von Willebrand disease but not in Bernard-Soulier syndrome.

In release reaction defects, ADP and epinephrine induce primary wave of aggregation but no secondary wave is produced (Table 13.6).

VerifyNow test: This commercially available point-of-care automated test is used to assess the level of platelet inhibition by antiplatelet agents (aspirin, clopidogrel) given for prevention of thrombosis. The test uses whole blood and assesses platelet aggregation by ADP after initiation of therapy. A baseline level of platelet aggregation by ADP is first established before beginning therapy. After initiation of therapy, the percent change from baseline is derived. Although resistance to antiplatelet agents may be detected in many patients, it is unclear whether results affect the clinical outcome.

Flow cytometry: Flow cytometry is widely used for (1) Diagnosis of Glanzmann's thrombasthenia by demonstration of reduced expression of platelet integrin $\alpha IIb\beta 3$ (CD41/CD61), and (2) Diagnosis of Bernard-Soulier syndrome by demonstrating absent expression of GP1b-IX-V (CD42a-d).

Tests of platelet secretion or release reaction: Secondary wave of aggregation with ADP or epinephrine is an indirect evidence of release reaction. Various direct tests for assessing release reaction are available. Dense granule secretion may be assessed by quantitation of serotonin, and measuring ATP concentration by firefly bioluminescence technique. Measurements of platelet factor 4 and β thromboglobulin released from α granules are sensitive indicators of platelet activation and have been applied in the study of hypercoagulable states.

Tests for detection of abnormalities in arachidonic acid metabolism: Arachidonic acid metabolism plays an important role in activation of platelets by generating thromboxane A2 (refer to Fig. 1.31). Defective platelet aggregation by arachidonic acid is indicative of abnormality in arachidonic acid metabolism. Techniques for quantitation of TxB2, malondialdehyde, and other intermediate products in arachidonate pathway are available. Their use can lead to the identification of deficiencies of phospholipases, cyclooxygenase, and thromboxane synthetase.

Tests for platelet procoagulant activity: Platelet procoagulant activity may be assessed by the prothrombin consumption test. This test assesses clotting activity or the amount of residual prothrombin remaining in serum after whole blood is allowed to clot completely. Prothrombin times of serum and of citrated plasma are performed and the result is expressed as their ratio. Presence of unconsumed prothrombin may be due to deficiency of coagulation factors or of platelet phospholipid.

Other platelet function tests: Clot retraction test: In this test citrated platelet-rich plasma is recalcified. The plasma clots, which subsequently, undergo retraction. Clot retraction is dependent upon adequate number and function of platelets. Poor clot retraction is observed in thrombocytopenia and in Glanzmann's thrombasthenia.

Specific Tests for Coagulation Phase

Mixing Study Based on PT or APTT

If a coagulation factor deficiency is suspected and if there is isolated prolongation of either PT or APTT, mixing study should be performed to determine whether factor deficiency or an inhibitor is present. In this test, abnormal PT or APTT is repeated using 50:50 mixture of normal and patients' plasma and whether normalization of previously prolonged test occurs should be noted. If deficiency of coagulation factor is present then the addition of normal plasma corrects prolonged clotting time. In the presence of inhibitors, result depends upon the type of inhibitor (Table 13.7). Inhibitors may be of immediate-acting or delayed-acting types. If immediate-acting inhibitor is present, APTT/PT performed using mixture of patient's plasma and normal plasma remains prolonged with no correction. If delayed-acting inhibitor is present, clotting time of the mixture immediately becomes normal; however, after incubation for 1 to 2 hours at 37°C, prolongation of clotting time is observed.

If mixing study indicates factor deficiency, it is necessary to identify the deficient factor. The deficient factor in patient's plasma can be identified by correction test using adsorbed normal plasma and aged normal human serum or by thromboplastin generation test.

Thromboplastin Generation Test (TGT)

This is a two-stage test.

Stage I (Generation of prothrombinase): Adsorbed plasma, serum, phospholipid, and calcium are incubated together. Adsorbed plasma supplies factors V and VIII; serum supplies factors IX and X, and both supply factors XI and XII. This leads to the generation of prothrombinase (F Xa-V-calcium-phospholipid complex).

Stage II (Assessment of adequacy of prothrombinase generated): The coagulant activity of the prothrombinase formed is measured by its ability to clot substrate (normal) plasma. If the prothrombinase generated is deficient, then abnormal result (i.e. prolonged clotting time) is obtained. In such a case, substitution studies are carried out to localize the defect. The test is performed using patient's adsorbed plasma and normal serum, and patient's serum and normal adsorbed plasma to detect which substitution produces normal or abnormal result.

Table 13.7: Interpretation of mixing study based on activated partial thromboplastin time.

Result of 50:50 mix	Cause
Correction	Factor deficiency
No correction	Lupus anticoagulant
Immediate correction, but prolongation after incubation	Factor inhibitor

Table 13.8: Interpretation of thromboplastin generation test.

History	Coagulation screen	TGT	Interpretation
Bleeding	PT-N, APTT-P	Plasma defect	F VIII deficiency
Bleeding	PT-P, APTT-P	Plasma defect	F V deficiency
Bleeding	PT-N, APTT-P	Serum defect	F IX deficiency
Bleeding	PT-P, APTT-P	Serum defect	F X deficiency
Bleeding	PT-N, APTT-P	Both plasma and serum defect	F XI deficiency
no bleeding	PT-N, APTT-P	Both plasma and serum defect	F XII deficiency

(APTT: activated partial thromboplastin time; N: normal; PT: prothrombin time; P: prolonged)

A presumptive diagnosis of a particular factor deficiency can be made by also considering the results of PT and clinical history (Table 13.8).

Quantitative Estimation of Fibrinogen

A number of methods are available for the estimation of plasma fibrinogen. Some of the methods are outlined below:
- Coagulable protein method based on thrombin time: This is the most widely used reference method. This method makes use of the reaction between fibrinogen and thrombin in which there is formation of a fibrin clot. Clauss modified the thrombin time screening test so that it could be applied for estimation of fibrinogen. If thrombin in excess is added to the diluted plasma, then the clotting time is inversely proportional to the concentration of fibrinogen. The modifications of higher reagent concentration and lower plasma concentrations provide a linear relationship between clotting time and concentration of fibrinogen. The clotting time obtained is compared with clotting times of known fibrinogen standards in the same system to get the result.
- Immunological methods: Immunologic procedures depend on reaction between plasma fibrinogen and antifibrinogen antibody. The methods include single radial immunodiffusion or radioimmunoassay. Immunologic methods, when applied together with functional (coagulable protein) method, are useful in diagnosing dysfibrinogenemias. In the presence of dysfunctional fibrinogen molecules, low values are obtained with functional method (i.e. coagulable protein method), while normal results are obtained with immunologic method.
- Other methods: Other methods of fibrinogen estimation are based on weighing of clot and precipitation of fibrinogen by heat (56°C) or by chemicals (sodium sulfite). Normal level of fibrinogen in plasma is 200 to 400 mg/dL.

Low levels of fibrinogen are seen in a- or hypofibrinogenemia, dysfibrinogenemia, and disseminated intravascular coagulation. Transient hyperfibrinogenemia occurs in inflammatory disorders, neoplasia, myocardial infarction, and trauma.

Coagulation Factor Assays

One-stage coagulation factor assays are commonly performed to diagnose factor deficiency and are based on APTT or PT. PT or APTT is performed using mixture of patient's plasma and factor-deficient plasma and the clotting time is noted (Factor-deficient plasma contains all the coagulation factors, except the one to be assayed). Clotting time obtained is compared with a previously prepared reference graph, which has clotting time in seconds on one axis and percentage activity of coagulation factor on the other. Reference graph is prepared using various dilutions of standard (or normal) plasma mixed with factor-deficient plasma; 1:10 dilution of standard plasma represents 100% activity.

Normal level of all coagulation factors is 50–150% or 50–150 units/dL.

FXIII Qualitative Assay

F XIII is a transglutaminase that catalyzes the formation of covalent bonds between fibrin monomers and imparts stability to the clot. In the absence of FXIII, fibrin clot is unstable and dissolves in 5M-urea solution or 1% monochloracetic acid.

In FXIII deficiency, all the screening tests of hemostasis are normal.

Paracoagulation Tests

Paracoagulation tests are employed for the detection of soluble (nonpolymerized) fibrin monomers in plasma. These include protamine sulfate or ethanol gelation tests. In these tests, ethanol or protamine sulfate is added to platelet-poor plasma and formation of a gel is noted. Positive test is indicative of active or ongoing intravascular coagulation. Positive result is also obtained in lobar pneumonia, liver disease, and after major surgery.

Reptilase Time

In this test, reptilase (a snake venom obtained from *Bothrops atrox*) is added to plasma and clotting time is noted. Clotting time is elevated in the same conditions in which thrombin time is elevated, but the test remains normal in the presence of heparin. This test is done if thrombin time is prolonged. It is most useful for evaluation of dysfibrinogenemia. Evaluation of thrombin time and reptilase time is shown in Figure 13.4.

Ecarin Time

Ecarin, obtained from venom of the saw-scaled viper *Echis carinatus*, directly activates prothrombin leading to clot formation. It is used for monitoring of antithrombin drug therapy like dabigatran.

Tests for Fibrinolysis

Detection of Fibrinogen/Fibrin Degradation Products by Latex Agglutination Test

Fibrin degradation products (FDPs) are fragments produced by proteolytic digestion of fibrinogen or fibrin by plasmin (refer to Figs. 1.41 and 1.42).

Test for FDPs is performed on serum. Venous whole blood is mixed with thrombin and either soybean trypsin inhibitor or epsilon-amino-caproic acid. Thrombin removes all fibrinogen by converting it into a fibrin clot. Soybean trypsin inhibitor or epsilon-amino-caproic acid are inhibitors of fibrinolysis that prevent in vitro breakdown of fibrin.

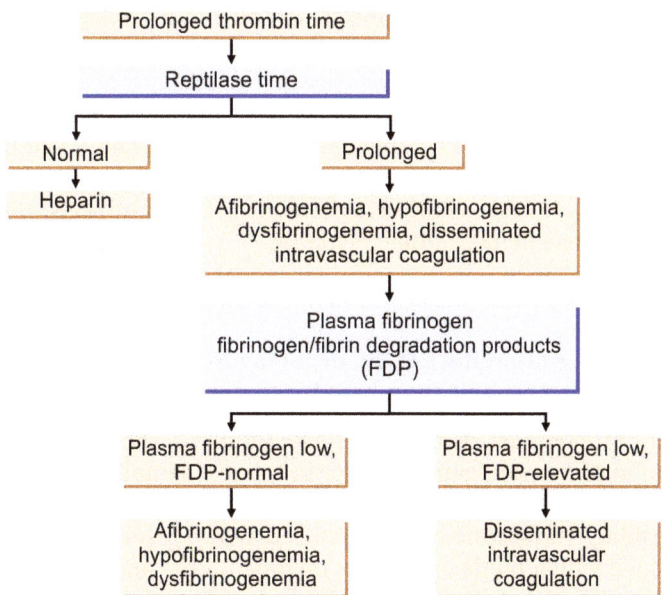

Fig. 13.4: Evaluation of prolonged thrombin time.

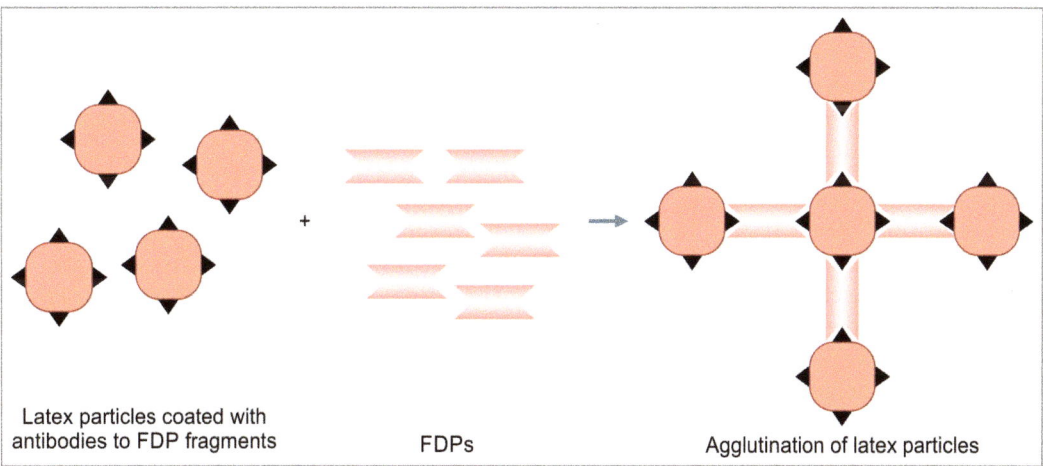

Fig. 13.5: Principle of latex agglutination test for fibrinogen/fibrin degradation products (FDPs).

A suspension of latex particles coated with antifibrinogen antibodies (FDPs share common antigenic determinants with fibrinogen) or with antibodies to specific FDPs is mixed with serum on a glass slide. If FDPs are present, then agglutination of latex particles occurs (Fig. 13.5). Apart from qualitative screening, a semiquantitative estimation of FDPs can also be done. These tests are simple, sensitive, and rapid but are expensive and false positive result with rheumatoid factor can occur.

Test for detection of FDPs are commonly employed for diagnosis of disseminated intravascular coagulation (DIC). Although FDPs are usually raised in most patients with DIC, FDP test may sometimes be negative. This is because of removal of clottable FDP fragments X and Y along with fibrinogen by thrombin in blood collection tubes. In early DIC in which circulating plasmin levels are low, FDP fragments are mostly X and Y and their removal can produce a false negative test.

Apart from DIC, FDPs are also detected in pulmonary embolism, deep venous thrombosis, severe pneumonia, and recent myocardial infarction.

Tests for D-dimer

D-dimer is the smallest end-product of the degradation of cross-linked fibrin by plasmin. Currently, ELISA-based and agglutination-based assays are available for D-dimer testing.

ELISA-based assay: Monoclonal antibody against D-dimer (called as "capture" antibody) is attached to the solid phase. Antigen (D-dimer in the test sample) is added and allowed to interact with the antibody. The antigen is 'captured' by the coated antibody. Unbound antigen is removed by washing. The second enzyme-labeled antibody (called as 'detection' antibody or detector) is added which binds to another epitope on the antigen. Unbound material is removed by washing. The labeled antibody is quantitated by measuring the amount of color developed after addition of the chromogenic substrate.

Agglutination-based assay: Latex or polystyrene particles are coated with monoclonal antibody against D-dimer antigen. Binding of D-dimer (if present in added test plasma) causes agglutination of these particles. The result is inspected visually and a semiquantitative result is obtained. Automated latex agglutination assays have been developed that can be performed on coagulation analyzers. In addition, point-of-care devices are also available which can generate a qualitative result for bedside diagnosis.

Applications of D-dimer testing: D-dimer is elevated in venous thromboembolism including pulmonary embolism, arterial thrombosis, and in disseminated intravascular coagulation or DIC. However, elevated D-dimer levels are also found in pregnancy, postoperative state, liver disease, and cancer. Therefore a positive test for D-dimer is not confirmatory for diagnosis of DVT, but a negative test excludes the diagnosis of DVT. The principle uses of D-dimer testing are (1) exclusion of venous thromboembolism and pulmonary embolism (high negative predictive value), and (2) diagnosis of DIC.

Thromboelastography

Thromboelastography (TEG) is considered as a global hemostatic test since it assesses both whole blood coagulation and fibrinolysis. The main use of TEG is in situations where blood loss can be extensive like liver transplantation, cardiac surgery, and trauma care unit. It provides information about lag time before beginning of clot formation, rate of clot formation, clot strength, and clot dissolution. This point of care device is mainly used to guide hemostatic therapy in bleeding patients.

BIBLIOGRAPHY

1. Allen GA, Gladers B. Approach to the bleeding child. Ped Clin North Am. 2002;49:1239-56.
2. Day HJ, Rao AK. Evaluation of platelet function. Semin Hematol.1986;23:89-101.
3. Greenberg CS, Devine DV, McCrae KM. Measurement of plasma fibrin antibody coupled to latex beads. Am J Clin Pathol. 1987;87:94-100.
4. Marder VJ, Matchett MO, Sherry S. Detection of serum fibrinogen and fibrin degradation products. Comparison of six technics using purified products and application in clinical studies. Am J Med. 1971;51:71-82.
5. Merskey C, Lalezari P, Johnson AJ. A rapid, simple, sensitive method for measuring fibrinolytic split products in human serum. Proc Soc Exp Biol Med. 1969;131:871.
6. Mhawech P, Saleem A. Inherited giant platelet disorders. Classification and literature review. Am J Clin Pathol. 2000;113:176-90.
7. Moreno A, Menke D. Assessment of platelet numbers and morphology in the peripheral blood smear. Clin Lab Med. 2002;22:193-213.
8. Triplett DA. Coagulation and bleeding disorders: Review and update. Clin Chem. 2000;46:1260-9.
9. Vora A, Makris M. An approach to investigation of easy bruising. Arch Dis Child. 2001;84:488-91.

CHAPTER 14

Bleeding Disorders Caused by Abnormalities of Blood Vessels (The Vascular Purpuras)

INTRODUCTION

Defective hemostasis occurs in a wide variety of vascular disorders (Table 14.1). In these diseases, clinical features are frequently distinctive, type of bleeding is superficial, and laboratory tests of hemostasis yield normal results (Box 14.1).

ANAPHYLACTOID PURPURA (HENOCH-SCHÖNLEIN PURPURA, ALLERGIC PURPURA)

This is an immune complex disease in which purpura results from vasculitis (due to deposition of IgA-containing complexes). Manifestations of allergic purpura include the following:
- Predominant occurrence in children (2–8 years). Frequently, there is a recent history of upper respiratory infection or of other inciting factor such as sensitivity to certain foods

Table 14.1: Vascular purpuras.

Acquired	Inherited
1. Anaphylactoid purpura	1. Hereditary hemorrhagic telangiectasia
2. Infections	2. Hereditary connective tissue disorders
3. Scurvy	– Ehlers-Danlos syndrome
4. Senile purpura	– Osteogenesis imperfecta
5. Purpura simplex	– Marfan's syndrome
6. Mechanical purpura	– Pseudoxanthoma elasticum
7. Drugs, e.g. corticosteroids	
8. Cushing's syndrome	
9. Factitious purpura	

Box 14.1: Diagnosis of vascular purpuras.
- Superficial, mild bleeding from skin and mucous membranes
- Bleeding from skin more in dependent portions of body
- Screening tests of hemostasis often normal
- Associated clinical features usually characteristic

- Rapid onset
- *Skin:* Palpable purpuric spots over extensor surfaces of extremities, associated with urticaria; sometimes hemorrhagic bullous and necrotic lesions occur
- *Gastrointestinal tract:* Abdominal pain (due possibly to mesenteric vasculitis), sometimes with bleeding
- *Joints:* Arthralgia
- *Kidneys:* Microscopic hematuria, proteinuria, acute glomerulonephritis, or nephrotic syndrome.

These features may occur in combination or one feature may predominate. The disease is self-limited but recurrent episodes are common. Chronic glomerulonephritis and CNS bleeding are rare complications.

Diagnosis is based on typical clinical presentation (palpable purpura, age of onset <20 years, acute abdominal pain) and granulocytic infiltrate in the walls of arterioles and venules.

Glucocorticoids are sometimes administered for symptomatic relief.

INFECTIONS

Infections can cause vascular damage by direct endothelial damage or by immune complex mechanism. Commonly responsible agents are meningococci, *Salmonella*, measles virus, and rickettsial organisms. Severe infections can also cause bleeding by other mechanisms such as thrombocytopenia or consumptive coagulopathy.

SCURVY

Vitamin C deficiency is frequently associated with hemorrhagic manifestations such as perifollicular hemorrhages, petechiae, bleeding gums, subperiosteal hemorrhages, and deep-seated hematomas, The cause of bleeding is defective synthesis of collagen. Bleeding tendency is readily corrected by oral administration of ascorbic acid.

SENILE PURPURA

Purpuric and ecchymotic lesions commonly develop in elderly persons over 70 years of age on forearms, hands, face, and neck. The lesions disappear after a few weeks leaving behind brown discoloration. There is atrophy of subendothelial collagen, subcutaneous fat, and elastic tissue due to aging which results in increased susceptibility of small blood vessels to trivial injury. No treatment is required.

PURPURA SIMPLEX

Mild bruising may develop spontaneously on lower legs in young women of reproductive age, with aggravation during menstruation. It requires no treatment.

MECHANICAL PURPURA

Violent and prolonged bouts of coughing may cause rupture of small blood vessels in face and neck area due to rise in local intravascular pressure. Prolonged upright posture in elderly may be associated with purpura in legs due to atrophy of perivascular connective tissue coupled with venous insufficiency (orthostatic purpura).

HEREDITARY HEMORRHAGIC TELANGIECTASIA (OSLER-WEBER-RENDU DISEASE)

This is a rare autosomal dominant disorder characterized by presence of multiple, small, telangiectatic lesions in skin, mucous membranes, and internal organs. Bleeding manifestations occur spontaneously or following minor trauma and are related to marked thinning of walls of dilated blood vessels. Onset of hemorrhages is usually in early adult life with recurrent epistaxis and gastrointestinal bleeding being common complaints. Bleeding tendencies increase with advancing age and commonly cause iron deficiency anemia. Topical hemostatics, embolization of pulmonary arteriovenous malformation, and administration of iron for correction of anemia are the usual forms of therapy.

BIBLIOGRAPHY

1. Kraft DM, McKee D, Scott C. Henoch-Schönlein Purpura: A review. Am Fam Physician. 1998;58: 405.
2. Lee GR, Bithell TC, Foerster J, Athens JW, Lukens JN (Eds). Wintrobe's Clinical Hematology, 9th edition. Philadelphia: Lea and Febiger; 1993.

CHAPTER 15

Bleeding Disorders Caused by Abnormalities of Platelets

Disorders of platelets include—(i) thrombocytopenia, (ii) thrombocytosis, and (iii) platelet dysfunction.

THROMBOCYTOPENIA

Thrombocytopenia refers to a decrease in the number of platelets in peripheral blood below normal (<1.5 lacs/mm³). It may result due to four main mechanisms (Table 15.1).
- Increased peripheral destruction of platelets
- Decreased production of platelets in the bone marrow
- Sequestration in enlarged spleen
- Artefactual thrombocytopenia.

The lower value of platelets is 150,000/mm³. Platelet count between 150,000/mm³ and 50,000/mm³ is generally not associated with clinically significant bleeding. Platelet counts between 50,000/mm³ and 20,000/mm³ usually cause bleeding with trauma or surgery or mild spontaneous bleeding. Platelet count below 20,000/mm³ is associated with risk of spontaneous, severe hemorrhage.

Immune Thrombocytopenia

Immune thrombocytopenia (ITP) is an acquired immune disorder in which premature platelet destruction occurs due to antibodies directed against platelets. It is classified as primary or secondary (Table 15.1).

International Working Group (Vicenza Consensus Conference) in 2009 introduced a standardized terminology for immune thrombocytopenia as follows:
- Threshold for diagnosis of thrombocytopenia: <100,000/mm³.
- Primary ITP: ITP without any associated cause (diagnosis of exclusion)
- Secondary ITP: ITP resulting from an underlying cause like infections, drugs, autoimmune disorders, lymphoproliferative disorders, etc.
- Newly diagnosed ITP: All cases within first 3 months from diagnosis
- Persistent ITP: All cases between 3 and 12 months from diagnosis
- Chronic ITP: Thrombocytopenia lasting for more than 12 months from diagnosis.

Section 4: Disorders of Hemostasis

Table 15.1: Causes of thrombocytopenia.

1. *Increased destruction of platelets*
   - Immune
     - Immune thrombocytopenia (ITP)
       » Primary immune thrombocytopenia
       » Secondary immune thrombocytopenia: Infections (e.g. HIV, HCV, *H. pylori*, EBV), Drugs (heparin, quinine, quinidine, etc.), autoimmune disorders, lymphoproliferative disorders
     - Neonatal alloimmune purpura
     - Post-transfusion purpura
   - Non-immune
     - Disseminated intravascular coagulation
     - Thrombotic microangiopathy: Thrombotic thrombocytopenic purpura, hemolytic uremic syndrome
     - Giant hemangioma
     - HELLP syndrome
2. Decreased production of platelets:
   - Hereditary
     - Congenital amegakaryocytic thrombocytopenia
     - Fanconi anemia
     - *MYH-9* related macrothrombocytopenia
     - Wiskott-Aldrich syndrome
   - Acquired
     - Aplastic anemia
     - Megaloblastic anemia
     - Bone marrow infiltration (leukemias, myelofibrosis, lymphoma, metastatic carcinoma)
     - Cytotoxic chemotherapy
3. Increased sequestration
   - Hypersplenism
4. Artefactual thrombocytopenia
   - Inadequate anticoagulation of blood sample
   - EDTA-dependent pseudothrombocytopenia
   - Giant platelets

ITP was previously called as idiopathic thrombocytopenic purpura, immune thrombocytopenic purpura, or autoimmune thrombocytopenic purpura. The term immune thrombocytopenia is appropriate as thrombocytopenia results from autoantibody-mediated mechanism, and bleeding is absent in a significant number of patients.

ITP can be acute or chronic. Acute ITP is a short-lasting illness of sudden onset which occurs in children often in the winter and spring following the incidence of viral infections. Chronic ITP is an indolent disorder of insidious onset with multiple remissions and relapses, occurs predominantly in adult women, and is not preceded by any infection and is not associated with any underlying disease.

Pathogenesis: In ITP, autoantibodies (predominantly IgG, less commonly IgM) bind to platelet glycoproteins GPIIb/IIIa and/or GPIb/IX. These antibody-coated platelets bind to Fc receptors on macrophages and are destroyed in spleen and liver. GPIIB/IIIa are sites for fibrinogen binding during platelet aggregation. Thus, in addition to causing destruction of platelets, these antibodies also induce platelet dysfunction by blocking GPIIb/IIIa receptors. Antibodies also react with megakaryocytes in bone marrow and interfere with platelet production.

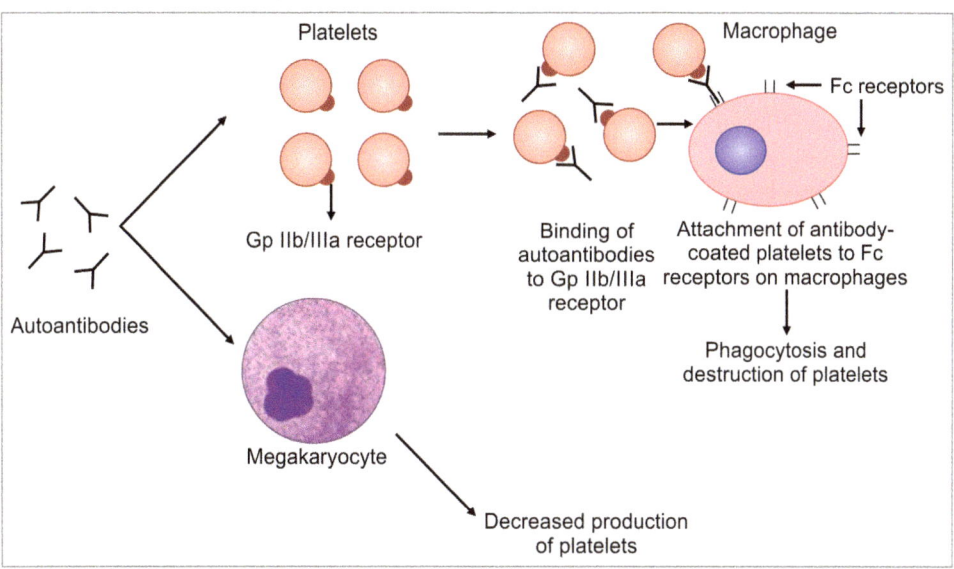

Fig. 15.1: Pathogenesis of idiopathic thrombocytopenic purpura (ITP).

Antibody-coated platelets are rapidly destroyed in reticuloendothelial organs particularly spleen and liver (Fig 15.1). Thrombocytopenia results when peripheral destruction of platelets exceeds compensatory increase in thrombopoiesis in bone marrow.

Cellular immunity is also perturbed in the form of abnormal regulatory T cells (TReg) that normally prevent autoimmune reactions, and loss of T-cell tolerance against platelet antigens with accumulation of autoreactive cytotoxic T cells. Cytotoxic T cells directly cause lysis and apoptosis of platelets as well as of megakaryocytes.

Clinical Features

Incidence of ITP increases with age.

Clinical presentation varies from severe thrombocytopenia and bleeding to asymptomatic mild thrombocytopenia detected incidentally.

Acute ITP predominantly affects children between 2 and 6 years of age with sex ratio being 1:1. The disease often follows viral respiratory infection or vaccination after an interval of 2 to 3 weeks. There is increased incidence during winter and spring. The disease starts suddenly with cutaneous and mucous membrane bleeding in the form of purpuric spots and ecchymoses (especially on legs), bleeding from gums, nose, gastrointestinal tract, and hematuria. Intracranial hemorrhage though rare can be fatal. Spleen tip may be palpable but significant splenomegaly is unusual. The disease is self-limited and spontaneous complete remissions usually occur within 2 to 6 weeks in more than 80% of patients. Recurrences are uncommon. In about 15 to 20% of children, thrombocytopenia persists beyond 6 months.

Chronic ITP occurs in young adults. It is more common in females (3F:1M). There is an insidious onset of superficial bleeding from skin and mucous membrane; menorrhagia is particularly common in women. Chronic bleeding can cause iron deficiency anemia. History of preceding viral infection or any underlying disease is lacking. Spleen is not palpable in chronic ITP and in the presence of splenomegaly, alternative diagnosis should be considered.

Table 15.2: Differences between acute and chronic immune thrombocytopenia (ITP).

	Parameter	Acute ITP	Chronic ITP
1.	Age	Childhood (2–5 years)	Adults (20–40 years)
2.	Sex	No sex preference (1:1)	More common in females (3:1)
3.	History of preceding viral infection or vaccination	Common (1–3 weeks before)	No
4.	Seasonal occurrence	Yes (winter, spring)	No
5.	Onset of bleeding	Sudden	Insidious
6.	Severity of bleeding	Severe (Hemorrhagic bullae in mouth indicate severe disease)	Mild to moderate
7.	Degree of thrombocytopenia (Initial)	Severe <20,000/mm^3	Mild to moderate (30,000–80,000/mm^3)
8.	Eosinophilia or lymphocytosis	Often	No
9.	Duration of disease	Self-limited (average 4–6 weeks)	Many years with remissions and exacerbation
10.	Spontaneous remission	Usual	Rare

Some patients have asymptomatic thrombocytopenia and are discovered incidentally during routine blood counts. Chronic ITP is an indolent disease with remissions and recurrences in bleeding occurring over many years.

Clinical features of acute and chronic ITP are contrasted in Table 15.2.

Laboratory Features

Examination of peripheral blood: Blood loss may lead to anemia. In children, lymphocytes and eosinophils are frequently increased. In acute ITP, platelets are markedly reduced (<20,000/mm^3) while in chronic ITP platelet count is variable (usually moderately low, i.e. around 50,000/mm^3). Morphologically, platelets are frequently large (megathrombocytes) (Fig. 15.2). In chronic ITP, bleeding manifestations are frequently mild as compared to the degree of thrombocytopenia; this is due to the presence of large, giant platelets in circulation, which are functionally hyperactive. The number of large platelets is proportional to megakaryocyte number in marrow. Blood film is also necessary to rule out nonimmune causes of thrombocytopenia (e.g. aplastic anemia, leukemia, myelodysplasia, megaloblastic anemia, pseudothrombocytopenia [see later], and inherited thrombocytopenia).

Bone marrow examination: In bone marrow, megakaryocytes are normal or increased in number (Fig. 15.3) and frequently show morphological changes such as hypogranularity of cytoplasm, vacuolization, lack of platelet budding, nuclear nonlobulation or hypolobulation, and dense nuclear chromatin. These morphologic abnormalities are seen in any condition associated with accelerated platelet destruction and are not specific for ITP.

If clinical features, complete blood count, and blood smear are indicative of ITP, bone marrow examination is not necessary for diagnosis of ITP. However, it should be carried out if presentation is unusual (e.g. presence of splenomegaly or hepatosplenomegaly) and morphological abnormalities of leukocytes are present.

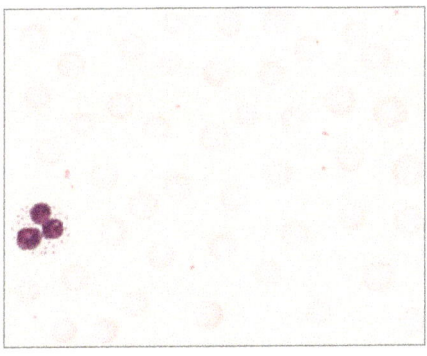
Normal platelets

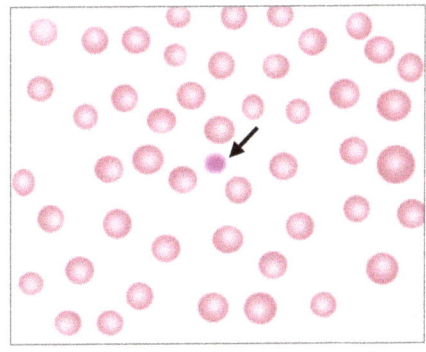
Large platelet in ITP

Fig. 15.2: Blood smear in idiopathic thrombocytopenic purpura (ITP). Blood smear on left shows normal number and size of platelets. Blood smear on right shows reduced number of platelets with only a single large platelet (megathrombocyte) (arrow) in ITP.

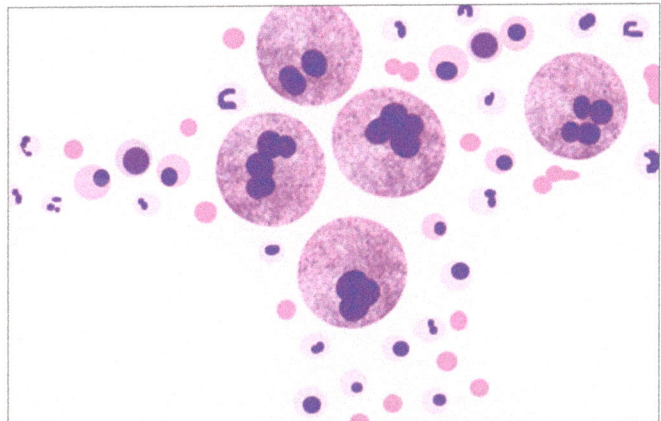

Fig. 15.3: Increased megakaryocytes in bone marrow in idiopathic thrombocytopenic purpura (ITP).

Coagulation profile: Prolonged bleeding time and deficient clot retraction are the usual abnormalities. Tests for blood coagulation are normal.

Platelet antibodies: Levels of platelet-associated immunoglobulins are raised in majority (more than 90%) of patients with ITP. This test, however, is neither sufficiently sensitive nor specific for ITP. Therefore, it is not necessary for diagnosis.

Differential Diagnosis (Table 15.3)

Diagnosis of ITP is one of exclusion since there are no specific clinical or laboratory features. In neonates and small children, maternal ITP, alloimmune neonatal thrombocytopenia, and inherited thrombocytopenia (Box 15.1) should be considered. Possibilities of drug-induced thrombocytopenia and post-transfusion isoimmune purpura are suggested by history. Isolated thrombocytopenia may be the initial manifestation of systemic lupus erythematosus and antinuclear and anticardiolipin antibody tests should be carried out. If immune hemolytic

Table 15.3: Differential diagnosis of idiopathic thrombocytopenic purpura.

Isolated thrombocytopenia	Thrombocytopenia associated with other hematological abnormalities
Secondary immune thrombocytopenia (HIV, HCV, *H. pylori*, autoimmune disorders) Drug-induced thrombocytopenia Inherited thrombocytopenia Pseudothrombocytopenia	Megaloblastic anemia HELLP syndrome/Pre-eclampsia Hypersplenism Hematologic malignancies Aplastic anemia Thrombotic thrombocytopenic purpura/hemolytic uremic syndrome Disseminated intravascular coagulation Evans syndrome Liver disease

(HCV: hepatitis C virus; HIV: human immunodeficiency virus)

Box 15.1: Causes of inherited thrombocytopenia.

- Small platelets: Wiskott-Aldrich syndrome
- Normal-sized platelets: Thrombocytopenia absent radii syndrome, congenital amegakaryocytic thrombocytopenia
- Giant platelets: MYH-9 syndrome (May-Hegglin anomaly, Fechtner syndrome, Epstein syndrome, Sebastian syndrome), Bernard-Soulier syndrome, Gray platelet syndrome, Montreal platelet syndrome

anemia is present along with thrombocytopenia, diagnosis of Evans' syndrome should be considered. Autoimmune thrombocytopenia can occur in lymphoproliferative disorders (lymphoma, chronic lymphocytic leukemia) and in diseases of thyroid and these possibilities should be excluded by appropriate investigations. Human immunodeficiency virus (HIV) infection is emerging as a common cause of thrombocytopenia and should be excluded in high-risk cases. Hereditary thrombocytopenia (Bernard-Soulier syndrome, Wiskott-Aldrich syndrome, May-Hegglin anomaly) may mimic ITP and should be considered when recurrent thrombocytopenia unresponsive to treatment is present since childhood and family history is positive. Fragmented red cells in peripheral blood or abnormal coagulation profile suggest disseminated intravascular coagulation or microangiopathic hemolytic anemia. Distinctive clinical and laboratory features allow one to make the correct diagnosis in various other hematologic diseases in which thrombocytopenia is a secondary feature (such as leukemias, lymphomas, myeloma, and aplastic anemia).

Diagnosis

Diagnosis of ITP is based on combination of following features:
- Mucocutaneous type of bleeding with abrupt onset (acute ITP) or insidious onset (chronic ITP)
- No other abnormality on physical examination with patient otherwise being normal
- Presence of isolated thrombocytopenia with no other abnormality on complete blood count
- Bone marrow examination is normal (not required for diagnosis unless clinical presentation and course are unusual)
- Exclusion of other causes of thrombocytopenia.

Treatment

Acute ITP: Acute ITP is a self-limited disorder with spontaneous remission occurring in majority of patients within 2 to 6 months. Therefore, the management of acute ITP is mainly supportive. In the absence of significant bleeding symptoms, simple observation without specific therapy to raise the platelet count is preferred. In children with severe bleeding symptoms, oral corticosteroids or intravenous immunoglobulins are given. Platelet transfusions along with high-dose intravenous steroids or intravenous immunoglobulin are indicated in life-threatening hemorrhage.

A few children go on to develop chronic ITP; even in these cases spontaneous remission is usual.

Chronic ITP: Patients with asymptomatic compensated thrombocytopenia should be observed without any treatment. Symptomatic patients and platelet count <30,000/mm^3 are indications for treatment. The initial therapy in chronic ITP is corticosteroids. (Mode of action of corticosteroids is suppression of phagocytosis of antibody-coated platelets by macrophages and suppression of antibody production.). In patients unresponsive to steroids, intravenous immunoglobulin can be tried (blocks Fc receptors of reticuloendothelial cells). Failure to respond to steroids, relapse, and very high doses of steroids to maintain remission are indications for splenectomy. With splenectomy, 75% of patients achieve remission. Intravenous immunoglobulin is usually administered before splenectomy to temporarily raise the platelet count.

See Box 15.2 for treatment of ITP and newer drugs available.

Approach for management of ITP is shown in Figure 15.4.

Box 15.2: Treatment of immune thrombocytopenia.

- First-line therapy: Corticosteroids, IV immunoglobulin, IV anti-D (only in Rh D+ve individuals)
- Second-line therapy: Rituximab, TPO receptor agonists (romiplostim, eltrombopag), splenectomy
- Life-threatening bleeding: IV immunoglobulin, platelet transfusions

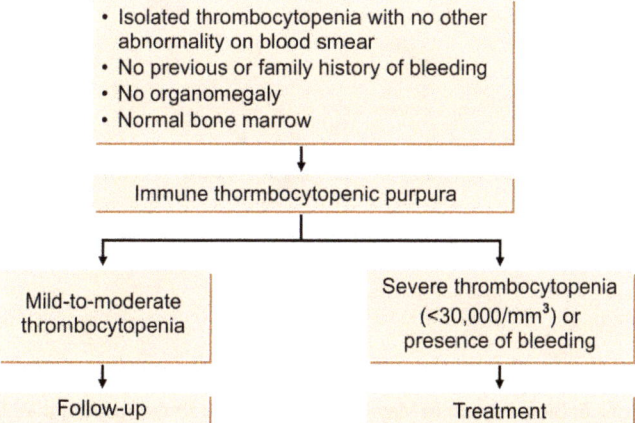

Fig. 15.4: Approach for management of immune thrombocytopenia.

Alloimmune Neonatal Thrombocytopenia

When the fetal platelets possessing paternally derived antigens lacking in the mother enter maternal circulation during gestation or delivery, formation of alloantibodies is stimulated. These maternal antibodies cross the placenta and cause destruction of fetal platelets. Firstborn babies are also frequently affected. The most common platelet antigen against which antibodies form is HPA-1a (PlAl). The condition is self-limited and usually resolves by 3 weeks (maximum 3 months) after delivery. There is a risk of intracranial hemorrhage due to trauma during vaginal delivery. In severe cases, purpura and hemorrhages are evident at birth or manifest within a few hours. Alloimmune neonatal thrombocytopenia should be distinguished from other causes of neonatal thrombocytopenia (Box 15.3).

Severe symptomatic thrombocytopenia is usually treated by transfusion of platelets obtained from the mother.

Box 15.3: Causes of neonatal thrombocytopenia.

Increased peripheral destruction of platelets
1. Immune destruction by maternal antibodies: Autoimmune antibodies (maternal ITP or SLE), alloimmune neonatal thrombocytopenia
2. Nonimmune mechanism: Disseminated intravascular coagulation, intrauterine infections, giant hemangioma.

Decreased production of platelets
1. Thrombocytopenia absent radii (TAR) syndrome
2. Wiskott-Aldrich syndrome
3. May-Hegglin anomaly (Fig. 15.5)
4. Bernard-Soulier syndrome
5. Fanconi anemia
6. Congenital malignancy

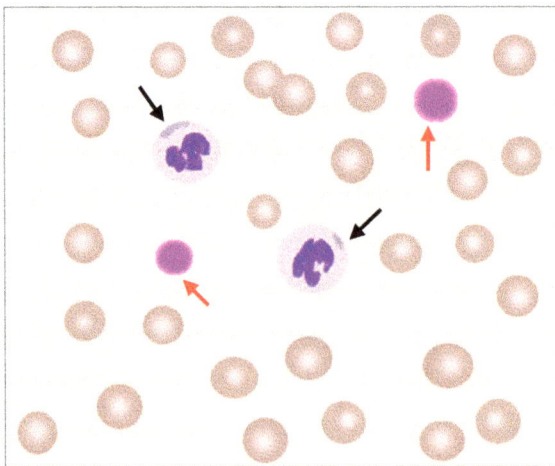

Fig. 15.5: Blood smear in May-Hegglin anomaly showing giant platelets (red arrows) and Dohle-like inclusions within neutrophils (black arrow).

Post-Transfusion Purpura

In this very rare but life-threatening disorder, sudden onset of thrombocytopenia and bleeding occurs about 1 week to 10 days following blood transfusion in some adult multiparous women. In all cases, donor platelets possess HPA-1a antigen while this antigen is lacking on patient's platelets. Patients are probably sensitized previously during pregnancy by fetal platelets having HPA-1a antigen. Following blood transfusion severe thrombocytopenia due to destruction of patient's platelets develops. However, why the anti-HPA-1a antibodies cause destruction of patient's own platelets, which are HPA-1a-negative, is unknown. It has been suggested that HPA-1a antigen in donor binds with an alloantibody and these immune complexes are nonspecifically adsorbed on patient's own platelets. Another explanation offered is HPA-1a antigen in donor plasma gets passively adsorbed on patient's platelets making them HPA-1a-positive and leading to their destruction by alloantibodies. The condition is treated by intravenous gamma globulin and plasmapheresis.

Thrombotic Microangiopathies

Thrombotic microangiopathies are characterized by microvascular thrombosis, microangiopathic hemolytic anemia (MAHA), and thrombocytopenia, and include thrombotic thrombocytopenic purpura (TTP) and hemolytic uremic syndrome (HUS).

Thrombotic Thrombocytopenic Purpura

This uncommon disorder is characterized by formation of hyaline microthrombi in microcirculation of various organs due to aggregation of platelets. In idiopathic TTP, autoantibodies against ADAMTS13 (A disintegrin and metalloprotease with thrombospondin type 1 motif 13) lead to deficiency of ADAMTS13 and accumulation of ultralarge vWF multimers that bind large number of platelets. In familial TTP (Upshaw-Schulman syndrome), ADAMTS13 deficiency results from mutations in *ADAMTS13* gene.

The disorder mainly affects young adults and is slightly more common in females. The pentad of manifestations includes: (i) Microangiopathic hemolytic anemia: hemolysis of red cells results from their passage across fibrin strands of microthrombi in circulation. Clinically patients have pallor and frequently icterus. Peripheral blood examination shows presence of fragmented and nucleated red cells and reticulocytosis (Fig. 15.6). Levels of lactate dehydrogenase and unconjugated bilirubin in serum are raised and indicate increased hemolysis; (ii) Bleeding manifestations secondary to severe thrombocytopenia such as petechiae, ecchymoses, epistaxis, and gastrointestinal/genitourinary bleeding. Coagulation studies (PT, APTT) are normal in most patients; (iii) Fluctuating neurologic dysfunction such as altered level of consciousness, seizures, visual field abnormalities, and hemiparesis, which may terminate in coma; (iv) Renal abnormalities: Proteinuria, hematuria, azotemia; (v) Fever. These five features may not be present in all patients. It is essential to make the correct diagnosis since platelet transfusions for correction of thrombocytopenia can aggravate the predisposition to thrombosis. Most patients respond to transfusions of fresh frozen plasma or to plasmapheresis. In those patients who fail to respond, antiplatelet drugs, corticosteroids, or vincristine may be tried.

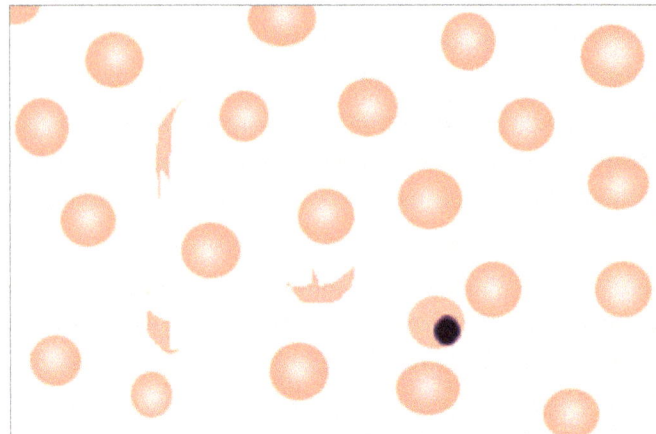

Fig. 15.6: Blood smear in thrombotic thrombocytopenic purpura showing schistocytes, thrombocytopenia, and a late normoblast.

Hemolytic Uremic Syndrome

HUS is characterized by triad of acute renal failure, thrombocytopenia, and microangiopathic hemolytic anemia. HUS is classified into two types: typical and atypical. Typical HUS occurs predominantly in children less than 5 years of age and is associated with Shiga toxin-producing *Escherichia coli* O157:H7; it is characterized by a prodrome of diarrheal illness followed by MAHA, thrombocytopenia, and renal failure. Atypical HUS has similar clinical features but is not preceded by diarrheal prodrome.

Differences between TTP and HUS are presented in Table 15.4. Microangiopathic hemolytic anemia and thrombocytopenia can also occur in pre-eclampsia, HELLP syndrome, autoimmune disorders, systemic infections, systemic malignancy, and malignant hypertension.

Table 15.4: Comparison of thrombotic thrombocytopenic purpura and hemolytic uremic syndrome.

Feature	Thrombotic thrombocytopenic purpura (TTP)	Hemolytic uremic syndrome (HUS)
1. Age	Adults	Children <5 years
2. MAHA	Present	Present
3. Thrombocytopenia	Present	Present
4. Fever	Present	Absent
5. Severe renal failure	Uncommon	Common
6. Major neurologic abnormalities	Common	Uncommon
7. Prodrome of bloody diarrhea	Absent	Present (in typical HUS)
8. Cause	Severe deficiency of ADAMTS13	Infection by *Escherichia coli* O157:H7 (in typical HUS)
9. Coagulation tests	Normal	Normal
10. Treatment	Plasma exchange	Supportive

(MAHA: microangiopathic hemolytic anemia)

Massive Transfusion

Stored whole blood is deficient in viable platelets and in labile coagulation factors (F, V, and F VIII). Transfusion of massive amounts of such blood to individuals with severe blood loss can lead to thrombocytopenia or coagulation factor deficiency by dilutional effect. Bleeding due to massive transfusion can be prevented by transfusion of fresh frozen plasma and platelet concentrates along with stored blood.

Thrombocytopenia due to Increased Platelet Sequestration or Pooling

Normally, about 30% of total platelets in the body are sequestered in the spleen. In conditions associated with enlargement of spleen, splenic platelet pool expands and may reach up to 90% in some cases. Due to compensatory increase in platelet production in bone marrow, thrombocytopenia is usually mild.

Pseudothrombocytopenia

When platelet counts are determined by electronic cell counters on blood samples collected in EDTA, sometimes a falsely low result may be obtained. Examination of a parallel peripheral blood smear made from EDTA anticoagulated blood, however, reveals large clumps of platelets and platelets rosetting around neutrophils (Figs. 15.7A to C). The platelet clumping results from presence of EDTA-dependent antiplatelet antibody in some patients. EDTA alters the conformation of GpIIb/IIIa complex and exposes neoantigen. The antibody reacts with this cryptic antigen and causes platelet clumping only in vitro. These antibodies do not have any clinical significance. Incorrect diagnosis of thrombocytopenia can be avoided by simultaneous examination of peripheral blood film along with determination of direct platelet count.

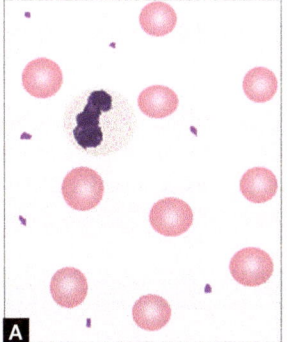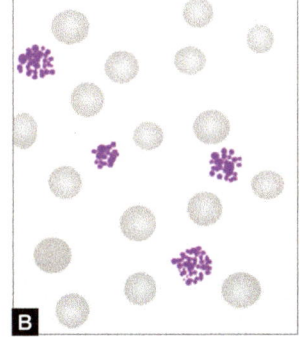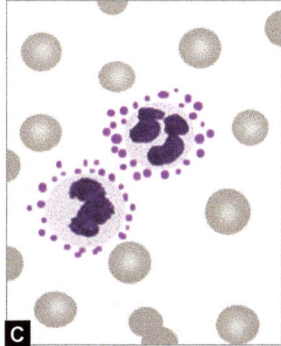

Figs. 15.7A to C: (A) Normal distribution of platelets on blood smear; (B) Blood smear showing aggregation of platelets; (C) Blood smear showing adherence of platelets to neutrophils (satellitism); Both (B) and (C) are examples of pseudothrombocytopenia reported on automated hematology analyzer in blood sample collected in EDTA anticoagulant.

EVALUATION OF A THROMBOCYTOPENIC PATIENT

A thrombocytopenic patient presents with purpuric spots, ecchymoses, or mucous membrane bleeding (epistaxis, gastrointestinal, genitourinary bleeding). The differential diagnosis is wide (Table 15.1: Causes of thrombocytopenia). To ascertain the cause of thrombocytopenia, complete clinical examination is essential including previous history of bleeding, family history, history of drug intake, presence of underlying disorder, and presence or absence of palpable spleen. Laboratory examination includes examination of peripheral blood smear, bone marrow examination, and coagulation screen. A scheme for evaluation of a thrombocytopenic patient is shown in Figure 15.8. Salient diagnostic features of platelet disorders are shown in Box 15.4.

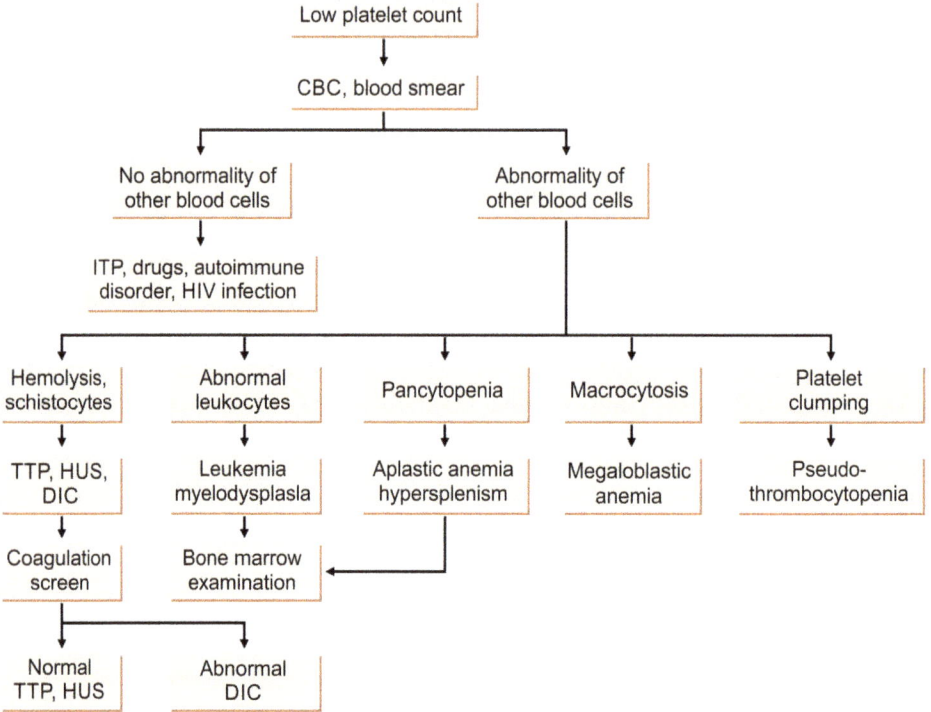

Fig. 15.8: Evaluation of thrombocytopenia.
(CBC: complete blood count; DIC: disseminated intravascular coagulation; ITP: immune thrombocytopenia; HUS: hemolytic uremic syndrome; TTP: thrombotic thrombocytopenic purpura)

Box 15.4: Diagnosis of bleeding due to platelet disorders.
- Superficial type of bleeding (mucocutaneous)
- Platelet count low (thrombocytopenia) or normal (platelet function defect); bleeding time may be prolonged
- Coagulation screen (PT, APTT): Normal
- Specific laboratory evaluation is directed by results of screening tests for primary hemostasis, i.e. whether indicative of thrombocytopenia (low platelet count) or platelet function defect (prolonged bleeding time with normal platelet count, abnormal PFA-100 test)

THROMBOCYTOSIS

This refers to increase in the platelet count above normal (>4 lacs/mm³). Causes of thrombocytosis are listed in Table 15.5.

Thrombocytosis due to myeloproliferative disorders is known as primary thrombocytosis. It can be usually distinguished from reactive (secondary) thrombocytosis by the presence in the former of leukocytosis and immature white cells and nucleated red cells in peripheral blood, defective platelet function (deficient epinephrine-induced platelet aggregation), and splenomegaly. Also, in secondary thrombocytosis features of underlying causative disorder are evident.

Thrombocytosis in essential thrombocythemia is associated with thromboembolic and bleeding manifestations. In reactive thrombocytosis, platelet count is modestly elevated and has no clinical significance. However, persistent thrombocytosis following splenectomy for chronic hemolytic anemia may result in increased risk of thromboembolic complications if hemolysis is not completely corrected.

Table 15.5: Causes of thrombocytosis.

- ***Reactive (Secondary):*** Hemorrhage, trauma, infections, iron deficiency, malignancy, splenectomy, chronic inflammatory disease
- ***Primary:*** Essential thrombocythemia, polycythemia vera, chronic myeloid leukemia, idiopathic myelofibrosis

DISORDERS OF PLATELET FUNCTION

Disorders of platelet function are classified into two broad categories: inherited and acquired (Table 15.6).

Inherited Disorders of Platelet Function

Bernard-Soulier Syndrome

This is a rare autosomal recessive congenital bleeding disorder. In this disease, adhesion of platelets to subendothelium is defective due to congenital absence of glycoprotein Ib receptor complex (which consists of GpIb, V, and IX) on platelet surface. This receptor is essential for binding of platelets to subendothelium via von Willebrand factor (*see* Fig. 15.10).

Table 15.6: Disorders of platelet function.

Inherited	Acquired
• Bernard-Soulier syndrome	• Hematopoietic stem cell disorders: myeloproliferative neoplasms, acute leukemias, myelodysplastic syndrome, paroxysmal nocturnal hemoglobinuria
• Glanzmann's thrombasthenia	
• Storage pool deficiency	
– Dense granule	
– Alpha granule	• Paraproteinemias
• Defective thromboxane synthesis	• Uremia
	• Cardiopulmonary bypass
	• Drugs

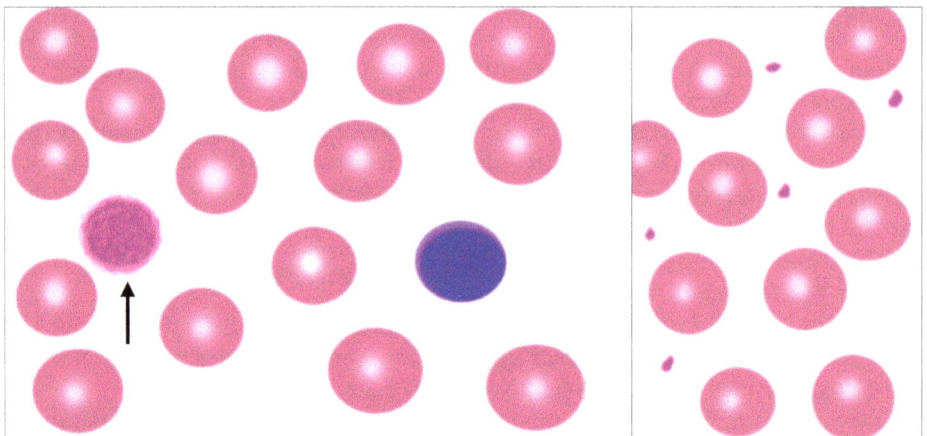

Fig. 15.9: Blood smear showing a giant platelet (arrow). Panel on right shows normal platelets for comparison.

It is caused by defects in *GP9* (located on 3q21.3), *GP1BB* (located on 22q11.21), and *GP1BA* (located on 17p13) genes.

The hemorrhagic manifestations usually begin in infancy or early childhood. They are of moderate to marked degree and consist of purpuric spots, easy or spontaneous bruising, and mucosal bleeding.

Characteristic laboratory abnormalities include giant platelets on peripheral blood smear (Fig. 15.9), mild-to-moderate thrombocytopenia not proportional to the severity of bleeding, abnormal platelet function studies (in the form of prolonged bleeding time, impaired platelet aggregation with ristocetin not corrected by addition of normal plasma, normal platelet aggregation with other agonists), and absence of GpIb, V, and IX (CD42a-d) on flow cytometry.

No satisfactory form of therapy is available. Severe hemorrhagic episodes are managed by platelet transfusions. Repeated platelet transfusions can induce alloimmunization and formation of antibodies against glycoproteins that are absent.

Glanzmann's Thrombasthenia

In this very rare autosomal recessive bleeding disorder, platelet aggregation is deficient due to absence of GpIIb/IIIa receptor complex on platelets. The disorder results from mutations in genes *ITGB3* (located on 17q21.32) or *ITGA2B* (located on 17q21.32). Normally upon activation of platelets, GpIIb/IIIa receptors become exposed on platelet surface and serve as binding sites for fibrinogen. Fibrinogen molecules form bridges between adjacent platelets during aggregation.

In Glanzmann's thrombasthenia, the absence of fibrinogen binding due to lack of receptors is responsible for deficient aggregation (Fig. 15.10).

On peripheral blood smear, platelets appear small and discrete (i.e. they are not in clumps due to lack of aggregation), platelet count is normal, platelet function studies are abnormal (in the form of prolonged bleeding time, poor clot retraction, platelet aggregation is absent with ADP, epinephrine, collagen, and arachidonic acid and normal with ristocetin), and lack of GpIIb/IIIa complex (CD41, CD61) on flow cytometry.

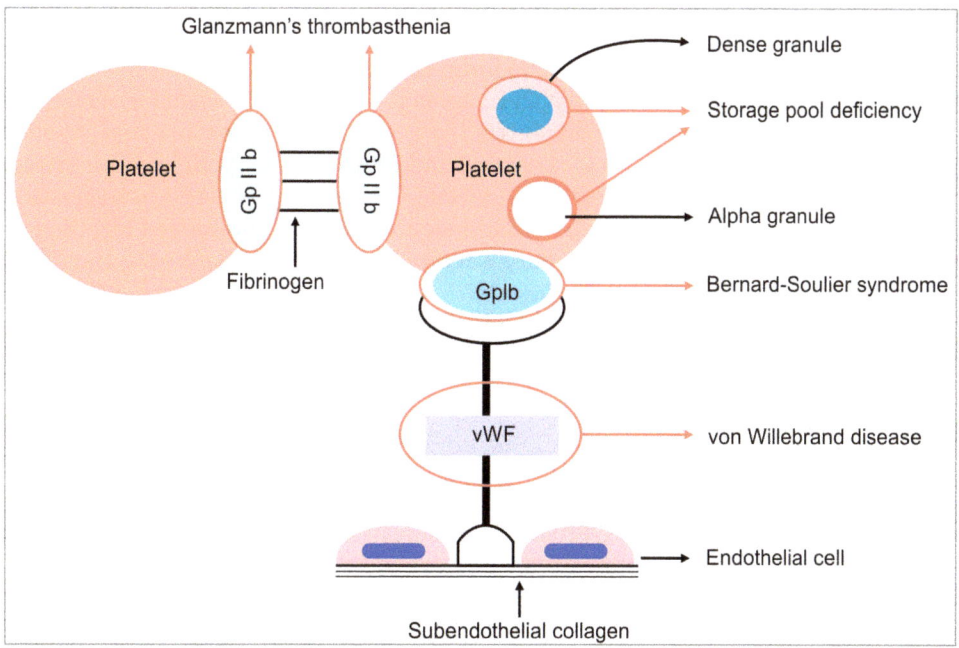

Fig. 15.10: Sites of defects in some platelet function disorders.

No effective form of therapy is available. Severe hemorrhages are treated by platelet transfusions.

Storage Pool Deficiency

Deficiency of intracellular granules of platelets is referred to as storage pool deficiency. It may involve dense granules, alpha granules, or both.

Dense granule storage pool deficiency: This is the most common type of hereditary platelet function disorder. Patients usually present with mild mucocutaneous bleeding. Electron microscopy reveals absence of dense granules (Fig. 15.10). Intraplatelet levels of ADP, serotonin, and calcium are diminished. Platelet aggregation studies with ADP and epinephrine reveal primary wave of aggregation but secondary wave is absent. Aggregation with collagen is defective. Ristocetin-induced aggregation is normal.

Dense granule storage pool deficiency occurs most commonly as a sole abnormality. Less commonly, it occurs in association with various congenital disorders such as Hermansky-Pudlak syndrome, Wiskott-Aldrich syndrome, etc. Hermansky-Pudlak syndrome is characterized by deficiency of dense granules, albinism, and presence of macrophages containing pigment (ceroid).

Bleeding episodes are managed with platelet concentrates.

Alpha granule storage pool deficiency (Gray platelet syndrome): In this condition, which has been described in only a few patients, alpha granules and their contents are diminished or absent (Fig. 15.10). These patients have a mild bleeding diathesis. Platelets are mildly decreased in number, are large in size, and appear pale-gray on stained blood smears. Defective platelet aggregation has also been described. Reticulin fibers are increased in bone marrow.

Defective Thromboxane Synthesis (Aspirin-like Defect)

Thromboxane A2 synthesized from arachidonic acid normally stimulates secretion from dense and alpha granules and is also a platelet agonist. Therefore, deficiencies of enzymes in arachidonic acid metabolism can impair release of granular contents from platelets (*refer to* Fig. 1.31). Congenital deficiencies of cyclooxygenase and thromboxane synthetase are extremely rare in which platelet secretion is defective. Ingestion of aspirin inhibits cyclooxygenase and induces a similar defect. Patients have a mild bleeding disorder, prolonged bleeding time, normal primary wave but absent secondary wave with ADP and epinephrine, and deficient aggregation with collagen and arachidonic acid.

Basic laboratory studies for diagnosis of inherited disorders of platelet function have been presented earlier (Chapter 13).

Acquired Disorders of Platelet Function

Drugs

Aspirin inhibits the enzyme cyclooxygenase by causing its irreversible acetylation. This results in inability of the platelets to synthesize thromboxane A2 and failure of platelet secretion. This forms the basis of use of aspirin as antiplatelet drug in practice. The inhibitory effect of aspirin on platelet function lasts for 7 to 10 days (lifespan of affected platelets). Aspirin should be withheld for at least 10 days before performing platelet function studies. Platelet aggregation studies with ADP and epinephrine after aspirin ingestion reveal primary wave of aggregation but no secondary wave. Aspirin should be avoided in persons with bleeding disorders. In a patient taking aspirin, aspirin should be discontinued for at least 7 days before any surgical procedure. Other drugs affecting platelet function are other nonsteroidal analgesic anti-inflammatory drugs, penicillin, cephalosporins, local anesthetics, dipyridamole, dextran, and heparin.

Myeloproliferative Neoplasms

Bleeding manifestations occur in myeloproliferative neoplasms in the presence of normal or increased platelet count. A variety of platelet functional abnormalities have been described, the most common being defective aggregation response to epinephrine. Aggregation may also be defective with ADP and collagen.

Paraproteinemias

Paraproteins in multiple myeloma and Waldenström's macroglobulinemia coat the platelet surface and inhibit adhesion and aggregation. Paraproteins also interfere with interaction of coagulation factors.

Uremia

The bleeding tendency associated with uremia is usually in the form of petechiae, ecchymoses, and gastrointestinal hemorrhages, and may be severe. Platelet functional abnormalities are thought to play a major role. The usual laboratory abnormalities are prolongation of bleeding time and impaired platelet aggregation with ADP and epinephrine. The hemostatic abnormalities in uremia are corrected by dialysis suggesting that a dialyzable substance causes them. The substances suspected include guanidinosuccinic acid, urea, and phenols. The usual form of treatment of bleeding diathesis in uremia is hemodialysis. Cryoprecipitate and DDAVP (Desmopressin) may also be of benefit.

BIBLIOGRAPHY

1. Bick AL. Platelet function defects associated with hemorrhage or thrombosis. Med Clin North Am. 1994;78:577-607.
2. British Committee for Standards in Haematology: Guidelines for the investigation and management of idiopathic thrombocytopenic purpura in adults, children, and pregnancy. Br J Haematol. 2003;120:574-96.
3. Bromberg ME. Immune thrombocytopenic purpura—The changing therapeutic landscape. N Engl J Med. 2006;355:1643-5.
4. Cines D, Bussel J, Liebman H, et al. The ITP syndrome: Pathogenic and clinical diversity. Blood. 2009;113:6511-21.
5. Cines DB, Blanchette VS. Immune thrombocytopenic purpura. N Engl J Med. 2002;346:995-1008.
6. Cooper N, Bussel J. The pathogenesis of immune thrombocytopenic purpura. Br J Haematol. 2006;133:364-74.
7. George JN, El-Harake MA, Raskob GE. Current concepts: Chronic idiopathic thrombocytopenic purpura. N Engl J Med. 1994;331:1207-11.
8. George JN. How I treat patients with thrombotic thrombocytopenic purpura: 2010. Blood. 2010;116:4060-9.
9. Hardisty AM and Caen JP. Disorders of platelet function. In: Bloom AL, Thomas DP (Eds). Haemostasis and Thrombosis, 2nd edition. Edinburgh: Churchill Livingstone; 1987.
10. Karpatkin S. Autoimmune thrombocytopenic purpura. Blood. 1980;56:329-43.
11. Karpatkin S. Autoimmune thrombocytopenic purpura. Semin Hematol. 1985;22: 260-88.
12. Kiefel V, Santos S, Mueller-Eckhardt C. Serological, biochemical, and molecular aspects of platelet autoantigens. Semin Hematol. 1992;l29:26-33.
13. Kunicki TJ, Newman PJ. The molecular immunology of human platelet proteins. Blood. 1992;80:1386-404.
14. McCrae KR, Samuels P, Schreiber AD. Pregnancy-associated thrombocytopenia: Pathogenesis and management. Blood. 1992;80:2697-714.
15. McMillan R. Chronic idiopathic thrombocytopenic purpura. N Engl J Med. 1981;304:1135.
16. Rao AK, Holmsen H. Congenital disorders of platelet function. Semin Hematol. 1986;23:102-18.
17. Rodeghiero F, Stasi R, Gernsheimer T, et al. Standardization of terminology, definitions, and outcome criteria in immune thrombocytopenic purpura of adults and children: Report from an International Working Group. Blood. 2009;113:2386-93.
18. Rutherford CJ, Frenkel EP. Thrombocytopenia. Issues in diagnosis and therapy. Med Clin North Am. 1994;78:555-75.
19. Stasi R, Provan D. Management of immune thrombocytopenic purpura in adults. Mayo Clin Proc. 2004;79:504-22.
20. Waters AH. Autoimmune thrombocytopenia: Clinical aspects. Semin Hematol. 1992;29:18-25.

CHAPTER
16

Disorders of Coagulation

INHERITED DISORDERS OF COAGULATION

HEMOPHILIA A

Hemophilia A (classical hemophilia) is the most common hereditary coagulation disorder. It occurs in approximately 1:10,000 individuals. It is caused by hereditary deficiency or dysfunction of Factor VIII. In India, about 1,300 hemophiliacs are born every year and currently there are about 50,000 patients with severe disease.

Inheritance

The mode of inheritance of hemophilia A is X-linked recessive (Fig. 16.1). The abnormal gene (or the gene coding the synthesis of F VIII) is located on the X chromosome. The disease manifests only in males because they lack the complementary normal X chromosome. Females are carriers but do not manifest the disease as they have a normal allele on the complementary

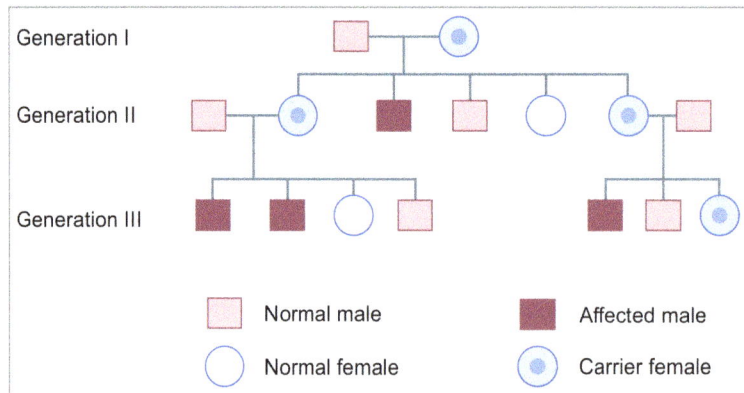

Fig. 16.1: An example of X-linked pattern of inheritance in hemophilia A. Only males are affected. History of hemorrhagic diathesis is obtained in uncles and male cousins on maternal side. Carrier females transmit the disease.

X chromosome. Typically, positive family history is obtained in maternal grandfather, maternal uncles, and maternal male cousins. If a carrier female marries a normal male, then the male offspring has a 50% chance of being affected while the female offspring has a 50% chance of becoming a carrier. If a hemophilic male marries a normal female, all his sons will be normal while all his daughters will be carriers.

Positive family history is not obtained in about 30% of patients with hemophilia. These cases probably arise from spontaneous mutation. Therefore, negative family history does not rule out the possibility of hemophilia.

Majority of female carriers of hemophilia A do not suffer from hemorrhagic diathesis. This is because FVIII synthesized by complementary gene on the normal X chromosome is adequate to achieve hemostasis. However, hemophilia may develop in carrier females when there is lyonization predominantly of normal X chromosomes during embryogenesis. Other mechanisms by which hemophilia can occur in females are homozygosity of hemophilic gene in the female offspring of carrier female and affected male, or hemizygosity of hemophilic gene due to chromosome anomalies such as Turner's (XO) syndrome. It should be noted, however, that a more common cause of F VIII deficiency in females is von Willebrand disease.

Pathogenesis of Bleeding in F VIII Deficiency

In vivo, extrinsic pathway controls bleeding after injury. Tissue factors—F VIIa complex activates F IX and F X and initiates a rapid but limited generation of thrombin on tissue injury. The initial formation of thrombin is subsequently amplified by a feedback mechanism in which thrombin activates F XI and F VIII of intrinsic pathway. In F VIII deficiency, inadequate amounts of thrombin are generated. Secondly, increased amount of thrombin is required for activation of TAFI (thrombin-activatable fibrinolysis inhibitor). Therefore, F VIII deficiency is associated with insufficient clot formation as well as rapid clot removal.

Clinical Features

Clinical severity of hemophilia A is variable and correlates with F VIII:C activity. Hemophilia A is classified into mild, moderate, and severe types based on the level of F VIII:C in patient's plasma (Table 16.1).

In addition to above three types, a fourth category has also been described by some investigators in which FVIII:C levels are greater than 25%; these patients usually have moderately excessive bleeding only when exposed to a severe hemostatic challenge such as major trauma or major surgery.

Table 16.1: Severity of hemophilia.

F VIII: C level	Type	Frequency	Clinical features
<1%	Severe	70%	Frequent and spontaneous deep tissue hemorrhages and hemarthrosis
1–5%	Moderate	15%	Excessive hemorrhage after mild to moderate injury; occasional hemarthrosis; spontaneous bleeding infrequent
>5%	Mild	15%	Excessive hemorrhage only after major trauma or surgery

Normal level of F VIII:C is 50–150%.

In patients with mild disease, disorder may not be diagnosed until middle age (e.g. prolonged bleeding after major surgery).

Insufficiency of F VIII (hemophilia A) or F IX (hemophilia B) results in similar symptoms since the two coagulation factors are involved in the same step in the coagulation mechanism.

Petechiae are absent in hemophilia.

Factor VIII level and severity of bleeding are fairly similar in affected members of a particular hemophilic kindred.

In severe hemophilia, bleeding manifestations often start when the child begins to crawl or learns to walk. They include deep-seated hematomas and hemarthroses; mucous membrane bleeding from lips and tongue can occur after eruption of deciduous teeth.

Bleeding into weight- or stress-bearing joints (hemarthroses) is a characteristic feature of hemophilia A. Commonly affected joints are knees, ankles, hips, and elbows. Hemarthroses are a major cause of incapacitation in hemophilia. Onset of bleeding into the joint is preceded by tingling sensation, mild discomfort, and slight restriction of movement. This is followed by pain, swelling, and stiffness of the affected joint. Blood induces inflammation of the synovium. Inflamed synovium, being hypervascular and friable, is vulnerable to re-bleeding following injury and a vicious cycle of repeated bleeding with progressive joint damage sets in. In the patient, often one specific joint is susceptible to repeated bleeding and damage and such a joint is called as target joint. Narrowing and irregularity of joint space due to destruction of cartilage, subchondral cysts, and osteoporosis develop and ultimately joint becomes disorganized and immobile. Cartilage and bone degeneration due to joint bleeding is known as hemophilic arthropathy.

Intramuscular hematomas are particularly common in muscles of calf, thigh, forearm, and buttocks. They can compress vital structures such as arteries (distal ischemic injury) or peripheral nerves (sensory or motor neuropathy) and cause pressure necrosis of adjacent tissue.

Intracranial hemorrhage can occur following trivial trauma and is a common cause of death in hemophilia. Hematuria frequently occurs in severe hemophilia and may induce colicky pain (clot colic). Severe bleeding can occur postoperatively or after dental extractions in unrecognized hemophilics; such bleeding is typically of delayed onset.

Laboratory Features

Coagulation Profile

Tests for primary hemostasis (platelet count, bleeding time) and for extrinsic and common coagulation pathway [prothrombin time (PT)] are normal. The only abnormality in coagulation profile is prolongation of activated partial thromboplastin time (APTT), i.e. a measure of intrinsic and common pathways. The sensitivity of APTT to F VIII deficiency depends on the reagents used. Most APTT systems are prolonged in severe and moderate deficiencies of F VIII but results are variable in mild cases and may sometimes be normal. Results of APTT must be viewed in the light of the patient's complaints and F VIII:C assay should be performed in indicated cases even though APTT is normal.

Clotting time is a crude screening test for coagulation disorders and prolonged values are obtained mostly in severe cases (F VIII: C<1%); it is often normal in mild/moderate cases. Therefore, clotting time has been replaced by APTT as a screening test for coagulation disorders.

Thromboplastin generation test (TGT) is a second-line test and reveals "plasma defect." The combination of normal PT, prolonged APTT, and plasma defect in TGT are highly suggestive of F VIII deficiency.

Factor VIII:C Assay

There are two main methods for F VIII assay: Clot-based one-stage assay based on APTT and chromogenic assay. The one-stage assay is most commonly used since it is simple, reagents are easy to obtain, and the test can be done on any automated coagulation analyzer. Serial dilutions of normal reference plasma (normal pooled plasma) are made. To each dilution, F VIII-deficient substrate plasma is added and APTT of the mixture is determined. A reference graph is prepared showing relationship between APTT and F VIII:C percent activity (1:10 dilution of reference plasma has 100% F VIII:C). APTT of mixture of diluted patient's plasma and substrate plasma is determined. From the APTT obtained F VIII:C content is derived from reference graph.

In chromogenic assay, patient's plasma is incubated with F IXa, F VIII, excess F X, calcium, and phospholipid. F X is converted to F Xa. F Xa cleaves chromogenic substrate to generate color. The intensity of color produced is proportional to the amount of F Xa and amount of F VIII in patient's plasma. As compared to one-stage assay, chromogenic assay is more sensitive to low level of F VIII, but is more expensive, and more complex to perform.

Normal F VIII: C level in plasma is 50 to 150%. It is affected by various factors such as venous stasis before collection of blood, prolonged storage of blood, severe exercise, pregnancy, inflammation, fever, liver diseases, hyperthyroidism, and hemolysis.

Apart from establishing the diagnosis of F VIII deficiency, F VIII: C assay is used to monitor F VIII replacement therapy.

Differential Diagnosis

Diagnosis of hemophilia A can be made when a male patient with appropriate family history presents with typical hemorrhagic manifestations, prolonged APTT with normal PT and bleeding time, and a plasma defect in TGT. F VIII:C assay should be carried out for confirmation of diagnosis (Box 16.1).

Causes of F VIII: C deficiency include hemophilia A, von Willebrand disease, combined hereditary deficiency of Factors V and VIII, and acquired disorders such as F VIII inhibitors, and disseminated intravascular coagulation (DIC). Causes of inherited deficiency of F VIII are shown in Box 16.2.

von Willebrand disease occurs in both sexes and bleeding manifestations are mainly in the form of mucocutaneous hemorrhages such as petechiae and epistaxis, though hemarthrosis may occur. Laboratory investigations usually show prolonged bleeding time, prolonged APTT, and defective ristocetin induced platelet aggregation.

Box 16.1: Diagnosis of hemophilia.
- Hematomas, hemarthrosis, excessive post-traumatic bleeding, delayed bleeding
- Presentation in early childhood; family history often +ve (X-linked recessive)
- Bleeding time, platelet count—normal
- APTT—prolonged
- Definitive diagnosis—Factor VIII assay

Box 16.2: Causes of inherited deficiency of F VIII.
- Hemophilia A
- von Willebrand disease (especially type 2N and type 3)
- Combined deficiency of F V and F VIII
- Some carriers of hemophilia A

Table 16.2: Comparison of hemophilia A, hemophilia B, and von Willebrand disease.

Parameter	Hemophilia A	Hemophilia B	von Willebrand disease
1. Prevalence in general population	1:10,000	1:30,000	1:100
2. Pathogenesis	F VIII deficiency	F IX deficiency	Deficiency or qualitative abnormality of vWF
3. Inheritance	X-linked recessive	X-linked recessive	Autosomal dominant
4. Function of deficient factor	Cofactor; enhances conversion of F X to F Xa	Enzyme; conversion of F X to F Xa	Adhesion of platelets to subendothelium, carrier of factor VIII
5. Nature of bleeding	Deep tissues	Deep tissues	Superficial ± Deep
6. Abnormal screening tests	APTT	APTT	APTT, bleeding time
7. Diagnosis	F VIII assay	F IX assay	Ristocetin-induced platelet aggregation
8. Treatment	Cryoprecipitate, F VIII concentrate, desmopressin	F IX concentrate, prothrombin complex concentrate	Desmopressin, vWF concentrate

In **combined deficiency of Factors V and VIII**, both PT and APTT are prolonged. Combined FV and FVIII deficiency is an autosomal recessive disorder in which bleeding occurs mainly in skin, mucous membranes, and as menorrhagia in females. It results from mutations in two genes *LMAN1* (lectin mannose binding 1) and *MCFD2* (multiple coagulation factor deficiency 2). Proteins encoded by these genes are involved in intracellular transport of FV and FVIII.

Presence of **F VIII inhibitors** can be excluded by mixing experiment, i.e. APTT is repeated using mixture of patient's and normal plasma.

In **disseminated intravascular coagulation**, clinical features are usually dominated by the underlying disease and investigations reveal multiple coagulation abnormalities and thrombocytopenia.

Clinically, F VIII deficiency (hemophilia A) and **F IX deficiency (hemophilia B)** are indistinguishable. Distinction between them is critical as treatment of the two conditions is different. Thromboplastin generation test and specific factor assays allow one to make the correct diagnosis.

Differences between hemophilia A, hemophilia B, and von Willebrand disease are shown in Table 16.2.

Therapy of Hemophilia A

Therapeutic Agents

Factor VIII concentrate, cryoprecipitate, and desmopressin (DDAVP) are the three therapeutic options in hemophilia A.

Factor VIII concentrate: They are of two types—plasma-derived and recombinant. Plasma-derived F VIII concentrate is derived by fractionation of pooled plasma obtained from multiple donors. It is available in the form of freeze-dried powder in vials labeled with the F VIII content. It is reconstituted by the addition of a diluent and administered intravenously. F VIII concentrates are sterilized by heating or solvent detergent treatment by their manufacturers to inactivate viruses. As compared to cryoprecipitate, F VIII concentrate is stable when stored at 4°C and is relatively easy to administer. Its major drawback is high cost. Double inactivation procedures are nowadays employed to improve the safety. A purification process employing monoclonal antibodies against F VIII can now prepare highly purified F VIII concentrates.

Recombinant F VIII concentrates prepared by genetic engineering technology have recently been introduced and are found to be as effective as plasma-derived F VIII concentrates. They have the advantages of being free from infectious agents and a potential of large-scale production.

Cryoprecipitate: Preparation of cryoprecipitate: Plasma is separated from whole blood within 6 hours of collection of blood. Individual bags of freshly separated plasma are frozen at −70°C and then thawed at 4°C. A mixture of plasma and a flocculent precipitate is obtained which is then centrifuged. Most of the supernatant plasma is removed leaving behind sediment of cryoprecipitate and residual 10 to 15 mL of plasma. When stored at −25°C or lower, cryoprecipitate remains stable for 1 year. Before infusion, required number of bags of cryoprecipitate are thawed at 37°C, and pooled together.

The cryoprecipitate has high content of F VIII:C, von Willebrand factor (vWF), fibrinogen, and fibronectin and also contains some amount of F XIII. On average, each bag of cryoprecipitate should have 80 units of F VIII:C.

As compared to F VIII concentrate, cryoprecipitate has low cost and is prepared from relatively few donors. However, cryoprecipitate is suitable mostly for hospitalized patients and cannot be used for treatment in home settings; in addition, viral attenuation of cryoprecipitate is difficult and F VIII content is variable from bag to bag. Hemolysis of recipient's red cells can occur due to the presence of anti-A or anti-B. Due to the availability of simpler and safer alternatives, cryoprecipitate is no longer used at major centers.

Desmopressin (DDAVP): This drug increases levels of F VIII and vWF in plasma by stimulating their release from endothelial cells and platelets. Desmopressin is helpful in mild and moderate hemophilia but not in severe cases.

Management

Bleeding episodes in hemophilia A are treated by F VIII replacement therapy. The aim is attainment of a critical level of F VIII in the body sufficient to arrest the bleeding. Administration of 1 unit/kg body weight of F VIII raises plasma level by 2 units/dL. The approximate minimum desired F VIII levels required to control bleeding are—(i) Mild bleeding: 30% (0.3 units/mL), (ii) Serious or major bleeding: 50% (0.5 units/mL), and (iii) Major surgery: 80–100% (0.8 units/mL). A formula for calculating units of F VIII to be infused to achieve the desired rise is as follows:

Units of F VIII to be administered = required rise in % units × weight in kg × 0.5

Where,

Required rise in units/mL = required level of F VIII in patient's plasma in units/mL − Actual F VIII level before infusion.

To maintain the desired levels repeated doses are necessary as half-life of F VIII is about 8 to 12 hours. Severity of bleeding decides the duration of therapy.

Aside from treatment of bleeding episodes, another form of therapy in hemophilia A is prophylactic therapy. In this form of treatment, F VIII is regularly and periodically administered (every 2–3 days) to maintain the concentration of F VIII greater than 1% that prevents serious, and spontaneous hemorrhages, i.e. a severe disease is converted to a moderate disease. This form of therapy has been shown to significantly reduce the joint disease. However, prophylactic therapy is not commonly employed due to the high cost and limited supply of F VIII concentrates.

Antifibrinolytic agents such as epsilon-aminocaproic acid and tranexamic acid inhibit fibrinolysis and are used to prevent or treat oral hemorrhages (such as following dental extractions). Saliva contains high concentration of fibrinolytic enzymes. Antiplatelet drugs (such as aspirin) and intramuscular injections should be avoided. Precautions should be observed to prevent injuries especially in children.

Complications of Replacement Therapy

Inhibitor antibodies against F VIII: Antibodies against F VIII develop in about 10 to 15% of patients with severe hemophilia who have received multiple transfusions. These antibodies may inactivate in fused F VIII with patient becoming resistant to replacement therapy. There are two types of inhibitors—one type shows rise to a low titer while the other type shows anamnestic response to a high titer after administration of F VIII. Inhibitors are usually quantitated by Bethesda method. One Bethesda unit is the quantity of inhibitor that leaves 50% of residual F VIII when the mixture of patient's and normal pooled plasma is incubated at 37°C for 2 hours. Low titer inhibitors are usually treated by high doses of F VIII concentrates. Treatment of high titer inhibitors is difficult; products available to manage bleeding in these patients are prothrombin complex concentrates, porcine F VIII concentrates, and F VIIa. (Also see section on "Acquired inhibitors of coagulation.")

Transmission of viral infections: Earlier generations of FVIII concentrates were associated with a significant risk of transmission of hepatitis B and C viruses (HBV and HCV) and human immunodeficiency virus (HIV). Before introduction of HIV screening tests for donor units and viral inactivation procedures for F VIII concentrates, about 60% of hemophilic patients got infected with HIV-1. Majority of these patients also were found to have developed antibodies to HCV. HBV and HCV infections carry the risk of chronic liver disease, cirrhosis, and hepatocellular carcinoma. Donor screening and viral inactivation procedures of F VIII concentrates (heat and solvent detergent treatment) have markedly reduced the risk of transmission of these agents. All newly diagnosed patients should receive HBV and HAV vaccines (if not immune).

Molecular Genetics of Hemophilia A

Genetic Defects in Hemophilia A

As in thalassemias, genetic defects in hemophilia A are diverse (Box 16.3). Human gene mutation database (2008) has reported 2320 mutations in *F8* gene. The most frequent mutation is intron 22 inversion (52%), followed by intron 1 inversion, both of which cause severe hemophilia. Mechanism of inversion of intron 22 is shown in Figure 16.2. Insertions or deletions causing severe hemophilia can be large or small. It has been suggested that hemophilic patients with large deletions, nonsense mutations, or intron 22 inversions are more likely to develop F VIII inhibitors

Box 16.3: F8 gene mutations.

- Severe hemophilia: Inversions, deletions, insertions, missense mutations, nonsense mutations
- Moderate/mild hemophilia: Missense mutations, single nucleotide deletions, splicing errors

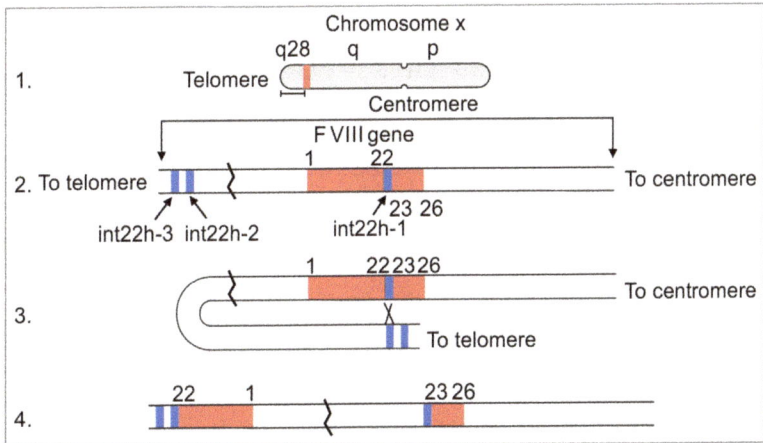

Fig. 16.2: Mechanism of inversion of intron 22 leading to splitting of F VIII gene and severe hemophilia A. (1) Location of F VIII gene on Xq28 toward telomere. (2) Expanded region showing F VIII gene (red) and the homologous repeats (blue) which are referred to as int22h-1, int22h-2, and int22h-3. (3) During meiosis in males, looping around of X chromosome occurs and homologous recombination can occur between two copies of int22h since the sequences are almost identical. (4) As a result of intrachromosomal recombination, 22 exons from 5′ end of F VIII gene are moved to the telomeric end of X chromosome, while exons 23 to 26 from 3′ end remain at the original position. This causes disruption of F VIII gene into two parts that cannot encode F VIII protein and severe hemophilia results.

than those with other molecular defects. Missense mutation (mutation which leads to the formation of a different amino acid) or small deletions have low risk of forming inhibitors. But these associations are not consistent. Some **point mutations** cause formation of a stop codon with premature termination of F VIII translation (nonsense mutation) and synthesis of a short nonfunctional protein; others lead to the formation of a complete but dysfunctional F VIII molecule due to single amino acid substitution. Genetic defects have not been identified in a significant proportion of hemophilia A pedigrees. The molecular lesions in hemophilia A are constant in a given kindred.

Detection of Carriers

All the daughters of a hemophilic father are obligate carriers as they receive their father's defective X chromosome. Carrier state is also established in a female if she has a diseased son and a diseased relative or if she has more than one diseased son. In approximately 30% of cases, family history is negative as spontaneous mutation during gametogenesis is responsible for hemophilic state. Family history will also be negative if hemophilia has been silent in previous generations there being no male offspring. Carrier testing may be done if carrier status of a female cannot be ascertained on the basis of family history alone. Documentation of carrier status of a woman provides the carrier and her spouse with options such as prenatal diagnosis or sterilization.

There are two basic methods of carrier detection—phenotypic and genotypic.

Phenotypic Methods

Factor VIII:C assay: Normal level of F VIII:C in plasma is 50 to 150%. In female carriers F VIII:C levels are expected to be around half the normal, i.e. 50%. This is because during the process of lyonization half of the normal and half of the abnormal X chromosomes would be inactivated by random chance. However, as lyonization is unpredictable, considerable overlap can occur between values obtained in normal and carrier females. Although the carrier state is suggested when F VIII:C level is 50% of normal or less, it cannot be ruled out even if F VIII:C levels are higher.

Determination of F VIII:C and vWF:Ag: Normally levels of vWF:Ag closely correlate with levels of FVIII:C. In carriers vWF:Ag levels are normal or slightly increased while F VIII:C levels are comparably less resulting in reduction of F VIII:C/vWF:Ag ratio. (F VIII: C/ vWF: Ag ratio less than 1.0).

As F VIII:C levels may be normal in carriers (due to the process of random lyonization) about 10 to 20% of carriers remain undetected by this method.

Genotypic Methods

A definitive method of establishing the carrier state is genotypic analysis. There are two methods—direct and indirect.

Direct methods: Identification of a specific defect in the F VIII gene may be accomplished by restriction enzyme analysis or by oligonucleotide probes. This analysis is suitable when the genetic abnormality in the affected kindred is known.

a. *Restriction endonuclease analysis:* When the point mutation in the F VIII gene alters (i.e. creates or abolishes) the cutting site of a particular restriction enzyme, then this method can be applied for detection of carriers. Steps of this analysis are—(1) DNA is isolated from leukocytes and separated into fragments by a restriction enzyme. (2) Fragments of DNA are separated by gel electrophoresis according to their size and then blotted on to the nitrocellulose membrane. (3) The fragments are hybridized with radioactive DNA probes followed by autoradiography. If cutting site of the restriction enzyme is altered due to a point mutation, then a fragment of a different size is produced.

   Alternatively, polymerase chain reaction (PCR) can be used to amplify DNA followed by digestion of DNA by restriction enzyme. As DNA is amplified, digest can be analyzed by direct inspection of the electrophoretically separated DNA fragments.

b. *Oligonucleotide probe analysis:* Desired normal and abnormal oligonucleotide probes are synthesized chemically and are radiolabeled. DNA isolated from leukocytes is digested by restriction enzyme and fragment to be analyzed is separated by electrophoresis. Hybridization is carried out with the labeled oligonucleotide probes followed by autoradiography. The normal and abnormal (mutant) probes hybridize with normal and mutant sequences, respectively.

Indirect method: If the genetic defect in the affected family is unknown, then the indirect method, i.e. restriction fragment length polymorphism (RFLP) can be employed. Although the coding regions of the gene (exons) are highly conserved, DNA sequence variations can occur in the noncoding extragenic regions as well as in introns. These DNA sequence variations frequently alter the recognition site of a particular restriction enzyme resulting in formation of fragments of different sizes. The polymorphic restriction enzyme site, if linked closely to the abnormal gene and co-segregates in affected families, can be used as a genetic marker of the disease in the particular family. Key family members should be heterozygous for the polymorphism. Sources of error in RFLP analysis are recombination or crossing-over of genetic material during meiosis and nonpaternity.

Three restriction enzymes, Bc I, Bgl I, and Xba I are used for RFLP analysis. Although Southern blot analysis can be used, polymerase chain reaction technology is a rapid method that requires no radioactive gene probes. In the PCR-based method, the segment of DNA, which contains the restriction enzyme polymorphism, is amplified and then digested with the restriction enzyme. This is followed by agarose gel electrophoresis, ethidium bromide staining, and visualization of fragments by ultraviolet fluorescence. If the cutting site of the restriction enzyme is altered, then a fragment of a different size is obtained. Presence or absence of a restriction site is used as a marker for tracking the hemophilia gene in pedigree analysis (Fig. 16.3).

Tests for detection of genetic abnormalities are shown in Box 16.4.

Prenatal Diagnosis

Prenatal diagnosis determines whether the fetus of female carrier is affected and thus offers the option of termination of pregnancy. Two methods of prenatal diagnosis are available—fetal blood sampling and genotypic analysis.

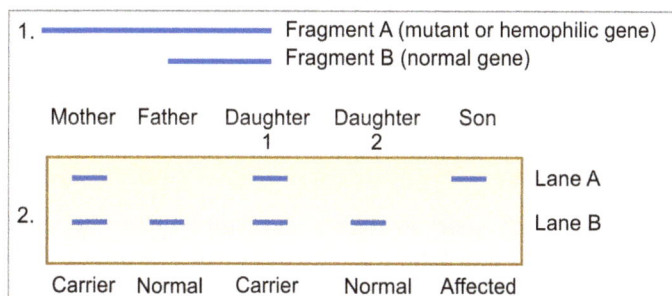

Fig. 16.3: Analysis of hemophilia A pedigree. 1: Restriction enzyme digestion produces DNA fragments of different size in mutant and normal genes. 2: DNA is separated by electrophoresis and hybridized with labeled probe. Here, fragment A (larger) is linked with hemophilia A gene while fragment B (shorter) is linked with normal gene. Thus, status of family members can be ascertained.

Box 16.4: Tests for detection of genetic abnormalities in hemophilia A.

Direct DNA testing
- Southern blot analysis: Detection of intron 22 and intron 1 inversion
- Amplification of regions of F VIII gene by polymerase chain reaction followed by agarose gel electrophoresis: Detection of insertions or deletions in F VIII gene
- Single-stranded conformational polymorphism (SSCP) analysis: Detection of point mutations

Indirect DNA testing
- Linkage analysis for detection of restriction fragment length polymorphisms, if exact genetic defect has not been identified (for tracking defective gene in family members).

Fetal sex is determined by amniocentesis around 14 to 15 weeks of gestation. Fetal blood is obtained at 18 to 20 weeks by fetoscopy. Level of F VIII:Ag is determined by immunoradiometric assay which is capable of detecting minute amounts. F VIII:Cag is undetectable in hemophilia A. However, this assay is not suitable in kindreds with positive cross-reacting material in plasma.

For genotypic analysis, fetal DNA can be obtained either by amniocentesis (14–15 weeks) or by chorionic villus biopsy (9–12 weeks). Various methods of genetic analysis are outlined under "Detection of carriers."

Prenatal diagnosis by genetic analysis using chorionic villus sampling is possible in the first trimester while fetal blood sampling can be applied only in the second trimester. Therefore genotypic analysis has the advantage of earlier (and thus safer) termination of pregnancy if required.

Preimplantation Diagnosis

Although prenatal diagnosis can avoid the birth of an affected child, it is traumatic for the parents due to the uncertainty involved during each pregnancy and the prospect of abortion of every affected fetus. Preimplantation diagnosis offers the genetic diagnosis in preimplantation embryos and thus eliminates the problem of termination of pregnancy. The advent of polymerase chain reaction and in vitro fertilization techniques has made preimplantation diagnosis feasible. In this technique, a single cell is removed from the embryo (6- to 10-cell stage) following in vitro fertilization and its DNA is amplified using polymerase chain reaction. Techniques for detection of mutation are applied on the amplified DNA. The unaffected embryo is implanted into the uterus. Preimplantation diagnosis has been applied to hemophilia A, β-thalassemia, sickle-cell anemia, cystic fibrosis, Lesch-Nyhan syndrome, Tay-Sachs disease, and some other monogenic diseases.

Noninvasive Prenatal Diagnosis

It is known that fetal cells (such as erythroblasts and lymphocytes) are present in maternal circulation during pregnancy. These fetal cells though small in number, can be isolated from maternal blood by a method utilizing antigenic differences between fetal and maternal cells. DNA is extracted from these fetal cells and analyzed by a sensitive technique (polymerase chain reaction). If a mutation is detected, then it can be confirmed by doing chorionic villus biopsy in early pregnancy. The technique, at present, is in investigational stage.

VON WILLEBRAND DISEASE

von Willebrand factor is synthesized by endothelial cells and megakaryocytes. The vWF gene is located on chromosome 12. The basic mature vWF molecule is a monomer composed of 2050 amino acids. vWF monomers associate with each other through disulfide bonds to form multimers of varying sizes. The large multimers of vWF are more effective in hemostasis as they have greater binding sites for mediating adhesion of platelets to subendothelium.

Most of the vWF is synthesized by endothelial cells from where they are secreted constitutively or are stored in Weibel-Palade bodies for later secretion. In megakaryocytes vWF is stored in α-granules and is secreted when platelets are activated. Soon after their secretion into the blood, vWF multimers are cleaved by the metalloprotease ADAMTS13 (a disintegrin and metalloprotease with thrombospondin type 1 motif 13.) ADAMTS13 cleaves a site within the A2 domain of vWF. In thrombotic thrombocytopenic purpura, degradation of large vWF multimers does not occur due to deficiency of ADAMTS13. Structure of vWF is shown in Figure 16.4. In plasma, vWF and F VIII circulate as a noncovalently bound complex (Fig. 16.5).

Functions of vWF: There are two major functions of vWF in hemostasis—(i) vWF mediates adhesion of platelets to subendothelium by binding to platelet glycoprotein receptor Gp Ib (and also to Gp IIb/III a when platelets are activated) and subendothelium; and (ii) vWF forms a noncovalent complex with F VIII in circulation and serves to prevent the degradation and rapid removal of F VIII from circulation.

The multimeric vWF consists of different functional domains, which bind F VIII, Gp Ib, Gp IIb/IIIa, and collagen.

Von Willebrand disease is a markedly heterogeneous congenital bleeding disorder characterized by deficiency or functional defect of vWF. Von Willebrand disease is the most

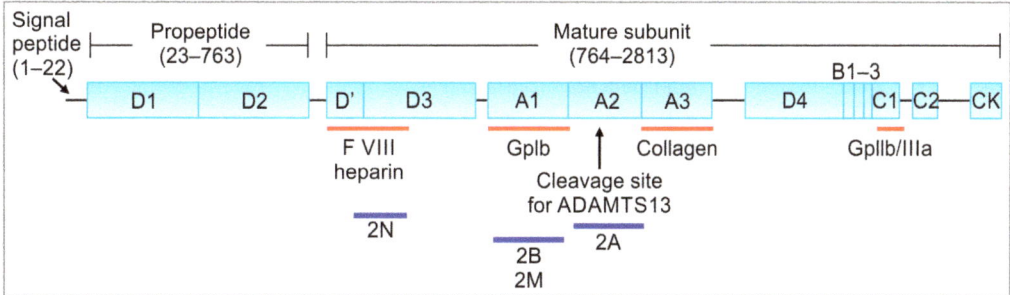

Fig. 16.4: Structure of von Willebrand factor. The vWF precursor consists of a signal peptide (amino acids 1–22), propeptide (amino acids 23–763), and mature vWF subunit (amino acids 764–2813). Various domains, binding sites for F VIII, heparin, GpIb, collagen, and GpIIb/IIIa, and cleavage site for ADAMTS-13 are shown. Mutations causing type 2 vWD are mainly located within specific domains: type 2A within A2; types 2B and 2M within A1; and 2N within D' and D3 domains.

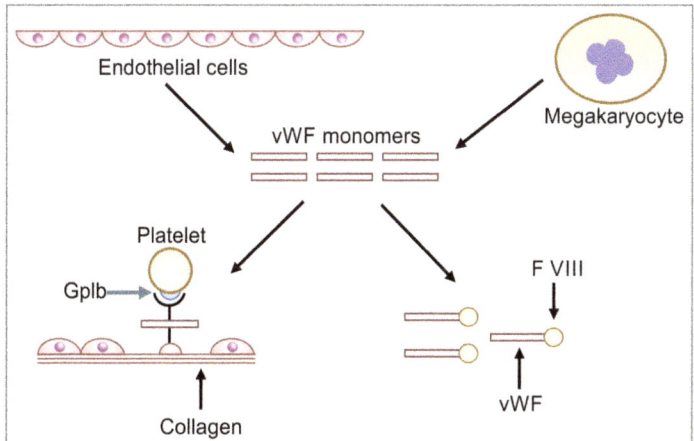

Fig. 16.5: Synthesis and functions of von Willebrand factor. Endothelial cells and megakaryocytes synthesize vWF. Main functions of vWF are mediation of adhesion of platelets to subendothelial collagen and carriage of F VIII in circulation.

Table 16.3: Classification of von Willebrand disease.

Parameter	Type 1	Type 2A	Type 2B	Type 2M	Type 2N	Type 3
1. Frequency of all vWDs	75–80%	~15%	~5%	Uncommon	Uncommon	Rare
2. Inheritance	AD	AD	AD	AD, AR	AR	AR
3. Bleeding	Mild	Mild to moderate	Mild to moderate	Mild to moderate	Mild to moderate	Severe
4. vWF:Ag	↓	↓ or N	↓ or N	↓ or N	↓ or N	Absent
5. vWF:RCo	↓	↓	↓	↓	↓ or N	Absent
6. F VIII	↓ or N	↓ or N	↓ or N	↓ or N	↓↓	↓↓↓
7. RIPA	Normal	↓	Normal	↓	Normal	Absent
8. LD-RIPA	Absent	Absent	↑↑↑	Absent	Absent	Absent
9. vWF multimer analysis	Mild ↓ of all multimers	Mild to moderate ↓ of intermediate and large multimers	Loss of large multimers + qualitative defect	Normal	Normal	Absence of all types of multimers

(↓,↓↓,↓↓↓: Relative decrease;↑↑↑: markedly increased; N: normal; AD: autosomal dominant; AR: autosomal recessive; vWF:Ag: vWF antigen; vWF:RCo: vWF ristocetin cofactor activity; RIPA: ristocetin-induced platelet aggregation; LD-RIPA: low-dose ristocetin-induced platelet aggregation)

common congenital bleeding disorder with overall prevalence in the general population being 1%.

Terminology related to vWF and F VIII is given in Chapter 1 "Overview of Physiology of Blood."

Classification

von Willebrand Disease is classified according to the criteria developed by The Working Party on von Willebrand Disease Classification (The International Society on Thrombosis and Hemostasis, 1994 and 2006) (Table 16.3).

Type 1 vWD (Classical vWD)

1. There is a mild to moderate quantitative deficiency of all types of vWF multimers (i.e. small, intermediate and large); relative proportion of multimers is normal (Fig. 16.6).
2. This is the most common type of vWD accounting for 70% of all cases; bleeding manifestations are mild to moderate. Mode of inheritance is autosomal dominant.
3. There is a corresponding reduction of vWF:Ag, vWF:RCo, and FVIII:C.

Type 2 vWD (Variant vWD)

In type 2 vWD, there is a qualitative abnormality of vWF with absence of large vWF multimers. Laboratory subclassification of type 2 vWD is based on multimeric analysis by electrophoresis (Fig. 16.6).

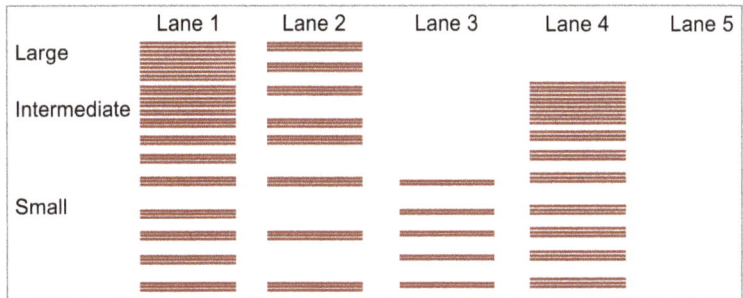

Fig. 16.6: Electrophoretic analysis of vWF multimer patterns in different types of von Willebrand disease. Lane 1: Normal multimers showing large multimers at the top followed by intermediate and small multimers; Lane 2: Type 1 vWD: mild quantitative deficiency of all types of multimers; Lane 3: Type 2A vWD: deficiency of large and intermediate sized multimers along with abnormality of multimer pattern; Lane 4: Type 2B: selective loss of large vWF multimers; Lane 5: Type 3 vWD: complete deficiency of all types of vWF multimers.

Type 2A:
1. Deficiency of large- and intermediate-size vWF multimers is due either to defective secretion into plasma or increased proteolysis of large vWF multimers after synthesis and secretion.
2. Type II A comprises about 15% of all cases of vWD. Mode of inheritance is autosomal dominant and bleeding is mild to moderate.
3. There is variable reduction in vWF:Ag, vWF:RCo, and FVIII:C.

Type 2B:
1. Large vWF multimers have inappropriately increased affinity to bind to platelets; the abnormality resides in the GpIb-binding domain of vWF. This causes clearance from circulation of large vWF multimers along with platelets (to which they are bound) from circulation; this leads to reduction in their levels in plasma and mild thrombocytopenia. Quantity of vWF multimers in platelets is normal.
2. This is an uncommon type of vWD with autosomal dominant mode of inheritance and mild to moderate bleeding tendency.
3. Laboratory abnormalities include variable reduction in vWF:Ag, vWF:RCo, and FVIII:C; increased responsiveness to small concentration of ristocetin in platelet aggregation studies, and mild thrombocytopenia.

Type 2M:
1. There is reduced vWF-dependent platelet adhesion without selective deficiency of high molecular weight vWF multimers.
2. Screening test results are similar in type 2M and type 2A vWD; distinction depends on multimer analysis.

Type 3:
1. There is a severe quantitative deficiency of all forms of vWF multimers.
2. This is a rare but severe bleeding disorder with autosomal recessive inheritance.
3. vWF:Ag, vWF:RCo, and F VIII:C are markedly diminished.

Platelet-type vWD (Pseudo-vWD):
1. There is an abnormal avidity of platelet membrane glycoprotein GpIb-IX complex to bind large vWF multimers leading to reduced levels of vWF multimers in plasma.
2. This is a rare, mild to moderate bleeding disorder with autosomal dominant inheritance.

3. Laboratory features are similar to type IIB vWD. Addition of cryoprecipitate (rich in vWF) to patient's platelet-rich plasma induces aggregation in platelet-type but not in type IIB vWD.

Type 2N:
1. There is a markedly reduced vWF binding affinity for F VIII due to a defect in the F VIII-binding domain of vWF.
2. F VIII:C levels in plasma are reduced. The disease is called as autosomal hemophilia due to its resemblance to hemophilia A of mild to moderate type.

Clinical Features

vWD types 1, 2A, and 2B are inherited in an autosomal dominant manner. Bleeding manifestations in these patients are mild to moderate and superficial in type, i.e. petechiae, ecchymoses, epistaxis, bleeding from gums and gastrointestinal tract, and menorrhagia. There is a marked heterogeneity in frequency, nature, and severity of bleeding. Often many patients are asymptomatic and come to attention because of abnormal bleeding time during a routine preoperative coagulation screen or because of excessive post-traumatic bleeding.

Type 3 vWD is a severe autosomal recessive disorder with onset in early childhood. Bleeding manifestations are related to defective primary as well as secondary hemostasis such as mucocutaneous bleeding, deep hematomas, and hemarthroses.

Laboratory Features

The typical diagnostic features of von Willebrand disease are prolonged bleeding time, reduction (or qualitative abnormality) of vWF:Ag, and decrease in vWF:RCo and F VIII:C levels.

However, there is a marked variability in the results of laboratory tests both among different individuals and in the same individual. The results of laboratory studies are influenced by many variables. Persons with blood group O have lower vWF values as compared to those with other blood groups. Higher vWF levels are obtained in older age, inflammatory states, pregnancy, physical exertion, and when estrogen levels are raised. Mild and heterogeneous clinical nature of the disorder and nonavailability of a specific and sensitive test for diagnosis further add to the difficulty. Frequently, repeated testing is required to unequivocally establish the diagnosis.

Bleeding time is prolonged in vWD, particularly in types 2 and 3. In type 1 vWD, a single bleeding time measurement may be normal and repeated testing is frequently necessary. Although platelet count is normal in most patients, it is slightly low in type 2B and platelet type vWD. Activated partial thromboplastin time (APTT) may be prolonged secondary to decreased F VIII:C levels in plasma (5–40%). In mild F VIII:C deficiency, APTT may be normal. Therefore, F VIII:C assay is required to definitively establish the deficiency.

vWF:Ag is commonly measured by Laurell rocket immunoelectrophoresis method. In this technique, antibody to vWF is incorporated into the agarose gel on a glass slide and patient's sample to be quantitated for vWF:Ag is placed in a well. After electrophoresis, immunoprecipitation develops in the form of rockets the length of which is proportional to the quantity of the antigen. The lower limit of normal for vWF: Ag is about 50%. In type 1 vWD, vWF:Ag is 20 to 50% while in type 2 it is markedly reduced or absent. The newer techniques for quantitation of vWF:Ag are ELISA and latex immunoassay.

The ristocetin-induced platelet aggregation (RIPA) is a commonly employed qualitative test for detection of von Willebrand disease. In this test ristocetin (1 mg/mL) is added to patient's platelet-rich plasma and aggregation response is observed. In vWD, RIPA is deficient, as it requires the presence of vWF-related ristocetin cofactor activity. In mild cases, however, this test may be normal; also it is not specific for vWD as positive test is also obtained in Bernard-Soulier syndrome and certain other conditions. In type 2B and platelet-type vWD, enhanced responsiveness to small concentration of ristocetin (0.5 mg/mL) is noted.

In the assay for ristocetin cofactor (RCoF) activity, ristocetin, formalinized normal platelets and patient's plasma are mixed, and extent of aggregation is determined. Ristocetin facilitates binding of vWF to GpIb on platelets causing their agglutination. This test quantitates ability of the patient's vWF to bind to platelets (GpIb) and cause aggregation. Degree of agglutination is proportional to the amount of vWF. vWF:RCo is decreased in vWD. The vWF:RCo assay has now been replaced with assays based on binding of vWF to recombinant GPIb, which does not require platelets or ristocetin. Another assay that assesses vWF function is vWF:CB (von Willebrand factor-collagen binding capacity).

In mild cases of vWD, bleeding time and APTT may be normal and assay for ristocetin cofactor activity inconclusive. Since many variables affect the laboratory results, repeated testing may be needed to establish the diagnosis.

vWF multimer analysis is done by sodium dodecyl sulfate-agarose gel electrophoresis. Normally, small, intermediate, and large multimers are present. Type 1 vWD shows mild to moderate decrease in all types of multimers, type 2 has deficiency of large vWF multimers while in type 3, severe deficiency of all multimer types is observed. Subclassification of type 2 vWD is based on this technique (Fig. 16.6).

Laboratory tests in vWD are shown in Table 16.4.

Acquired von Willebrand disease: vWD can occur in various acquired disorders such as hypothyroidism, congenital heart disease, autoimmune diseases, lymphoproliferative disorders, monoclonal gammopathies, myeloproliferative disorders, and Wilms tumor. The underlying pathogenic mechanism may be autoantibodies directed against high molecular weight multimers of vWF, increased degradation of high molecular weight multimers by enzymes, or adsorption of vWF by tumor cells.

Treatment

For mild mucous membrane bleeding, antifibrinolytic agents—tranexamic acid or ε-aminocaproic acid can be used. For significant bleeding, two treatment options in vWD are desmopressin and plasma-derived F VIII concentrate rich in high molecular weight multimers

Table 16.4: Laboratory tests in von Willebrand disease.

Initial tests

1. vWF:Ag (Laurell rocket immunoelectrophoresis, ELISA): Measures concentration of vWF protein in plasma
2. vWF:RCo (ELISA): Functional assay that measures binding of vWF (patient's plasma) to normal platelets in the presence of ristocetin
3. F VIII assay (one-stage assay based on APTT): Measures concentration of FVIII in plasma (in vWD, it assesses the ability of vWF to maintain F VIII in circulation)

Further tests

4. Low-dose ristocetin-induced platelet aggregation (platelet aggregation with < 0.6 mg/mL ristocetin): Measures aggregation response when patient's plasma is mixed with normal platelet-rich plasma and ristocetin
5. vWF multimer analysis (SDS electrophoresis): Assesses distribution of different vWF multimers

or cryoprecipitate. Desmopressin or 1-deamino-(8-D-arginine)-vasopressin (DDAVP), a synthetic vasopressin analog, is the treatment of choice in type 1 vWD. It can be administered intravenously or as a nasal spray. Desmopressin raises vWF and F VIII:C levels by stimulating their release from storage sites. It is not much effective in vWD types 2A and 3. Desmopressin is contraindicated in type 2B as it aggravates thrombocytopenia.

Plasma-derived F VIII concentrate rich in vWF or cryoprecipitate is the treatment of choice in those cases not responsive to desmopressin such as type 2 variant and type 3 vWD. The former preparation is preferred as it can be virus-inactivated.

In platelet-type vWD, platelet concentrates may be tried as both desmopressin and cryoprecipitate can induce thrombocytopenia.

HEMOPHILIA B

Hemophilia B (also known as Christmas disease, after the first patient described) is a hereditary F IX deficiency state with X-linked recessive mode of inheritance. The incidence is about 1:60,000 populations.

Clinical features and inheritance pattern are similar to hemophilia A. It is essential to distinguish between hemophilia A and B in the laboratory because of different therapeutic products required.

Coagulation profile shows selective prolongation of activated partial thromboplastin time (APTT). In mild cases, APTT may be normal and in such cases if clinical features are suggestive then specific F VIII and IX assay should be performed (F VIII assay should always be performed first). Thromboplastin generation test shows serum defect as against plasma defect in F VIII deficiency. F IX assay should be done in all cases; its principle is similar to that of F VIII assay. About 1 to 2% of patients with severe hemophilia B develop inhibitor antibodies against F IX.

The therapeutic products for hemophilia B are recombinant F IX (treatment of choice), fresh frozen plasma (for mild/moderate cases), and prothrombin complex concentrate (for severe cases). As half-life of infused F IX is about 24 hours, it is administered once per day. Prothrombin complex concentrate (PCC) contains all vitamin K-dependent coagulation factors, i.e. F II, VII, IX, and X. However, presence of minute amounts of activated coagulation factors in PCC may trigger the coagulation cascade leading to thromboembolic phenomena. Due to this potential risk, use of prothrombin complex concentrates is restricted to severe cases and is administered along with small amount of heparin.

Various genetic defects including gene deletions and point mutations are responsible for hemophilia B. Inhibitor antibodies against F IX develop more commonly in patients with gene deletions. Carrier detection in hemophilia B follows the same general principles as outlined for hemophilia A.

In contrast to hemophilia A, most cases of hemophilia B result from point mutations.

Hemophilia B Leiden: In this form of hemophilia B, F IX levels in blood increase at the time of puberty followed by resolution of bleeding manifestations. It is seen in 3% of hemophilia B patients and results from specific F IX promoter mutations.

INHERITED DISORDERS OF FIBRINOGEN

Hereditary disorders of fibrinogen are of two types—(i) deficiency: afibrinogenemia or hypofibrinogenemia, and (ii) dysfunction: dysfibrinogenemias.

Hereditary Afibrinogenemia

This rare autosomal recessive disorder is characterized by almost complete absence of fibrinogen in plasma. In the neonatal period there may be bleeding from the umbilical stump; afterward common manifestations are excessive bleeding following trivial trauma, easy bruisability, and bleeding from nose and gums. Intracranial hemorrhage is a frequent cause of death. Some patients present with hemarthrosis.

Coagulation profile reveals marked prolongation of all the screening tests of coagulation such as clotting time, PT, activated partial thromboplastin time, and thrombin time. Estimation of fibrinogen (outlined in Chapter 13: "Approach to the diagnosis of bleeding disorders") reveals total absence or trace amounts (<5 mg/dL) of fibrinogen. Platelet function abnormalities are common and include prolongation of bleeding time and defective platelet aggregation with ADP, epinephrine, and collagen. Fibrinogen level of 50–100 mg/dL is usually sufficient for control of bleeding.

Treatment of bleeding episodes consists of administration of fibrinogen concentrate, fresh frozen plasma or cryoprecipitate.

Hypofibrinogenemia

In this condition, fibrinogen concentration in plasma is less than 100 mg/dL. Mode of inheritance is autosomal recessive or dominant. The condition may be asymptomatic or may manifest as a mild bleeding disorder. Thrombin time is usually prolonged and quantitative estimation of fibrinogen shows reduced levels. The condition should be differentiated from acquired causes of hypofibrinogenemia such as disseminated intravascular coagulation, liver disease, and fibrinolytic therapy.

Bleeding, if present, may be managed by cryoprecipitate or fresh frozen plasma.

Dysfibrinogenemias

Dysfibrinogenemias are characterized by qualitative (or functional) abnormality of the fibrinogen molecule. Functional defects in dysfibrinogenemias are diverse. Numerous dysfunctional fibrinogen molecules have been described which impair the formation of the fibrin clot by interfering in the formation of fibrin monomers (cleavage of fibrinopeptides by thrombin), spontaneous polymerization of fibrin monomers, or cross-linking of fibrin monomers by F XIIIa.

Patients with dysfibrinogenemia may be asymptomatic or may have mild bleeding tendency, a predisposition to thrombosis, or poor wound healing.

Prothrombin time, thrombin time, and reptilase time are frequently prolonged while activated partial thromboplastin time is variable. Typically, estimation of fibrinogen by functional or clot-based assay shows reduced quantity of fibrinogen while immunologic method shows normal levels. Bleeding tendencies respond to cryoprecipitate.

ACQUIRED DISORDERS OF COAGULATION

Acquired disorders are more common than hereditary disorders of coagulation. They are usually secondary to some underlying disease and are frequently associated with multiple hemostatic defects. Some acquired coagulation disorders are presented in Table 16.5.

Table 16.5: Acquired coagulation disorders.

1. Disseminated intravascular coagulation	2. Liver disease
3. Vitamin K deficiency	4. Acquired inhibitors of coagulation
5. Heparin, oral anticoagulation, thrombolytic therapy	6. Renal disease
7. Paraproteinemias	8. Cardiopulmonary bypass
9. Massive transfusion of stored blood	

VITAMIN K DEFICIENCY

Vitamin K is a fat-soluble vitamin that is absorbed in the proximal small intestine in the presence of bile salts. Green leafy vegetables are a good source of vitamin K. It is also synthesized by bacterial flora in the large intestine. It is stored in small amounts in the liver.

Vitamin K is required for gamma carboxylation of glutamic acid residues of four vitamin K-dependent factors II, VII, IX, and X (*see* Fig. 16.11). This post-translational modification is essential for binding of these coagulation factors to phospholipid in the presence of calcium. In the absence of vitamin K gamma carboxylation fails to occur and nonfunctional forms of vitamin K-dependent factors circulate in blood. These are called as acarboxy forms or PIVKAs (proteins induced by vitamin K absence or antagonism). Vitamin K is also necessary for gamma carboxylation of two natural anticoagulant proteins C and S.

Causes of vitamin K deficiency are hemorrhagic disease of newborn, poor dietary intake, impaired absorption due to obstructive jaundice or malabsorption syndromes, and drugs such as oral anticoagulants and broad-spectrum antibiotics.

Hemorrhagic Disease of the Newborn

In the normal newborn, levels of vitamin K-dependent clotting factors are depressed and show a further fall at 2 to 3 days of life. In premature infants levels are even lower. After a few days the levels gradually begin to rise. Vitamin K deficiency exaggerates the fall of these coagulation factors and causes bleeding.

Three forms of hemorrhagic disease of newborn are distinguished—early, classic, and late (Table 16.6). Early type is associated with maternal ingestion of oral anticoagulants or phenytoin and bleeding manifests at birth. Classic hemorrhagic disease of newborn typically occurs in exclusively breast-fed infants (breast milk is a poor source of vitamin K) and bleeding usually

Table 16.6: Hemorrhagic disease of newborn.

Parameter	Early	Classic	Late
1. Time of bleeding after birth	Within 24 hours	2–7 days	After 7 days to few months
2. Contributory factors	Maternal ingestion of anticonvulsants, oral anticoagulants, anti-TB drugs	Exclusive breastfeeding, low placental transfer of vitamin K, sterile gut	Malabsorption, chronic diarrhea, prolonged breastfeeding with no supplementation, antibiotics
3. Nature of bleeding	Severe	Bruising, bleeding from GIT, umbilical stump or postcircumcision	Intracranial bleeding common

manifests at 2 to 3 days of life. Late type develops usually after 1 month and is associated with underlying disorder such as malabsorption or biliary atresia.

F VII falls quickly due to its short half-life leading to prolongation of PT. As factors IX and X subsequently decline, prolongation of activated partial thromboplastin time also occurs.

It is recommended that all neonates be administered prophylactic 0.5 to 1 mg of vitamin K at birth to prevent hemorrhagic disease of newborn. Treatment consists of parenteral vitamin K supplementation. If bleeding is severe and life-threatening, fresh frozen plasma may be administered.

LIVER DISEASE (CIRRHOSIS OF LIVER)

The liver has a major role in hemostasis (Table 16.7). Because of this, chronic liver disease often produces complex coagulation abnormalities.

Causes of bleeding in liver disease (cirrhosis) include—(i) Esophageal varices (secondary to portal hypertension) and peptic ulcer; (ii) Thrombocytopenia (due to splenomegaly secondary to portal hypertension); (iii) Deficient synthesis of coagulation factors; (iv) Deficient utilization of vitamin K; (v) Synthesis of dysfunctional fibrinogens (dysfibrinogenemia) which leads to defective fibrin polymerization; (vi) Defective platelet function due to raised FDPs; (vii) Disseminated intravascular coagulation due to inefficient clearance of activated coagulation factors and decreased synthesis of coagulation inhibitors-antithrombin III and protein C; and (viii) Increased fibrinogenolysis due to deficient clearance of plasminogen activators and α2-antiplasmin.

Laboratory abnormalities include prolongation of PT, activated partial thromboplastin time, and thrombin time (due to reduced synthesis of coagulation factors and production of dysfunctional fibrinogen). F VII, a vitamin K-dependent factor is the earliest to fall owing to its short half-life. Protein C, an anticoagulant also falls along with F VII. This is followed by decrease in the level of other coagulation factors. F VIII:C and von Willebrand factor levels are normal.

In advanced disease, fibrinolytic activity is increased leading to increase in the level of FDPs. Thrombocytopenia due to splenomegaly, and platelet dysfunction due to inhibitory action of FDPs are also noted. Laboratory abnormalities in DIC in liver disease include reduction of F VIII:C, increased D-dimer, and raised thrombin-antithrombin complexes.

Therapy is given if bleeding especially from gastrointestinal tract is present and as a cover if surgery/biopsy is being considered. Various modes of therapy for hemostatic correction

Table 16.7: Role of the liver in hemostasis.

1. Synthesis of proteins
    - Coagulation system—Factors I, II, V, VII, VIII, IX, X, XI, XII, XIII, prekallikrein, high molecular weight kininogen
    - Natural anticoagulants—Antithrombin III, protein C, protein S
    - Fibrinolytic system—Plasminogen, α–2 antiplasmin
2. Utilization of vitamin K for synthesis of vitamin K-dependent proteins (vitamin K is required for post-translational gamma carboxylation of Factors II, VII, IX, and X and proteins C and S)
3. Clearance of activated coagulation factors and plasminogen activators by reticuloendothelial cells of liver

are—(i) Fresh frozen plasma: This provides all the coagulation factors. However, treatment of hemostatic defect needs large amounts of FFP, which can cause circulatory overload. (ii) Prothrombin complex concentrates: They supply vitamin K-dependent factors. They contain activated coagulation factors and thus may initiate DIC. (iii) Fibrinolytic inhibitors may be used if fibrinolysis is the major cause of bleeding and there is no DIC. Due to the risk of DIC, these agents have a limited role. (iv) Vitamin K is useful in liver disease with obstructive element.

DISSEMINATED INTRAVASCULAR COAGULATION

Synonyms—Defibrination syndrome, Consumptive coagulopathy

Disseminated intravascular coagulation (DIC) is an acquired disorder occurring in a wide spectrum of underlying diseases and characterized by (i) widespread systemic activation of coagulation with formation of microthrombi in small blood vessels and (ii) bleeding diathesis secondary to depletion of coagulation factors and platelets (Fig. 16.7).

Etiology

Important causes of DIC are listed in Table 16.8. Mechanisms initiating DIC in these conditions are as follows:
- **Sepsis and severe infections:** Membrane components of microorganisms, such as lipopolysaccharides and endotoxins, or release of bacterial exotoxins cause release of inflammatory cytokines from mononuclear cells and endothelial cells.
- **Severe trauma:** Release of fat and phospholipids from damaged tissue, hemolysis, and endothelial damage cause systemic activation of coagulation. In patients with head trauma, DIC is especially common due to release of large amount of tissue factor from cerebral injury.
- **Obstetric conditions:** Leakage of thromboplastin-like material from placenta into the maternal circulation.

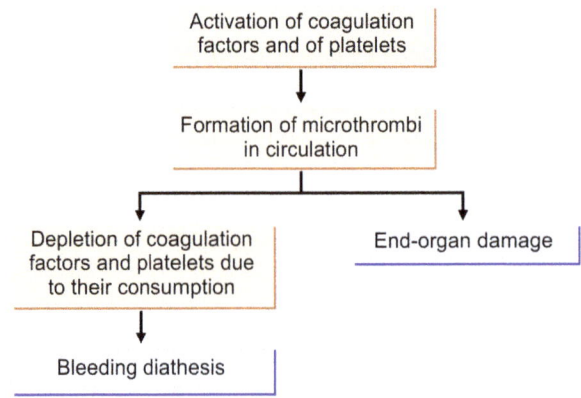

Fig. 16.7: General mechanism of DIC.

Table 16.8: Causes of DIC.

1. Sepsis or severe infections
2. Trauma especially of brain or crush injury
3. Obstetric conditions: Amniotic fluid embolism, abruptio placentae, septic abortion, eclampsia, intrauterine retention of dead fetus
4. Malignancy: Disseminated solid cancers, acute promyelocytic leukemia
5. Severe hemolytic transfusion reactions
6. Thermal injury: Heat stroke, extensive burns
7. Snake bite, e.g. Russell's viper
8. Severe liver disease
9. Giant hemangioma (Kasabach-Merritt syndrome)

- **Malignancy:** Expression of tissue factor on malignant cells; release of procoagulant substances from promyelocytes in acute promyelocytic leukemia.
- **Vascular disorders (Kasabach-Merritt syndrome):** Local activation of coagulation with consumption of coagulation factors and platelets.
- **Snakebite:** Proteolytic activation of coagulation factors. Envenomation by Russell's viper and Echis carinatus induces DIC.

Pathogenesis

Disseminated intravascular coagulation is a systemic thrombohemorrhagic disorder characterized by (1) intravascular activation of extrinsic pathway of coagulation with generation of thrombin and fibrin, (2) reduction in levels of endogenous anticoagulants (antithrombin, protein C, and tissue factor pathway inhibitor), and (3) suppression of fibrinolytic system which causes delayed and inadequate removal of fibrin. These three factors in combination lead to generalized deposition of fibrin (with formation of microthrombi) in circulation (Fig. 16.8). End-organ damage from generalized thrombotic occlusion of small blood vessels is responsible for most of the morbidity and mortality.

Depletion of coagulation factors and platelets results from their consumption in widespread microthrombi formation. This produces hemorrhagic diathesis. There is secondary activation of fibrinolysis (though insufficient to remove all fibrin) that leads to generation of fibrinogen/fibrin degradation products. Plasminogen bound to platelet-fibrin thrombi is converted to plasmin by plasminogen activators. Plasmin cleaves fibrinogen as well as fibrin to generate fibrinogen/fibrin degradation products (FDPs). Fibrinogen degradation products are X, Y, D, and E fragments (refer to Fig. 1.41). Fibrin degradation yields different fragments due to the presence of cross-linkages. A unique fibrin degradation product is D-dimer (refer to Fig. 1.42). Circulating FDPs inhibit fibrin polymerization and contribute to bleeding.

Mechanical damage to red cells by fibrin strands in circulation leads to microangiopathic hemolytic anemia.

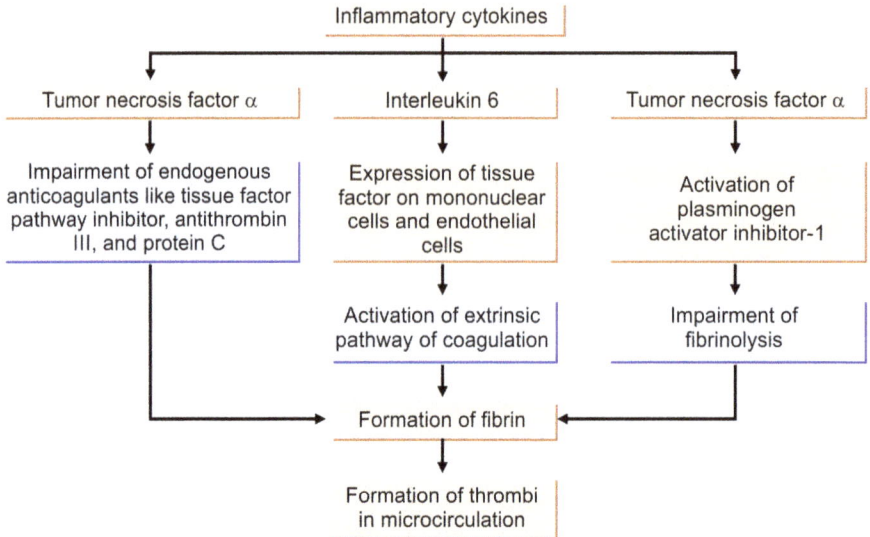

Fig. 16.8: Pathogenesis of intravascular fibrin formation in DIC. Tissue factor is expressed on the surface of mononuclear cells and endothelial cells. This leads to initiation of extrinsic pathway of coagulation and generation of thrombin and fibrin. There is simultaneous inhibition of natural anticoagulants (antithrombin, protein C, and tissue factor pathway inhibitor) that further amplifies thrombin generation. At the same time fibrinolytic mechanism is suppressed by increased plasma levels of plasminogen activator inhibitor type 1 (PAI-1) that causes further propagation of fibrin formation. Inflammatory cytokines released from activated mononuclear cells and endothelial cells mediate these effects.

Clinical Features

Clinical features are largely determined by underlying disease that causes DIC. Two types of DIC are distinguished: Acute and chronic.

1. ***Acute or decompensated DIC:*** There is a rapid and extensive activation of coagulation leading to significant bleeding from consumption of coagulation factors and widespread microvascular thrombosis with consequent end-organ damage. Examples are DIC induced by sepsis and trauma.
2. ***Chronic or compensated DIC:*** There is slow activation of coagulation in small amounts with slow consumption of coagulation factors; coagulation factor levels are normal or increased as they are replenished by enhanced synthesis. In chronic DIC, clinical features are minimal or absent and laboratory abnormalities are the only evidence of DIC. Examples of diseases initiating chronic DIC are intrauterine retention of dead fetus, liver disease, giant hemangioma, eclampsia, and malignancy.

In acute, fulminant DIC there is a sudden onset of spontaneous bleeding from multiple sites, such as skin (petechiae, ecchymoses), gastrointestinal tract, urinary system (hematuria), epistaxis, and oozing from venepuncture sites. Intracranial hemorrhage can occur. Purpura fulminans (patchy areas of hemorrhagic skin necrosis) is a typical sign of fulminant DIC and results from thrombosis of small vessels of skin. Thrombotic occlusion may also affect vasculature of CNS, kidneys, heart, liver, lungs, or adrenals.

Chronic DIC is a mild and protracted disease, which manifests usually with venous thrombosis; bleeding and microvascular thromboses are uncommon.

Laboratory Features

There is no single test that is diagnostic of DIC. Diagnosis is usually based on combination of clinical and laboratory features. Often multiple and frequent testing is required.

Acute DIC

In typical cases, all the coagulation screening tests (PT, APTT, and TT) are prolonged due to consumption of coagulation factors and inhibitory effect of FDPs (Box 16.5). It should be noted, however, that these tests might sometimes be normal. This is due to the presence of activated coagulation factors in circulation that cause rapid clot formation in the test system or the presence of X and Y FDP fragments which are coagulable by thrombin.

Quantitation of fibrinogen reveals hypofibrinogenemia. Peripheral blood examination shows fragmented red cells (schistocytes, helmet cells) on blood film and thrombocytopenia (Fig. 16.9). Soluble fibrin monomers can be detected by "paracoagulation tests." In DIC, fibrin monomers combine with circulating FDPs to form soluble fibrin monomers. This inhibits fibrin monomer polymerization. When ethanol or protamine sulfate is added to patient's plasma, fibrin monomers dissociate from FDPs and spontaneously polymerize to form a gel. This test is positive in early DIC but is

Box 16.5: Typical findings in acute DIC.
- Presence of underlying disease known to be associated with DIC
- Low platelets or falling platelets on repeat testing
- Prolonged PT and APTT
- Low fibrinogen or falling levels on repeat testing
- Low plasma levels of coagulation inhibitors: ATIII or protein C
- Schistocytes (fragmented red cells) on blood smear
- FDP and D-dimer: Increased

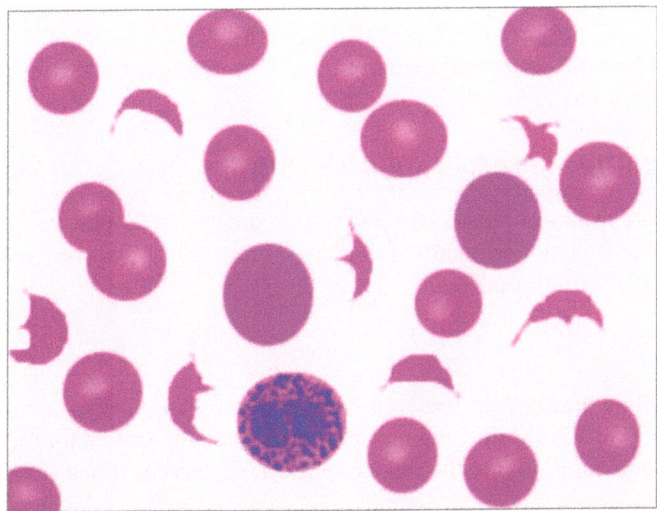

Fig. 16.9: Blood smear in DIC. Schistocytes, polychromatic cells, a neutrophil with toxic granules, and thrombocytopenia are present.

not sufficiently sensitive. Positive test is also obtained in liver disease, lobar pneumonia, and after major surgery.

Proteolytic action of plasmin on fibrinogen/fibrin generates FDPs. Latex agglutination test is commonly used for detection and quantitation of FDPs. This test has been outlined earlier. (*see* Chapet 13: "Approach to the diagnosis of bleeding disorders.") FDPs are raised in most patients with DIC. However, FDP test may sometimes be negative.

Proteolysis of cross-linked fibrin by plasmin produces D-dimer fragments (refer Fig. 1.41). Detection of D-dimers indicates both thrombin and plasmin generation. Latex particles coated with a monoclonal antibody against D-dimer are mixed with patient's serum and observed for agglutination. Amongst the currently available tests for DIC, D-dimer test is the most specific.

Chronic DIC

In chronic DIC, coagulation screening tests (PT, APTT, TT) are usually normal and platelet count is normal or slightly reduced. Test for FDPs and for fibrin monomers are abnormal (Box 16.6).

> **Box 16.6:** Typical findings in chronic DIC.
> - Platelet count: Normal
> - PT and APTT: Normal
> - FDP and D-dimer: Increased

General Principles of Therapy

1. Treatment of DIC depends on underlying cause and severity of clinical manifestations.
2. Management of the underlying disease process is the most effective measure in controlling DIC.
3. Transfusion of platelets or plasma components:
   - ***Platelets:*** In patients with DIC and bleeding and a platelet count < 50,000/mm^3
   - ***Fresh frozen plasma:*** In patients with DIC and bleeding and prolonged PT and APTT
   - ***Fibrinogen concentrate or cryoprecipitate:*** Severe hypofibrinogenemia (<1 g/L) that persists despite FFP replacement
4. ***Heparin:*** In DIC, where thrombosis predominates (arterial or venous thromboembolism, purpura fulminans with acral ischemia).
5. ***Recombinant human-activated protein C:*** In severe sepsis with DIC; it should not be given to patients at high-risk of bleeding.

ACQUIRED INHIBITORS OF COAGULATION (CIRCULATING ANTICOAGULANTS)

Acquired inhibitors of blood coagulation are substances that impair coagulation either by inactivating specific coagulation factors (specific inhibitors) or by interfering in coagulation reactions (nonspecific inhibitors).

Specific Inhibitors

These are antibodies that inhibit the activity of specific coagulation factors. They include inhibitors against F VIII, F IX, fibrinogen, vWF, prothrombin, and factors V, XI, XIII, VII, XII, and X. Inhibitors against F VIII are the most common followed by those against F IX.

F VIII Inhibitors

F VIII inhibitors develop in about 10 to 15% of patients with severe hemophilia A who have been exposed to multiple transfusions. They are uncommon in mild hemophilia. Their development causes refractoriness to F VIII replacement therapy. F VIII inhibitors are not restricted to hemophilic patients. They also occur in autoimmune disorders (rheumatoid arthritis, systemic lupus erythematosus), postpartum females, malignancy, and during drug therapy especially penicillin. They also occur in elderly persons without any apparent cause. F VIII inhibitors in these patients cause bleeding but hemarthroses and deep hematomas are rare.

Coagulation profile reveals isolated prolongation of APTT. APTT performed using both patient's plasma and normal plasma (50:50) shows progressive (time-dependent) prolongation when incubated at 37°C for 2 hours.

The inhibitor antibodies against F VIII are commonly expressed in terms of Bethesda units. Patient's plasma (containing F VIII inhibitor) is mixed with normal pooled plasma (contains 100% F VIII activity), incubated at 37°C for 2 hours and residual F VIII activity in the mixture is assayed. The result is expressed as Bethesda units of inhibitor present per ml depending upon the reduction in the F VIII concentration in the incubation mixture.

Management of F VIII inhibitors is difficult. Various treatment options for F VIII inhibitors are: (i) High doses of F VIII concentrates along with plasmapheresis to remove inhibitor antibodies; (ii) Porcine F VIII concentrates which have low cross-reactivity against F VIII antibodies; (iii) Prothrombin complex concentrates and anti-inhibitor coagulant complex (Autoplex) which bypass F VIII; (iv) Immunosuppressive therapy and immunomodulation (IV immunoglobulin).

Nonspecific Inhibitors

They are not directed against specific coagulation factors. The prototype example is lupus anticoagulant.

Lupus anticoagulant (Lupus inhibitor): Lupus anticoagulants are acquired autoantibodies directed against phospholipid-protein complexes that can cause antiphospholipid syndrome. Antiphospholipid syndrome is an autoimmune disease characterized by venous or arterial thrombosis and/or recurrent fetal loss and presence of antiphospholipid antibodies in plasma. Types of antiphospholipid antibodies include anticardiolipin antibodies, anti-β2-glycoprotein I antibodies, and lupus anticoagulant. Anticardiolipin and anti-β2-glycoprotein I antibodies are detected by ELISA while lupus anticoagulant is identified by clot-based coagulation tests.

Antiphospholipid antibodies are encountered in systemic lupus erythematosus and other autoimmune diseases, neoplasia, lymphoproliferative disorders, viral infections particularly human immunodeficiency virus, in association with certain drugs, and in otherwise normal persons.

According to current guidelines, definite antiphospholipid syndrome is present if at least one clinical and one laboratory criteria are met:
1. ***Clinical criteria:*** Vascular thrombosis, pregnancy morbidity
2. ***Laboratory criteria:*** Anticardiolipin antibody, anti-β2-glycoprotein I antibody, lupus anticoagulant (laboratory test should be positive on ≥2 occasions at least 12 weeks apart).

Rarely, patients with antiphospholipid syndrome present with multiorgan failure of rapid onset that is associated with high mortality (catastrophic antiphospholipid syndrome). Acute thrombotic microangiopathy develops in multiple organs especially kidneys, lungs, central nervous system, heart, and skin.

Pathogenesis of thrombosis is unknown. Probably antiphospholipid antibodies activate endothelial cells, monocytes, and platelets causing increased synthesis of tissue factor and thromboxane A2. Activation of complement cascade by antiphospholipid antibodies may trigger inflammatory reaction on the vessel wall or trophoblast surface. Interaction of antibodies with proteins like protein C, annexin 5, and plasmin may inhibit inactivation of procoagulant factors and impede fibrinolysis. A "second hit" is possibly required for thrombosis or fetal loss to occur (like traumatic injury to vessel, infections, estrogens, etc.).

The name "lupus anticoagulant" is a misnomer since (i) most patients do not have systemic lupus erythematosus, and (ii) there is association with thrombosis rather than bleeding. The risk of fetal loss is high after 10th week of gestation.

Criteria for diagnosis of lupus anticoagulant are shown in Box 16.7 and Figure 16.10.

Box 16.7: Criteria for diagnosis of lupus anticoagulant (International Society on Thrombosis and Hemostasis).

- Prolongation of phospholipid-dependent screening test of coagulation*
- Failure of correction of prolonged screening test by mixing patient's plasma with normal platelet-poor plasma
- Correction of shortening of prolonged screening test by addition of excess phospholipids
- Exclusion of other coagulopathies like F VIII inhibitor or heparin

*At least two different screening tests (e.g. APTT, dilute Russell's viper venom time, kaolin clotting time, hexagonal phospholipids test) should be used before considering the sample as negative.

Note: For confirmation of diagnosis, re-testing of positive results is necessary after ≥12 weeks.

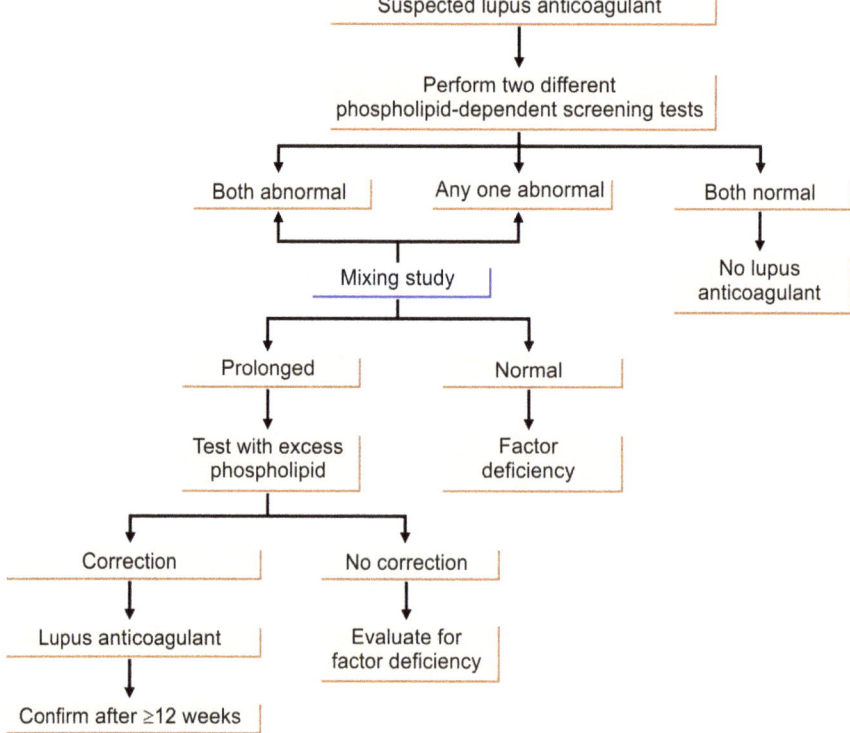

Fig. 16.10: Strategy for laboratory identification of lupus anticoagulant.

Incidental detection of lupus anticoagulant in an asymptomatic patient usually requires no treatment. Long-term anticoagulant therapy is frequently required in patients with thrombosis. In repeated fetal loss, encouraging results have been reported with low-dose subcutaneous heparin and/or aspirin.

HEPARIN THERAPY

Heparin is a widely used, rapidly acting, and potent anticoagulant drug prepared from bovine intestinal mucosa or lung or from porcine intestinal mucosa. It is not a homogeneous substance but a mixture of glycosaminoglycans of different molecular weights. The basis of anticoagulant effect of heparin is potentiation of action of antithrombin III (AT III), which is an inhibitor of thrombin (F IIa), F Xa, and F IXa.

Major clinical application of heparin is prophylaxis and treatment of thromboembolism. For prophylaxis low-dose heparin while for treatment of thrombosis full-dose heparin is given.

Low-dose heparin (5,000 units two to three times per day) given subcutaneously is effective in preventing deep vein thrombosis in (i) patients >40 years who have to undergo elective abdominal or pelvic surgery, and (ii) medical diseases such as congestive cardiac failure or myocardial infarction.

Full-dose intravenous heparin (5,000 units loading dose followed by infusion of 1,000–2,000 units per hour) is employed for treatment of acute thrombosis and is given either as continuous infusion or intermittent injections.

Full-dose intravenous heparin therapy for treatment of acute thrombosis is monitored usually by APTT to maintain the dose within the therapeutic range. Therapeutic range is the level of anticoagulation that is sufficient to prevent thrombosis but does not cause spontaneous bleeding. Heparin level of 0.2 to 0.4 units/mL is considered as adequate anticoagulation. It is recommended to maintain the APTT of the patient between 1.5 and 2.5 times the control result to cover the therapeutic range.

Complications of heparin therapy include hemorrhage, thrombocytopenia, thrombosis, and osteoporosis.

Heparin-induced thrombocytopenia occurs in a small proportion of patients receiving standard heparin or low molecular weight heparin (LMWH). It occurs in two forms—type I and type II.

Type I is a mild form of thrombocytopenia (platelets >1 lakh/mm^3) which occurs early, i.e. during first few days of therapy and is often asymptomatic. It appears to be caused by aggregating effect of heparin on platelets.

Type II thrombocytopenia is more severe (platelets < 40,000/mm^3), of delayed onset (usually develops after 4th day of treatment) and mediated by immune mechanism. Bleeding is rare despite marked thrombocytopenia. Paradoxically many patients with type II thrombocytopenia develop thrombosis [heparin-induced thrombocytopenia with thrombosis (HITT)]. Thrombotic events include acute myocardial infarction, thrombotic stroke, peripheral arterial thromboses, and deep venous thrombosis.

The pathogenesis involves binding of IgG-heparin-platelet factor IV complex to Fc receptors on platelets that causes activation and aggregation of platelets as well as clearance of coated platelets by macrophages of reticuloendothelial system. Diagnosis is made by excluding other causes of thrombocytopenia, by noting rise in platelet count after heparin withdrawal, and by demonstrating heparin-dependent platelet antibody by special tests. Platelet count gradually improves after cessation of heparin, but thrombocytopenia develops on re-exposure. Treatment of thrombosis consists of immediate discontinuation of heparin and administration of inhibitors of thrombin like hirudin or danaparoid.

Low Molecular Weight Heparins

Low molecular weight heparins (LMWHs) are prepared by enzymatic or chemical digestion of standard heparin. The anticoagulant action of LMWH is due to AT III-mediated inhibition predominantly of F Xa. The antithrombin action of LMWH is relatively weak. Duration of anticoagulation with LMWH is considerably longer than standard unfractionated heparin. LMWH is now the standard form of treatment in majority of patients since risk of heparin-induced thrombocytopenia and thrombosis is low. Monitoring by APTT is not required. Because of longer duration of action, LMWH can be administered once daily. It is indicated for prevention and treatment of venous thrombosis and in acute coronary syndrome.

ORAL ANTICOAGULANTS

Vitamin K is required for gamma carboxylation of coagulation factors II, VII, IX, and X. Oral anticoagulants interfere with the recycling of reduced vitamin K by inhibiting vitamin K epoxide reductase and also vitamin K reductase. This decreases availability of reduced form of vitamin K and thus inhibits gamma carboxylation (Fig. 16.11).

In the absence of vitamin K, functionally inactive forms of these coagulation factors circulate in plasma, which are unable to bind calcium. Such inactive forms are called as a carboxy forms or PIVKA (proteins induced by vitamin K absence or antagonism). These inactive coagulation factor precursors retain their antigenicity as detected by immunological assays but are unable to participate in the coagulation cascade.

Apart from factors II, VII, IX, and X, oral anticoagulants also inhibit two natural anticoagulant proteins C and S.

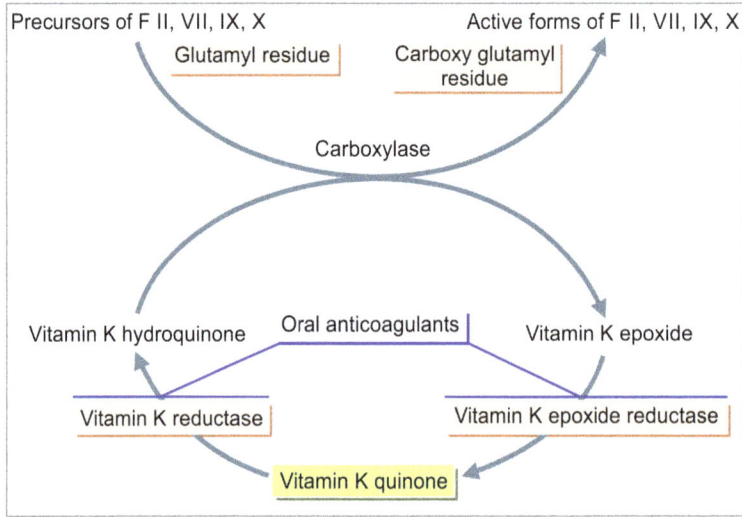

Fig. 16.11: Vitamin K cycle. Oral anticoagulants inhibit vitamin K epoxide reductase and vitamin K reductase.

Time required for suppression of vitamin K-dependent coagulation factors depends on their half-lives. F VII, which has the shortest half-life (6 hour), disappears first followed by F IX (24 hour), F X (30 hour), and prothrombin (60 hour). Effective anticoagulation does not occur until all the pre-existing vitamin K-dependent coagulation factors are cleared from the circulation (3–4 days).

Oral anticoagulants are of two types—coumarins and the indanediones. Indanediones are rarely used due to the high-risk of side effects. The most commonly used coumarin anticoagulant is warfarin sodium. A wide variety of drugs potentiate or inhibit the action of oral anticoagulants. This can increase the risk of bleeding or may reduce the anticoagulant effect. Dosage of oral anticoagulants may have to be adjusted when certain drugs are being given simultaneously.

Drugs may potentiate the action of oral anticoagulants by various mechanisms: (1) Impairment of platelet function (e.g. aspirin, nonsteroidal anti-inflammatory drugs); (2) Impairment of warfarin metabolism (e.g. disulfiram); (3) Inhibition of recycling of vitamin K (cephalosporins); (4) Reduction of availability of vitamin K by interference with bacterial flora (broad-spectrum antibiotics); (5) Anticoagulant action (heparin); and (6) Acceleration of clotting factor metabolism (thyroxine).

Drugs may inhibit the action of oral anticoagulants by: (1) Stimulating the hepatic microsomal enzymes and increasing the metabolism of warfarin (e.g. barbiturates, rifampicin, and griseofulvin); and (2) Reducing the absorption of warfarin from the gut (cholestyramine).

Indications for oral anticoagulants are—(i) *Treatment of deep vein thrombosis (DVT):* DVT is a significant risk factor for pulmonary embolism. Initial treatment of DVT consists of immediate anticoagulation by intravenous heparin, which is given for 7 to 10 days. This is followed by warfarin which is started at least 2 to 3 days before discontinuing heparin. (ii) *Prevention of DVT in high-risk patients,* e.g. patients with previous history of venous thrombosis, patients undergoing hip surgery or surgery for cancer. (iii) *Cardiac conditions* such as myocardial infarction (for prevention of recurrence and stroke), valvular prostheses (to reduce the risk of thromboembolism), and atrial fibrillation (to decrease systemic embolization) and (iv) *Recurrent thromboembolic phenomena.*

Oral anticoagulant therapy is regularly monitored by PT that is a measure of three of the four vitamin K-dependent factors. The result is usually reported as ratio of PT of patient to PT of control. However, responsiveness of tissue thromboplastins (PT reagent), which are obtained from rabbit, bovine, or human sources, to decreased vitamin K-dependent factors is variable and the result of PT depends on type of thromboplastin used. Thus level of anticoagulation can vary widely even though identical PT results are obtained with different tissue thromboplastins. The therapeutic range with one thromboplastin reagent cannot be directly applied to another reagent. To achieve standardization among laboratories, it is recommended to report the result of PT as International Normalized Ratio (INR) that is derived from the formula:

$$INR = \frac{(PT \text{ of patient})^{ISI}}{(PT \text{ of control})}$$

International Sensitivity Index (ISI) of a particular tissue thromboplastin is derived by comparing it with reference thromboplastin of known ISI.

The recommended therapeutic range depends on the indication for anticoagulation; for most cases, INR of 2.0 to 3.0 (commonly 2.5) is advised. Side effects of warfarin include: (1) Bleeding, (2) skin necrosis due to microvascular thrombosis in subcutaneous tissue (protein C deficiency is thought to play a role), and (3) Teratogenic effect on the fetus if given during pregnancy.

OTHER ACQUIRED COAGULATION DISORDERS

Renal Diseases

Excessive urinary loss of coagulation factor IX and antithrombin III may occur in nephrotic syndrome. Thrombotic tendencies in these patients are probably related to deficiency of antithrombin III.

Hemostatic abnormalities commonly develop in uremia such as defective platelet function (which manifests as prolonged bleeding time and deficient platelet aggregation with ADP and epinephrine) and impairment of fibrin monomer polymerization. These abnormalities are reversed by dialysis and are probably caused by a dialyzable substance. Bleeding diathesis usually responds to hemodialysis. Desmopressin and cryoprecipitate are other modes of therapy.

Paraproteinemias

Paraproteinemias are frequently associated with thrombocytopenia, impairment of platelet function (due to coating of platelet surface by paraproteins causing blocking of platelet receptors), and defective fibrin monomer polymerization. Treatment of primary disease with lowering of paraprotein level is followed by improvement.

Amyloidosis

Amyloid deposits in tissues avidly bind F X and can cause its secondary deficiency.

Cardiopulmonary Bypass

Hemostatic defects are frequent during and after cardiopulmonary bypass surgery and include platelet dysfunction, thrombocytopenia, inadequate inactivation of heparin by protamine, and disseminated intravascular coagulation. Bleeding can be treated by platelet concentrates, desmopressin, and fresh frozen plasma or cryoprecipitate.

Massive Transfusion of Stored Blood

Massive transfusion refers to the transfusion equal to or greater than patient's blood volume within 24 hours. Stored blood is usually deficient in platelets and some coagulation factors (F V and VIII). Hemostatic defects in massively transfused patients are caused by dilution of platelets and coagulation factors. Disseminated intravascular coagulation secondary to shock and underlying disease is probably a more important cause of major bleeding in these patients than dilutional effect.

BIBLIOGRAPHY

1. Aledort LM. Treatment of von Willebrand's disease. Mayo Clin Proc. 1991;66:841-46.
2. Antonarakis SE, Waber PG, Kittur SD, et al. Hemophilia A. Detection of molecular defects and of carriers by DNA analysis. N Engl J Med. 1985;313:842-48.
3. Baglin T. Disseminated intravascular coagulation: Diagnosis and treatment. BMJ. 1996;312:683-87.
4. Bakshi S, Arya LS. Diagnosis and treatment of disseminated intravascular coagulation. Indian Pediatrics. 2003;40:721-30.

5. Barrowcliffe TW. Low molecular weight heparin(s). Br J Haematol.1995;90:1-7.
6. Bick RL, Baker WF. The antiphospholipid and thrombosis syndromes. Med Clin North Am. 1994;78: 667-84.
7. Bick RL. Disseminated intravascular coagulation: Objective criteria for diagnosis and management. Med Clin North Am. 1994;78:511-43.
8. Bloom AL, Peake IR. Haemophilia. Diagnosis and management. In: Poller L (Ed). Recent Advances in Blood Coagulation. No. 5. Edinburgh: Churchill Livingstone; 1991.
9. Bowen DJ. Haemophilia A and Haemophilia B: Molecular insights. Mol Pathol. 2002;55:127-44.
10. Chong BH. Heparin-induced thrombocytopaenia. Br J Haematol. 1995;l89:431-39.
11. Furie B, Limentani SA, Rosenfield CG. A practical guide to the evaluation and treatment of hemophilia. Blood. 1994;84:3-9.
12. Ginsburg D, Walter Bowie EJ. Molecular genetics of von Willebrand disease. Blood. 1992;79:2507-19.
13. Graham JB, Green PP, McGraw RA, et al. Application of molecular genetics to prenatal diagnosis and carrier detection in the hemophilias: Some limitations. Blood. 1985;66:759-64.
14. Greaves M, Preston FE. Clinical and laboratory aspects of thrombophilia. In: Poller L (Ed). Recent Advances in Blood Coagulation. No. 5. Edinburgh: Churchill Livingstone; 1991.
15. Hanly JG. Antiphospholipid syndrome: An overview. CMAJ. 2003;168:1675-82.
16. Hembleton J, Leung LL, Levi M. Coagulation: Consultative hemostasis. American Society of Hematology. Hematology. 2002;335-52.
17. Hirsh J, Dalen JE, Deykin D, et al. Heparin: mechanism of action, pharmacokinetics, dosing considerations, monitoring, efficacy, and safety. Chest. 1992;102:337S-351S.
18. Hirsh J, Dalen JE, Deykin D, et al. Oral anticoagulants—Mechanism of action, clinical effectiveness, and optimal therapeutic range. Chest. 1992;102:312S-326S.
19. Hirsh J. Oral anticoagulants. N Engl J Med. 1991;324:1865-75.
20. Hoyer LW, Carta CA, Golbus MS, Hobbins JC, Mahoney MJ. Prenatal diagnosis of classic hemophilia (Hemophilia A) by immunoradiometric assays. Blood. 1985;65:1312-7.
21. Hoyer LW. Hemophilia A. N Engl J Med. 1994;330:38-47.
22. Kanavakis E, Traeger-Synodinos J. Preimplantation diagnosis in clinical practice. J Med Genet. 2002;39: 6-11.
23. Kashyap R, Choudhury VP. Hemophilia. Indian Pediatrics. 2000;37:45-53.
24. Kogan SC, Doherty M, Gitschier J. An improved method for prenatal diagnosis and carrier detection of genetic diseases by analysis of specifically amplified polymorphic sequences: Application to haemophilia A. N Engl J Med. 1987;317:985-90.
25. Levi M, Cate HT. Disseminated intravascular coagulation. N Engl J Med. 1999;341:586-92.
26. Mammen EF. Coagulation defects in liver disease. Med Clin North Am. 1994;78:545-54.
27. Mannucci PM, Tuddenham EGD. The hemophilias—From royal genes to gene therapy. N Engl J Med. 2002; 344:1773-79.
28. McVey JH, Pattinson JK, Tuddenham EGD. Molecular biology in blood coagulation. In: Poller L (Ed). Recent Advances in Blood Coagulation. No. 5. Edinburgh: Churchill Livingstone; 1991.
29. Miyakis S, Lockshin MD, Atsumi T, et al. International consensus statement on an update of the classification criteria for definite antiphospholipid syndrome (APS). J Thromb Haemost. 2006;4:295-306.
30. Morrision AE, Ludlam CA. Acquired haemophilia and its management. Br J Haematol. 1995;89:231-6.
31. Newland AC, Evans TGJR. ABC of clinical haematology: Haematological disorders at the extremes of life. BMJ. 1997;314:1262.
32. Nilsson IM, Lethagen S. von Willebrand's disease. Indian J Pediatr. 1993;60:167-86.
33. Report of a WHO Scientific group: Control of hereditary diseases. WHO Technical Report series. 865. World Health Organization, Geneva. 1996.
34. Rick ME. Diagnosis and management of von Willebrand's syndrome. Med Clin North Am. 1994;78:609-23.
35. Risberg B, Andreasson S, Eriksson E. Disseminated intravascular coagulation. Acta Anaesthesiol Scand. 1991;35 (suppl 95):60-71.

36. Ruggeri ZM, Zimmerman TS. von Willebrand factor and von Willebrand disease. Blood. 1987;70:895-904.
37. Sadler JE. A revised classification of von Willebrand disease. For the Subcommittee on von Willebrand Factor of the Scientific and Standardization Committee of the International Society on Thrombosis and Hemostasis. Thromb Hemost. 1994;71:520-5.
38. Sadler JE, Budde U, Eikenboom JC, et al. Update on the pathophysiology and classification of von Willebrand disease: A report of the Subcommittee on von Willebrand factor. J Thromb Hemost. 2006;4:2103-14.
39. Smock KJ, Rodgers GM. Laboratory identification of lupus anticoagulants. Am J Hematol. 2009;84:440-2.
40. Toh CH, Dennis M. Disseminated intravascular coagulation: Old disease, new hope. BMJ. 2003;327:974-7.
41. Triplett DA. Laboratory diagnosis of von Willebrand's disease. Mayo Clin Proc. 1991;66:832-40.
42. White GC II, Shoemaker CB. Factor VIII gene and hemophilia A. Blood. 1989;73:1-12.

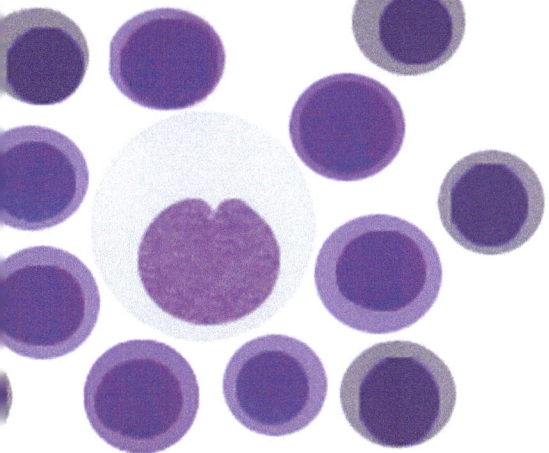

Blood Transfusion

Section Outline

17. Blood Group Systems 497
18. Serologic and Microbiological Techniques 504
19. Collection of Donor Blood, Processing, and Storage 517
20. Whole Blood, Blood Components, and Blood Derivatives 526
21. Transfusion of Blood to the Recipient 536
22. Adverse Effects of Transfusion 541
23. Autologous Transfusion 551
24. Alternatives to Blood Transfusion 554

SECTION 5

CHAPTER 17

Blood Group Systems

International Society of Blood Transfusion (ISBT) Working Party recognizes 36 blood group systems (Table 17.1). Red cell antigens that are produced by alleles (alternative forms of a specified gene) at a single gene locus or very closely linked loci constitute a blood group system.

Blood group genes are inherited in a Mendelian manner and are mostly located on autosomes. Most of the blood group genes are expressed in a codominant manner (i.e. the two allelic forms are expressed equally if inherited in a heterozygous state). The particular alleles at a specified gene locus in an individual constitute the genotype. Phenotype is the outward expression of the genotype.

Table 17.1: Blood group systems (The International Society of Blood Transfusion or ISBT, 2015).

Traditional name	ISBT no.	ISBT symbol	Traditional name	ISBT no.	ISBT symbol
ABO	001	ABO	Kx	019	XK
MNS	002	MNS	Gerbich	020	GE
P1Pk	003	P1	Cromer	021	CROM
Rh	004	RHD, RHCE	Knobs	022	KN
Lutheran	005	LU	Indian	023	IN
Kell	006	KEL	Ok	024	OK
Lewis	007	LE	Raph	025	RAPH
Duffy	008	FY	John Milton Hagen	026	JMH
Kidd	009	JK	I	027	I
Diego	010	DI	Globoside	028	GLOB
Yt	011	YT	GIL	029	GIL
Xg	012	XG	RHAG	030	RHAG
Scianna	013	SC	Forsmann	031	FORS
Dombrock	014	DO	Jr	032	JR
Colton	015	CO	Lan	033	LAN
Landsteiner-Wiener	016	LW	Vel	034	VEL
Chido/Rodgers	017	CH/RG	CD59	035	CD59
Hh	018	H	Augustine	036	AUG

Section 5: Blood Transfusion

In blood transfusion practice, most important blood group systems are ABO and Rh. This is because A, B, and RhD antigens are the most immunogenic (i.e. capable of eliciting a strong antibody response on stimulation) and their alloantibodies can cause destruction of transfused red cells or induce hemolytic disease of newborn (HDN). ABO antigens are also important in organ transplantation.

Next to A and B, other antigens important in transfusion medicine due to their immunogenicity are D, K, C, Fy^a, c, E, k, e, Jk^a, S, and s.

ABO SYSTEM

In ABO system, there are four main types of blood groups—A, B, AB, and O. Identification of these four blood groups is based on presence or absence of A and/or B antigens on red cells. According to Landsteiner's law, anti-A and/or anti-B antibodies are always present in plasma of individuals who lack corresponding antigen(s) on their red cells (Table 17.2). There are two major subgroups of A: A1 (80%) and A2 (20%). Thus, ABO system comprises of six groups. Antigens and antibodies of these groups are—**A1**: Anti-B; **A2**: Anti-B, and in 1–8% cases Anti-A1; **B**: Anti-A; **A1B**: Nil; **A2B**: Anti-A1 in 22–35% cases; **O**: Anti-A, Anti-B. Usually, Anti-A1 antibodies are weak and are of little clinical significance in routine practice.

Antigens of the ABO System

Antigens of the ABO system are A (A1, A2), B, and H. In addition to red cells, they are also expressed on white cells, platelets, and various body tissues. They are also present in a soluble form in various body secretions (in secretors).

ABO antigens are carbohydrate structures on glycoproteins and glycolipids. ABO antigens are poorly expressed at birth, increase gradually in strength and become fully expressed around 1 year of age. In older age, they become slightly weak.

Formation of ABH antigens: The *H* gene (genotype *HH or Hh*) produces a transferase enzyme, which changes precursor substance (present on red cells) into H substance. The A and B genes produce specific transferase enzymes which convert H substance into A and B antigens, respectively. Some amount of H antigen remains unchanged on red cells. The *O* gene produces an inactive transferase so that H antigen persists unchanged on red cells (Fig. 17.1).

The difference between A and B antigens is one sugar molecule. A sugar that makes one antigen different from other is termed as immunodominant sugar.

Table 17.2: ABO blood groups.

Blood group	Approximate Indian frequency	Genotype	Antigen(s) on red cells	Antibody in plasma
A	27%	AA or AO	A	Anti-B
B	31%	BB or BO	B	Anti-A
AB	8%	AB	AB	Nil
O	34%	OO	Nil	Anti-A and anti-B

Note: *A* and *B* genes are dominant while *O* gene is recessive

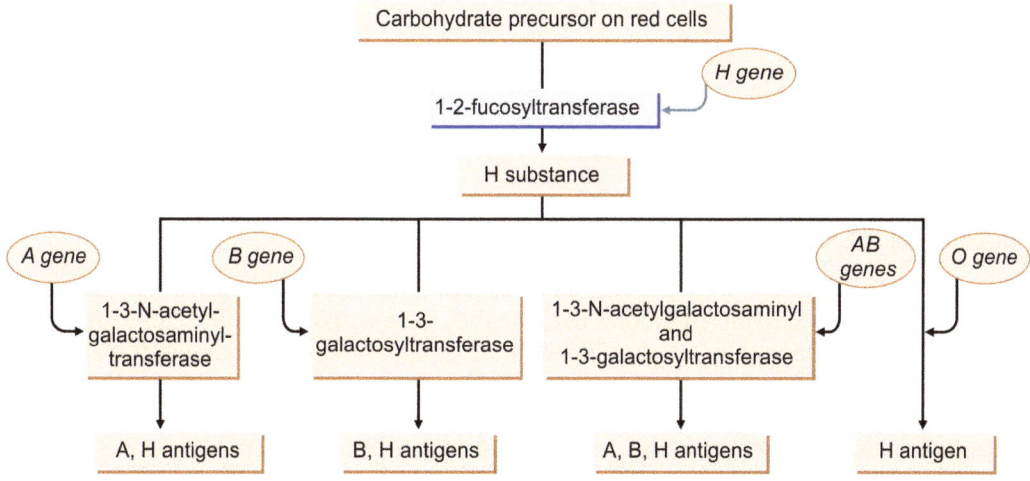

Fig. 17.1: Formation of antigens of the ABO system.

The immunodominant sugars for H, A, and B antigens are as follows:
H antigen: L-fucose
A antigen: N-acetyl-D-galactosamine
B antigen: D-galactose

Some persons do not inherit the *H* gene (genotype *hh*) and thus cannot synthesize H substance. Such persons may inherit the *A* or *B* gene but cannot express it, as they are unable to produce the H substance. Such individuals are said to have Bombay phenotype or Bombay blood group (Oh). Their red cells type as group O; however, unlike group O individuals, Oh persons have no H antigen on their red cells and their plasma contains strong anti-H in addition to anti-A and anti-B. Therefore, Bombay group persons should be transfused only with Oh blood.

Secretors and nonsecretors: Secretors are persons who secrete A, B, and H antigens into body fluids (such as plasma, gastric juice, saliva, sweat, tears, semen, milk, etc.). This ability is dependent on presence of a dominant secretor gene (*Se*). About 80% of individuals are secretors (genotype *Sese* or *SeSe*) and remaining are nonsecretors (genotype *sese*). Both secretors and nonsecretors express ABO antigens on red cells.

Antigens secreted by different ABO blood groups are as follows:
- Group A: A, H
- Group B: B, H
- Group AB: A, B, H
- Group O: H

Antigens secreted in to body fluids are called as ABH substances. Testing for ABH substances in saliva may be helpful when red cell grouping yields uncertain results. Determining secretor status in saliva and semen can be helpful in forensic studies (e.g. semen sample collected from a rape victim revealing a soluble ABH antigen that does not match with the ABO blood group of the accused). *Inhibitor tests* are used to detect the presence of soluble blood group antigens in body secretions. If saliva contains a soluble antigen, and if corresponding antibody is added, the activity of the antibody is neutralized due to binding of antibody to antigen. When red cells carrying the appropriate antigens are subsequently added to the mixture, there will be inhibition of agglutination (i.e. the person is a secretor). If agglutination occurs, then the individual is a nonsecretor.

Example:
   Blood group: B
   Step 1: Saliva + anti-B
   Step 2: Add B cells
   Result: No agglutination
   Interpretation: Secretor

Antibodies of the ABO System

The most important antibodies in transfusion practice are anti-A and anti-B. They are also called as naturally occurring antibodies because they arise without immune stimulation (i.e. transfusion or pregnancy) by relevant blood group antigens. They are not detectable in the blood of newborn infants due to their underdeveloped immune system and appear around 3-6 months of life. It is thought that they are produced in response to A- and B-like antigens of bacteria which are present in the intestine and certain foods. If anti-A and/or anti-B are present at birth, they are of maternal origin (IgG). Anti-A and anti-B antibodies are usually of IgM class. They can efficiently fix the complement. Naturally occurring ABO antibodies can cause the following:
- Hemolytic transfusion reaction in case of ABO—mismatched blood transfusion
- Acute graft rejection in case of ABO—incompatible solid organ transplantation
- Hemolysis of donor red cells following ABO—incompatible bone marrow transplantation.

Less commonly, some individuals have large amounts of ABO antibodies of immune nature. Usually, group O individuals following immune stimulation by transfusion, pregnancy, or injection of certain vaccines or toxoids (that contain bacterial A- and B-like antigens) produce them in large amounts. These antibodies are of IgG class, of high titer, and cannot be neutralized by soluble blood group antigens. If blood of such group O individuals (called dangerous universal group O donors) is transfused to group A or B individuals, serious hemolysis of recipient's red cells can occur. Therefore, group O donors should not be employed as universal donors. (Note: Red cells of group O donors are devoid of A and B antigens and cannot be agglutinated by anti-A and anti-B antibodies. Therefore, group O persons are traditionally considered as universal donors.) In addition to causing hemolytic transfusion reaction, these IgG antibodies can cross the placenta and induce hemolytic disease of newborn.

THE RH SYSTEM

When Rhesus monkey red cells were injected into rabbits and guinea pigs, antibody which was raised, was found to react with Rhesus monkey red cells as well as with 85% of human red cells. The antigen involved was called as Rh factor. Subsequently, it was shown that the original antibody was different from anti-D antibody discovered later. The name of the antigen, however, has remained as Rhesus. According to the recent nomenclature by ISBT, the system has been named as Rh.

The Rh system is only next in importance to ABO system in transfusion practice. The importance of this system lies in the high immunogenicity of RhD antigen which readily induces formation of anti-D antibodies in RhD-negative individuals. Anti-D antibodies can cause hemolytic transfusion reaction or in pregnant women, Rh hemolytic disease of newborn.

Antigens of the Rh System

The important antigens of the Rh system are C, D, E, c, and e. D antigen is the most immunogenic. There are various nomenclature systems for Rh antigens. Fisher-Race or CDE nomenclature system is simpler and is outlined below:

According to Fisher and Race, three closely linked genes are inherited together on one chromosome (haplotype) from each parent. Allelic forms of these genes are *C* and *c*, *D*, and *d*, and *E* and *e* with eight possible haplotypes—*CDe, cde, cDE, cDe, cdE, Cde, CDE,* and *CdE*. As an individual inherits one haplotype from each parent, 36 genotypes are possible, such as Cde/cde, Cde/cDe, CDE/cde, etc. The presence of D in either homozygous (D/D) or heterozygous (D/d) state makes that individual **Rh-positive**, while **Rh-negative** persons are homozygous for d(d/d). It was thought that d gene was an amorph. Results of current genetic studies are consistent with Fisher-Race theory. It has been found that the *RH* locus is located on chromosome 1 and consists of two closely linked genes—*RHD* and *RHCE*. The alleles of *RHCE* are *CE, Ce, ce,* and *cE* (Fig. 17.2). In Rh-negative persons, deletions, point mutations, or partial mutations of D gene have been found. Rh antigens are expressed only on red cells and not on any other tissues. They are also not secreted in body fluids. In contrast to ABO antigens, Rh antigens are fully expressed on red cells before birth and also on red cells of early fetuses.

Depending on the presence or absence of antigen D on red cells, a person is grouped either as Rh-positive (when red cells express antigen D) or Rh-negative (when D antigen is absent on red cells). Frequency of D antigen varies in different populations. **In India, approximately 95% of the people express D antigen on their red cells (RhD-positive), while 5% are Rh D-negative.** Other forms of D antigen are weak D and partial D. Red cells having **weak D antigen** were formerly called as D^u cells, which react weakly with anti-D reagent. There is a quantitative reduction in the number of D antigen sites on such red cells. D^u recipients do not make anti-D antibodies following stimulation by D antigen (e.g. following D+ve blood transfusion). D^u donors should be considered as Rh-positive and their blood should not be transfused to Rh-negative donors. In red cells having **partial D antigen,** parts of D antigen are missing. Variants

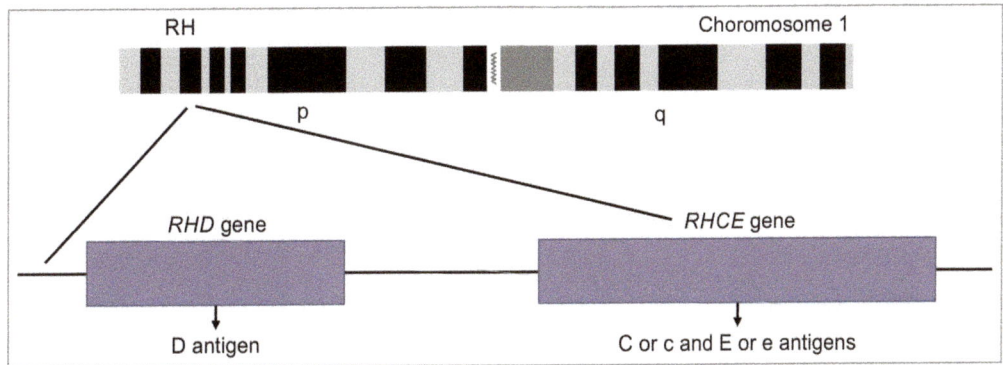

Fig. 17.2: Genes of the Rh system. There are two genes of the Rh system: *RHD* gene that codes for D antigen and *RHCE* gene that codes for C or c and E or e antigens (giving rise to CE, Ce, cE, and ce antigen combinations). Presence of *RHD* gene confers RhD positive phenotype, while its absence RhD negative phenotype.

of partial D antigen exist. Individuals with D^{VI} variant are able to produce anti-D antibody against the missing part of the antigen if exposed to D+ve antigen. Such recipients should be considered as Rh-negative, while donors should be regarded as Rh-positive. However, in practice, individuals with partial D antigen are typed as D negative and are identified only after they have produced anti-D antibodies.

Complete absence of all Rh antigens on red cells (Rh null cells) is associated with stomatocytosis (red cells have a slit-like area of central pallor, reminiscent of mouth) and compensated hemolysis.

Rh Antibodies

In general, most Rh antibodies are of immune type, i.e. they are the result of immunization by blood transfusion or pregnancy. Most of these antibodies are of IgG class. Comparison of ABO and RhD groups is given in Table 17.3.

In practice, Rh antibodies can cause hemolytic transfusion reaction or hemolytic disease of newborn. Since Rh antibodies do not activate complement, hemolysis is extravascular and predominantly occurs in spleen. Due to high immunogenicity of D antigen, Rh-negative persons (especially women of childbearing age) should be transfused only with Rh-negative blood. During pregnancy, IgG anti-D can cross the placenta and induce hemolytic disease of newborn by causing immune hemolysis of fetal red cells. Rh hemolytic disease of newborn can be prevented by prophylactic administration of Rh immune globulin to all Rh-negative women during mid pregnancy and within 72 hours of delivery. Anti-D and anti-c can cause severe HDN. Anti-C, anti-E, and anti-e usually do not cause HDN or cause mild HDN.

Table 17.3: Comparison of ABO and RhD groups.

Parameter	ABO group	RhD group
1. Location of gene	Chromosome 9	Chromosome 1
2. Antigens	A, B, AB	D
3. Distribution of antigens	Red cells, platelets, many tissues, body fluids	Red cells only
4. Development of antigens	Weak expression at birth	Fully developed at birth
5. Dosage effect*	No	Present
6. Nature of antibodies	Naturally occurring	Immune
7. Antibody class	IgM	IgG
8. Whether antibodies fix complement	Yes	No
9. Optimal reaction temperature of antibody	4°C	37°C
10. Optimal reaction medium	Saline	Antihuman globulin

* Dosage effect: A situation where antibody reacts more strongly with red cells having double the dose of antigen (due to homozygous state) than those having single dose (heterozygous state).

BIBLIOGRAPHY

1. Contreras M, Lubenko A. Antigens in human blood. In Hoffbrand AV and Lewis SM (Eds). Postgraduate Haematology, 3rd edition. London: Heinemann Professional Publishing Ltd.; 1989.
2. Kelton JG, Heddle NM, Blajchman MA. Blood transfusion—A conceptual approach. New York: Churchill Livingstone; 1984.
3. Knowles SM. Blood cell antigens and antibodies: erythrocytes, platelets and granulocytes. In: Lewis SM, Bain BJ, Bates I (Eds). Dacie and Lewis Practical Haematology, 9th edition. London: Churchill Livingstone; 2001.
4. World Health Organization. (2009). World Health Organization: Safe blood and blood products. Module 3. Blood group serology.

CHAPTER 18

Serologic and Microbiological Techniques

SEROLOGIC TECHNIQUES

ABO Grouping

In transfusion practice, test for ABO grouping is essential because of the consistent occurrence of hemolytic, naturally occurring antibodies in plasma of persons lacking the corresponding antigen on red cells (Box 18.1). There are two methods for ABO grouping—cell grouping (forward grouping) and serum grouping (backward or reverse grouping). Both cell and serum grouping should be done since each test acts as a check on the other thus reducing the risk of error in grouping. In cell grouping, red cells are tested for the presence of A and B antigens employing known specific anti-A and anti-B sera. In serum grouping, serum is tested for the presence of anti-A and anti-B antibodies by employing known group A and group B reagent red cells. Serum grouping should not be carried out in infants below 4 months since infants start producing anti-A and anti-B antibodies by 4 to 6 months of age. Elderly persons may also have depressed antibody levels. In both these cases, ABO grouping is reliably performed by cell grouping method.

There are five methods for blood grouping: Slide, tube, microplate, column agglutination or gel technology, and solid phase adherence technology.

Box 18.1: Blood grouping.
- Routinely ABO and Rh grouping are done
- Importance of ABO grouping: Consistent presence of hemolytic, naturally occurring reciprocal antibodies in the plasma of all individuals lacking the corresponding antigen on red cells
- Importance of Rh grouping: RhD antigen is highly immunogenic (next to A and B antigens) and induces formation of anti-D antibodies in persons lacking D antigen. Immune anti-D antibodies (IgG) can cause hemolytic transfusion reaction and hemolytic disease of newborn.

Slide Test (Forward Grouping or Cell Grouping)

Principle: Red cells from the specimen are tested for A and/or B antigens by using known reagent antisera (anti-A and anti-B). Agglutination of red cells indicates presence of corresponding antigen on red cells.

Specimen: Specimen may be either capillary blood from finger prick or venous blood collected in EDTA anticoagulant.

Reagents:
Antisera: Antisera are used to detect antigens on red cells. Previously, polyclonal anti-A, anti-B, and anti-AB sera obtained from humans were used for cell grouping. (Polyclonal antiserum contains many different antibodies directed against different epitopes of an antigen and are produced by different clones of plasma cells). These now have been replaced by anti-A and anti-B monoclonal antisera. (Monoclonal antiserum contains specific antibodies against a specific antigenic epitope and is produced by a single clone of plasma cells). Polyclonal antisera are obtained from human donors immunized with soluble antigens. Monoclonal antibodies are obtained by hybridoma technology. (Specific antibodies producing mouse B-lymphocytes from immunized mice are artificially fused with mouse myeloma cells which are able to grow indefinitely in culture. The resulting hybrid cell, called hybridoma, is cloned and cultured to get large amounts of monoclonal antibodies). Monoclonal antisera are specific, avid, sensitive, and can detect weak antigens. Anti-A is color-coded blue and anti-B is color-coded yellow. A third antiserum called anti-A, B is also used in some blood banks (especially for grouping in newborns and to resolve ABO discrepancies); anti-A, B is colorless. Antisera also contain a preservative (0.1% sodium azide) to prevent growth of bacteria. They are stored at 2–8°C. Monoclonal antisera are free from infectious agents like HIV, HBV, or HCV, unlike sera obtained from humans. If monoclonal antisera are being used, third antiserum anti-AB is not required.

Method:
1. Divide a clean and dry glass slide into two sections with a glass marking pencil. Label the sections as anti-A and anti-B (Fig. 18.1).
2. Place one drop of anti-A and one drop of anti-B antiserum in the center of the corresponding section of the slide.
3. Add one drop of blood sample to be tested to each drop of antiserum.
4. Mix antiserum and blood by using a separate stick for each section.
5. By tilting the slide from side to side, observe for agglutination after exactly 2 minutes.

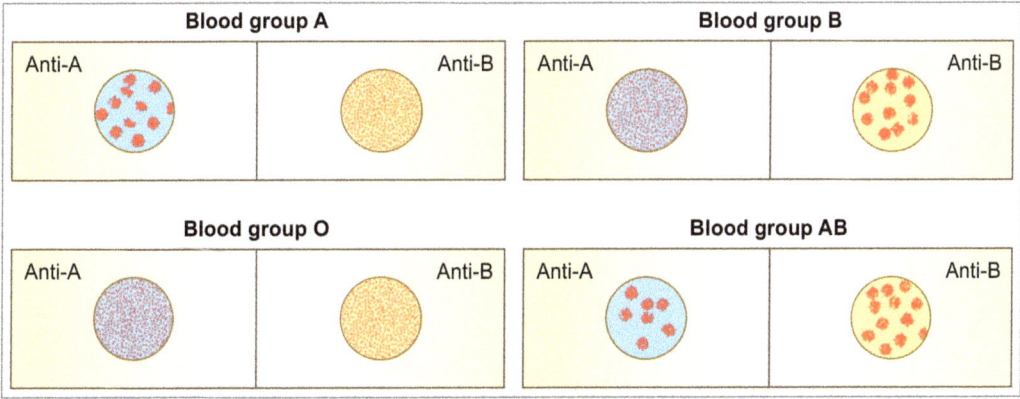

Fig. 18.1: ABO blood grouping by slide method.

Table 18.1: Interpretation of cell grouping by slide test.

Anti-A	Anti-B	Blood group
+	−	A
−	+	B
+	+	AB
−	−	O

6. Result:
   Positive (+): Small clumps of red cells are seen floating in a clear liquid.
   Negative (−): Uniform suspension of red cells.
7. Interpretation: Interpret the result as shown in Table 18.1.

Note: Slide test is rapid and simple. In practice, it is used: (1) As a preliminary grouping test before blood donation, (2) In blood donation camps, and (3) In case of an emergency. Results of slide test should always be confirmed by cell and serum grouping by tube method.

Weakly reactive antigens (like A1) may be missed by slide method. Slide test is also not suitable for serum grouping. Drying of the antiserum-blood mixture around the edges can be misinterpreted as agglutination. If the result is read before 2 minutes, weak antigens may be missed.

Tube Method

For cell grouping, known antiserum and patient's red cells are mixed in a test tube, incubated at room temperature for 5 minutes, and then centrifuged. In **serum or reverse grouping**, serum from the patient and reagent red cells of known group (available commercially or prepared in the laboratory) are used. Following centrifugation, a red cell button (sediment) will be seen at the bottom of the tube. Cell button is resuspended by gently tapping the base of the tube.
   Positive (+) test: Clumps of red cells suspended in a clear fluid.
   Negative (−) test: Uniform suspension of red cells (Fig. 18.2).

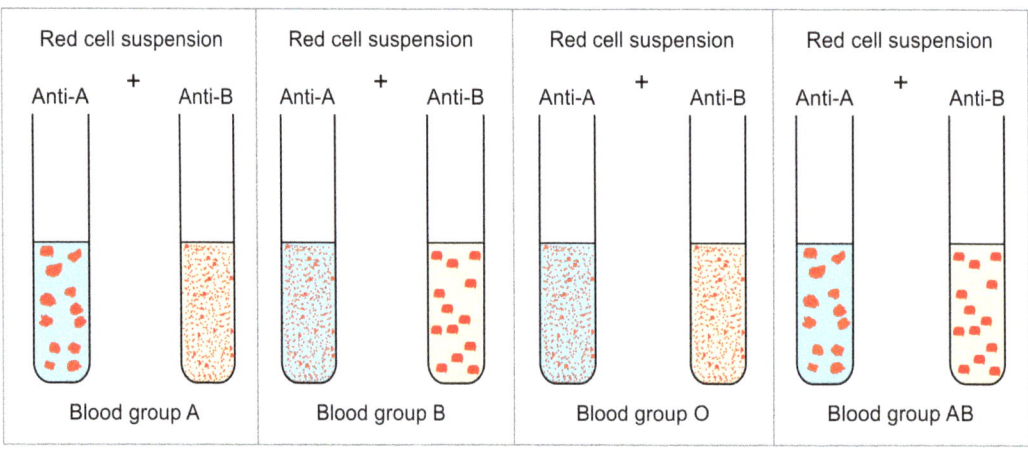

Fig. 18.2: ABO grouping by tube method.

Separate tubes of autocontrol, positive control, and negative control should always be set up along with the test sample tube.

Autocontrol is necessary to rule out autoagglutination of patient's red cells which occurs when autoantibodies are present in patient's serum. In autocontrol tube, patient's red cells are mixed with patient's own serum and the tube is centrifuged; if agglutination occurs, it is autoantibody-induced. Autocontrol test is particularly essential when ABO grouping is being done only by forward method and blood group is typed as AB.

In two positive control tubes, anti-A serum is mixed with group A red cells and anti-B is mixed with group B red cells, respectively. In two negative control tubes, anti-A serum is mixed with group B red cells and anti-B serum is mixed with group A red cells, respectively. These controls are necessary to confirm that reagents are working properly.

Test tube method of blood grouping is more reliable than slide method. This is because centrifugation brings antigen and antibodies closer together and allows detection of weaker antigen-antibody reactions.

Microplate method: This technique is commonly used in many blood bank laboratories. A microwell plate consists of 96 small wells (U- or V- or flat-bottom) (Fig. 18.3). U-type is preferable since results are easier to read. Microplate method is more cost-effective since far less antisera is required as compared to the test tube method; also multiple samples can be tested at the same time because of 96 wells.

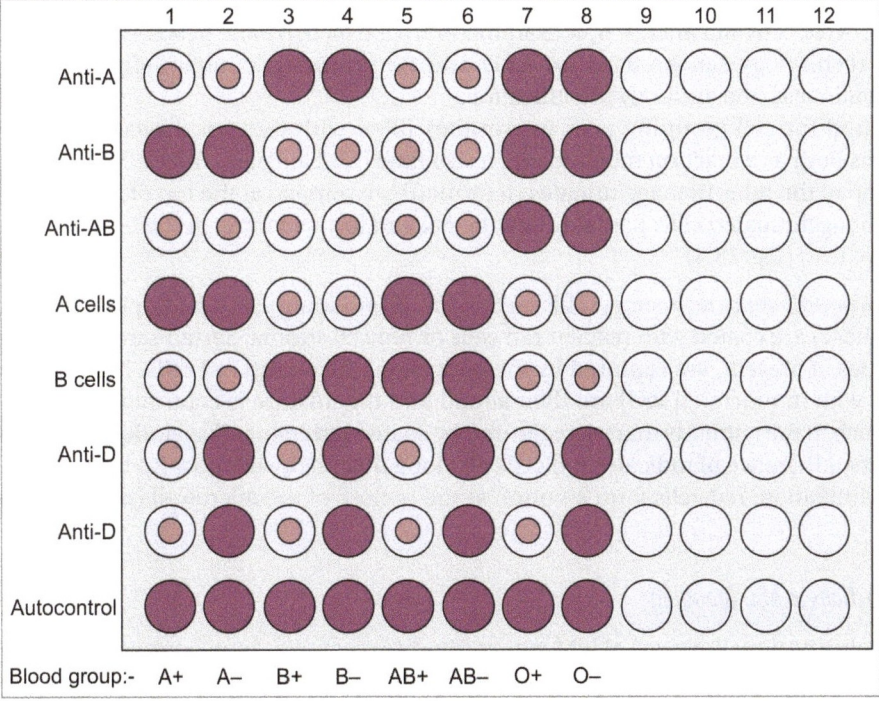

Fig. 18.3: Microplate (96 well) method for blood grouping. Numbers 1 to 12 represent patient identification numbers. Reagents added to the patient sample are written on left, while interpretation (blood group of patient) is written at the bottom. Red compact button indicates agglutination, while uniform suspension indicates no agglutination.

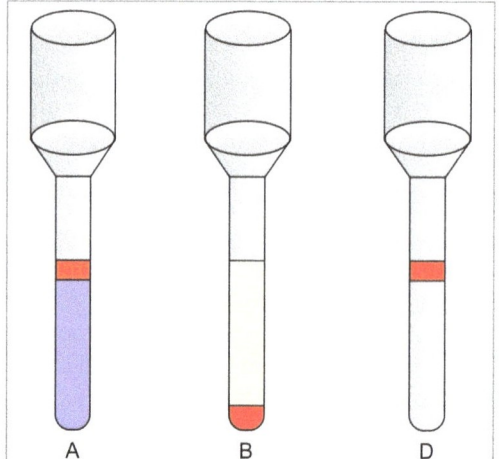

Fig. 18.4: Gel or column agglutination technology for ABO and RhD grouping. If cells settle at the bottom it indicates a negative result and if cells remain at the top of the column it indicates positive result. The above example shows positive reaction with anti-A (blue) and anti-D, and a negative reaction with anti-B (yellow). The group is A RhD+ve.

Column agglutination or gel technology: This method is easy, accurate, standardized, needs small sample volume, and reduces exposure to biohazardous samples. It does not require washing of red cells and microscopic examination. It is expensive and needs a special centrifuge.

Gel technology can be used for ABO and Rh grouping, compatibility testing, direct antiglobulin test, and antibody identification.

Method for cell grouping uses microtubes filled with dextran acrylamide gel (which functions both as a reaction medium and a size filter) and antisera. After addition of red cells to the top of the tube, hemagglutinates (if formed) are trapped at the top of the tube (positive test). Nonagglutinated cells pass through the gel and form a button at the bottom of the tube (negative test) (Fig. 18.4).

Solid phase adherence technology: This method of cell grouping uses a microplate in which wells (solid phase) are coated with reagent red cells or red cell stroma. Serum sample is added and antibodies, if present, are captured by the antigen on the coated red cells. Indicator red cells (coated with monoclonal IgG) are then added and the mixture is centrifuged. Indicator red cells attach to the antibody that was captured by coated red cells and agglutination is indicated by diffuse adherence of indicator red cells all along the microwell (positive test). If there is no hemagglutination, red cells form a button at the bottom of the microwell (negative test) (Fig. 18.5).

False Reactions in ABO Grouping

Autoagglutination: Presence of IgM autoantibodies reactive at room temperature in patient's serum can lead to autoagglutination. If autocontrol is not used, blood group in such a case will be wrongly typed as AB. Therefore, for correct result, if autocontrol is also showing agglutination, cell grouping should be repeated after washing red cells with warm saline (to remove autoantibodies), and serum grouping should be repeated at 37°C.

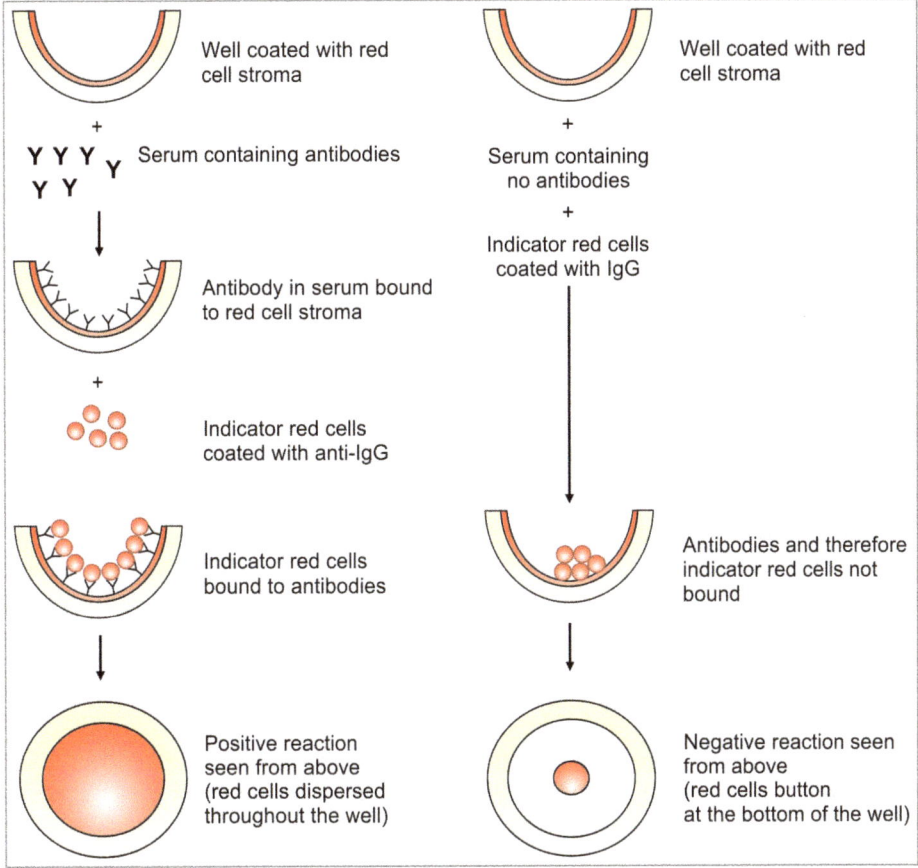

Fig. 18.5: Principle of solid phase adherence test for blood grouping.

Rouleaux formation: In rouleaux formation, red cells adhere to each other like a stack of coins. Rouleaux formation may be due to high levels of paraproteins in blood or intravenous administration of dextran. Rouleaux can be mistaken for agglutination during blood grouping test. Rouleaux formation is noted during serum grouping or if unwashed red cells are used for cell grouping. Rouleaux, but not agglutination, disappear on addition of normal saline.

False negative result due to inactivated antisera: Use of inactivated antisera or deterioration of reagent red cells will cause false negative result in ABO grouping. Antisera are inactivated if they are left at room temperature for long and are not kept stored at proper temperature.

Unexpected Results in Blood Grouping

Problems with cell grouping:
1. *Acquired B antigen:* Microbial enzyme D-acetylase can modify A antigen on red cells so that it resembles the terminal sugar (galactose) of B antigen. This is seen in Gram-negative septicemia, carcinoma of colon/rectum, and intestinal obstruction.

2. *Chimerism:* A blood sample containing more than one population of red cells can result from (i) transfusion of ABO-compatible but not ABO-identical blood, (ii) bone marrow transplantation (when blood group of donor is different from that of recipient), and (iii) fetomaternal hemorrhage.
3. *Polyagglutinable red cells:* Polyagglutination (agglutination of red cells by almost all normal adult human sera) results when certain antigens (like T or Tk) are exposed on red cells following action by some microorganisms. The cells return to normal following clearance of infection.
4. *Coating of red cells by Wharton's jelly of umbilical cord:* This can cause nonspecific agglutination of red cells if blood sample is collected from umbilical cord of the newborn.
5. *Weakening or loss of red cell antigens:* This can occur in malignancies like leukemia and some solid cancers giving rise to a false negative result.
6. *Excessive amounts of blood group substances:* Certain cancers are associated with excessive amounts of blood group substances in plasma; this can inhibit anti-A and anti-B sera causing a weak or negative result.
7. *ABO subgroups:* Anti-A1 is produced by a small proportion of patients with A2 and A2B group; this antibody agglutinates A1 and A1B red cells but not A2 and A2B cells.

Problems with serum grouping:
1. *Lack of expected antibodies:* This occurs in immunosuppression, hypogammaglobulinemia, neonates, and elderly.
2. *Unexpected antibodies* are observed in cold-reacting auto- or alloantibodies, paraproteinemia, and following transfusion of plasma components.

Causes of unexpected results in ABO grouping are listed in Table 18.2.

Table 18.2: Causes of unexpected results in blood grouping.

Unexpected positive	Unexpected negative
Cell grouping	
Acquired B antigen (gastric or colonic cancer, intestinal obstruction)	ABO subgroup
Bone marrow transplantation	Antigen suppression in leukemia or cancer
Out-of-group transfusion	High levels of soluble blood group substances
Fetomaternal hemorrhage	
Coating of red cells by Wharton's jelly of umbilical cord	Improperly stored antisera
Polyagglutinable red cells	
Serum grouping	
Cold-reacting agglutinins	Newborns and elderly
Monoclonal immunoglobulins	ABO subgroup
Transfusion of plasma components	Hypogammaglobulinemia
	Immunosuppression

RhD Grouping

Out of the various antigens of the Rh system, D antigen is the most immunogenic and therefore, red cells are routinely tested for D. Individuals with D antigen on their red cells are called as Rh-positive, while those without D antigen are called as Rh-negative. If Rh-negative individuals are transfused with Rh-positive blood, 90% of them will produce anti-D antibodies. In such sensitized individuals, re-exposure to D antigen can cause hemolytic transfusion reaction or, in pregnant women, hemolytic disease of newborn. Rh grouping is especially important in young girls and in women of reproductive age group due to the risk of Rh hemolytic disease of newborn.

RhD grouping is done only by forward or cell grouping method. Serum or reverse grouping is not carried out because of the absence of anti-D in majority of Rh-negative persons. Anti-D antibodies are not naturally occurring and develop only after exposure to RhD-positive red cells following transfusion or pregnancy.

Method of RhD grouping is similar in principle to ABO grouping. Since serum or reverse grouping is not possible, each sample is tested in duplicate in blood banks. Autocontrol (patient's red cells + patient's serum) and positive and negative controls are included in every test run. With polyclonal antisera, if anti-D testing is negative, further testing for weak D should be performed. Positive reaction with either labels the unit as RhD-positive. Blood units negative with both D and weak D are labeled as Rh-negative. Monoclonal IgM anti-D antiserum should be used for cell grouping, which allows Rh grouping to be carried out at the same time as ABO grouping at room temperature. With monoclonal antisera, most weak forms of D antigen are detected and further testing for weak forms of D antigen (D^u) is not required.

Compatibility Test (Cross-Match)

Compatibility testing refers to a set of procedures that are carried out before issuing blood for transfusion to the patient and consists of:
1. Checking of patient's blood request form and blood bank records for reason for transfusion, history of previous transfusions, result of previous blood grouping test, any clinically significant antibodies detected, and significant adverse effects to transfusion.
2. Performing ABO and Rh grouping of patient's blood sample and checking against previous results.
3. Antibody screening and identification.
4. Confirmation of ABO and Rh blood group of donor unit.
5. Crossmatching: This is the final serologic compatibility test. This consists of testing patient' serum against donor red cells to detect any antibodies in patient reacting with donor red cells (major cross-match) and testing patient's red cells against donor serum to detect any donor antibodies reacting with patient's red cells (minor cross-match). Donor blood is considered to be compatible if there is no agglutination or hemolysis in major or minor cross match.

   Crosmatching is performed to:
   - Confirm compatibility between ABO blood groups of the donor and the recipient, and
   - Detect any irregular antibodies present in recipient's serum reactive against donor red cells. (Those antibodies other than anti-A and anti-B are called as irregular or unexpected antibodies. They are capable of destroying transfused red cells carrying

> **Box 18.2:** Tests for crossmatching.
> - Saline test at room temperature and 37°C: For detection of clinically significant IgM antibodies
> - Indirect antiglobulin test (IAT) at 37°C, low ionic strength solution test at 37°C, or enzyme-treated red cell test at 37°C: For detection of clinically significant IgG antibodies
>
> **Note:**
> (1) If agglutination or hemolysis is not observed in any of the above stages, donor unit is considered to be compatible with recipient's serum. Agglutination or hemolysis at any stage is indicative of incompatibility.
> (2) The commonly used major cross match test is a saline test at 37°C followed by conversion to IAT at 37°C.

the relevant antigen [like D, C, c, E, e, K, k, Fya, Fyb]. They may be naturally occurring or immune).

The name "cross-match" originated from the past practice of testing the recipient's serum against donor's red cells (major cross-match) and donor's serum against recipient's red cells (minor cross match). However, minor cross-match is considered as less important since antibodies in donor blood unit get diluted or neutralized in recipient's plasma. Also, if antibody screening and identification is being carried out, minor cross matching is not essential.

6. Labeling of blood product with identifying information of the recipient and compatibility test result.

Tests for crossmatching are listed in Box 18.2.

The aim of compatibility testing is to prevent hemolytic transfusion reaction in the recipient. Before compatibility testing, ABO and Rh groups of the recipient are determined and group-compatible donor blood is selected. (In well-equipped blood banks, antibody screening of donor and recipient's blood is also carried out before cross matching to detect unexpected or irregular antibodies).

A single tube cross match consisting of three stages is recommended. Recipient's serum is tested against donor's red cells under three different conditions; agglutination or hemolysis in any one of the three stages indicates incompatibility. The three stages of compatibility test are as follows:

1. Compatibility test at room temperature
2. Compatibility test at 37° C
3. Indirect antiglobulin test

Compatibility test at room temperature (Immediate spin cross-match): The purpose of this test is to detect ABO incompatibility. Saline-suspended red cells of the donor and recipient's serum are mixed in a test tube, incubated briefly at room temperature, and centrifuged. Agglutination or hemolysis indicates incompatibility. If agglutination or hemolysis is absent, next step is performed.

Compatibility test at 37°C: The above test tube is incubated at 37° C for 20 minutes, centrifuged again, and examined for agglutination. If absent, perform the last stage.

Indirect antiglobulin test: The above mixture is incubated at 37°C for 30 to 60 minutes, washed in saline, and antiglobulin reagent is added. Following re-centrifugation, examine for agglutination or hemolysis. This test detects most of the clinically significant IgG antibodies. Principle of antiglobulin test has been described earlier in chapter on "Immune hemolytic anemias".

If agglutination or hemolysis is not observed in any of the above stages, donor unit is considered to be compatible with recipient's serum. Agglutination or hemolysis at any stage is indicative of incompatibility.

False Reactions in Compatibility Testing

1. Autoagglutination: If autoantibodies are present in the recipient's serum, they can cause agglutination of recipient's own red cells as well as red cells of all donors. Autoantibodies are usually cold-reacting, and therefore, agglutination will be observed in saline stage at room temperature. To distinguish whether agglutination is due to auto- or alloantibodies, an autocontrol test is usually set up simultaneously. If autoantibodies are present, agglutination will also be observed in autocontrol. If agglutination disappears by keeping the tube at 37°C for 10 minutes, presence of cold agglutinins is confirmed.
2. Rouleaux formation: Rouleaux may be mistaken for agglutination. Rouleaux have a characteristic "stack of coins" appearance when seen under the microscope. Rouleaux (seen in multiple myeloma and after administration of dextran) disappear after addition of a drop of saline to the slide.

Limitations of Cross-Match

Crossmatching will not prevent sensitization of recipient to new red cell antigens. This is because only those red cell antigens are detected for which corresponding antibodies are present in the recipient's serum. Also, all ABO and Rh grouping errors will not be detected.

Emergency Cross-Match

If blood is required urgently, ABO and Rh grouping are carried out by rapid slide test and immediate spin cross match (saline test) is performed (to exclude ABO incompatibility). If the blood unit is compatible, then after issuing it, remaining stages of the cross match are completed. If any incompatibility is detected in these two tests, the concerned physician is immediately notified and transfusion is discontinued.

Antibody Screening and Identification

Screening for unexpected or irregular antibodies is carried out before transfusion in recipient's serum and in donor's blood (and during antenatal period in women). Sera of majority of recipients do not contain unexpected antibodies and are compatible with donor blood of same ABO and Rh type. Only about 1–3% of recipients demonstrate irregular antibodies for whom selection of blood lacking the corresponding red cell antigen is essential.

Antenatal patients should be screened for antibodies apart from anti-D which can cause hemolytic disease of newborn (e.g. anti-c, anti-Kell, etc.). For antibody screening, serum of the recipient is tested against a set of three group O screening red cells of known antigenic type. Agglutination or hemolysis indicates presence of antibody reactive against red cell antigen.

MICROBIOLOGIC TECHNIQUES

Microbiological agents that can be transmitted through transfusion are listed in Table 18.2. Donor blood should be screened for those pathogenic organisms that are frequent in a

particular geographic region and which are transmissible by transfusion. In India, currently, it is mandatory to screen donor blood for following organisms:
- Hepatitis B virus (HBV)
- Hepatitis C virus (HCV)
- Human immunodeficiency virus types 1 and 2
- Syphilis
- Malaria

Hepatitis B Virus

Blood samples from all donations are routinely tested for hepatitis B surface antigen (HbsAg). This antigen was previously called as "Australia antigen" because it was first detected in the serum of an Australian aborigine. Screening of all blood donations for HbsAg has greatly reduced the risk of transmission of HBV through transfusion; the risk, however, is not completely eliminated. HbsAg-negative donor may transmit HBV when blood is collected in early incubation period or when very low levels of HbsAg, not detectable by presently employed methods, are present. This possibility, however, is very small.

An individual who has received HBV vaccine will have hepatitis B surface antibody but not HBsAg in blood.

Tests for screening donor blood for HbsAg are:
- Reverse passive hemagglutination assay (RPHA)
- Enzyme-linked immunosorbent assay (ELISA)
- Radioimmunoassay (RIA)

Commercial test kits for detection of HbsAg are available and the exact test procedure is provided with each kit. General principles of these tests are outlined below.

Reverse passive hemagglutination assay: In RPHA, red cells that are coated with anti-HBs antibody are mixed with donor's serum. If HbsAg is present in the serum, it will bind to the red cells and induce agglutination. Lack of agglutination indicates negative test. The test is called as "reverse" agglutination because antibody, and not antigen is coated onto the red cells. The test is called as "passive" because the anti-HbsAg antibody coated onto the red cells is not an intrinsic component of the red cells and is coated onto the red cells artificially. The test is performed in U- or V-shaped wells of a microtiter plate.

Enzyme-linked immunosorbent assay: Serum sample to be tested is added to a well of the microtiter plate (which has been coated with anti-HbsAg antibody). A microtiter plate, wells of which have been precoated with anti-HBs is called as solid phase support system. This is followed by a period of incubation (specified by the manufacturer) during which binding of antigen from serum (if present) and antibody (attached to the well) occurs. Washing of the solid phase removes the unbound antigen but not the antigen bound to the antibody on the surface of the well. This is followed by the addition of an enzyme-linked anti-HBs antibody (called as conjugate) which will combine with the bound antigen. After further incubation, a second wash is given to remove any unbound conjugate. A chromogenic substrate (for the enzyme) is then added and the mixture is incubated in the dark. If enzyme is present (bound to the antigen), then its action on the substrate will lead to the color development. A stopping solution (an acid) is added to prevent any further reaction between the enzyme and substrate. The result is read in a spectrophotometer at the specified wavelength. The cut-off value is obtained from the absorbance of negative-and low positive controls [negative control + (low positive control × 0.2)]. If the absorbance of test sample is greater than the cut-off value, the sample is considered as positive for HbsAg.

Radioimmunoassay: In principle, RIA is similar to ELISA. Serum samples to be tested are added to the wells of the microplate which have been coated with anti-HBs antibody. If HbsAg is present in the test serum, it will bind to the coated antibody. This is followed by addition of radioactive iodine (I^{125})-linked anti-HBs antibody. A gamma counter measures the amount of bound radiolabeled anti-HBs. The mean for negative controls is also calculated. If the value of the test sample exceeds that of mean for negative controls, the sample is positive for HbsAg.

Hepatitis C Virus

Amount of HCV antigen released in bloodstream is small and cannot be detected readily. Therefore, screening of donor blood for HCV infection relies on detection of anti-HCV antibody in serum (which becomes detectable after 6–8 weeks of infection).

ELISA test for anti-HCV antibody is available from various commercial manufacturers. Sensitivity and specificity of these tests are variable. The earlier tests (first-generation ELISAs) used recombinant proteins complementary to the NS4 region of the HCV genome. Second-generation ELISAs incorporated recombinant or synthetic antigens from NS4 as well as NS3 regions of the genome resulting in improvement in sensitivity and specificity over first-generation tests. The third-generation ELISAs, in addition to NS3 and NS4, also include antigens from NS5 region.

ELISA test for detection of antibody to HCV is expensive. It can detect about 95% of chronic infections and 50–70% of acute infections. False positive reactions are also known to occur. In clinical practice (but not in transfusion practice), a positive ELISA screening test for HCV needs to be confirmed by a recombinant immunoblot assay (RIBA) or by polymerase chain reaction.

Human Immunodeficiency Virus (HIV)

All blood units are routinely tested for antibodies against HIV-1 and HIV-2. Although many tests are available for detection of anti-HIV antibodies, ELISA test is usually employed for screening of blood donors.

Enzyme-linked Immunosorbent Assay (ELISA)

In antiglobulin or indirect ELISA, serum to be tested is added to microwells of a microtiter plate which have been coated with HIV antigens. If anti-HIV antibodies are present in the test serum, they will bind to antigens. After washing which removes unbound material, antihuman globulin antibody coupled to an enzyme is added which attaches to HIV antibodies. An appropriate enzyme substrate is added which gives a color reaction. The intensity of color developed is read in a spectrophotometer (Fig. 18.6).

Nucleic Acid Testing (NAT)

Nucleic acid testing is rapidly becoming a standard method for detection of pathogens before the appearance of antibodies. It narrows the window period (during which patient is infected but antibodies have not yet appeared) thereby increasing the blood safety. It has been reported that with NAT, window for HIV has been shortened to 11 days as compared to 22 days with antibody testing, and window for HCV has been shortened to 10 days from 82 days as compared to antibody testing. In this technique, nucleic acid is extracted from donor plasma, amplified, and the viral genetic sequence is identified. Very low amounts of viral copies can be detected

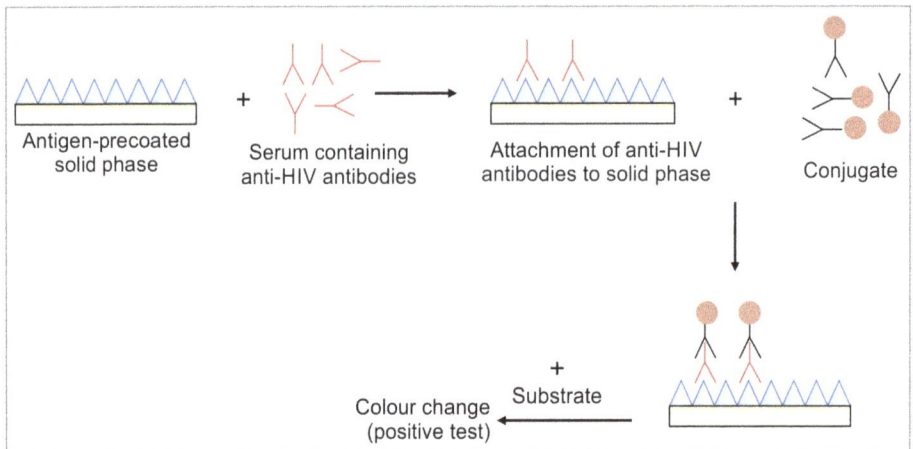

Fig. 18.6: Principle of ELISA test for HIV.

before the appearance of antibodies. NAT can detect HIV RNA, HCV RNA, West Nile Virus RNA, and HBV DNA.

HIV NAT testing can be done by 2 methods: (1) polymerase chain reaction, and (2) transcription-mediated amplification. HIV NAT testing is expensive and is initially done on pools of 16-24 donor samples (minipool NAT); if a particular pool is positive, individual donor NAT is carried out from the pool to identify the donor sample(s) causing the positive NAT result. After the advent of NAT testing, test for p24 antigen of HIV was discontinued as it no longer provided added advantage in reducing the risk of transfusion transmission of HIV.

The window periods for HIV and HCV according to the screening tests are as follows:
- HIV: Enzyme immunoassay 21 days, Minipool NAT 9 days
- HCV: Enzyme immunoassay 51-58 days, Minipool NAT 7 days.

Syphilis

Screening of donor blood for antibody to *Treponema pallidum* is usually carried out by venereal disease research laboratory (VDRL) test. In this nonspecific test, donor serum (which has been heated to 56°C to inactivate the complement) is mixed with cardiolipin-lecithin-cholesterol antigen. If flocculation is observed, the test is reported as reactive.

Malaria Parasite

Sensitivity of blood smear for detection of malaria parasite is low. At least 100 parasites/μL of blood should be present for them to be detected on the blood smear.

BIBLIOGRAPHY

1. Cheesbrough M. District Laboratory practice in Tropical Countries. Part 2. Cambridge:Cambridge University Press; 2000.
2. World Health Organization. (2003). Manual of Basic Techniques for a Health Laboratory. 2nd Edition.

CHAPTER 19

Collection of Donor Blood, Processing, and Storage

Collection of blood is a process whereby one unit (350 mL) of whole blood is collected from a suitable donor in an anticoagulant solution. Since all blood components and blood products are obtained from donor blood, safe transfusion practice begins with the proper selection of blood donors.

Risk of transmission of infectious diseases through transfusion depends on incidence and prevalence of infections in the blood donor population, effectiveness of donor selection process, and use of sensitive screening tests for infectious diseases.

A national comprehensive blood transfusion policy and a voluntary blood donation program, should be implemented, which will serve as a foundation for safe blood supply. Blood donation should be entirely voluntary and nonremunerated.

TYPES OF BLOOD DONORS

There are three main types of blood donors:
1. Voluntary
2. Professional
3. Replacement

A voluntary blood donor donates blood out of his/her own free will and does not expect to receive any financial or other reward as an alternative to money. Voluntary donors donate blood on humanitarian grounds or out of sense of duty or responsibility toward community. Voluntary donors have lower incidence and prevalence of infections transmissible by transfusion as compared to paid or replacement donors. Since there is no monetary gain, they are not likely to hide any significant information or high-risk behavior through which they might have been infected with transmissible microorganisms. Voluntary donors often donate blood on regular basis, which helps in maintaining adequate blood supply. Voluntary blood donors are also more likely to come forward in response to an appeal for blood donation in an emergency.

Paid or professional donors donate blood for financial gain or other benefit that can be substituted for money. They donate blood solely for money and not because of any sense of duty or social commitment. Most of these blood sellers are alcoholics and drug abusers and sell their blood to earn money to engage in these vices. Paid donors have a very high incidence of infections transmissible by transfusion. They often donate blood at short intervals that puts them at risk of iron deficiency anemia. Because of monetary benefit, they also conceal important medical information or their high-risk behavior.

A replacement blood donor is a friend or a relative of the recipient whose donated blood unit is credited to the patient. Blood unit that has been donated replaces the blood unit used for the patient. The practice of replacement donation is carried out in many blood banks since blood supply through voluntary donation falls short of requirements. Replacement donation, however, is less suitable than voluntary donation. If relatives of the patient are unable to find a suitable blood donor known to them, they search for professional donors in order to meet the requirement. Also, because of pressure, replacement donor may hide significant medical information.

Directed donors are types of replacement donors who specifically request that their blood be given to a named patient; this is probably because of concerns regarding safety of blood from unknown donors. However, directed donation from mother to her child can induce transfusion-associated lung injury (due to formation in the mother of HLA antibodies to fetal antigens during pregnancy). Also, transfusion of blood from close relatives to prospective recipients of hematopoietic stem cell transplant carries the risk of HLA immunization and graft rejection.

Practice of replacement donation is helpful where voluntary donation is inadequate. However, this practice is stressful for patient's relatives who have to find replacement donors at a time when they are already under stress due to patient's illness. Blood needs of the patient may not be met as the amount of blood donated may fall short of requirements.

CRITERIA FOR SELECTION OF BLOOD DONORS

Careful selection of blood donors is an essential requirement for safe transfusion practice. It is necessary to ensure well-being of both the donor and the recipient. Selection of blood donors should be carried out by a qualified physician or by a person working under his supervision. Donor selection process consists of four parts:
1. Predonation counseling
2. Medical history
3. Physical examination
4. Hemoglobin estimation

The prospective donor should be assured that the personal information revealed shall be kept confidential.

Criteria for selection of blood donors are given below in short.

Predonation Counseling

This is an education program in which information about health condition, high-risk behavior, self-exclusion/self-deferral, and procedures involved in blood donation is given, donor's questions are answered, informed consent is obtained, and reassurance is given in case of anxiety.

Medical History

Age

The lower and higher age limits for blood donation are 18 and 60 years, respectively. These age limits are set because of:
- Age of consent and increased iron needs of the adolescents
- Risk of cardiovascular and cerebrovascular disease in old age following removal of large quantity of blood.

Donation Interval

The interval between two consecutive blood donations should be at least 3 months. This is to avoid iron depletion in the donor.

Volume of Donation

An individual weighing 45 kg or more can safely donate blood up to 350 mL. This limit intends to preclude the risk of vasovagal attack.

Pregnancy and Lactation

Pregnant women and lactating mothers (up to 1 year postpartum) should not donate blood.

Infectious Diseases

HIV-1 and HIV-2: Blood should not be collected from donors who give history suggestive of HIV infection (unexplained fever, weight loss, swollen lymph nodes, uncontrolled diarrhea, or unusual skin lesions).

To eliminate the "window period" (early antibody-negative period in individuals infected with HIV) donations, individuals who have been exposed to the risk of HIV infection should be requested not to donate blood (such as homosexuals; intravenous drug abusers; or individuals having contact with commercial sex workers, with multiple sexual partners, or with known AIDS or HIV positive persons). Intention of this policy of "self-exclusion" of high-risk donors is elimination of donors in early (HIV antibody-negative) stage of HIV infection. Such individuals can be offered the choice of HIV antibody testing and counseling.

Hepatitis

An individual with history of jaundice within last 1 year or a positive test for HBsAg or anti-HCV antibodies should not be accepted for blood donation.

Malaria

In endemic areas, a donor may be accepted after 3 months of asymptomatic period following malarial attack and after full treatment.

Illness

Individuals with diabetes mellitus, hypertension, heart disease, renal disease, liver disease, lung disease, cancer, epilepsy, bleeding disorder, or allergic disease are not accepted.

Drugs

Many donors who are taking drugs are excluded because of their underlying disease. Other donors are excluded because of the nature of the drug they are taking, e.g. aspirin or other nonsteroidal inflammatory drugs (which affect platelet function), and drugs with teratogenic action like finasteride, isotretinoin, acitretin, and etretinate, or cytotoxic drugs (like cyclophosphamide). Patients receiving human pituitary-derived growth hormone are permanently unfit due to the risk of Creutzfeldt-Jakob disease.

Dentistry

Due to the possibility of bacteremia following tooth extraction or fillings, a 72-hour deferral period before donation is necessary.

Skin Piercing

Donors with history of tattooing, electrolysis, ear piercing, accidental needle stick in healthcare workers, or acupuncture during last 12 months should not be accepted.

Blood Transfusion

A person should not be accepted as blood donor for 6 months after receiving blood transfusion.

Immunization

Donors who have received killed viral vaccines are acceptable as blood donors. Nature of vaccine received and respective deferral period are as follows:
- Attenuated live virus vaccine for measles, mumps, yellow fever, Sabin polio: 2 weeks
- German measles: 4 weeks
- Rabies: 1 year
- Passive immunization with animal sera: 4 weeks
- Hepatitis B immuneglobulin: 1 year.

Physical Examination

This should consist of:
- Weight: It should be minimum 45 kg
- Blood pressure: Systolic blood pressure should be 100–180 mm Hg and diastolic: 50–100 mm Hg
- Pulse: Pulse rate should be 50–100/min and regular
- Temperature: It should be normal.

Donor should be in good general health. Inspect donor's arms for possible evidence of intravenous drug abuse such, as scars or infection at venepuncture site. Clinical examination of cardiovascular system, respiratory system, and abdomen should be normal.

Laboratory Test for Anemia

Screening of donors for anemia in blood bank is done by copper sulfate specific gravity method. This method is as follows:

A drop of blood is allowed to fall in copper sulfate solution of specific gravity 1.053 from a height of 1 cm. Specific gravity of 1.053 is equivalent to hemoglobin concentration of 12.5 g/dL. The drop of blood gets covered with copper proteinate and remains discrete for 15–20 seconds. If the drop sinks within this time, its specific gravity is higher than that of copper sulfate solution (i.e. hemoglobin is >12.5 g/dL) and hemoglobin level is acceptable for donation. If it floats, hemoglobin level is unacceptable. However, specific gravity of whole blood is also affected by total leukocyte count and concentration of plasma proteins. In the presence of leukocytosis (e.g. as in chronic myeloid leukemia) or hypergammaglobulinemia (e.g. multiple myeloma), hemoglobin value will be misleadingly high.

COLLECTION OF DONOR BLOOD

In the blood bank, donor blood should be collected in a well-ventilated, hygienic, and air-conditioned room. Donor should be bled by a qualified physician or by an assistant who is well trained and is working under his supervision.

Equipment and Materials

1. Blood bag: Blood from a donor is collected in a sterile, disposable plastic bag (single, double, triple, or quadruple bag system) with capacity to hold 350 mL of blood. These bags contain a standard amount of anticoagulant preservative solution for specified amount of blood. Whole blood transfusion is still practiced in many blood banks, and therefore single bag is the most common type of blood bag used. Double, triple, and quadruple bag systems are used at places where facilities for separation of components are available.
2. Anticoagulant-preservative solution: The solution in the blood bag usually contains citrate phosphate dextrose adenine -1 (CPDA-1) (49 mL for 350 mL of blood). This solution prevents clotting of blood and also provides nutrients to maintain metabolism and viability of red cells. In CPDA-1, blood can be kept stored at 2–6°C for maximum of 35 days. Function of each component of this solution is as follows:
   - Citrate: Anticoagulation by binding of calcium in plasma
   - Phosphate: Acts as a buffer to minimize the effects of decreasing pH in blood
   - Dextrose: Maintenance of red cell membrane and metabolism
   - Adenine: Generation of ATP (energy source)
3. Sphygmomanometer, weighing balance, sealing clips or sealer, artery forceps
4. 70% ethanol, sterile cotton gauze, adhesive tape
5. Emergency drugs and equipment

6. Blood tubes for collection of blood for testing (grouping, crossmatching, screening for infectious diseases).

Technique

Blood bag should be labeled with the identification number of the donor before withdrawal of blood.

Blood is collected from a vein in the antecubital fossa. To make the veins prominent and palpable, a sphygmomanometer cuff is applied to the arm and inflated to 60–80 mm Hg. The area selected for venepuncture is thoroughly cleansed with 70% ethanol and allowed to dry.

The blood collection bag is placed on a weighing balance that has been kept about 30 cm below the level of the arm. A loose knot is tied in the tubing near the venepuncture needle.

Venepuncture is performed, and the needle is secured in place with an adhesive tape after ensuring free flow of blood.

The pressure is reduced to 40 to 60 mm Hg. The donor is asked to squeeze a rubber ball or a similar object slowly for the duration of donation. The blood and the anticoagulant are mixed at short intervals in the blood bag. The amount of blood collected should be monitored on the weighing balance. When the blood bag weighs 400–450 g, the required amount of blood has been collected.

The pressure cuff is completely deflated and the tubing is clamped with forceps about 10 cm away from the needle. The knot made earlier (close to the needle) is tightened or a sealing clip is applied.

The tubing is cut between the clamp and the knot/sealing clip. The clamp is removed from the tubing and blood samples (for grouping, crossmatching, infectious disease screening) are collected in appropriate tubes. The tubing is then reclamped.

Needle is removed from the vein and pressure is applied over the puncture site with sterile cotton gauze. The needle is disposed of in a special "sharps" container.

Blood remaining in the tubing is nonanticoagulated and is forced back ("stripped") into the blood bag. Bag is inverted gently several times to mix the blood and the anticoagulant. Anticoagulated blood is then allowed to run back into the tubing.

Time required for blood collection should be between 7 minutes and 10 minutes.

Blood sample tubes should be labeled with the donor identification number.

After cessation of bleeding, the venepuncture site is covered with sterile gauze and an adhesive tape. After a few minutes, the donor is allowed to sit up and taken to the refreshment area, where liquids are given. The donor is thanked for donation and is issued a donation card. Donor is given information about need to drink fluids, activities permissible, and care of venepuncture site.

Blood bag is stored in the refrigerator at 2 to 6°C.

At no time during the donation period, donor should be left unattended.

Donor Reactions

Occurrence of donor reactions is rare. One relatively common problem is a fainting attack or loss of consciousness due to sudden deprivation of blood supply to the brain *(syncope or vasovagal attack)*. It is due to the action of the autonomic nervous system and is induced by anxiety, sight of blood, or pain. Its features are sweating, slowing of pulse rate, pallor, coldness of skin, sudden hypotension, and sometimes fainting or vomiting. In such a case, donation should be discontinued. Legs should be elevated above the level of the head to augment the venous return and increase blood flow to the brain. Oral fluids are given if the donor is conscious. If there is prolonged hypotension, intravenous fluids may have to be administered. A severe vasovagal reaction is a contraindication for future donations.

If the donor is highly apprehensive, he may hyperventilate which may cause excessive loss of carbon dioxide and respiratory alkalosis. This may result in tonic-clonic muscle contractions. **Hyperventilation** can be corrected by breathing in a paper bag.

Other reactions include formation of a bruise, hematoma, infection at venepuncture site, thrombophlebitis, and puncture of an artery.

It is necessary to mention occurrence of any adverse reaction on the card issued to the donor.

Collection of Blood by Apheresis

Apheresis is a procedure in which a particular blood component is collected and the remainder of the blood is returned back to the donor by an automated machine. Blood is separated into components based on their specific gravity by centrifugal force. In a closed system, blood flows from the donor's arm into the centrifuge bowl, a specific component is removed, and the remaining blood is returned to the donor. The procedure may take 30 minutes to 2 hours. Apheresis may be continuous or intermittent flow. In intermittent flow, blood is removed through a venepuncture, centrifuged, and returned in alternating steps through the same venepuncture. In continuous flow, blood is removed by one venepuncture in one arm, centrifuged, and returned through another venepuncture in another arm.

This technique allows collection of larger volume of a specific component and decreases exposure of the patient to the number of donors. Donor apheresis is of two main types: Plasmapheresis and cytapheresis. Donor requirements vary with the procedure.

Plasmapheresis: Plasma is harvested from the donor and the cellular components are returned to the donor. For occasional plasmapheresis (once every 12 weeks), criteria are same as for whole blood donors. For frequent plasmapheresis (more than once every 12 weeks), donor testing is necessary before every procedure (hemoglobin >12 g/dL, serum proteins ≥6.0 g/dL). Volume of plasma for a donor weighing ≥55 kg should not exceed 500 mL during one procedure.

Cytapheresis: Individual cellular components are harvested from whole blood by cell separator machine. Cell components that can be collected include:
- Red cells (red cell apheresis): Two units can be collected from donors who are larger and have higher hematocrit than for single red cell donations. Red blood cells are collected in acid citrate dextrose solution. There is deferral period of 16 weeks between double red cell donations.
- Plateletpheresis: This is also known as single donor platelets. For plateletpheresis once every 4 weeks, criteria are same as for whole blood donors. If interval between donations is less than 4 weeks, platelet count must be atleast 150,000/µL before collection. For plateletpheresis, atleast 48 hours gap should be there between two donations and donors should not donate more than two times in week, and should not exceed 24 times in a year. The advantage of this procedure is HLA-matched platelets can be collected for patients who are refractory to random donor platelets due to development of anti-HLA antibodies.

Apheresis platelets can be leucoreduced during the procedure. One unit of apheresis platelets should contain a minimum of 3×10^{11} platelets (equivalent to a pool of 5-6 platelets prepared from whole blood).
- Leucapheresis: This is collection of granulocytes by apheresis. For collection of adequate numbers of granulocytes from donor, drugs or sedimenting material may be given to the donor. This procedure is not widely used.

Stem cell collection: Hematopoietic stem cells can be collected from peripheral blood of donor by apheresis for reconstitution of bone marrow in patients with hematologic malignancies, aplastic anemia, and hemoglobinopathies.

PROCESSING OF DONOR BLOOD

This refers to various tests and procedures carried out on the donor blood after collection but prior to cross matching. Tests done on donor blood are listed in Table 19.1.

STORAGE OF DONOR BLOOD UNIT

Whole blood is stored at a temperature between 2°C and 6°C in a refrigerator specifically designed for blood storage. These temperature limits are set because:
- At temperatures below 2°C, freezing and lysis of red cells will occur; transfusion of such hemolyzed blood will lead to disseminated intravascular coagulation and acute renal failure in the recipient
- Proliferation of any contaminating bacteria, which may have gained entry during venepuncture, is kept at a minimum level (up to 6°C)
- Glycolysis in red blood cells is kept at a minimum level in this temperature range so that dextrose in anticoagulant preservative solution is not utilized rapidly.

Changes which Occur in Stored Blood

Certain changes occur in blood with increasing duration of storage. These are:
- **Loss of viability of red cells:** Viability refers to the ability of red blood cells to survive following transfusion in recipient's circulation. It gradually decreases with increasing length of storage. A proportion of red cells is removed from the circulation within the first 24 hours post-transfusion. Storage conditions should be such that, after transfusion, at least 75% of

Table 19.1: Tests done on donor blood.

- Grouping
  - ABO grouping—cell and serum grouping
  - RhD grouping
- Screening and identification of unexpected antibodies
- Screening tests for infectious organisms:
  - Hepatitis B surface antigen
  - Anti-HCV antibodies
  - HIV-1 and HIV-2 antibodies
  - VDRL test
  - Blood smear for malaria parasite

transfused red cells should survive at 24 hours in the recipient's circulation. Shelf-life of the stored whole blood is based on this criterion. For whole blood stored in CPDA-1 and maintained at 2 to 6° C, shelf-life is 35 days.

- **Loss of ATP:** Loss of ATP (energy source) occurs with increasing duration of storage leading to spherocytic shape change, membrane lipid loss, and increasing rigidity. Such cells have reduced survival. Adenine in CPDA-1 solution provides ATP and improves viability of red cells.
- **Depletion of 2,3-diphosphoglycerate (2,3-DPG):** Appropriate levels of 2,3-DPG in red cells are essential for a low oxygen affinity of hemoglobin and ready release of oxygen to the tissues. Progressive reduction of 2,3-DPG with storage increases oxygen affinity and reduces release of oxygen at tissue level. Restoration of 2,3-DPG in red cells occurs within 24 hours of transfusion; therefore, depleted 2,3-DPG levels are likely to be of significance mainly in patients with severe anemia.
- **Loss of granulocyte function** occurs within 24 hours and **loss of platelet function** occurs within 48 hours of blood collection.
- **Decrease in pH of blood**
- **Increase in plasma potassium level**
- **Decrease in factor VIII level** to 10 to 20% of normal occurs within 48 hours of blood collection.
- **Formation of microaggregates:** In stored blood, tiny aggregates of cell debris, aged platelets, leukocytes, fibrin strands, and cold insoluble globulin form.

BIBLIOGRAPHY

1. Cheesbrough M. District Laboratory Practice in Tropical Countries. Part 2. Cambridge: Cambridge University Press; 2000.
2. Saran RK, Makroo RN. Transfusion Medicine Technical Manual. Directorate General of Health Services. 1991.

CHAPTER 20

Whole Blood, Blood Components, and Blood Derivatives

In the past, whole blood was the only preparation that could be administered to replace red cells, platelets, coagulation factors, etc. in a patient. In addition to what patient required, this caused unnecessary administration of unwanted cell or plasma constituents. Large volume of whole blood needed to achieve satisfactory replacement of a particular component also posed an important limitation. A significant advance in transfusion medicine was made when techniques became available for separation of blood components in a closed system and patient could be administered specific replacement therapy. One unit of donor blood can be utilized for preparation of different components and thus can benefit more than one patient.

Nowadays, whole blood can be separated into various blood components and further derivatives can be obtained from plasma by fractionation (Box 20.1 and Fig. 20.1). This permits administration of specific replacement therapy as per the patient's requirements, and avoids transfusion of unwanted constituents of blood. One unit of donor blood can benefit more than one patient after its separation into plasma, red cell, and platelet components.

Separation of blood components from one another by centrifugation is possible due to differences in their specific gravities. Preparation of blood components has been greatly facilitated by the introduction of double and triple bags having closed integral tubing. After their separation, various components can be transferred from one bag to another in a closed circuit thus maintaining the sterility (Fig. 20.2). Venepuncture should be clean with little trauma to tissues. Blood and anticoagulant should be mixed constantly, and blood collection should be completed within 8 to 10 minutes. Blood should be processed for component separation within 6 hours of collection.

Box 20.1: Blood products.

Whole blood
One unit of donor blood collected in a suitable anticoagulant-preservative solution and which contains blood cells and plasma.
Blood components
A constituent separated from whole blood by differential centrifugation of one donor unit or by apheresis.
Blood derivatives
A product obtained from multiple donor units of plasma by fractionation.

Chapter 20: Whole Blood, Blood Components, and Blood Derivatives

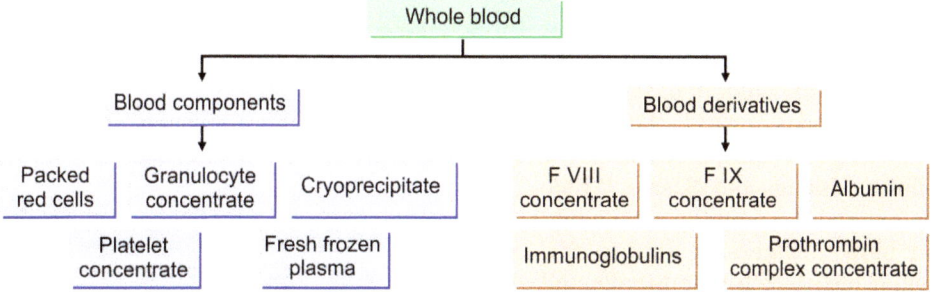

Fig. 20.1: Blood components and derivatives that can be made from whole blood.

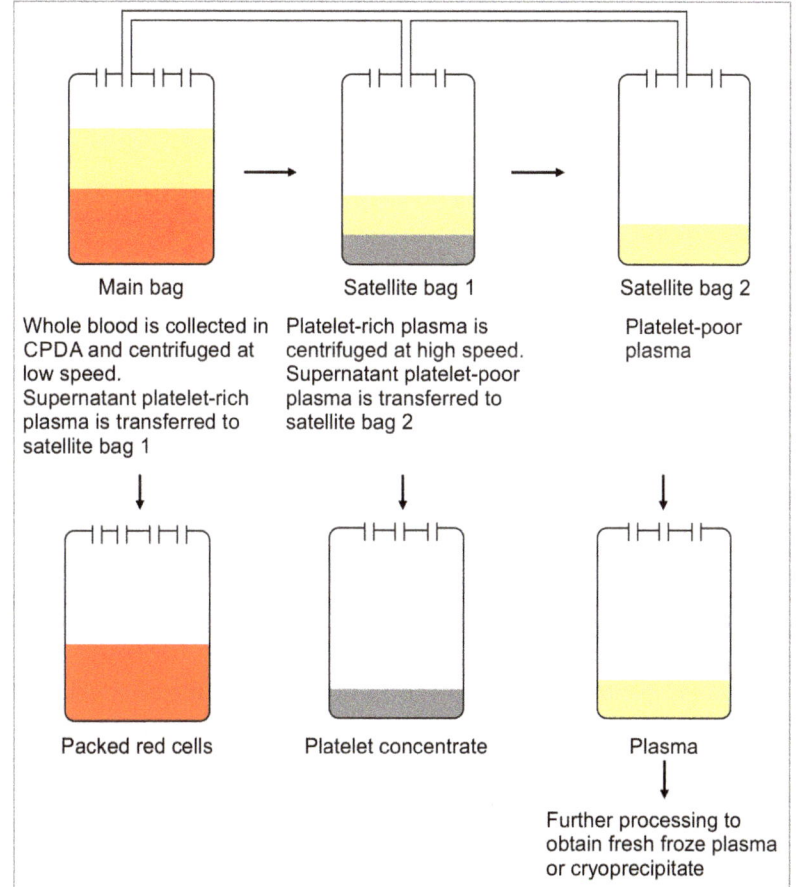

Fig. 20.2: Principle of preparation of blood components from a single unit of whole blood. Packed red cells, platelet concentrate, and plasma thus obtained can be utilized for three different patients.

WHOLE BLOOD

Whole blood still remains a commonly employed blood product at some places because of the lack of facility for component separation.

Whole blood is one unit of donor blood collected in a suitable anticoagulant-preservative solution. Its total volume is about 400 mL (350 mL of blood + 49 mL of anticoagulant). It consists of cellular elements and plasma. Whole blood is stored in a properly maintained blood bank refrigerator at 2 to 6°C and shelf-life of such blood (collected in CPDA anticoagulant) is 35 days (Box 20.2).

Before ordering whole blood transfusion, following should be noted:
- Transfusion of one unit raises hemoglobin by 1 g/dL or hematocrit by 3%.
- Whole blood stored at 2 to 6°C does not contain functionally effective platelets after 48 hours of collection and also labile coagulation factors (i.e. F V and F VIII). Therefore, stored whole blood should not be used to replace platelets, granulocytes, or coagulation factors.
- Whole blood transfusion is associated with the risk of volume overload in patients with chronic severe anemia and compromised cardiovascular function.

Box 20.2: Whole blood.
- One unit of blood collected in a suitable anticoagulant solution
- Hematocrit 35–45% and hemoglobin 12.0 g/dL
- Contains no functionally effective platelets and no labile coagulation factors
- Storage temperature: 2–6°C in appropriate blood bank refrigerator
- Shelf-life: 35 days (in CPDA-1)
- Indication: Acute massive blood loss, exchange transfusion, nonavailability of packed red cells
- Risk of volume overload in patients with chronic anemia and compromised cardiovascular function

Transfusion of whole blood to the recipient should commence within 30 minutes of removing the blood bag from the refrigerator and should be completed within maximum of 4 hours of starting transfusion.

Many times, the clinician requests "fresh" blood (i.e. one which is less than 24 hours old). After collection, blood can be issued only after all the necessary tests are completed (which may take 24 hours). Such "fresh" blood can be utilized for infants, thalassemics (who need red cells with maximal survival), and bleeding disorders (since platelets and labile coagulation factors become functionally ineffective after 48 hours of storage). However, if available, packed red cells, plasma components, or platelet concentrates are more effective and preferred forms of therapy for such patients.

In this era of blood component therapy, the only indication for whole blood transfusion is acute massive blood loss, i.e. correction of both hypovolemia and red cell mass. (In these patients also, packed red cells along with a crystalloid solution are preferable). For all other indications, specific component therapy is administered.

BLOOD COMPONENTS

Blood components can be separated from one another by centrifugation due to differences in their specific gravities. Separation of blood components is carried in double or triple bags with closed integral tubing. After collection from donor, blood should be processed for component separation within 6 hours. Blood components are listed in Box 20.3. Storage temperatures and duration of storage of some blood products are shown in Box 20.4.

Red Cell Components

Packed Red Cells

Packed red cells are prepared by removing most of the plasma from one unit of whole blood. Whole blood is either allowed to sediment overnight in a refrigerator at 2 to 6°C or is spun in a refrigerated centrifuge. Supernatant plasma is then separated from red cells in a closed system by transferring it to the attached empty satellite bag. Red cells and a small amount of plasma are left behind in the primary blood bag.

Main indication for packed red cells is replacement of red cells in anemia (chronic anemia, severe anemia with congestive cardiac failure, anemia in elderly).

Transfusion of packed red cells lowers the risk of volume overload. In contrast to whole blood, for a given volume, double the amount of red cells can be infused, i.e. total volume of whole blood is 400 mL (150 mL red cells + 250 mL plasma) while that of packed red cells is 250 mL (150 mL red cells + 100 mL plasma). Hematocrit of whole blood is about 40% while that of packed red cells is 55 to 75%. Normal saline can be added using Y-pattern infusion set to increase the speed of transfusion by reducing the viscosity. Packed red cells have a high viscosity and therefore the rate of infusion is slow.

Transfusion of one unit of red cells increases hemoglobin by 1 g% (or increases PCV by 3%). This rise becomes detectable 24 hours after transfusion (Box 20.5).

Box 20.3: Blood components.

Red cells
- Packed red cells
- Red cells in additive solution
- Leukocyte-poor red cells
- Washed red cells
- Frozen red cells
- Irradiated red cells

Platelets
- Platelet concentrate

Granulocytes
- Granulocyte concentrate

Plasma
- Fresh frozen plasma
- Cryoprecipitate

Box 20.4: Temperature and duration of storage of blood products.

- Whole blood, packed red cells: 2–6°C for 35 days
- Platelet concentrates: 20–24°C for 3 days with continuous agitation
- Fresh frozen plasma: Below –25°C for 1 year
- Cryoprecipitate: Below –25°C for 1 year

Box 20.5: Packed red cells (red cell concentrate).

- Red cells from which most of plasma has been removed
- Hematocrit 55–75% or hemoglobin 20 g/dL
- Raises hemoglobin by 1 g% or hematocrit by 3%
- Storage temperature: 2–6°C and shelf-life 35 days (in CPDA)
- Indication: Replacement of red cells in anemia and in acute/massive blood loss (along with crystalloid or colloid)
- Volume: 250 mL

Red Cells in Additive Solution (Red Cell Suspension)

Commonly used additive solution is SAGM (which contains saline, adenine, glucose, and mannitol). After collection of whole blood in the primary collection bag (containing CPDA-1), maximum amount of plasma is removed (after centrifugation) and transferred to one satellite bag. The additive solution from the second satellite bag is transferred into the primary collection bag (containing packed red cells) in a closed circuit.

Advantages of this method are:
- Maximum amount of plasma can be removed for preparation of plasma components
- Red cells with improved viability are obtained (shelf-life increases from 35 to 42 days)
- Flow of infusion is improved due to reduction in viscosity

Indications for red cells in SAGM are similar to those for packed red cells. Red cells in SAGM are contraindicated for exchange transfusion in neonates.

Leukocyte-poor Red Cells

These are the red cells from which most of the white cells have been removed. By definition, leukocyte-depleted red cells should contain less than 5×10^6 white cells per bag. They are obtained by passing blood through a special leukocyte-depletion filter at the time of transfusion; they can also be prepared in the blood bank.

Leukocyte-poor red cells are indicated:
- To avoid sensitization to HLA antigens (e.g. in patients with severe aplastic anemia who are likely to receive allogeneic bone marrow transplant)
- To avoid febrile transfusion reactions in persons who require repeated transfusions or who have earlier been sensitized to white cell antigens
- To reduce the risk of transmission of cytomegalovirus (CMV) in certain patients (if CMV-seronegative blood is not available)

Leukocyte-depleted red cells cannot prevent graft-versus-host disease.

Washed Red Cells

Packed red cells can be washed with normal saline to remove plasma proteins, white cells, and platelets. Use of such red cells is restricted for IgA-deficient individuals who have developed anti-IgA antibodies.

Frozen Red Cells

Red cells can be stored frozen for up to 10 years. To prevent hemolysis of red cells during freezing and thawing, a cryoprotective agent, such as glycerol is added. Donor red cells with rare blood groups can be stored frozen for recipients who have developed antibodies against frequently occurring red cell antigens. Similarly, red cells can be stored frozen for future autologous transfusion, if blood group is rare. Before transfusion, red cells are thawed and glycerol removed gradually by using progressively less hypertonic solutions. Such red cells are virtually free from leukocytes, platelets, and plasma and thus their use is associated with low-risk of nonhemolytic transfusion reactions.

Irradiated Red Cells

Transfusion of gamma-irradiated red cells is indicated for prevention of graft-versus-host disease in susceptible individuals like:
- Immunodeficient individuals
- Patients receiving blood from first-degree relatives.

Lymphocytes from donor blood react against the tissues of the recipient. Gamma irradiation (25 Gy) inhibits replication of donor lymphocytes.

Platelets

There are two methods for obtaining platelets (Box 20.6) for transfusion:
- Differential centrifugation of a unit of whole blood (platelet concentrate)
- Plateletpheresis (Box 20.7 for principle of pheresis).

Platelet Concentrate (Random Donor Platelets)

Platelet concentrate is prepared by differential centrifugation of one unit of whole blood within 6 hours of donation and before refrigeration. One unit of whole blood is centrifuged at low speed to obtain platelet-rich plasma (PRP). PRP is then transferred to the attached satellite bag and spun at high speed to get platelet aggregates (at the bottom) and platelet-poor plasma or PPP (at the top). Most of the PPP is returned back to the primary collection bag or to another satellite bag, leaving behind 50 to 60 mL of PPP with the platelets.

Platelets are stored at 20 to 24°C with continuous agitation (in a storage device called platelet agitator). Maximum period of storage is 3–5 days.

Box 20.6: Platelets.
- Obtained either from single donor units of whole blood by centrifugation or by plateletpheresis.
- Platelets prepared from whole blood donation are supplied either as a single unit or as a pooled unit (i.e. platelets obtained from 4 to 6 donor whole blood units are "pooled" together in one bag). Platelets obtained from plateletpheresis are supplied as one pack of single donor platelets.
- Storage: 20–24°C with constant agitation up to 72 hours.
- Common indications are thrombocytopenia due to decreased platelet production and hereditary platelet function defect.

Box 20.7: Pheresis.
- Donor pheresis is a procedure in which a suitable donor is connected to an automated cell separator machine through which whole blood is withdrawn, the desired blood component is retained, and the remainder of the blood is returned back to the donor. Depending on the component that is separated and removed, the procedure is called as plateletpheresis, leukapheresis, or plasmapheresis.
- Therapeutic pheresis consists of removing the undesirable blood component and returning the remaining blood portion to the patient's circulation. The undesirable component is discarded. Examples are therapeutic plasmapheresis in hyperviscosity syndrome in plasma cell dyscrasias, and leukapheresis in hyperleukocytosis in AML or CML.

One unit of platelet concentrate contains more than 45×10^9 platelets. Transfusion of one unit will raise the platelet count in the recipient by about 5,000/μL.

The usual adult dose is 4 to 6 units of platelet concentrate (or 1 unit/10 kg of body weight). These units (which are from different donors) are pooled into one bag before transfusion. This dose will raise the platelet count by 20,000 to 40,000/μL.

Plateletpheresis (Single Donor Platelets)

In plateletpheresis, a donor is connected to a blood cell separator machine in which whole blood is collected in an anticoagulant solution, platelets are separated and retained, and remaining components are returned back to the donor. With this method, a large number of platelets can be obtained from a single donor (equivalent to 6 units). This method is especially suitable if HLA-matched platelets are required (i.e. if patient has developed refractoriness to platelet transfusion due to the formation of alloantibodies against HLA antigens).

Platelets are administered for prevention and treatment of bleeding due to thrombocytopenia or platelet dysfunction. The usual indications are:
- Thrombocytopenia due to decreased platelet production, e.g. aplastic anemia, hematologic malignancies, following chemotherapy or radiotherapy, etc.
- Hereditary disorders of platelet function
- Massive blood transfusion.

Most of the adverse reactions associated with platelet transfusions are due to the presence of contaminating leukocytes or plasma (e.g. febrile nonhemolytic transfusion reactions, allergic reactions, etc.).

Platelet concentrates are contraindicated in thrombotic thrombocytopenic purpura and in hemolytic uremic syndrome.

Transfusion of multiple platelet concentrates from random donors can induce alloimmunization to HLA antigens. This causes resistance to further platelet transfusions and predicted post-transfusion rise in platelet count fails to occur due to rapid clearance of infused platelets by anti-HLA antibodies. Such patients should receive HLA-compatible platelets obtained from a single donor by plateletpheresis.

Bacterial proliferation can occur in platelet concentrates since they are stored at room temperature; consequently septicemia can occur in the recipient.

As platelet concentrates also contain a small amount of red cells, it is preferable to transfuse platelet concentrates of same or compatible ABO group and same Rh group; this precaution is especially important if recipient is a woman of child-bearing age.

Granulocyte Concentrate

Granulocyte concentrates are rarely used because:
- Most infections can be effectively controlled by appropriate antibiotic therapy
- A granulocyte concentrate prepared from a single donor unit has insufficient granulocytes and is also heavily contaminated with red cells
- Transfusion of granulocyte concentrate is associated with significant risks (like nonhemolytic transfusion reactions, lung infiltrates, transmission of cell-associated viruses like cytomegalovirus, etc.).

Granulocytes for transfusion can be obtained either from a single donor unit by differential centrifugation or by leukapheresis. Leukapheresis is preferred because of better granulocyte yield, which can further be enhanced by administration of corticosteroids to the donor.

Administration of granulocyte concentrates can be considered in a patient with severe neutropenia with documented bacterial or fungal infection, which is not responding to appropriate antibiotic therapy.

Plasma Components

Plasma can be obtained either by centrifugation of a unit of whole blood or by plasmapheresis. Various components can be prepared from plasma, the important ones being fresh frozen plasma and cryoprecipitate.

Fresh Frozen Plasma (FFP)

For preparation of FFP, plasma is separated from whole blood by centrifugation, transferred into the attached satellite bag, and rapidly frozen at −25°C or at lower temperature. This process is carried out within 6 hours of collection because after this time, labile coagulation factors (F V and F VIII) are lost. Volume of FFP is 200 to 250 mL. FFP contains all the coagulation factors (Box 20.8).

Fresh frozen plasma can be stored for 1 year if temperature is maintained below −25°C. When required for transfusion, FFP is thawed between 30°C and 37°C and then stored in the refrigerator at 2 to 6°C. Since labile coagulation factors rapidly deteriorate, FFP should be transfused within 2 hours of thawing.

Box 20.8: Fresh frozen plasma
- Plasma separated from whole blood within 6 hours of collection and then rapidly frozen to −25°C or lower
- Contains all the coagulation factors
- Storage: At −25°C or lower up to 1 year
- Volume: 200–300 mL
- Indications: Multiple coagulation factor deficiencies (liver disease, warfarin overdose), disseminated intravascular coagulation, and massive blood transfusion

Indications for FFP are:
- Deficiency of multiple coagulation factors as in liver disease, massive transfusion, disseminated intravascular coagulation, and thrombotic thrombocytopenic purpura
- Reversal of warfarin overdose
- Inherited deficiency of a coagulation factor for which no specific concentrate is available.

FFP should not be used for volume expansion alone, for which synthetic crystalloids or colloids are safer alternatives.

FFP should be administered in a dose of 15 mL/kg of body weight over 1 to 2 hours. ABO-compatible FFP is preferred to avoid the risk of hemolysis of recipient's red cells by antibodies in donor plasma.

Cryoprecipitate

Cryoprecipitate is prepared by slowly thawing 1 unit of FFP at 4 to 6°C. Plasma and a white precipitate are obtained. After centrifugation, most of the supernatant plasma is removed leaving behind sediment of cryoprecipitate suspended in 10–20 mL of plasma. The unit is then refrozen (−25°C or colder) for storage and can be kept for 1 year at this temperature. When required for transfusion, cryoprecipitate is thawed at 30 to 37°C and then kept in the refrigerator at 2 to 6°C till transfusion (for maximum of 6 hours).

Cryoprecipitate contains F VIII (about 80 units), von Willebrand factor, fibrinogen, F XIII, and fibronectin. If specific factor concentrates are not available, cryoprecipitate can be used for treatment of F VIII deficiency, von Willebrand disease, F XIII deficiency, and hypofibrinogenemia.

BLOOD DERIVATIVES

Blood derivatives are manufactured by fractionation of large pools (obtained from many thousand donations) of human plasma. Some form of viral inactivation treatment is incorporated during manufacturing process to reduce the risk of viral transmission. Important plasma derivatives are listed in Box 20.9.

Box 20.9: Blood derivatives.
1. Human albumin solutions
2. F VIII concentrate
3. F IX concentrate
4. Prothrombin complex concentrate
5. Immunoglobulins

Human Albumin Solutions

Albumin is prepared by cold ethanol fractionation of pooled plasma and is available as 5% and 20% solutions. Albumin solutions are heat-treated (at 60° C for 10 hours) to inactivate any contaminating viruses.

Physiological functions of albumin are maintenance of normal colloid osmotic pressure of plasma and to act as a carrier protein for certain substances in circulation.

Albumin is used as a replacement fluid in therapeutic plasma exchange, and for treatment of diuretic-resistant edema of hypoproteinemia.

F VIII Concentrate

F VIII concentrate, prepared by fractionation from large pools of donated plasma, is supplied as a freeze-dried powder in vials. During manufacturing process, it is treated with heat or chemicals to destroy lipid-enveloped viruses like HIV, HBV, HCV, and HTLV. It is stored in the refrigerator at 2 to 6° C. Before administration, it is reconstituted as per manufacturer's directions and given intravenously.

F VIII concentrate is indicated for treatment of:
- Hemophilia A
- Severe von Willebrand disease.

Apart from plasma-derived F VIII concentrate, F VIII prepared by recombinant DNA technology is now commercially available. It is free from infectious viruses and thus safer than plasma-derived F VIII.

F IX Concentrate

Both plasma-derived and recombinant F IX concentrates are available for treatment of hemophilia B.

Prothrombin Complex Concentrate (PCC)

Prothrombin complex concentrate contains factors II, IX, and X, and sometimes also F VII. PCC contains trace amounts of activated coagulation factors and can induce thrombotic complications in patients with liver disease and in patients prone to thrombosis.

Indications for PCC are:
- Inherited deficiency of F IX, II, or F X
- Hemophilia A with inhibitor antibodies against F VIII and who are nonresponsive to F VIII concentrate.

Immunoglobulins

Immunoglobulins are prepared by cold ethanol fractionation of pooled plasma and are used for passive immunization against infections. They are of two main types—(i) nonspecific ("normal") immunoglobulins and (ii) specific immunoglobulins.

Nonspecific or "Normal" Immunoglobulins

These are prepared from the pooled plasma of nonselected donors and are composed of antibodies against infectious agents that are prevalent in the donor population. Some preparations are only for intramuscular administration, while others can be given intravenously.

Indications for nonspecific immunoglobulins are:
- Passive prophylaxis against hepatitis A
- Congenital or acquired hypogammaglobulinemia
- Autoimmune thrombocytopenic purpura to temporarily raise platelet count.

Specific Immunoglobulins

They are prepared from donors who have specific high titer IgG antibodies (e.g. from patients convalescing from infectious diseases or who are already immunized).

Specific immunoglobulins include:
- Specific immunoglobulins for passive prophylaxis against hepatitis B, varicella zoster, cytomegalovirus, or tetanus.
- Anti-RhD immunoglobulin, which is used for prevention of immunization against RhD antigen in RhD-negative mothers during pregnancy. It is obtained from Rh-negative persons immunized to RhD antigen.

BIBLIOGRAPHY

1. Nanu A. Blood components: Preparation and quality control. Indian J Hematol Blood Transf. 1991;9: 159-70.
2. World Health Organization. 2002. Blood Transfusion Safety: The Clinical Use of Blood.

CHAPTER 21

Transfusion of Blood to the Recipient

Once it is decided that blood transfusion is required for a particular patient, a properly filled blood requisition form accompanied with labeled blood samples from the prospective recipient should be sent to the blood bank. It is the responsibility of the attending clinician to properly fill the request form. It should provide the following information:
1. Name of the patient
2. Hospital registration number
3. Age/sex
4. Ward number
5. Clinical diagnosis
6. Indication for transfusion, number of blood units required
7. Nature of product required, whether whole blood, packed red cells, platelets, fresh frozen plasma, cryoprecipitate, etc.
8. Date and time when required
9. Blood group of the patient, if known
10. Previous history of transfusion, transfusion reactions.

Before withdrawing blood sample, the prospective recipient should be positively identified. Blood is collected in a plain tube (for serum grouping and compatibility testing) and also in a tube containing EDTA anticoagulant (for cell grouping). Sample tubes should be carefully labelled at the bedside. It should be kept in mind that **the most common cause of a hemolytic transfusion reaction is clerical error,** i.e. collecting blood from the wrong patient and incorrect labeling of sample tubes.

SELECTION OF DONOR BLOOD FOR WHOLE BLOOD OR PACKED RED CELL TRANSFUSION

The first choice is the donor blood of the same ABO group as that of the recipient. If blood supply is inadequate, blood of the same ABO group may occasionally be not available; in such a case, if blood transfusion is likely to be potentially lifesaving and urgent, blood of an alternate but compatible group may be transfused (Table 21.1). Possible benefits and risks should be carefully assessed before considering such a transfusion.

To reduce the risk of hemolysis in a case of nonidentical but compatible ABO transfusion, packed red cells instead of whole blood should be transfused (i.e. most of the plasma which

Table 21.1: Selection of donor blood group for transfusion of whole blood or packed red cells.

Recipient blood group	Donor blood group	
	First choice	Alternative
A	A	O
B	B	O
AB	AB	A, B, O (in this order)
O	O	Nil

contains anti-A and/or anti-B should be removed). This is especially important with group O donor blood, which can contain immune anti-A and anti-B antibodies that will cause serious hemolysis in a nongroup O recipient.

For AB group recipients, if red cells of group AB are not available, group A donor blood is preferred over other alternatives since anti-B in group A is weaker than anti-A in group B.

Transfusion of Rh-positive blood to Rh-negative persons carries the risk of evoking the formation of anti-D antibodies (after about 3 months). Subsequent transfusion of Rh-positive blood to such sensitized individuals will cause hemolytic transfusion reaction. In the Rh system, **individuals with Rh-negative blood group should be transfused only with Rh-negative blood,** especially Rh-negative females of child-bearing age and young girls (to prevent Rh immunization and future hemolytic disease of newborn). In an emergency, Rh-positive blood may be transfused to nonimmunized Rh-negative men and older women, if Rh-negative blood is not available and if blood transfusion will be potentially lifesaving. However, if such individuals are likely to need regular transfusions in future also, they should preferably be not exposed to Rh-positive blood.

Although persons with Rh-positive group can receive either Rh-positive or Rh-negative blood, they should be transfused with Rh-positive blood (owing to the rarity of Rh-negative blood which should be reserved only for Rh-negative recipients). Currently, enzymatic removal of A and/or B antigens from red cells of A, B, and AB groups is being tried experimentally to convert all A, B, and AB donor units to group O unit. Since group O is a universal donor group, success in this strategy will hopefully make finding ABO-compatible blood less of a problem and will also reduce the risk of ABO mismatched transfusion reactions.

SELECTION OF DONOR PLASMA

For transfusion of plasma and plasma components, selection of blood group of donor is given in Table 21.2.

Table 21.2: Selection of donor blood group for transfusion of plasma.

Donor blood (plasma) group	Recipient blood group
AB plasma (contains neither anti-A nor anti-B antibodies)	AB, A, B, O
A plasma (contains anti-B)	A, O
B plasma (contains anti-A)	B, O
O plasma (contains both anti-A and anti-B)	O only

ANTIBODY SCREENING AND IDENTIFICATION

In well-equipped blood banks, screening for unexpected or irregular antibodies against red cell antigens is carried out before transfusion in both recipient's and donor's sera. For recipients demonstrating irregular antibodies, selection of donor blood lacking the corresponding antigen is selected.

COMPATIBILITY TEST

The final check of compatibility between recipient and donor blood is cross-matching or compatibility test. There are two types of compatibility test: major and minor. The aim of cross-matching is detection of ABO incompatibility and presence of clinically significant unexpected antibodies. If cross-match is compatible, a compatibility label should be attached to the blood bag showing patient's (recipient's) name, hospital registration number, ward number, blood group, donation identification number, date of expiry of unit, and date of compatibility test.

ISSUE OF DONOR BLOOD UNIT

Before issuing the blood unit for the recipient, information on the blood bag, request form, and compatibility label should be checked by the blood bank for any discrepancy.
Blood bag should be inspected for the following (Fig. 21.1):
- Evidence of hemolysis (pink discoloration of plasma or red coloration of plasma just above the red cell layer)
- Large clots in plasma
- Black or purple discoloration of red cells indicative of bacterial contamination
- Leakage.

The physician at the bedside should also carry out similar inspection before beginning transfusion. If any abnormality is detected, blood should not be transfused and blood bank is notified.

Blood bag should be procured from the blood bank only at the time of transfusion (i.e. when the intravenous line is in place in the recipient). Transfusion should commence within

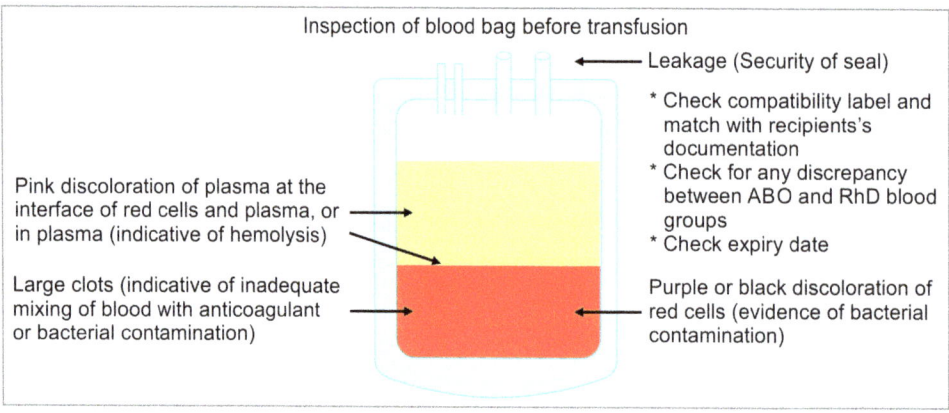

Fig. 21.1: Checking of blood bag is essential on its arrival in ward or operating room and before beginning transfusion.

30 minutes of removing the blood bag from the refrigerator of the blood bank. Blood unit should not be transfused if the blood bag is out of refrigerator for more than 30 minutes, since it increases the risk of proliferation of contaminating bacteria.

Do not transfuse blood unit if it shows evidence of hemolysis, clots, discoloration of red cells, or leakage.

TRANSFUSION OF BLOOD UNIT

Before beginning transfusion, it is necessary to check the label on the blood bag, compatibility label, blood bag itself (for evidence of hemolysis, clots, discoloration of red cells, or leakage), and identity of the recipient. Check ABO and Rh D groups of both the recipient and donor written on the blood bag and the date of expiry of the blood unit.

It is necessary to correctly identify the recipient during sample collection and before beginning transfusion.

Blood should be transfused through a sterile, disposable administration set incorporating a standard filter (170-μm pore size). This filter retains small clots or cellular aggregates but permits passage of single cells and microaggregates. The usual needle size is 18 or 19 gauge. Microaggregate or leukocyte depletion filters are available which are used to prevent or decrease the febrile transfusion reactions in multiply transfused patients.

It is not necessary to warm blood before transfusion when rate of infusion is slow. However, rapid infusion of large volume of cold blood can induce ventricular arrhythmias or cardiac arrest. Blood warmer is used to warm blood in such cases. Blood should be warmed only by blood warmer and not by any other means, such as hot water bowl, since high temperature will induce hemolysis and release of potassium from red cells, which may prove fatal for the recipient.

No drugs of any kind should be added to the blood. Ringer's lactate (which contains calcium) or 5% dextrose causes formation of clots and hemolysis, respectively. If fluids are to be added, the only acceptable one is normal saline. Normal saline is used for starting transfusion and also can be added to packed red cells to reduce viscosity. Addition of a drug may induce hemolysis; also if a reaction occurs, it may be difficult to decide whether it is drug induced or is related to blood transfusion.

The patient should be monitored closely during transfusion (by regularly noting general appearance, pulse, respiratory rate, temperature, and blood pressure). The patient should be closely observed, especially during first 15 minutes, as most life-threatening hemolytic transfusion reactions are likely to occur during this period. Following this, patient is observed every hour, at the end of transfusion, and 4 hours after the end of transfusion.

Transfusion should be initiated within 30 minutes of removing blood unit from the storage refrigerator in the blood bank. Transfusion of whole blood or packed red cells should be completed within maximum of 4 hours of starting transfusion. If ambient temperature is high, infusion should be completed within a shorter period. This is because of the risk of bacterial proliferation in the blood unit, which increases with time at room temperature. (Bacteria may have gained entry into the blood unit during blood collection, storage, or transfusion.)

After transfusion is over, details of transfusion such as time of starting and completion, nature of blood product transfused, donation identification number, and any adverse reactions should be recorded in the case records of the recipient.

BIBLIOGRAPHY

1. Boral LI, Weiss ED, Henry JB. Transfusion medicine. In: Henry JB (Ed). Clinical Diagnosis and Management by Laboratory Methods, 20th edition. Philadelphia: WB Saunders Company; 2001.
2. World Health Organization. (2002). Blood Transfusion Safety: The Clinical Use of Blood. [online] Available from https://www.who.int/bloodsafety/clinical_use/en/Handbook_EN.pdf?ua=1 [Last Accessed March 2019].

CHAPTER 22

Adverse Effects of Transfusion

INTRODUCTION

Blood transfusion is a lifesaving but a potentially hazardous procedure. It should be considered only if there are no alternative means (like intravenous fluids, specific treatment of anemia) of treating the condition. Before contemplating transfusion, risks and benefits should be assessed. This is because even with best possible blood banking standards, transmission of infections or other complications can occur. Benefits of blood transfusion include improvement of oxygen-carrying capacity and replacement of coagulation factors, platelets, immunoglobulins, and other proteins. Potential risks of transfusion are transmission of infections like hepatitis and AIDS, transfusion reactions, and immunization to antigens. Fluids such as saline or dextrose should be used when only volume replacement is required. Adverse effects of transfusion are listed in Box 22.1. At many places, blood transfusion consists of giving a single unit of blood

---

Box 22.1: Adverse effects of transfusion.

Immediate
Immunological
- Febrile nonhemolytic transfusion reactions
- Hemolytic transfusion reactions
- Allergic reactions
- Anaphylactic reactions
- Transfusion-associated lung injury

Non-immunological
- Circulatory overload
- Bacterial contamination of donor blood unit

Delayed
- *Immunological*
- Hemolytic transfusion reactions
- Post transfusion purpura
- Graft-versus-host disease

Nonimmunological
- Transmission of infectious organisms
- Iron overload

Complications associated with massive transfusion

(which in most cases is unnecessary) and whole blood (for which there are very few indications and which exposes the recipient to unwanted components). Risks of such practice should be realized before undertaking single unit transfusion.

IMMEDIATE COMPLICATIONS

Febrile Nonhemolytic Transfusion Reaction (FNHTR)

This manifests with fever, and sometimes with chills, flushing, headache, anxiety, itching, and tachycardia. The reaction begins 30 to 60 minutes following start of transfusion. FNHTR is common in recipients of multiple transfusions and in women who have had multiple pregnancies (due to previous sensitization).

Febrile non-hemolytic transfusion reaction is caused by:
- Release of cytokines from leukocytes during storage of blood, and
- Reaction of alloantibodies in the recipient with transfused white cells leading to release of pyrogens.

Diagnosis of FNHTR is based on eliminating other causes of fever such as hemolytic transfusion reaction, bacterial contamination of donor blood unit, transfusion associated lung injury, or underlying disease in the patient.

Management consists of:
- Stopping transfusion
- Workup for hemolytic transfusion reaction (see below) and for bacterial contamination of blood unit
- Administration of oral or rectal antipyretics (paracetamol) and IM/IV antihistaminic.

In regularly transfused patients, prevention of FNTHR involves slow speed of transfusion (up to 4 hours for 1 unit of whole blood) and administration of antipyretics before starting transfusion. If these measures are unsuccessful, leukocyte-depleted blood should be given (i.e. prior removal of buffy coat or transfusion through leukocyte depletion filters).

Hemolytic Transfusion Reaction (HTR)

Acute intravascular hemolysis is caused by transfusion of incompatible red cells. Binding of antibodies in patient's circulation to donor red cells leads to activation of full complement cascade and hemolysis (Fig. 22.1).

Acute HTR most often results from ABO incompatibility and is mediated by IgM (or sometimes IgG) anti-A or anti-B antibodies. ABO incompatibility almost always results in HTR because of consistent occurrence of potent and lytic IgM antibodies in plasma of patients lacking corresponding antigen on their red cells.

Mismatched ABO blood transfusion usually results from clerical error. This error may be:
- Incorrect identification of recipient during sample collection or during transfusion.
- Incorrect labeling of sample tubes or incorrect filling of request form.

Signs and symptoms of acute HTR usually appear within minutes of starting transfusion since only a small amount of blood (5–10 mL) can trigger the reaction.

Patient complains of pain or heat at the infusion site, substernal pain, restlessness, and loin or back pain. There is development of fever, rigors, breathlessness, tachycardia, hypotension, and bleeding manifestations. In severe cases, renal failure may follow. The

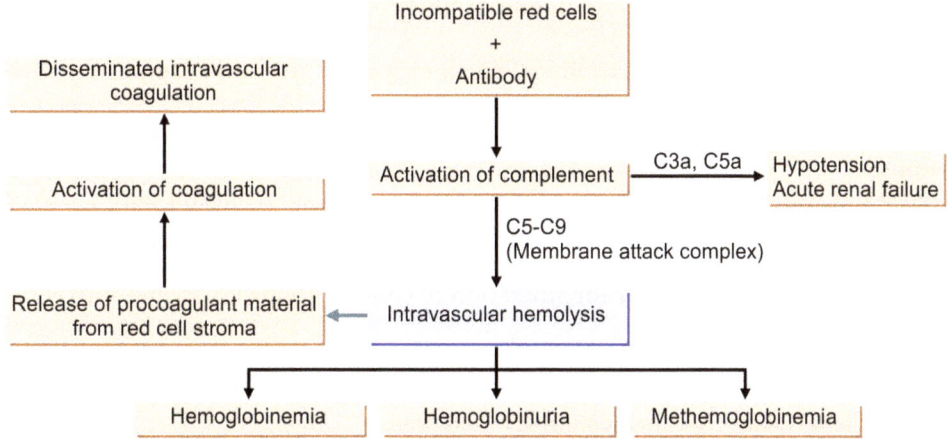

Fig. 22.1: Pathogenesis of intravascular acute HTR following ABO incompatibility.

reaction may be fatal and patient may die from shock, acute renal failure, or disseminated intravascular coagulation.

In unconscious or anesthetized patients, the only indicators of HTR may be hypotension and excess bleeding.

Acute HTR is an emergency. Treatment consists of:
- Immediate discontinuation of transfusion
- Maintenance of intravenous access with normal saline
- Management of hypotension, renal failure, and disseminated intravascular coagulation.

Investigation of a Hemolytic Transfusion Reaction

If acute HTR is suspected, blood transfusion should be immediately stopped. This is because severity of reaction partly depends on the amount of incompatible red cells transfused. The transfusion set should be removed, but the intravenous line should be maintained with normal saline. The concerned physician is immediately notified. As the clerical error is the most common cause of HTR, the label on the blood bag and the affixed compatibility label should be checked against the identity of the recipient. If there is a discrepancy, blood bank should be immediately notified since another patient may be involved in the possible mix up.

Diagnosis of acute HTR depends on demonstration of intravascular hemolysis in the recipient and of ABO incompatibility between the donor and the recipient.

Following samples should be collected from the recipient:
1. Venous blood in a plain tube and in a tube containing EDTA anticoagulant, and
2. First urine passed following transfusion.

Diagnosis of intravascular hemolysis is based on the presence of following findings in the posttransfusion sample from the recipient:
- Pink coloration of plasma (after centrifugation of EDTA blood sample)
- Spherocytes and fragmented red cells on a stained blood smear
- Hemoglobinuria
- Reduced haptoglobin in blood
- Increased indirect serum bilirubin in blood.

Demonstration of blood group incompatibility between the donor and the recipient depends on following investigations:
- Repeat ABO blood grouping and Rh typing on recipient's pre- and posttransfusion blood samples and on donor blood unit
- Repeat cross matching of donor blood against recipient's pretransfusion and posttransfusion samples
- Direct antiglobulin test (DAT) on recipient's pre- and posttransfusion samples. Positive DAT with posttransfusion sample and negative DAT with pretransfusion sample indicate occurrence of antigen-antibody reaction.

In addition, **investigations for identification of complications** associated with HTR can be carried out as follows:
- Tests for disseminated intravascular coagulation: Coagulation screen, platelet count, fibrin degradation products
- Tests for renal failure: Serum creatinine, blood urea.

It is to be noted that hemolysis of donor red cells can also result from following causes:
1. Bacterial contamination of donor unit: Infected blood shows black or purple discoloration of red cells and evidence of hemolysis. Blood from the donor unit should be sent for Gram's stain and bacterial culture.
2. Thermal damage: Keeping the blood bag in the freezer compartment of the ward refrigerator or keeping the blood unit in the hot water bowl for warming result in hemolysis.
3. Addition of drugs to the donor unit.

If no cause of hemolysis is found, possibility of a hemolytic anemia like paroxysmal nocturnal hemoglobinuria or glucose-6-phosphate dehydrogenase deficiency should be considered.

Allergic Reactions

Mild urticaria, rash, and pruritus may develop within minutes of initiating transfusion. This results from reaction between some plasma proteins and corresponding IgE antibodies in recipient's plasma (with local release of histamine). Rate of transfusion should be slowed and an antihistamine given.

Anaphylactic Reaction

Anaphylactic reaction is rare and characterized mainly by hypotension, shock, and breathlessness. There is no fever. The reaction develops within minutes of starting transfusion. A very severe anaphylaxis occurs in individuals with IgA deficiency; in these patients, anti-IgA antibodies react with IgA of donor plasma leading to activation of complement and generation of anaphylatoxins (C3a and C5a). Transfusion should be immediately stopped and patient is given adrenaline and hydrocortisone.

Transfusion-associated Lung Injury (TRALI)

Transfusion-associated lung injury manifests within 1 to 4 hours of starting transfusion and is characterized by fever, chills, respiratory distress, and dry cough. X-ray shows diffuse pulmonary infiltrates.

Potent leukoagglutinins in donor blood incompatible with granulocytes of the recipient react with leukocytes in recipient's circulation leading to the formation of leukocyte aggregates. After lodging in pulmonary microcirculation, they cause increase in vascular permeability.

Donors are generally multiparous women who develop leukoagglutinins at the time of pregnancy.

Treatment is supportive.

Circulatory Overload

Circulatory overload can develop if the rate of transfusion is too rapid (before compensatory fluid redistribution can occur), or is excessive, or if there is impairment of renal or cardiac function. It results in cardiac failure and pulmonary edema.

It is especially likely to occur in patients with chronic severe anemia and in patients with compromised cardiovascular function.

Treatment consists of propping up the patient in a sitting position, and administration of oxygen and intravenous diuretics.

Bacterial Contamination of Donor Unit

Transfusion of blood that is contaminated with bacteria can cause septicemic shock. Bacterial contamination is more common with platelet concentrates (1–2% cases) than with whole blood or packed red cells (0.4%). This is because platelet concentrates are stored at a higher temperature (20–24°C) that favors proliferation of contaminating bacteria.
Causes of bacterial contamination of a blood unit are:
- Incomplete sterilization of skin during venipuncture for blood collection
- Asymptomatic bacteremia in the donor at the time of blood collection (especially occurs with *Yersinia enterocolitica*)
- Tiny breaks in plastic bag leading to the entry of bacteria during storage
- Thawing of cryoprecipitate or fresh frozen plasma in a water bath.
  The usual contaminating organism in blood stored at 2 to 6°C is *Pseudomonas*. *Staphylococcus* is the common contaminant in platelet concentrates.
  Clinical features resemble those of an acute hemolytic transfusion reaction. After starting transfusion, patient rapidly develops high-grade fever with rigors, hypotension, and shock. Treatment consists of high doses of intravenous antibiotics and supportive measures.
  Diagnosis depends on Gram staining and culture of blood from blood bag.

DELAYED COMPLICATIONS

Delayed Hemolytic Transfusion Reaction

Delayed HTR occurs in individuals who have been sensitized earlier to certain red cell antigens by previous transfusion or pregnancy. The concentration of antibody, however, is so low that it cannot be detected by tests before transfusion. On re-exposure to the same red cell antigen, there is a secondary immune response that causes destruction (predominantly extravascular) of transfused red cells bearing the particular antigen.

Clinically, patient develops fever, anemia, and jaundice about 5 to 10 days after transfusion. Severe reaction is rare. Direct antiglobulin test is positive.

The usual antigens implicated are Rh and Kidd.

Post-transfusion Purpura

Severe thrombocytopenia can rarely develop in some adult multiparous women about 5 to 10 days following blood transfusion. There is previous sensitization of the recipient to a platelet antigen (HPA-1a or PlA1) during pregnancy; following re-exposure to the same antigen through transfusion, the antibodies paradoxically cause destruction of patient's own platelets (which are negative for HPA-1a or PlA1).

The condition is potentially fatal. Treatment consists of plasma exchange and intravenous immunoglobulins.

Transfusion-Associated Graft-versus-Host Disease

Graft-versus-host-disease can develop following:
- Blood transfusion in immunodeficient individuals (e.g. recipients of bone marrow transplant, premature infants, etc.), or
- Blood transfusion from a first-degree relative in immunocompetent individuals GVHD results from engraftment in the recipient of donor lymphocytes that react against host tissues.

About 10 to 12 days following transfusion, patient develops fever, skin rash, vomiting, diarrhea, hepatitis, and pancytopenia (bone marrow suppression). The condition is usually fatal.

Irradiation of blood (25 Gy) before transfusion is recommended to prevent proliferation of donor lymphocytes and avoid GVHD.

Transmission of Infectious Organisms

The organisms likely to be transmitted by transfusion are usually those, which are prevalent in a particular geographic area or population. Organisms transmissible by transfusion are listed in Box 22.2.

In India, pretransfusion testing of donor blood for following agents is currently mandatory (i.e. prior consent of prospective donor is not necessary) for:
- Hepatitis B virus (HBV)
- Hepatitis C virus (HCV)
- HIV-1 and HIV-2
- *Treponema pallidum* (Syphilis)
- Malaria parasite.

Infection by hepatitis B and C viruses and HIV-1 and HIV-2 is characterized by:
- Persistence of organisms in circulation for prolonged duration without necessarily causing clinical manifestations
- Long incubation period
- Ability to cause chronic carrier state
- Viability of organisms in blood stored at 4 to 6°C.

Box 22.2: Microorganisms transmissible by transfusion.

Viruses
- Hepatitis viruses
  - Hepatitis A virus
  - Hepatitis B virus
  - Hepatitis C virus
- Human immunodeficiency virus (HIV)
  - HIV-1
  - HIV-2
- Cytomegalovirus (of significance in immunocompromised recipients)
- Epstein-Barr virus (rare)
- Human T cell leukemia virus (HTLV) (endemic in Japan and the Carribbean)
  - HTLV-I
  - HTLV-II
- Human parvovirus B 19 (of significance in patients with chronic hemolysis)

Prions
- Creutzfeldt-Jakob disease (CJD) and variant CJD (not proven)

Bacteria
- *Treponema pallidum* (syphilis)
- Bacterial contamination of donor unit (*Pseudomonas*, Staphylococci)
- Brucellosis (rare)

Parasites
- Malaria parasites
- *Trypanosoma cruzi* (prevalent in Latin America)
- *Toxoplasma gondii* (of significance only in immunocompromised recipients receiving granulocyte transfusion)
- *Babesia microti* (prevalent in North America)
- *Leishmania donovani* (rare)

Following two principal measures can prevent transmission of infection through transfusion:
- Blood should be collected only from voluntary, nonremunerated donors. All high risk (intravenous drug abusers, homosexuals, prostitutes, and sexual partners of such persons) and professional donors should be excluded. Standard criteria for selection of blood donors should be followed.
- All blood donations should be tested for infectious agents by screening tests.

Reliance solely on laboratory screening tests to exclude infections transmissible by transfusion is inadequate to ensure safe blood supply.

Hepatitis B Virus

Hepatitis B virus is a partially double-stranded DNA virus of 42 nm diameter. It can cause:
- Acute hepatitis
- Chronic hepatitis
- Asymptomatic carrier state
- Cirrhosis
- Hepatocellular carcinoma.

According to WHO, more than 10% of potential blood donors in developing countries are HBV carriers. HBV is highly infectious (50-100 times more so than human immunodeficiency virus). It is transmitted through all blood components and most of the blood derivatives.

Infected hepatocytes release large amounts of hepatitis B surface antigen (HbsAg) into the bloodstream. Presence of HbsAg indicates active infection.

Screening of all blood donations for HbsAg has greatly reduced the risk of transmission of HBV through transfusion; the risk, however, is not completely eliminated. HbsAg-negative donor may transmit HBV when blood is collected in early incubation period or when very low levels of HbsAg, not detectable by presently employed methods, are present.

An individual who has received HBV vaccine will have hepatitis B surface antibody but not HbsAg in blood.

Hepatitis C Virus

Hepatitis C virus is a single-stranded RNA virus of flaviviridae family, which was first identified in 1989. Prior to its discovery, it was known as non-A, non-B (NANB) hepatitis virus. Incubation period following infection is about 8 weeks. Most cases of HCV infection are asymptomatic. Following infection, chronic hepatitis develops in majority of cases. Cirrhosis (10–20% cases) and hepatocellular carcinoma (1–5% cases) are late sequelae in patients with chronic infection.

According to estimates of WHO (1999), prevalence rate of HCV in Southeast Asia is 2.15%.

Amount of HCV antigen released in bloodstream is small and cannot be detected readily. Therefore, screening of donor blood for HCV infection relies on detection of anti-HCV antibody in serum (which becomes detectable after 6–8 weeks of infection).

Human Immunodeficiency Virus

Human immunodeficiency virus or HIV is RNA retrovirus, which causes slowly progressive immunodeficiency in infected persons. HIV infects CD4+ T lymphocytes, which play a central role in immune system. Infection leads to destruction of CD4+ lymphocytes with slowly progressive impairment of the immune system. The infected individual becomes susceptible to a range of opportunistic infections and malignancies. The most advanced stage of HIV disease is acquired immune deficiency syndrome or AIDS. HIV also infects nerve cells and causes neurological damage. HIV infection is lifelong and the infected individual remains infectious for life.

There is a wide variation in the prevalence of HIV infection between and within countries. Majority (95%) of cases of HIV infection occurring in the world are in the developing countries, the most affected region being sub-Saharan Africa. Southeast Asia is the second most affected region in the world, with majority of cases occurring in India, Myanmar, and Thailand.

According to the estimates of India's National AIDS Control Organisation (NACO), adult prevalence of HIV infection is 0.7% with approximately 4 million HIV infections, 90% of which are in the age group of 15 to 45 years.

In industrialized nations, HIV infection occurs chiefly in homosexual men and intravenous drug abusers.

In developing countries, HIV is transmitted mainly by following routes:
- Heterosexual intercourse (80% cases)

- Parenteral (i.e. transfusion of infected blood or blood products; use of blood-contaminated needles, syringes, or other skin-piercing instruments)
- Mother to child (during delivery or breastfeeding).

There are two types of HIV—HIV-1 and HIV-2.
i. *HIV-1:* This is the most common type found worldwide. It is divided into two groups—M and O. There are eight subtypes of M (A to H). In India, subtype C is prevalent.
ii. *HIV-2:* This is found mainly in West Africa, India, and Sri Lanka.

Following HIV infection, viremia becomes detectable after a few days and lasts for several weeks. During this period, the infected person may remain asymptomatic or develop a glandular fever-like illness. Anti-HIV antibodies appear 6 to 12 weeks after infection (called as seroconversion). **Window period** is the period between the onset of HIV infection and appearance of detectable antibodies in serum; it is the infectious but seronegative period (i.e. the test for anti-HIV antibodies is yet to become positive). Transfusion of donor blood collected during the window period will transmit HIV to the recipient. Collection of blood from the donor during the window period of HIV infection is, however, a rare event.

Following are main measures for the prevention of transmission of HIV through blood transfusion (Box 22.3):
- Recruitment only of voluntary, nonpaid donors and exclusion of all professional or high-risk donors
- Self-exclusion of high-risk donors
- Screening test of donor blood for anti-HIV antibodies
- Avoidance of unnecessary blood transfusions.

Box 22.3: Measures to prevent transmission by transfusion of hepatitis and HIV infections

- Transfuse only when essential. Avoid single unit transfusions
- Exclusion of all high-risk donors such as homosexuals, bisexuals, intravenous drug abusers, prostitutes, and sexual partners of these persons
- Reliance solely on voluntary donations. Exclude all professional donors
- Screening of all blood donations for HbsAg, anti-HCV, and anti-HIV before transfusion
- Use autologous transfusions wherever possible
- Viral inactivation of blood components and derivatives
- Patients requiring regular transfusion therapy (e.g. hemophilics and thalassemics) should be given HBV vaccine

Treponema Pallidum

Transmission of *Treponema (T.) pallidum* through blood transfusion causes syphilis. However, only fresh blood or platelet concentrates can transmit these organisms since storage of donor blood unit at 2 to 6°C for 48 to 72 hours inactivates *T. pallidum*. Transfusion-transmission of syphilis is, therefore, rare. The main value of testing donor blood for *T. pallidum* is to identify and exclude donors with high-risk behavior and thus who are at risk of having sexually transmitted infections.

Plasmodium Species

Malaria parasite can be transmitted through all blood components. In endemic areas, testing of all blood units for malaria parasite is not feasible; it is also not practical to reject all potential donors who have had malaria in the past. Therefore, it is essential to maintain a high degree of suspicion if a transfusion recipient develops symptoms suggestive of malaria and appropriate treatment should be given.

Iron Overload

Each unit of blood contains about 200 mg of iron, while the daily physiologic loss of iron is only 1 mg. There is no physiologic mechanism for removal of excess iron. Therefore, patients receiving regular long-term blood transfusion therapy (such as thalassemics) inevitably develop iron overload. Deposition of excess iron in heart, liver, and endocrine glands can cause respective organ failure. Iron chelating therapy with desferrioxamine should be instituted early in these patients to minimize iron accumulation.

COMPLICATIONS ASSOCIATED WITH MASSIVE BLOOD TRANSFUSION

Massive blood transfusion refers to the replacement of patient's blood loss with transfusion of stored blood equivalent to total blood volume within 24 hours. The need for massive transfusion is usually an emergency that arises following an accident or an obstetric problem. Rapid loss of large amount of blood needs urgent correction to restore blood volume and to maintain tissue perfusion, oxygenation, and hemostasis. Morbidity and mortality in these patients is usually due to the underlying condition coupled with major hemorrhage. In addition, massive blood transfusion is also associated with certain complications. Storage of blood at 2 to 6°C for 48 hours is associated with loss of platelet function and loss of labile coagulation factors (F V and F VIII). Therefore, rapid infusion of large volumes of stored blood will lead to dilution of platelets and coagulation factors. Prolongation of prothrombin time, activated partial thromboplastin time, thrombocytopenia, or bleeding manifestations are indications for platelet transfusions or fresh frozen plasma.

Hyperkalemia (due to release of potassium from stored red cells), hypocalcemia (due to binding of calcium by citrate anticoagulant), and hypothermia (due to rapid infusion of large quantity of cold blood) can induce cardiac arrhythmias.

Microaggregates composed of platelets and leukocytes form gradually in stored blood. Following massive transfusion, these microaggregates can migrate to the lungs and induce adult respiratory distress syndrome. Microaggregates can be removed during transfusion through special filters.

BIBLIOGRAPHY

1. Contreras M (Ed). ABC of Transfusion, 3rd edition. London: BMJ Books; 1998.
2. Regan F, Taylor C. Recent developments. Blood transfusion medicine. BMJ. 2002;325: 143-7.
3. World Health Organization. (2002). Blood Transfusion Safety: The Clinical Use of Blood. [online] Available from https://www.who.int/bloodsafety/clinical_use/en/Handbook_EN.pdf?ua=1 [Last Accessed March 2019].

CHAPTER 23

Autologous Transfusion

In autologous transfusion, patient's blood is collected and is reinfused back subsequently when required. Although having a limited scope, autologous transfusion has certain advantages as shown in Box 23.1.

There are three methods of autologous transfusion:
- Predeposit (preoperative blood donation)
- Acute normovolemic hemodilution
- Blood salvage

Box 23.1: Advantages of autologous transfusion.
- Avoids transmission of infectious organisms
- Avoids immunologic complications associated with homologous transfusion (such as hemolysis, alloimmunization, graft-versus-host disease, TRALI, allergic reactions)
- Reduces need for blood from homologous donors
- Avoids problem of finding compatible blood for a patient with a rare blood group or multiple red cell antibodies

PREDEPOSIT AUTOLOGOUS BLOOD TRANSFUSION

This technique is applicable to those patients who are posted for elective surgery, are otherwise fit, and are likely to need blood since significant operative blood losses are expected. Patient's blood is collected in a blood bag before elective surgery, stored in the blood bank, and is reinfused back after surgery to replace the operative blood losses. Blood collection from the patient starts 5 weeks before surgery. One unit of blood is collected every 7 days. Patient should be living near the transfusion center. Maximum of total 4 units can be collected, with the number depending on the nature of surgery. The last donation is collected at least 4 days before operation to allow restoration of plasma volume. Patient is put on oral iron supplements to maintain hemoglobin level. Before each donation, hemoglobin level should be more than 11.0 g/dL. Blood bag(s) should be properly labelled and stored in the blood bank refrigerator. Pre-transfusion testing is carried out as for other homologous blood units.

If patient's blood group is rare or multiple antibodies against common red cell antigens are present, compatible blood may be difficult to find. In such cases, patient's red cells can be stored frozen for many years for any future requirement.

This technique is contraindicated in patients with cancer, significant cardiovascular disease, anemia, trauma, uncontrolled hypertension, epilepsy, and pregnancy. Patients with bacteremia should be excluded because proliferation of bacteria during storage can induce septicemic shock following transfusion. Patients having infections transmissible by transfusion should also not be considered since clerical or administrative error may cause blood to be transfused inadvertently to the wrong recipient.

Wastage of donated blood unit(s) can occur in the event of cancellation of surgery or if the amount of blood donated exceeds the required amount. Unused blood is often not suitable for other donors because strict criteria for selection of donors are not followed.

Predeposit autotransfusion cannot prevent the risk of circulatory overload, clerical error leading to hemolytic transfusion reaction, and bacterial contamination (during collection).

Close coordination between patient, surgeon, and blood bank is required. Implementation of this technique requires considerable planning and organization.

ACUTE NORMOVOLEMIC HEMODILUTION

Immediately before beginning surgery, patient's whole blood (1 or 2 units) is collected in blood bag(s) containing suitable anticoagulant. To maintain the blood volume, equivalent amount of crystalloid (at least 3 mL for every 1 mL of blood collected) or colloid (1 mL for every 1 mL collected) solution is infused. During surgery, the artificially created acute normovolemic hemodilution will reduce the red cell loss for the given amount of bleeding. The collected blood units are returned back to the patient after surgical bleeding is controlled. Blood collected from the patient is labelled and kept near the patient. It remains at room temperature for only a short period so that there is minimal loss of coagulation factors and platelets. Testing and cross-matching are not carried out. Keeping the blood bag near the patient minimizes the risk of administrative error (i.e. transfusing blood to the wrong patient). This procedure can be carried out if significant blood loss is anticipated during surgery, i.e. greater than 1000 mL or 20% of blood volume. It should not be carried out in patients who will be unable to tolerate reduction in oxygen supply due to hemodilution (e.g. those having cardiopulmonary disease). Careful monitoring of the patient during surgery is essential.

BLOOD SALVAGE

Blood salvage consists of collection of blood that is shed during surgery (intraoperative blood salvage) or following surgery (postoperative blood salvage) and subsequent re-infusion of the recovered blood to the same patient.

Blood salvage can be carried out in elective as well as emergency surgery when expected blood loss is extensive, for example, cardiac surgery, total knee replacement, trauma surgery, ruptured ectopic pregnancy, or ruptured spleen. This procedure should not be carried out if salvaged blood is contaminated with bowel contents, urine, bacteria, amniotic fluid, or malignant cells. Re-infusion of blood that was collected more than 6 hours back can be harmful due to red cell lysis, hyperkalemia, and bacterial contamination.

In intraoperative blood salvage, blood lost during surgery is aspirated from the operative field, anticoagulated, filtered to remove clots and debris, centrifuged, washed, and suspended in sterile saline before re-infusion. A red cell product free of contaminants is thus obtained. The technique requires an expensive automated blood salvage device and for each patient costly disposable materials.

In postoperative blood salvage, blood is recovered from wound drains and re-infused back directly through a filter.

BIBLIOGRAPHY

1. Vanderlinde ES, Heal JM, Blumberg N. Autologous transfusion. BMJ. 2002;324: 772-5.
2. World Health Organization. (2002). Blood Transfusion Safety: The Clinical Use of Blood. Geneva. World Health Organization.

CHAPTER 24

Alternatives to Blood Transfusion

INTRODUCTION

Although blood transfusion can be lifesaving; it is associated with a risk of serious complications and of transmission of infections (see "Adverse effects of transfusion"). Therefore, blood transfusion should be considered only if there are no alternative means of therapy and there is a likelihood of significant morbidity or mortality without transfusion. Blood transfusion can be avoided or its use can be minimized through the following measures:

- **Avoidance of single unit transfusions**. One unit of blood raises hemoglobin only by 1 g/dL and rarely provides clinical benefit in chronic anemia
- **Avoidance of unnecessary administration of blood** (e.g. before surgery to raise hemoglobin level, to effect early discharge from hospital, etc.)
- **Early diagnosis and specific treatment of anemia**
- **Use of safer alternatives,** like synthetic crystalloids or colloids if only volume replacement is required
- **Meticulous surgical and anesthetic techniques** to minimize operative blood losses
- **Consideration of autologous transfusion** in healthy patients undergoing elective surgery
- **Use of drugs to reduce bleeding during surgery** like aprotinin, tranexamic acid, fibrin glues, and sealants
- **Exploration of alternatives to blood transfusion:** (a) hematopoietic growth factors, (b) recombinant blood coagulation factors, or (c) red cell substitutes.

HEMATOPOIETIC GROWTH FACTORS

Hematopoietic growth factors (HGFs) are polypeptides that regulate proliferation, differentiation, and maturation of hematopoietic progenitor cells. Erythropoietin, granulocyte macrophage-colony stimulating factor (GM-CSF), and granulocyte-colony stimulating factor (G-CSF) are the HGFs that are currently available commercially. They are produced by recombinant DNA technology.

Erythropoietin

This is produced in the kidneys (90%) and in the liver (10%). It stimulates erythroid precursors to proliferate, differentiate, and mature. Recombinant erythropoietin is the treatment of choice in anemia of chronic renal failure and significantly reduces the need for red cell transfusions in end-stage renal disease. It is also helpful in anemia of cancer and in anemia in HIV-positive patients receiving zidovudine. Desirable response is obtained after several weeks of therapy with erythropoietin. Therefore, it is not helpful in acutely developing anemias.

Granulocyte Macrophage-Colony Stimulating Factor

Granulocyte macrophage-colony stimulating factor (GM-CSF) stimulates proliferation, differentiation, and maturation of precursor cells of neutrophil and monocyte/macrophage cell lines. Recombinant GM-CSF accelerates myeloid recovery following bone marrow transplantation, and shortens duration of neutropenia after chemotherapy-induced myelosuppression.

Granulocyte-Colony Stimulating Factor

Granulocyte-colony stimulating factor (G-CSF) stimulates myeloid progenitor cells to form mature neutrophils. Recombinant G-CSF is used to shorten the period of neutropenia following myelosuppressive chemotherapy.

RED CELL SUBSTITUTES

Red cell substitutes are being developed which will transport oxygen from the lungs to the tissues similar to red cells. To be effective, red cell substitutes should bind oxygen in the lungs, readily release oxygen at the tissue level, should be non-toxic and non-immunogenic, sterilizable, and should remain functional in circulation for long duration. Currently, hemoglobin solutions and perfluorocarbons are undergoing clinical trials, but their major problem is short half-lives in circulation.

Red cell substitutes include the following :
- Hemoglobin solutions
- Perfluorocarbons.

Hemoglobin Solutions

Hemoglobin solutions are obtained from various sources, such as the following:
- Human red cells (outdated blood units)
- Bovine red cells

Hemoglobin solutions prepared from human and bovine sources carry the risk of transmission of infections
- Transgenic animals: Hemoglobin gene is introduced into the embryo of animals like mice or pigs at an early stage of development. This leads to the synthesis of human hemoglobin in the transgenic animal
- Recombinant DNA technique.

Disadvantages of Hemoglobin Solutions

- *Short survival in circulation*: Free hemoglobin molecules rapidly disintegrate into smaller fragments in circulation, which are then cleared by the kidneys. To increase the survival of hemoglobin in circulation, following modifications have been tried: (1) intramolecular cross-linking of a hemoglobin molecule; (2) intermolecular cross-linking of many hemoglobin molecules to form large polymers of hemoglobin; (3) attaching hemoglobin to a polymer; and (4) enclosure of hemoglobin molecule in a lipid membrane (encapsulated hemoglobin).
- *Kidney damage*: Hemoglobin solutions contaminated with red cell stroma or fragmented molecules of hemoglobin can induce disseminated intravascular coagulation and renal damage.
- *Vasoconstriction* with marked rise in blood pressure and reduction in cardiac output.
- *Increased oxygen affinity:* Once outside the red cell, hemoglobin loses its ability to bind 2,3-DPG with consequent increase in oxygen affinity. To decrease the oxygen affinity of free hemoglobin molecule, hemoglobin is treated with pyridoxal-5-phosphate.

Perfluorocarbons (PFCs)

These are organic molecules in which hydrogen atoms have been replaced by fluorine. They can dissolve large amount of oxygen molecules. Oxygen dissociation curve of PFCs is linear (not sigmoid like that of hemoglobin). They are emulsified before infusion since they are not miscible with water and blood.

They circulate in blood for only a short duration and are considered as a temporary red cell substitute. One indication is maintaining oxygenation of distal myocardium during balloon angioplasty.

BIBLIOGRAPHY

1. Boral LI, Weiss ED, Henry JB. Transfusion medicine. In: Henry JB (Ed). Clinical Diagnosis and Management by Laboratory Methods, 20th edition. Philadelphia: WB Saunders Company; 2001.
2. Lowe KC. Red Cell Substitutes. In: Contreras M (Ed). ABC of Transfusion, 3rd edition. London: BMJ Books; 1998.

APPENDICES

APPENDIX A
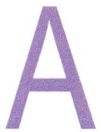

Reference Ranges

Reference ranges differ in different populations and also vary from laboratory to laboratory. Values obtained in an individual patient are best compared with the reference range established locally and interpreted in the context of clinical features and other investigations. Following reference values should be considered only as a rough guideline.

Hemoglobin:
- Adult males: 13.0–17.0 g/dL
- Adult females (nonpregnant): 12.0–15.0 g/dL
- Adult females (pregnant): 11.0–14.0 g/dL
- Children 6–12 years: 11.5–15.5 g/dL
- Children 6 months to 6 years: 11.0–14.0 g/dL
- Infants 2–6 months: 9.5–14.0 g/dL
- Newborns: 13.6–19.6 g/dL

Packed cell volume:
- Adult males: 40–50%
- Adult females (nonpregnant): 38–45%
- Adult females (pregnant): 36–42%
- Children 6–12 years: 37–46%
- Children 6 months to 6 years: 36–42%
- Infants 2–6 months: 32–42%
- Newborns: 44–60%

Red cell count:
- Adult males: 4.5–5.5 million/mm^3
- Adult females: 3.8–4.8 million/mm^3

Red cell indices:
- Mean cell volume (MCV): 80–100 fL
- Mean corpuscular hemoglobin (MCH): 27.0–32.0 pg
- Mean corpuscular hemoglobin concentration (MCHC): 32.0–36.0 g/dL

Reticulocyte count:
- Reticulocyte percentage: 0.5–2.5%
- Absolute reticulocyte count: 50,000–100,000/mm³

Relative proportions of hemoglobins:
- HbA: 95–97%
- HbA2: 1.5–3.5%
- HbF: <1%

Erythrocyte sedimentation rate (Westergren) (Upper limits):
- Adult males: 15 mm
- Adult females: 20 mm
- Children: 10 mm
- Elderly: Males—14 mm; females—20 mm

Osmotic fragility of red cells:
- Starts at 0.5% of sodium chloride or lower
- Complete at 0.3% of sodium chloride

Total leukocyte count (adults): 4,000–11,000/mm³

Differential leukocyte count (Adults):
- Neutrophils: 40–75%
- Lymphocytes: 20–40%
- Monocytes: 2–10%
- Eosinophils: 1–6%
- Basophils: <1%

Neutrophil alkaline phosphatase (NAP) score: 40–100

Platelet count: 150,000–400,000/mm³

Iron studies:
- Serum iron: 50–150 µg/dL
- Total iron binding capacity (TIBC): 300–400 µg/dL
- Percent transferrin saturation: 20–55%
- Free erythrocyte protoporphyrin (FEP): <80 µg/dL
- Serum transferrin receptor: 2.8–8.5 mg/L
- Serum ferritin: 15–300 µg/L

Vitamin B_{12} and folate studies:
- Serum vitamin B_{12}: 150–700 ng/L
- Serum folate: 3–20 µg/L
- Red cell folate: 150–700 µg/L

Coagulation studies:
- Bleeding time (BT):
  - Ivy method: 2–7 minutes
  - Template method: 2.5–9.5 minutes

- Prothrombin time (PT): 11–16 seconds
- International normalized ratio (INR): 0.8–1.2
- Activated partial thromboplastin time (APTT): 30–40 seconds
- Thrombin time (TT): ±3 seconds of control
- Plasma fibrinogen: 200–400 mg/dL
- Fibrinogen/fibrin degradation products (FDPs): <10 μg/mL
- D-dimer: <200 mg/L
- Factors II, V, VII, VIII, IX, X, XI, XII (percent activity): 50–150%
- vWF:Ag: 50–150%
- vWF:RCo: 50–200 IU/dL.

Differential count in bone marrow in adults:

- Myeloblasts: 0–3%
- Promyelocytes: 2–5%
- Neutrophil myelocytes: 8–15%
- Metamyelocytes: 9–24%
- Neutrophils (including band forms): 14–26%
- Erythroblasts: 15–36%
- Lymphocytes: 5–20%
- Plasma cells: 0–3%
- Myeloid:Erythroid (M:E) ratio: 2:1 to 4:1

Iron staining of bone marrow smears:

- Sideroblasts 30–50% of all erythroblasts
- No ringed sideroblasts

Biochemical studies:
- Serum bilirubin:
    - Total: <1.0 mg/dL
    - Direct: 0–0.2 mg/dL
- Total serum proteins: 6.0–8.0 g/dL
- Serum albumin: 3.5–5.0 g/dL
- Serum immunoglobulins:
    - IgG: 700–1,500 mg/dL
    - IgA: 100–500 mg/dL
    - IgM: 50–250 mg/dL
- Serum creatinine: 0.5–1.2 mg/dL
- Serum lactate dehydrogenase: 200–450 IU/L
- Serum uric acid: 3.0–8.0 mg/dL
- Serum calcium (total): 9.0–11.0 mg/dL
- Serum β2 microglobulin: 1.2–2.4 mg/L
- Serum haptoglobin: 0.8–2.7g/L
- Serum methylmalonic acid (MMA): 0–0.4 micromol/L
- Serum homocysteine: 4–15 micromol/L

APPENDIX B

Selected Cluster of Differentiation Antigens

The cluster of differentiation (CD) antigen system is a nomenclature system for the differentiation of antigens on the surface of white blood cells and certain other cells. Each CD antigen is ascribed a number (CD1, CD2, etc.). A variety of monoclonal antibodies bearing different names are available commercially for identification of these antigens. Functions of some of these molecules are cell adhesion, signaling, cell protection, etc. while those of other molecules are unknown.

Applications of CD antigen analysis in hematology are summarized here.

Hematologic Neoplasms

The main applications of flow cytometry in neoplastic hematopathology are:
- Diagnosis and classification of hematological neoplasms,
- Distinction of neoplastic from non-neoplastic processes,
- Identification of prognostic markers,
- Identification of potential therapeutic targets (e.g. monoclonal antibody rituximab directed against CD20 antigen), and
- Identification of minimal residual disease after therapy through aberrantly expressed antigens.

Lineage assignment markers are (WHO, 2008):
- *Acute lymphoblastic leukemias (ALL):* Antigens employed for B-lineage assignment are—(1) strong CD19 with at least one of the following strongly expressed markers: CD79a, cytoplasmic CD22, CD10; *or* (2) weak CD19 with at least two of the following strongly expressed markers: CD79a, cytoplasmic CD22, CD10.

  Antigens used for lineage assignment in T-ALL are—(1) cytoplasmic CD3 *or* (2) surface CD3.
- *Acute myeloid leukemia:* Antigens employed for myeloid lineage assignment are—(1) myeloperoxidase *or* (2) monocytic differentiation (at least two of the following markers: Nonspecific esterase, CD11c, CD14, CD64, lysozyme).

  Aberrant antigen expression in hematological neoplasms: Aberrant expression of antigen refers to expression of an antigen which is inappropriate for a lineage. Identification of such markers is helpful for identification of a neoplastic process and also helps in early detection of relapse and in detection of minimal residual disease. Examples: (1) Expression of CD19,

Appendix B: Selected Cluster of Differentiation Antigens

a pan-B marker, in AML with t(8;21); (2) Expression of CD7, a pan-T marker, in AML, acute promyelocytic leukemia, and monocytic leukemia.
3. *Mature B- and T-lymphoid neoplasms*: Mature lymphoid neoplasms are identified by an immunophenotype identical to mature lymphoid cells along with lack of expression of antigens of immaturity like TdT, CD34, and a weak expression of CD45.

Applications of flow cytometry in mature lymphoid neoplasms are:
- Identification of clonality: Immunoglobulin light chain class restriction (either kappa or lambda) is often used as a surrogate marker of clonality in mature B cell neoplasms.
- Diagnosis of mature B cell neoplasms.
- Prognosis of CLL/SLL: Expression of CD38 and ZAP-70 has prognostic importance in CLL/SLL.
- Identify targets for potential antibody-directed therapy.
- Detection of minimal residual disease: Aberrant antigen expression on neoplastic cells is helpful in monitoring patients following chemotherapy, e.g. expression of CD5, a pan-T cell marker in CLL and mantle cell lymphoma.
- Analysis of DNA ploidy, proliferation (S-phase), and programmed cell death (apoptosis).

Non-neoplastic Conditions

Leukocyte analysis:
- *Enumeration of lymphocyte subsets:* (1) The absolute CD4 count (CD3+ CD4+ subset) is used for predicting, staging, and monitoring disease progression and response to treatment in HIV+ve individuals. An inverted ratio (less than 1.0) is the usual finding in AIDS. (2) Total lymphocyte count (CD45+, CD14-), T lymphocytes (CD3+), cytotoxic T cells (CD3+CD8+), B lymphocytes (CD19+ or CD20+), and NK cells (CD16+ CD56+ CD3-) can be analyzed for evaluation of other immunodeficiency disorders.
- *Enumeration of CD34+ hematopoietic stem cells:* CD34 is a marker of hematopoietic stem cells and their (CD34+ CD45^{dim} cells with low side scatter) enumeration in peripheral blood or bone marrow is done in hematopoietic stem cell transplantation. This provides an estimate of the capacity of the stem cell product for repopulation after stem cell transplant. The numbers are used to decide the amount of product to be used for infusion.
- *Evaluation of neutrophil function:*
    - *Chronic granulomatous disease*: In chronic granulomatous disease, respiratory burst activity is deficient. Dihydrorhodamine 123 (DHR123) is a dye that is taken up by neutrophils, and when respiratory burst is stimulated, it is reduced and emits a strong fluorescent signal. In the absence of respiratory burst, the dye is non-fluorescent.
    - *Leukocyte adhesion deficiency*: In leukocyte adhesion deficiency, there is a congenital deficiency of leukocyte β2 integrin receptor complex (CD11/CD18) on the surface of neutrophils; this receptor is essential for neutrophil adherence to endothelial cells and transendothelial migration. Deficiency of CD11/CD18 antigen complex can be detected by flow cytometry.
- *Detection of intracytoplasmic myeloperoxidase in leukocytes:* MPO is an enzyme present in primary granules of neutrophils necessary for intracellular killing of microorganisms. Flow cytometry is a sensitive test for detection of MPO deficiency.
- *Detection of antileukocyte antibodies:* Antineutrophil antibodies, either free or bound to neutrophils, can be readily detected by flow cytometry and thus identify the cause of neutropenia.

Erythrocyte analysis:
- *Paroxysmal nocturnal hemoglobinuria (PNH)*: PNH can be diagnosed by identification of deficiency of GPI-anchored proteins like CD55 and CD59 on both erythrocytes and white blood cells, CD14 on monocytes, and CD66b on granulocytes. Another reagent fluorescent aerolysin (FLAER) binds specifically to GPI linkage and can identify GPI-deficient cells.
- *Detection and enumeration of red cells containing fetal hemoglobin*: Fetal red cells are identified by their high content of HbF and are readily distinguished from F cells (red cells containing intermediate amounts of HbF along with adult hemoglobin) and normal adult cells. Detection of HbF can be done using monoclonal antibodies against HbF. Applications include detection and quantification of fetal red cells in maternal circulation, quantification HbF in red cells of adults with hemoglobinopathies, and monitoring the effect of drugs stimulating HbF production in sickle cell anemia and thalassemia.
- *Reticulocyte counting*: Reticulocytes are young red cells containing residual RNA. Certain dyes like thiazole orange, thioflavin T, and ethidium bromide bind to RNA allowing detection and enumeration of these cells with precision by flow cytometry. Reticulocyte count is helpful in assessing the rate of production of red cells in bone marrow in hypoproliferative anemias like iron deficiency anemia, megaloblastic anemia, aplastic anemia, etc. and in assessing response to specific treatment.

Platelet analysis:
- *Diagnosis of inherited disorders of platelet function* due to deficiency of platelet receptors: Flow cytometry is a rapid method for detecting deficiency of platelet receptors in inherited platelet disorders: GpIIb/IIIa (Glanzmann's thrombasthenia), GpIb/IX/V (Bernard-Soulier syndrome), GpIa/IIa or GpVI (collagen receptor deficiency), and GpIba (platelet-type von Willebrand disease).
- *Reticulated platelets*: Immature or reticulated platelets can be identified and quantified by using a dye like thiazole orange which binds RNA. Immature platelets are increased in peripheral blood in thrombocytopenia due platelet destruction and decreased in thrombocytopenia due to reduced platelet production.
- *Antiplatelet antibodies*: Antibodies against platelets (immune thrombocytopenic purpura, neonatal alloimmune thrombocytopenia) can be detected by flow cytometry.
- *Platelet activation*: Flow cytometric determination of platelet activation can be clinically important in cardiac bypass surgery, and in treatment of patients with atherosclerotic coronary, cerebral, and peripheral vascular disease. Activated platelets express certain antigens (such as CD62P, CD63) which can be detected by flow cytometry. In addition, platelet activation results in formation of platelet-platelet, platelet-granulocyte, and platelet-monocyte aggregates which also can be detected.

Appendix B: Selected Cluster of Differentiation Antigens

Designation	Main reactivity	Use(s)
CD antigens		
CD1a	Cortical thymocytes, Langerhans cells	Langerhans cell histiocytosis; T-ALL; Thymoma
CD2	T lymphocytes (Pan T-cell marker), NK cells	T-ALL; Peripheral T cell lymphoma; NK cell neoplasms; Aberrant expression in CLL, HCL, microgranular type of acute promyelocytic leukemia, and in mast cell neoplasms
CD3	T lymphocytes (Pan T-cell marker; most specific marker for T cells)	T-ALL; Mature T-cell neoplasms
CD4	T helper cells, monocytes, dendritic cells	Peripheral T-cell lymphoma; Monocytic AML; angioimmunoblastic T-cell lymphoma; mycosis fungoides; Sézary syndrome; anaplastic large cell lymphoma; blastic plasmacytoid dendritic cell neoplasm
CD5	T lymphocytes	T-ALL; Mature T-cell neoplasms,; CD5+ mature B cell neoplasms (CLL/SLL, mantle cell lymphoma)
CD7	T lymphocytes	Mature T-cell neoplasms including T-PLL; T-ALL; aberrant expression in AML
CD8	Cytotoxic suppressor T lymphocytes	Mature T-cell neoplasms including T-large granular lymphocytic leukemia
CD10	Precursor B lymphocytes, neutrophils	B-ALL; follicular lymphoma; Burkitt lymphoma
CD11c	Monocytes, granulocytes, activated T lymphocytes	Hairy cell leukemia; acute monoblastic leukemia
CD13	Pan-myeloid antigen	Most cases of AML
CD14	Monocytes	Acute myelomonocytic leukemia (monocytic component); chronic myelomonocytic leukemia
CD15	Monocytes; granulocytes	Reed-Sternberg cells in classical Hodgkin lymphoma; AML with maturation
CD19	Pan B-cell marker	B-ALL; mature B-cell neoplasms
CD20	Pan B-cell marker	Mature B-cell neoplasms
CD22	Pan B-cell marker	B-ALL; hairy cell leukemia
CD23	B lymphocyte subsets	CLL/SLL
CD25	Activated B and T lymphocytes	Hairy cell leukemia; peripheral T cell lymphoma; adult T-cell leukemia/lymphoma; anaplastic large cell lymphoma

Contd...

Contd...

Designation	Main reactivity	Use(s)
CD30	Activated B and T lymphocytes	Reed-Sternberg cells in classical Hodgkin lymphoma; anaplastic large cell lymphoma
CD33	Pan myeloid marker	Acute myeloid leukemia
CD34	Stem cell or blast marker	AML; ALL
CD38	Plasma cells, activated T and B cells	Plasma cell neoplasms; prognostic marker in CLL
CD41	Megakaryocytes	Acute megakaryoblastic leukemia; also used to identify deficiency of GpIIb (CD41) in Glanzmann's thrombasthenia
CD42	Megakaryocytes	Acute megakaryoblastic leukemia
CD45*	Leukocyte common antigen (LCA)	AML (moderate+); B-ALL (dim+); Mature B-cell neoplasms (bright+)
CD55	Multilineage	Decay accelerating factor; absent on PNH cells
CD56	NK cells; T cell (subset); monocytes (subset)	Large granular lymphocytic leukemia; blastic plasmacytoid dendritic cell neoplasm; Plasma cell myeloma; Extranodal NK-T cell lymphoma
CD59	Multilineage	Membrane inhibitor of reactive lysis (MIRL); absent on PNH cells
CD61	Megakaryocytes; platelets	Acute megakaryoblastic leukemia; also used to identify deficiency of GpIIIa (CD61) in Glanzmann's thrombasthenia
CD64	Monocytes; macrophages	Acute leukemias with monocytic differentiation
CD71	Transferrin receptor	Pure erythroid leukemia
CD79a	B lymphocytes; plasma cells	B ALL; plasma cell myeloma
CD103	-	Hairy cell leukemia; hairy cell leukemia variant
CD117	C-kit; stem cell factor	AML; acute myelomonocytic leukemia; acute megakaryoblastic leukemia; mast cell neoplasms; plasma cell neoplasms; gastrointestinal stromal tumor
CD123	Plasmacytoid dendritic cells; hematopoietic progenitors	AML; hairy cell leukemia; blastic plasmacytoid dendritic cell neoplasm
CD138	Plasma cells	Plasma cell neoplasms
CD200	T lymphocytes, B lymphocytes, thymocytes	CLL/SLL (negative in mantle cell lymphoma); hairy cell leukemia; B-ALL; AML
CD235a (glycophorin A)	Erythropoietic precursors	Pure erythroid leukemia

Contd...

Contd...

Designation	Main reactivity	Use(s)
\multicolumn{3}{c}{**Other immunostains**}		
MPO	Granulocytes and precursors	AML
HLA-DR	Hematopoietic progenitor cells, and myeloid, erythroid, and megakaryocytic precursors; B-cells at different stages; immature T cells	Precursor and mature B-cell neoplasms; AML (negative in acute promyelocytic leukemia and plasma cell neoplasms)
TdT	Precursor marrow cells, cortical thymocytes	B cell and T-cell ALL; thymoma; hematogones; subset of AML (minimally differentiated)
Ki67	Proliferating cells	Assessment of mitotic activity in B-cell lymphomas
MUM1	Plasma cells	Plasma cell neoplasms
PAX-5	B cells	B-cell lymphomas including lymphoblasts; Hodgkin lymphoma

Note: (1) *CD45 is a general marker for hematopoietic neoplasms (pan-hematopoietic marker). Hematopoietic neoplasms that are CD45-negative: plasma cell myeloma, classical Hodgkin lymphoma, a subset of B-and T-lymphoblastic lymphomas, anaplastic large cell lymphoma, myeloid sarcoma (variable). CD45 is a part of a first-line panel for distinguishing hematopoietic from non-hematopoietic neoplasms. (2) Precursor markers: CD34, CD117, TdT. (3) Pan B-cell markers: CD19, CD20, CD22, CD79a, PAX-5. (4) Pan T-cell markers: CD2, CD3, CD5, CD7. (5) NK cell markers: CD3e, CD56, Perforin, Granzyme. (6) Myeloid markers: MPO, CD13, CD33. (6) Monocytic markers: CD68, CD163, Lysozyme, CD4, CD14. (7) Megakaryocytic markers: CD41, CD42a, CD61, vWF. (8) Erythroid markers: Glycophorin A, Hemoglobin, Spectrin.

APPENDIX C

Critical Values in Hematology

Critical values (also called as action values or callback values) refer to the laboratory results that need to be notified urgently to the concerned clinician since they may be indicative of a critical or sometimes life-threatening condition of the patient and thus need for urgent clinical intervention. Hematological critical values are listed here.

Critical values in hematology	
Laboratory test result	Interpretation/risk
1. Activated partial thromboplastin time ≥75 sec	Bleeding
2. D-dimer: Positive	Disseminated intravascular coagulation
3. Plasma fibrinogen <100 mg/dL	Bleeding
4. Fibrin monomer: Positive	Disseminated intravascular coagulation
5. Hemoglobin <7.0 g/dL	Myocardial ischemia
6. Hemoglobin >20 g/dL	Hyperviscosity syndrome
7. Total leukocyte count <2,000/mm^3	Infection especially if absolute neutrophil count <500/mm^3
8. Total leukocyte count >50,000/mm^3	Leukemoid reaction, leukemia
9. Prothrombin time >30 sec or >3 times control	Bleeding
10. Platelet count <20,000/mm^3	Bleeding
11. Platelet count >1 million/mm^3	Thrombosis
12. Blood smear showing blast cells	Leukemoid reaction, leukemia
13. Blood smear showing sickle cells	Crises
14. Blood smear showing *Plasmodium falciparum* ring forms	Cerebral malaria
15. New diagnosis of aplastic anemia	
16. New diagnosis of hematological malignancy	

APPENDIX D

Association of Morphology, Special Stains, and Laboratory Tests with Disease

MORPHOLOGY

Abnormal localization of immature precursors (ALIP): Myelodysplastic syndrome.

Acanthocyte: McLeod phenotype, severe liver disease (spur cell hemolytic anemia), abetalipoproteinemia, following splenectomy.

Anisocytosis: Variation in size of red cells; a common nonspecific abnormality in hematological disorders.

Atypical lymphocyte (Turk cell, Downey cell, reactive lymphocyte): Viral infections (especially infectious mononucleosis), following intake of certain drugs, postimmunization, and in autoimmune disorders.

Auer rod (John Auer, US physician, 1875–1948): Acute myeloid leukemia; also seen in RAEB-T subtype of myelodysplastic syndrome.

Autoagglutination of red cells: Cold antibody hemolytic anemia (paroxysmal cold hemoglobinuria, cold hemagglutinin disease).

Basket cell (Smudge cell): Chronic lymphocytic leukemia.

Basophilic stippling (Punctate basophilia): Megaloblastic anemia, lead poisoning, thalassemia, hereditary deficiency of pyrimidine 5'-nucleotidase.

Birbeck granules (Michael S Birbeck, 20th century British cancer researcher): Langerhans cells on electron microscopy.

Bite cell (keratocyte, degmacyte): G6PD efficiency.

Blister cell (hemighost cell): G6PD deficiency.

Boat-shaped cell: Sickle cell disease.

Botryoid nuclei (resembling bunch of grapes) of neutrophils: Heatstroke, burns, hyperthermia

Burr cell (echinocyte, crenated cell): Uremia.

Cabot's rings (Richard Clarke Cabot, US physician, 1868–1939): Megaloblastic anemia.

Contracted red cell (pyknocyte): G6PD deficiency.

Dacryocyte. *See* Teardrop red cell.

Dimorphic red cells: Presence of two distinct red cell populations; most commonly mixture of microcytic hypochromic red cells plus normochromic (normocytic or macrocytic) red cells; causes include iron deficiency anemia after administration of iron or blood transfusion; sideroblastic anemia, macrocytic anemia after blood transfusion, combined deficiency of iron and folate/vitamin B_{12}.

Döhle body in neutrophils (Karl GP Döhle, German histologist and pathologist, 1855–1928): Infections, burns, pregnancy, administration of some cytokines, and anticancer drugs. Döhle-like inclusion bodies are seen in May-Hegglin anomaly.

Downey cell (Hal Downey, US hematologist, 1877–1959): *See* atypical lymphocyte.

Drepanocyte: *See* Sickle cell.

Drumstick appendage in neutrophils: Seen in 2–3% of mature neutrophils in peripheral blood of females; represents one inactivated X chromosome.

Dutcher body (Thomas F Dutcher, 20th century US pathologist): Intranuclear inclusions in plasma cells in multiple myeloma and in Waldenström macroglobulinemia.

Dwarf megakaryocyte: Chronic myeloid leukemia.

Echinocyte: Previously called "Burr cell"; seen in chronic renal failure (uremia), storage artifact.

Elliptocyte: Numerous in hereditary elliptocytosis; a few elliptocytes in iron deficiency anemia.

Faggot cells: Acute promyelocytic leukemia (AML M3).

Flame cells: IgA-secreting plasma cell myeloma, reactive plasma cells.

Fragmented red cell (schistocyte): Microangiopathic hemolytic anemias, mechanical hemolytic anemias, hereditary pyropoikilocytosis, burns.

Fried-egg appearance: Appearance on bone marrow biopsy in hairy cell leukemia.

Gasser cells (Konrad J Gasser, 20th century Swiss pediatrician): Lymphocytes that contain large basophilic granules made of mucopolysaccharides; seen in mucopolysaccharidoses.

Gaucher cell (Philippe Charles Ernest Gaucher, French physician, 1854–1918): Gaucher's disease.

Gelatinous transformation of bone marrow (serous atrophy of bone marrow): Anorexia nervosa, cachexia (due to AIDS, cancer, lymphoma, tuberculosis).

Giant band forms: Megaloblastic anemia.

Giant metamyelocyte: Megaloblastic anemia.

Giant platelets: Bernard-Soulier syndrome, MYH-9 syndromes, and myeloproliferative neoplasms.

Hairy cell: Hairy cell leukemia.

Half ghost cell (hemighost cell): G6PD deficiency.

Hand mirror cell: Acute lymphoblastic leukemia.

HbH inclusions: Hemoglobin Bart's hydrops fetalis syndrome, hemoglobin H disease, α thalassemia carrier states.

Heinz body (Heinz-Ehrlich bodies, Ehrlich bodies) (Robert Heinz, German pathologist, 1865–1924): G6PD deficiency, unstable hemoglobin disease.

Heinz-Ehrlich bodies (Robert Heinz, German pathologist, 1865–1924; Paul Ehrlich, German physician and biochemist, 1854–1915): *See* Heinz bodies.

Helmet cell (keratocyte): Microangiopathic hemolytic anemias.

Hematogones: Normal B-cell precursors (lymphoblasts) in bone marrow whose morphology and immunophenotype are similar to lymphoblasts of ALL; they are present in small numbers in marrow of normal children and are increased during regeneration of marrow after chemotherapy or bone marrow transplantation.

Howell-Jolly bodies (William H Howell, US physiologist, 1860–1945, Justin Jolly, French histologist, 1870–1953): Megaloblastic anemia, following splenectomy.

Hypersegmented neutrophils: Neutrophils with 5 or more lobes in peripheral blood that are greater than 5% of all neutrophils are seen in megaloblastic anemia; also seen in myelokathexis, iron deficiency anemia, uremia, and myelodysplastic syndrome.

Hyperchromia: Red cells stained more intensely than normal like spherocytes and irregularly contracted cells.

Hypochromia: Causes similar to microcytosis.

Hyposegmentation of neutrophils: Hereditary Pelger-Huët anomaly, acquired Pelger-Huët anomaly (myelodysplastic syndrome, AML), specific granule deficiency.

Irregularly contracted cell: G6PD deficiency, unstable hemoglobin disease, Wilson disease.

Juvenile cell: Metamyelocyte.

Keratocyte (horned cell): Previously called helmet cell, bite cell; seen in microangiopathic hemolytic anemia, cardiac valve prosthesis, disseminated intravascular coagulation, G6PD deficiency.

L and H cell (popcorn cell): Abbreviation for lymphocytic and histiocytic cell; a variant of Reed-Sternberg cell seen in nodular lymphocyte predominant Hodgkin's lymphoma.

Lacunar cell: A variant of Reed-Sternberg cell seen in nodular sclerosis type of Hodgkin's lymphoma.

LD body (Leishman-Donovan body) (Sir William Boog Leishman, Scottish pathologist and British Army Medical Officer, 1865–1926, Charles Donovan, British surgeon, 1863–1951): Visceral leishmaniasis (Kala-azar).

LE cell: Abbreviation for lupus erythematosus cell; seen in systemic lupus erythematosus.

Leptocyte (wafer cell): Thalassemia, obstructive jaundice.

Leukemoid reaction (lymphoid type): Viral infections, tuberculosis, whooping cough.

Leukemoid reaction (myeloid type): Severe bacterial infection, acute hemolysis, hemorrhage, cancer metastatic to marrow.

Leukoerythroblastic reaction: Military tuberculosis, cancers metastatic to bone marrow, myelofibrosis, severe hemolysis, lymphoma, myeloma, Gaucher's disease, Niemann-Pick disease.

Macrocytosis: Alcoholism, liver disease, hypothyroidism, megaloblastic anemia, hemolytic anemia, myelodysplastic syndrome.

Macro-ovalocyte: Megaloblastic anemia, myelodysplastic syndrome.

Macropolycyte: An unusually large neutrophil (twice the size of normal neutrophil) with a multisegmented nucleus (>5 lobes) seen in megaloblastic anemia.

Maturation arrest: Increased numbers of early erythroid precursors in bone marrow as compared to more mature precursors; seen in megaloblastic anemia.

Maurer's dots (Maurer's clefts) (Georg Maurer, 20th century German physician in Sumatra): Red dots (stained with Leishman stain) that occur in red cells infected with *Plasmodium falciparum.*

Microcytosis: Iron deficiency, thalassemia, anemia of chronic disease, secondary acquired sideroblastic anemia.

Micromegakaryocytes: Myelodysplastic syndrome, acute myeloid leukemia with trilineage dysplasia, myelofibrosis, chronic myeloid leukemia.

Morula cell (Grape cell, Mott cell): An abnormal plasma cell with intracytoplasmic globular inclusions containing immunoglobulins; seen in multiple myeloma and in CSF in African trypanosomiasis.

Myeloid:Erythroid ratio (M:E ratio): The ratio of myeloid to erythroid precursors in bone marrow; normal ratio is 2:1–4:1; increased in myeloid hyperplasia (infections, myeloid leukemias) and in erythroid suppression; decreased in suppression of myeloid series or in erythroid hyperplasia.

Myelokathexis: A rare autosomal dominant disease with severe peripheral neutropenia but bone marrow neutrophilic hyperplasia.

Napoleon hat cell: Hemoglobin S-Oman disease.

Nurse cell: A specialized macrophage in bone marrow around which erythroblasts are grouped and that helps in development of red cells.

Pappenheimer bodies (AM Pappenheimer, US pathologist, 1878–1955): Iron-containing granules in red cells in sideroblastic anemia, following splenectomy.

Pelger-Huet anomaly (Karel Pelger, Dutch physician, 1885-1931; GJ Huët, early 20th century Dutch physician): An inherited autosomal dominant disorder characterized by inhibition of lobe development in granulocytes; neutrophils are monolobed or bilobed; can be confused with shift to left in neutrophil series; acquired (pseudo) Pelger-Huet anomaly occurs in AML, CML, and myelodysplasia.

Pencil cell: Iron deficiency anemia.

Pincer cell (mushroom-shaped red cell): Hereditary spherocytosis due to band 3 deficiency.

Platelet size abnormalities: (1) Normal: 1.5–3 µm, (2) Large: 4–7 µm; seen in conditions with increased peripheral platelet destruction; (3) Giant: More than size of mature red cell or of small lymphocyte; seen in Bernard-Soulier syndrome, MYH-9 syndromes, and myeloproliferative neoplasms (4) small: <1.5 µm; seen in Wiskott-Aldrich syndrome.

Poikilocytosis: Increased proportion of red cells with abnormal shape; common, nonspecific abnormality in many hematological disorders; marked or extreme poikilocytosis is seen in myelofibrosis, hereditary pyropoikilocytosis, hemoglobin H disease, and congenital dyserythropoietic anemia; in addition poikilocytes of certain shape have significance (e.g. sickle cells, spherocytes, elliptocytes).

Polychromasia (polychromatophilia): Pinkish-blue red cells that are slightly larger than normal; represent immature reticulocytes that are seen in acute blood loss, hemolytic anemia, following specific therapy for nutritional anemia.

Popcorn cell: *See* L and H cell.

Pseudo-Gaucher cell (Gaucher-like cells): Chronic myeloid leukemia, acute leukemia, thalassemia, multiple myeloma, lymphomas, and myelodysplastic syndrome; probably result from increased load of glucosylceramide derived from increased leukocyte turnover.

Pyknocyte: *See* Contracted red cells.

Reed-Sternberg cell (Dorothy M Reed, US pathologist, 1874–1964; George M Sternberg, US bacteriologist, 1838–1915): Hodgkin's lymphoma.

Ribosome-lamellar complexes: Seen on electron microscopy in some cases of hairy cell leukemia.

Rieder cell (Hermann Rieder, German pathologist, 1858–1932): A myeloblast occurring in acute myeloid leukemia that has widely and deeply indented nucleus.

Ring or doughnut nuclei of neutrophils: CML, AML, chronic neutrophilic leukemia, myelodysplastic syndrome, megaloblastic anemia.

Ring sideroblasts: Myelodysplastic syndrome.

Rouleaux formation: Hypergammaglobulinemia, plasma cell myeloma.

Russell bodies (William Russell, Scottish physician and pathologist, 1852–1940): Plasma cells in chronic inflammation or in multiple myeloma.

Schistocyte: *See* Fragmented red cell.

Schizocyte: *See* Fragmented red cell.

Schuffner's dots (Schuffner's granules) (Wilhelm Schüffner, German pathologist, 1867–1949): Numerous, fine, round, red or red-yellow dots as seen with Romanowsky stains in red cells infected with *Plasmodium vivax* or *Plasmodium ovale*.

Sea-blue histiocytes: Sea-blue histiocyte disease (primary), and as a secondary phenomenon in myeloproliferative neoplasms, myelodysplastic syndrome, hyperlipidemia, lysosomal storage disease, lymphoma, total parenteral nutrition, idiopathic thrombocytopenic purpura, and viral disorders.

Serous atrophy: *See* Gelatinous transformation.

Sézary cell (Albert Sézary, French dermatologist, 1880–1956): Sézary syndrome.

Shift to left: Physiological during pregnancy; common causes are infectious and inflammatory conditions.

Shift to right: Megaloblastic anemia, uremia.

Sickle cell (drepanocyte): Sickle cell disease.

Sideroblast: An erythroblast containing aggregates of nonheme iron which are demonstrable by Prussian blue stain; three types: Type I (iron-containing granules are small and few; normally about 30–50% of erythroid precursors in bone marrow are sideroblasts), II (iron-containing granules are numerous and large and seen in hemolytic states and iron overload), and III [iron-containing granules are 10 or more in number, arranged in the form of a ring around the nucleus (deposited in mitochondria that are located around the nucleus), covering atleast one-third of nuclear periphery and seen in sideroblastic anemias and myelodysplastic syndrome].

Siderocyte: A red cell that contains granules that react with Perl's Prussian blue stain for iron; these granules are known as Pappenheimer bodies on Romanowsky-stained smears. Seen in thalassemias, hemoglobinopathies, and following splenectomy.

Smudge cell: *See* Basket cell.

Spherocyte: Numerous spherocytes are seen in hereditary spherocytosis, warm autoimmune hemolytic anemia, delayed hemolytic transfusion reaction, ABO hemolytic disease of newborn, *Clostridium perfringens* sepsis, burns, fresh-water drowning or intravenous infusion of water.

Spur cell: Alcoholic liver disease.

Stab cell: Band neutrophil.

Starry sky appearance: Histological feature seen in Burkitt and other high grade lymphomas resulting from scattered pale-staining macrophages in the background of darkly stained neoplastic lymphocytes.

Stomatocyte: Hereditary stomatocytosis, alcoholism, alcoholic liver disease, Southeast Asian ovalocytosis, Rh-null syndrome.

Target cell (Mexican hat cell, codocyte): Thalassemia, hemoglobin C disease, sickle cell anemia, hemoglobin C disease, hemoglobin D disease, obstructive jaundice, hereditary LCAT (lecithin-cholesterol acyltransferase) deficiency.

Tart cell: A monocyte that contains ingested nucleus of other cells in which structure is still well-preserved. It may be confused with LE cell.

Teardrop red cell (dacryocyte): Myelofibrosis (primary or secondary to metastatic deposits), megaloblastic anemia, thalassemia major.

Thesaurocyte: A large plasma cell containing large amounts of homogeneous material that stains red or pink; seen in reactive states as well as in multiple myeloma.

Toxic granulation in neutrophils: Severe inflammatory conditions, infections, pregnancy,

Turk cell (Wilhelm Türk, Austrian internist, 1871–1916): SYN atypical lymphocyte.

Vacuolated lymphocyte: Mucopolysaccharidoses, Jordan's anomaly, I cell disease, Niemann-Pick disease, Wolman's disease, Tay-Sachs disease, Pompe's disease, and various rare congenital disorders of metabolism.-

Villous lymphocyte: Splenic marginal zone lymphoma.

Ziemann dots (Ziemann's stippling) (Hans RP Ziemann, German pathologist, 1865–1939): Tiny dots seen (under certain staining conditions) in erythrocytes in malaria caused by *P. malariae*.

SPECIAL STAINS

Acid phosphatase: A cytochemical reaction that is positive in a focal manner in T-ALL, AML-M6, and AML-M7.

Chloroacetate esterase (CAE) (Leder stain): A cytochemical stain that is positive in all cells of neutrophil series; commonly used in combination with nonspecific esterase (double esterase reaction) for diagnosis of leukemia with both myeloid and monocytic components.

Crystal violet stain: A supravital stain used for staining of reticulocytes.

Double esterase stain: Combination of CAE stain (for granulocytic cells) and nonspecific esterase stain (for monocytic cells) for diagnosis of acute myelomonocytic leukemia.

Kleihauer-Betke stain: This stain is used to (1) detect and quantify fetal red cells in maternal circulation (done in Rh-negative mother to calculate the dose of RH immunoglobulin, and (2) distinguish between hereditary persistence of fetal hemoglobin and dβ thalassemia.

Leukocyte alkaline phosphatase (LAP) score: A scoring system used in patients with raised leukocyte count to differentiate between chronic myeloid leukemia (low score) and leukemoid reactions and other myeloproliferative disorders.

Myeloperoxidase (MPO): The main aim of MPO is to distinguish between AML (positive) and ALL (negative); flow cytometry is more sensitive than cytochemistry for demonstration of MPO.

New methylene blue: A supravital stain (a basic thiazine dye) that is used mainly for staining of reticulocytes in peripheral blood.

Nonspecific esterase (Alpha naphthyl acetate esterase or alpha naphthyl butyrate esterase): Positive in cells of monocytic lineage and is used for demonstration of monocytic leukemia. The reaction is inhibited by sodium fluoride in monocytic cells.

Oil red O: Positive in Burkitt lymphoma (lipid vacuoles).

Periodic acid Schiff: Positive (block-like) in 70% cases of acute lymphoblastic leukemia. This stain is also positive in erythroblasts of AML-M6 and in megakaryoblasts.

Perls stain (Max Perls, German pathologist, 1843–1881): A stain used for demonstration of ferric iron in bone marrow samples. It is used for diagnosis of iron deficiency anemia and demonstration of ring sideroblasts in myelodysplastic syndrome.

Peroxidase stain: *See* Myeloperoxidase stain.

Prussian blue stain: *See* Perls stain.

Reticulin stain: To detect and grade reticulin fibrosis on bone marrow biopsy.

Sudan black B: Positive in AML and negative in ALL.

Tartrate-resistant acid phosphatase (TRAP): One of the isoenzymes of alkaline phosphatase detection of which is used for diagnosis of hairy cell leukemia.

Toluidine blue: A metachromatic stain that stains nucleic acids blue, and sulfated polysaccharides purple; commonly used for staining of mast cells and basophils.

LABORATORY TESTS IN HEMATOLOGY

Acidified glycerol lysis time (AGLT): Hereditary spherocytosis.

Acidified serum test (Ham's test): Paroxysmal nocturnal hemoglobinuria.

Activated partial thromboplastin time (APTT): Prolonged in deficiency of FVIII, FIX, circulating inhibitors of coagulation, disseminated intravascular coagulation, heparin therapy, and vitamin K deficiency.

Alkali denaturation test: Estimation of fetal hemoglobin.

Antiglobulin test, Direct (Coombs test, direct): Positive in hemolytic disease of newborn, autoimmune hemolytic anemia (warm type), immune hemolytic transfusion reaction, drug-induced immune hemolytic anemia.

Antiglobulin test, indirect (Coombs test, indirect): Used for cross-matching, antibody screening, and investigation of a transfusion reaction in blood bank, and in antenatal antibody screening.

Apt test (Leonard Apt, 20th century US pediatric ophthalmologist): Differentiating fetal or neonatal blood from maternal blood to—(1) identify the source of bloody stools in newborn infant, and (2) determine maternal (placenta previa) or fetal blood (vasa previa) in vaginal bleeding during late pregnancy.

Autohemolysis test: Hereditary spherocytosis.

Bleeding time: Prolonged in disorders of platelets, some vascular disorders, von Willebrand disease, and afibrinogenemia.

Buffy coat smear: Buffy coat is grayish-white layer obtained after centrifugation of anticoagulated whole blood; composed of white blood cells and platelets; thick buffy coat layer is obtained in leukocytosis and thrombocytosis; blood smears prepared from this layer are examined for parasites and abnormal cells, if they are scarce in peripheral blood.

Capillary fragility test (Hess test, Rumpel-Leede test): Thrombocytopenia, vitamin C deficiency.

Clot retraction time: Prolonged in thrombocytopenia and Glanzmann's thrombasthenia.

Clot solubility test (Urea clot solubility test): Factor XIII deficiency.

D-dimer test: Disseminated intravascular coagulation, thrombosis.

Deoxyuridine suppression test: A sensitive test for diagnosis of vitamin B_{12} or folate deficiency (used in research only).

Differential absorption test: *See* Paul-Bunnell-Davidsohn test.

Dilute Russell viper venom time (DRVVT): Test for detection of lupus anticoagulant.

Donath-Landsteiner test (Julius Donath, Austrian physician, 1870–1950, Karl Landsteiner, Austrian-American immunologist, pathologist, and Nobel laureate, 1868–1943): Test used for diagnosis of paroxysmal cold hemoglobinuria.

Ecarin clotting time: A test for monitoring anticoagulant therapy with hirudin.

Eosin-5-maleimide (EMA) binding test: A rapid flow cytometry screening test for diagnosis of hereditary spherocytosis.

Ethanol gelation test (paracoagulation test): Screening test for disseminated intravascular coagulation.

Euglobulin clot lysis time: A test for fibrinolysis.

Fibrinogen/fibrin degradation product (FDP): Disseminated intravascular coagulation.

Field stain (John William Field, Physician and Medical researcher, Malaysia, 1899–1981): A two stage rapid stain for thick and thin blood smears for detection of malaria parasites.

Flow cytometry: A procedure used for measuring multiple cellular and fluorescent properties of cells when they flow as a single cell suspension through a laser beam in a specialized instrument called as a flow cytometer; commonly used for immunophenotyping of leukemias and lymphomas.

Fluorescent in situ hybridization (FISH): A combination of cytogenetic and molecular techniques used to identify and localize the presence or absence of specific chromosomes or chromosomal regions through hybridization of fluorescent probes that bind specifically to its complementary target sequence.

Fluorescent spot test: A screening test for G6PD deficiency recommended by International Committee for Standardization in Haematology.

Formol gel test: Visceral leishmaniasis.

Glutathione stability test: A test for diagnosis of G6PD deficiency.

Heat instability test: Test for demonstration of unstable hemoglobins.

Heinz bodies: Inclusions within red cells attached to cell membrane that represent precipitated hemoglobin and demonstrated with supravital dyes (e.g. crystal violet); seen in G6PD deficiency and unstable hemoglobins; also called as Heinz-Ehrlich bodies, Ehrlich bodies.

Heterophile agglutination test: *See* Paul-Bunnell test.

High performance liquid chromatography: Screening test for hemoglobinopathies and thalassemias.

Hypertonic cryohemolysis test: Hereditary spherocytosis.

Immunofixation: Demonstration and identification of M protein in plasma cell neoplasms.

Immunophenotyping A technique that uses monoclonal antibodies and flow cytometry to detect antigens on cell surface or in cell cytoplasm so that information about cell lineage or clonality can be obtained; used along with morphology for diagnosis of leukemias and lymphomas.

International normalized ratio (INR): The standardized method for reporting prothrombin time ratio for patients receiving oral anticoagulant therapy.

Isopropanol precipitation test: Used for the detection of unstable hemoglobins.

Kaolin clotting time: A coagulation test for screening of lupus anticoagulant.

Liley's graph: Used to categorize severity of hemolytic disease of newborn.

Lymphocytotoxicity test: A test for detection of class I and II HLA antigens.

Mean corpuscular hemoglobin concentration (MCHC): Raised in hereditary spherocytosis, and is decreased in hypochromic anemia.

Mean corpuscular hemoglobin: Decreased in microcytic hypochromic anemia, and increased in macrocytic anemia and in newborns.

Mean corpuscular volume (MCV): Increased in megaloblastic anemia, chronic alcoholism, liver disease, hypothyroidism, and myelodysplastic syndrome, while decreased in iron deficiency anemia and thalassemia.

Mean platelet volume: Increased in thrombocytopenia due to peripheral destruction of platelets and normal or low when thrombocytopenia is due to impaired platelet production.

Mentzer index: Ratio of mean cell volume to red cell count; increased (>13) in iron deficiency, and decreased (<13) in thalassemia.

Metabisulfite test: A screening test for presence of sickle hemoglobin.

Methemoglobin elution method: A screening test for identification of female heterozygotes for G6PD deficiency.

Methemoglobin reduction test: A test used for screening of G6PD deficiency.

Mixed lymphocyte culture: A histocompatibility test for class II antigens.

Monospot test: A rapid slide test for diagnosis of infectious mononucleosis.

Motulsky dye reduction test (Arno G Motulsky, 20th century American medical geneticist): A screening test for deficiency of glucose-6-phosphate dehydrogenase deficiency.

Multimeric analysis: An electrophoretic technique to separate different multimers of von Willebrand factor according to size; the test is performed if screening tests suggest von Willebrand disease for correct classification of von Willbrand disease into a specific type.

NESTROFT: Abbreviation for Naked Eye Single Tube Red cell Osmotic Fragility Test; *See* Single tube osmotic fragility test.

Neutrophil alkaline phosphatase (NAP) score: *See* Leukocyte alkaline phosphatase score.

Nitroblue tetrazolium dye reduction test: Chronic granulomatous disease.

Osmotic fragility test: A screening test for hereditary spherocytosis.

Paracoagulation tests: Tests employed for detection of gel or fibrin strand formation when ethanol or protamine sulfate is added to plasma; the tests are used to differentiate between primary fibrinolysis (negative test) and disseminated intravascular coagulation (positive test). *See* Ethanol gelation test, Protamine sulfate test.

Paul-Bunnell test (John R Paul, US physician, 1893–1971; Walls W Bunnell, US physician, born 1902–1966): Test for detection of heterophile antibodies in sera of patient's with infectious mononucleosis.

Paul-Bunnell-Davidsohn test: A test to distinguish heterophile antibodies occurring in infectious mononucleosis from those occurring in other disorders.

Pentagastrin test: A test for determination of maximum or peak acid output following subcutaneous or intramuscular injection of pentagastrin; usually indicated in gastric analysis for Zollinger-Ellison syndrome, gastric or duodenal ulcer, and achlorhydria (pernicious anemia).

Platelet aggregation studies: Characteristic aggregation patterns are observed in Glanzmann's thrombasthenia, von Willebrand disease, Bernard-Soulier syndrome, storage pool deficiency, and following administration of aspirin and some anti-inflammatory agents.

Platelet distribution width (PDW): A measure of degree of variation of platelet size present in a blood sample; high PDW is seen in myeloproliferative disorders; while PDW is normal in reactive or secondary thrombocytosis.

Platelet function analyzer-100 (PFA-100) assay: Screening test for platelet function defect.

Primed lymphocyte typing (PLT): A test used for detection of HLA-Dw and HLA-DPw antigens.

Protamine neutralization assay: A test to calculate the dose of protamine sulfate necessary for neutralization of circulating heparin after cardiopulmonary bypass or for rapid reversal of heparinization, and to control heparin therapy.

Protamine sulfate test: Detection of early disseminated intravascular coagulation.

Prothrombin time (Quick's): Assesses the activity of extrinsic (Factor VII) and common pathways (Factors X, V, II, and I) of coagulation.

Red cell distribution width (RDW): A parameter of the variation in the red cell size in a blood sample that is measured by hematology analyzers; high RDW with low MCV occurs in iron deficiency anemia; while RDW is normal with low MCV in thalassemia minor.

Ristocetin cofactor (RCoF) assay: von Willebrand disease.

Ristocetin-induced platelet aggregation: von Willebrand disease.

Russell's viper venom time (Stypven time): Factor X deficiency.

Schilling test (Victor Theodor Adolf Georg Schilling, German hematologist, 1883–1960): Test used for evaluation of absorption of vitamin B_{12} in the gastrointestinal tract.

Schumm's test (Otto Schumm, German chemist, 1874–1958): Test in which a distinctive absorption band of methemalbumin is detected at 558 nm on spectrophotometry; methemalbumin is observed in plasma in intravascular hemolysis.

Serum free light chain assay: Plasma cell myeloma.

Serum haptoglobin: Decreased or absent in hemolysis.

Serum homocysteine: A test for evaluation of megaloblastic anemia; elevated in vitamin B_{12} deficiency and normal in folate deficiency.

Serum methylmalonic acid: A test for evaluation of megaloblastic anemia; elevated in vitamin B_{12} deficiency and normal in folate deficiency.

Serum/urine lysozyme: Acute monocytic leukemia.

Single tube osmotic fragility test: A test used for detection of thalassemia carriers in which red cells are suspended in 0.36% buffered saline and observed for hemolysis; red cells in thalassemia are more resistant to osmotic lysis than normal red cells. SYN NESTROFT (Naked eye single tube red cell osmotic fragility test).

Solubility test: A screening test for sickle cell hemoglobin (Hb S).

Soluble transferrin receptor: Transferrin receptor present in serum that is derived from proteolysis of cell membrane transferrin receptors during red cell maturation and its level correlates with number of cellular transferrin receptors; raised in iron deficiency and hemolytic anemia.

Stypven time: Differentiation between deficiency of factor VII and deficiency of factor X.

Sucrose hemolysis test: The standard screening test for paroxysmal nocturnal hemoglobinuria (PNH).

Telomere length assay: Dyskeratosis congenita.

Tetrazolium linked cytochemical method: A test for detection of heterozygotes for G6PD deficiency.

Textarin/ecarin ratio: A confirmatory test for lupus anticoagulant.

Thrombin time: Prolonged in deficiency of fibrinogen or in the presence of heparin.

Thrombin time: Prolonged in disorders of fibrinogen, heparin therapy, chronic liver disease, and presence of fibrinogen/fibrin degradation products.

Thromboelastography: A point of care device used in the surgical setting (trauma, cardiovascular) to guide transfusion practices.

Thromboplastin generation test (TGT): A two stage test for detection of deficiencies of factors VIII, IX, V, X, XI, and XII.

Tissue thromboplastin inhibition test: A test used for detection of lupus anticoagulant.

Total iron binding capacity (TIBC): The iron binding sites of all the circulating transferrin that is an indirect measure of transferrin level in blood; increased in iron deficiency anemia and decreased in anemia of chronic disease.

Transferrin saturation: Ratio of serum iron to total iron binding capacity expressed as a percentage and indicates proportion of transferrin to which iron is bound; average normal is 30%; reduced in iron deficiency anemia.

Watson-Schwartz test (Cecil J Watson, US physician, 1901–1983; Samuel Schwartz, 20th century US physician, born 1916): A screening test to distinguish between urobilinogen and porphobilinogen.

Index

Page numbers followed by *b* refer to box, *f* refer to figure, and *t* refer to table.

A

ABO group 498*t*, 502*t*, 504, 508, 536
    test for 504
ABO hemolytic disease 136, 218, 219*t*
ABO incompatibility 212, 543*f*
    detection of 538
ABO subgroups 510
ABO system 498
    antibody of 500
    antigens of 498, 499*f*
Acanthocyte 567
Achlorhydria 104
Acid
    elution test 151*f*, 164
    pH 115
    phosphatase 248, 249, 572
Acidified glycerol lysis time 139, 572
Acidified serum test 224, 572
Acidosis 217
Acquired aplastic anemia, pathogenesis of 111*f*
Acquired immunodeficiency syndrome 371, 401, 408, 413, 548
Activate cryptic splice sites 156
Activated partial thromboplastin time 431, 432*f*, 436*t*, 437, 464, 476, 573
    causes of prolongation of 431
Acute leukemia 235, 236, 238*t*, 246*f*, 249*t*, 253, 253*b*, 254, 255*b*, 256*b*, 257*b*, 277, 278, 321
    characterization of 253*t*
    classification of 240
    clinical features of 244
    diagnosis of 244, 244*b*, 245, 245*f*, 245*b*, 253*t*, 258*f*
    myelofibrosis 117
Addison's disease 32, 104
Adenosine deaminase deficiency 409
Adherence technology, solid phase 508
Adhesion 43
    molecules 184
Adipocytes 8
Adjunctive therapy 217
Adriamycin 376
Afibrinogenemia 424
    hereditary 479
Agammaglobulinemia, X-linked 410
Agarose gel electrophoresis 344, 347*f*
Agranulocytosis 394
Albers-Schönberg disease 392
Albumin
    infusion of 217
    physiological functions of 534
Alder-Reilly anomaly 397

Aldrich syndrome protein 412
Alemtuzumab 335
Alkali denaturation test 188, 573
Alkaline hematin method 63
Alkylating drugs 291
Allele-specific oligonucleotide probe 174
    analysis 191
Allergic
    diseases 395
    disorders 394
    purpura 442
    reactions 541, 544
Alloantibodies 35
Allogeneic bone marrow transplantation 226
Allogeneic hematopoietic transplantation 312
Alloimmune
    hemolytic anemia 200
    neonatal thrombocytopenia 452
Allopurinol 110, 269
Alopecia 415
Alpha granule storage pool deficiency 459
Alpha naphthyl
    acetate esterase 278, 575
    butyrate esterase 575
Alpha thalassemia 66, 159, 167
    syndrome 162
Ambiguous lineage, acute leukemias of 254
Amino acids 472
Ammonium oxalate 427
Amniotic villus 175
Amplification refractory mutation system 175
Amyloidosis 349, 492
Amylophagia 86
Analgesics 197
Anaphylactic reaction 541, 544
Anaphylactoid purpura 442
Androgens 116
Anemia 59, 61, 65, 67, 74, 81, 127, 129, 133, 160, 350
    acute
        blood loss 127
        megaloblastic 108
        posthemorrhagic 75
    causes of 65*b*, 73, 81
    classification of 70, 70*t*, 73
    congenital dyserythropoietic 128, 129*t*, 130*f*, 224
    determine cause of 64
    diagnosis of 61, 62, 122*b*
    differential diagnosis of 72*t*
    dimorphic 92
    etiological classification of 65*t*
    evaluation of 72, 72*f*
    exacerbation of 135

general clinical features of 86
grading of 63b
inherited 65
moderate 135
morphological classification of 71t
severe 74, 99, 119
    chronic 4
severity of 62, 91
signs of 64
symptoms of 64
treatment of 361
types of 68f, 79
Anisocytosis 567
Anisopoikilocytosis 163f, 165f
Ann Arbor staging system 386
Antacids 82
Antagonism 490
Antecubital vein 429
Antenatal laboratory testing 213b
Anthracycline 271
    addition of 268
Antibody 33
    coated platelets 447
    deficiencies, predominantly 409
    detection of 213, 440
    screening and identification 513, 538
Anticoagulant-preservative solution 521
Anticonvulsants 65, 100
Anti-D antibody 500
Antiepileptics 108, 110
Antigens 502
    development of 502
    distribution of 502
    expression, aberrant 560
    nonexpression of 254f
    presenting cells 25
    weakly reactive 506
Antiglobulin test 202, 573
    causes of positive direct 204b
    interpretation of 204f
    negative 204
    principle of indirect 203f
Anti-HLA antibodies, development of 523
Antihypertensive drug 210
Anti-inflammatory drugs 110
Antileukocyte antibodies, detection of 561
Antilymphocyte 116
Antimosquito agents 240
Antiphospholipid
    antibodies 487
    syndrome 487
Antiplatelet
    antibodies 562
    drugs 44f
Antirheumatics 110
Antithrombin 56
Antithymocyte 116
    globulin 116
Antithyroids 110
Aorta-gonad-mesonephros 3
    region 3

Aplastic anemia 109, 111, 112, 116, 127, 219, 448, 450
    acquired 109
    causes of 109t
    constitutional 118
    determine cause of 113
    diagnosis of 113
    differential diagnosis of 114
    evaluation of 110t
    grading of 114t
    management of 117f
    severe 114, 117
Aplastic crisis 135, 140, 185
Apoptosis, abnormal 289
Apotransferrin 84
Apt test 573
Arachidonic acid 434, 435, 458
    metabolism 435
Arrhythmias, cardiac 108
Aspergillus 413
Aspirin 197, 460
    inhibits 460
    like defect 435, 460
    low dose 323
    secondary 65
Asynchronous antigen expression 285
Ataxia telangiectasia 412
Atomic power plant accidents 288
Australia antigen 514
Autoagglutination 508
Autoantibody 35
    cold reacting 205, 206
    tests for 113
    warm-reacting 201
Autohemolysis test 138, 573
Autoimmune 8
    cytopenias 409
    diseases 487
    disorders 115, 321, 410
    hemolytic anemia 139, 200, 201, 202f, 205
        classification of 201b
        laboratory diagnosis of 204b
    thrombocytopenic purpura 446
Autoinflammatory disorders 409
Autologous transfusion 551
    advantages of 551b
    consideration of 554
Autosomal dominant disorders 424
Autosomal recessive disease 424
Azotemia 453
Azurophilic granules 20, 283f

B

B genes 11
B lymphocyte 24, 24t, 25, 221
    functions of 27, 408
    precursors 266
Babesia microti 547
Bacteremia 551
Bacterial proliferation 532
Balance polymorphism 160

Banding technique 256
Barr's body 19
Bart's hydrops fetalis 153
    syndrome 151, 172
Basket cells 329, 567
Basophil 22, 305
Basophilia 310, 311, 354, 396
Basophilic stippling 67, 567
B-cell 333, 413
    acute lymphoblastic leukemia 240
    development 378
        normal stages of 27f
    immunity 411
    lymphocytosis, persistent polyclonal 330, 404
    lymphomas 331t, 332, 378
    neoplasms, mature 265, 379, 381t
    ontogeny 26
    phenotype 265
    precursors 266
    prolymphocytic leukemia 325
Beef red cells 406
Bernard-Soulier syndrome 43, 44, 428, 435, 450, 452, 457, 477, 576
Beta thalassemia 153, 160
    displays 154
    inheritance of 165
    intermedia 166
    major 160, 161f, 164f
    minor 164, 164f, 166
Beta-globin gene 12f
Bilirubin
    concentrations, determination of 215
    formation of 77f
Bilobed nucleus, typical 283f
Bite cell 567
Blackwater fever 197
Blast
    cell 254
    different types of 247b
    gate 252
Bleeding
    disorders 423, 433t, 443b, 442, 445
        clinical evaluation 423
        congenital 424b
        diagnosis of 423
        investigation of 432f
        laboratory evaluation 425
        mild 43
        screening tests 426
    during surgery, reduce 554
    gastrointestinal 453
    genitourinary 453
    terminology 425b
    time 573
        prolongation of 426
Bleomycin 376
Blind loop syndrome 104, 105
Blister cell 567

Blood
    bank 539
        standards 541
    cell 221
        formation of 3
        production 3
    coagulation
        factors 46t
        mechanism of 50
    collection of 517, 523
    components 526, 529, 529b
        preparation of 526, 527f
        separation of 526
        therapy, era of 528
    derivatives 526, 534, 534b
    donation 506
    donors 520
        dentistry 520
        drugs 520
        hepatitis 519
        illness 520
        immunization 520
        infectious diseases 519
        malaria 519
        medical history 519
        physical examination 520
        predonation counseling 518
        selection of 518
        skin piercing 520
        test for anemia 521
        types of 517
    flow velocity 215
    group
        demonstration of 544
        genes 497
        substances, excessive amounts of 510
        system 211, 497, 497t
    grouping 213, 214, 504b
        causes of 510t
        method for 507f
        test for 509f
        unexpected results in 509
    hemoglobin 218
    in infectious mononucleosis 405f
    loss 65
        causes of 92
        chronic 64
        excess 65
    physiology of 1, 3
    pressure 539
    products 526b
        storage of 529b
    salvage 552
        intraoperative 552
    sample
        anemic 64f
        collection of 429

handling of 429
normal 64f
smear 129, 136f, 165f, 197f, 207f, 208, 216f, 219f, 227f, 390f, 391f, 399f, 428, 449f, 452
  examination 136
  normal peripheral 10f
transfusion 178, 192b, 495, 520, 541, 554
  mismatched 197
  therapy 179
unit, transfusion of 539
unnecessary administration of 554
urea nitrogen 126
vessels
  abnormalities of 442
  role of 40f
  walls of dilated 444
viscosity 315
Bloom's syndrome 235, 271
Blue-colored iron granules 123f
B-lymphoid neoplasms, mature 561
Boat-shaped cell 187, 567
Body iron
  compartments 82b
  load, assessment of 180
  stores 83
Bone lesions 350
  pathogenesis of 352f
Bone marrow 9f, 10f, 74, 79, 98f, 99, 265, 266, 310, 319, 343t, 392
  aplasia 110
  aplastic 113f
  aspiration 291
    smear 89f, 261f, 323f
  biopsy 127, 293, 322, 337, 354
  cellularity 113f
  erythroblasts 129
  examination 88, 100, 112, 137, 164, 260, 277, 291, 305, 320, 342, 358, 392, 448
  failure syndrome 118, 272
    causes of 115
    inherited 117
  fibrosis 293, 319
    causes of 321, 321t
  gelatinous transformation of 115, 115f, 568
  harvesting 419
  hyperplasia of 109
  infiltration 328f
  injury 110
  organization of 8, 9f
  plasmacytosis, reactive 357
  role of 72
  serous atrophy of 568
  smear 354f
  transplantation 414
  trephine biopsy 245
Bone mineral density, reduced 162
Bortezomib 361
Bothrops atrox 438
Brown-black malarial pigment 399f
Brucellosis 547
Bruise 425
Bruton's disease 410
Bruton's tyrosine kinase 410
Budd-Chiari syndrome 222
Buffy coat
  layer 64f
  smear 573
Bulky disease 260
Burkitt's cells 260
Burkitt's leukemia 243, 260
Burkitt's lymphoma 243, 260, 378, 383, 387
  advanced stage of 266
  pathogenesis of 378f
Burr cells 67, 126f, 567
Burst-forming unit
  erythroid 5
  megakaryocyte 5

C

Cabot's rings 98, 567
Calcium 50
Canalicular system, surface connected 42
Cancers metastatic 392
Candidiasis 412
Capillary fragility test 573
Carbamazepine 110
Carbohydrate 20, 41
Carboxy forms 480, 490
Carboxyhemoglobin 62
Carcinomas after radiotherapy 395
Cardiopulmonary bypass 492
Castleman's disease 357
Cataracts 179
Catastrophic antiphospholipid syndrome 487
Celiac disease 32, 65, 101
Cell
  grouping 504, 506, 510, 536
    interpretation of 506t
  lymphoma, small cleaved 330
  mature 299
  reactive 370
  surface
    antigens 26
    receptors, cytoplasmic domains of 314f
  tumors, small round blue 265
  turnover 101
Cellular
  dehydration 134
  immunity 447
  infiltrate, abnormal 112
Cellulose acetate 148, 344
  electrophoresis 145f
Central nervous system
  disease, status of 259b
  prophylaxis 269
Cerebral ischemia 322
Chain termination codon 157
Chediak-Higashi syndrome 397
Chemical agents 228

Chemotaxis 21*f*
Chemotherapy 284
    cytotoxic 408
    high-dose 416
Chest syndrome 186, 192, 193
Chimerism 510
Chipmunk facies 162
Chloramphenicol 65
Chloroacetate esterase 248-250, 573
Chloroma 272, 275
Chlorpromazine 110
Chorionic villus 175
Chromatin modifiers 238, 240
Chromosomal material
    gain of 294
    loss of 294
Chromosome 11q23 236
Chronic granulomatous disease 398, 409, 561
Chronic lymphocytic leukemia 27, 260, 325, 327*f*, 331, 333*t*, 335, 413
    atypical 329
    cell of origin 325
    clinical features 326
    complications of 332
    diagnosis of 327, 329
    differential diagnosis 330
    immunological studies 329
    laboratory features 326
    prognosis 332
    staging systems for 332
    treatment 332
Chronic myeloid leukemia 235, 236, 271, 299, 300, 305*f*-307*f*, 308*b*, 310*t*, 392
    accelerated phase of 308
    blast phase 309, 311
    course and prognosis of 311
    differential diagnosis of 309
    incidence 304
    natural history of 311
    pathogenesis 301, 302
    phase of 304
    stages of 304
Chronic renal failure 125, 126*f*
    anemia of 125
    pathogenesis 125
    treatment 126
Chronic transfusion therapy 162
Cirrhosis 179, 357
Citrate
    agar electrophoresis 146
    anticoagulant 550
Cladribine 340
Clonal neoplastic disorders 299
Clostridium
    perfringens 229
    welchii infection 197
Clot retraction time 573
Clot solubility test 573

Coagulation
    acquired
        disorders of 479
        inhibitors of 486
    cell based model of 53*f*
    disorders 425*f*, 462
        acquired 480*t*, 492
    factor assays 437
    inherited disorders of 427, 462
    natural inhibitors of 56, 56*f*, 57*t*
    phase, tests for 436
    profile 449
    protein, number of 45
    system 45
Cohesin complex 240
Cold agglutinin disease 205, 206*f*, 208*t*
Collagen vascular diseases 346
Colony-forming unit 4
    erythroid 5
    granulocyte 5
    mast cell 5
    megakaryocyte 5
Color deoxyribonucleic acid amplification 191
Coma 179
Compatibility test 511, 512, 538
Complete blood count 72*f*, 320, 407, 428, 456
Constitutional pure red cell aplasia 119
Conventional cytogenetic analysis 294
Cooley anemia 152
Coombs' test 79, 202
Cordocentesis 215
Coronary syndrome, acute 490
Cosmetologists 351
Cotrimoxazole 399
Cranial irradiation, combination of 269
C-reactive protein 324
Creutzfeldt-Jakob disease 520, 547
Cryoprecipitate 486, 529, 533
    preparation of 467
Cryptic splice site, activation of 156*f*
Crystal violet stain 573
Crystalloid solution 528
Cubam 94
    dysfunction of 94
Cyanmethemoglobin method 62, 63
Cyclophosphamide 387, 520
Cyclosporine 116
Cystitis, hemorrhagic 415
Cytapheresis 523
Cytochemical reactions 240, 250*f*, 251*f*
    applications of 248
    principles of 248
Cytochemical stains 261
Cytochemical techniques 248
Cytochemistry 245, 248, 249*t*, 293
Cytogenetic 295
    abnormalities 295
    analysis 263, 280, 294, 299, 306, 316, 321, 329
    classification 267

response 312
role of 294*b*
studies 255
Cytokines, types of 371
Cytomegalovirus 265, 532
Cytopenia 230, 288, 291, 428
   manifestations of 339
Cytoplasm 26
   basophilic 281*f*
   hemoglobinization of 88
Cytosine arabinoside 108, 271
Cytotoxic cells 28, 404
Cytotoxic drugs 65, 110

D

D antigen 217
   partial 501
Dacarbazine 376
Dacryocyte 568, 572
Dapsone 197
Daunorubicin 268
D-dimer 440
   test 440, 573
      applications of 440
Deafness 179
Deep vein thrombosis, treatment of 491
Deficient cytoskeletal protein, identification of 139
Degmacyte 567
Dehydrogenase
   deficiency 119
   enzymes 15
Dendritic cells 22, 23, 25
Dense granule 42
   storage pool deficiency 459
Deoxynucleotides 173
Deoxyribonucleic acid
   analysis 189
   methylation genes 240
   ploidy studies 255, 257
Deoxythymidylate monophosphate 96, 97
Deoxythymidylate triphosphate 97
Deoxyuridine
   monophosphate 95
   suppression test 573
Deoxyuridylate monophosphate 96, 97
Desmopressin 461, 467
Dexamethasone, intravascular 285
Diabetes mellitus 32
   insulin dependent 104
Diamond-Blackfan anemia 118
Diamond-Blackfan syndrome 119, 235
Diarrhea 412, 415
Diathesis, hemorrhagic 462*f*, 463
Diclofenac 110
Diepoxybutane 118
Dietary folates 96
Differential absorption test 406, 573
DiGeorge syndrome 411
Dihydrofolate 96, 108
Dilute Russell viper venom time 573

Diphtheria 408
Diphyllobothrium latum 105
Direct antiglobulin test 208, 209, 215, 546
   principle of 203*f*
Directantiglobulin test 80
Disseminated intravascular coagulation 272, 430, 466, 482, 456, 482*f*
   acute 484, 485, 485*b*
   causes of 483*t*
   chronic 484, 486
   clinical features 484
   compensated 484
   decompensated 484
   diagnosis of 440
   etiology 482
   laboratory features 485
   pathogenesis 483
Distal myocardium 556
Divalent metal transporter 83
Döhle inclusion bodies 390
Donath-Landsteiner test 208, 573
Donor blood
   collection of 517, 521
   group 537
      selection of 537*t*
   processing of 524
   selection of 536
   tests done on 524*t*
   issue of 538
   storage of 524
Donor unit, bacterial contamination of 541, 545
Dot blot analysis 175*f*
Double esterase stain 573
Down's syndrome 235, 243, 255, 271, 272, 274-276
Downey cell 567, 568
Doxorubicin 268, 387
Drabkin's solution 62
Drepanocyte 568, 571
Drug adsorption 209
Drumstick appendage 568
Duncan's syndrome 405
Duodenal cytochrome 82
Durie and Salmon staging system 360
Dutcher body 364, 568
Dye decolorization test 199
Dysfibrinogenemia 479, 481
Dyskeratosis congenita 111, 113, 114, 118
Dysmyelopoietic syndrome 287
Dysphagia 86
Dysplasia, hematopoietic 292
Dyspnea 291
   severe 272

E

Ecarin clotting time 573
Ecchymosis 425
Echinocyte 126, 568
Echis carinatus 438
Ectopic pregnancy, ruptured 552

Ehrlich bodies 569
Elane gene 394
Electron microscopy 249, 252
Electrophoresis, capillary 147, 346
Elliptocyte 568
Elliptocytosis, hereditary 133
Embden-Meyerhof pathway 15
Embryogenesis 195
Endosome, formation of 84f
Endothelial cells 8, 40, 47, 472, 473f, 484f
Endothelium 51
Enterocytes 95
Enzyme linked immunosorbent assay 514, 515
    test, principle of 516f
Enzyme replacement 401
    therapy 401
Eosin-5-maleimide binding test 139, 573
Eosinophil 10f, 22, 305, 395f
    cationic protein 22
    derived neurotoxin 22
    peroxidase 22
Eosinophilia 394
    causes of 395b
Epilepsy 551
Epinephrine 427
Epipodophyllotoxins 236, 271
Epistaxis 363
Epoetin alfa 8
Epsilon-amino-caproic acid 438
Epstein syndrome 397, 450
Epstein-Barr
    nuclear antigen 406
    virus 265, 371, 404, 413
        role of 371
Erythroblasts 84f, 123f, 216f, 247
    abnormalities of 130f
Erythrocyte
    analysis 562
    functions of 11
    protoporphyrin 90
    sedimentation rate 121
    structure of 11
Erythroid 306
    cells 221
    colonies 10f
    hyperplasia 76, 129, 292
    island 10f
    leukemia, pure 247, 275, 279
    multinuclearity, hereditary 224
    precursors 85
        cytoplasm of 85
    progenitors 10f
Erythropoiesis 83
    ineffective 99, 101
    inhibition of 125
    stages of 9
Erythropoietin 7, 8, 314, 555
    receptors 314f
Escherichia coli 101, 184, 399
Esophageal web 86

Esterase, nonspecific 23, 248-250, 575
Ethanol gelation test 574
Etoposide 236
Evans' syndrome 201, 202
    diagnosis of 450
Extranodal marginal zone lymphoma 382
Extravascular hemolysis 77, 78t, 209
    mechanism of 77f

F

Faggot cells 568
False-negative test, causes of 149
False-positive test, causes of 149
Fanconi's anemia 115, 118, 235, 271, 452
Fat cells 112, 328f
Fava beans, ingestion of 197
Febrile nonhemolytic transfusion reaction 541, 542
Fecal occult blood, tests for 91
Fechtner syndrome 397, 450
Ferrochelatase 125
Ferroportin 1 83
Ferrous gluconate 93
Ferrous sulfate 92
Fetal anemia 215
Fetal blood 172
    analysis 190
    group 211
        incompatibilities 211t
Fetal deoxyribonucleic acid analysis 172, 190
Fetal hemoglobin 150, 184
    estimation of 150
    hereditary persistence of 184
Fibrin
    degradation products 54, 55f, 431, 438, 439f, 483
    generation of 484f
    polymer 51
Fibrinogen 45, 46, 341, 431, 439f, 474
    concentrate 486
    degradation products 53, 55f
    disorders of 431
    estimation, methods of 437
    hereditary disorders of 478
    in plasma, level of 437
    inherited disorders of 478
    quantitative estimation of 437
Fibrinolysis 39
    inhibitor of 53
    tests for 438
Fibrinolytic inhibitors 54
Fibrinolytic system 52, 53f
    components of 54t
Fibroblasts 8, 370
Figlu excretion test 102
Filgrastim 8
Fine needle aspiration cytology 384
Fish tapeworm 105
Five Q-syndrome 291
Flame cells 568
Flow cytometry 216, 293, 355, 435, 574
    role of 278b, 305

Fluorescence histogram 225f
Fluorescent in situ hybridization 307f, 329, 574
Fluorescent spot test 198, 574
Folate
    deficiency 65, 97, 99-101, 103f, 105, 107, 107t
        causes of 100, 100b
        treatment of 103
    functions 97
    metabolism, normal 96
    role of 96f
    sources of 96
Follicular lymphoma 330, 331, 378, 382
    pathogenesis of 379f
Formiminoglutamate excretion test 102
Formol gel test 574
Fragmented cells 197f, 568
Frank leukemiam, development of 237
Free erythrocyte protoporphyrin 87, 92
French-American-British classification 240, 289
French-American-British Cooperative Group Classification 241t, 272
Fresh frozen plasma 486, 529, 533, 533b
    indications for 533
Fried-egg appearance 568
Frozen red cells 529, 530
Furosemide 110

G

Gallstones 136
Gamma-irradiated red cells, transfusion of 531
Gasometric method 63
Gasser cells 568
Gastrectomy 104
Gastric
    atrophy 104
    blood loss 65
Gastritis, chronic atrophic 104
Gastrointestinal tract 86, 106, 484
Gaucher's cells 400, 401, 568
    cytoplasm of 401f
    demonstration of 401
Gaucher's disease 392, 400, 401
    clinical features 400
    diagnosis 400, 402
    symptoms of 401
    treatment 401, 402
Gel electrophoresis methods 346
Gel technology 508
Gelatinous transformation 117
Genes 11, 31
    location of 31, 502
    mutations 242, 274, 279
        acquired 288
Genetic 195
    abnormality
        detection of 471
        primary 350
    counseling 170
    defect, direct detection of 175

    disease 271
    tests 286
Genitourinary system 186
Genome
    guardian of 239
    sequencing 237
Ghosts 199
Giant band forms 568
Giant cell 372
Giant metamyelocyte 99, 568
Giant platelets 322f, 450, 452f, 458f, 568
    causes of 429b
Gilbert syndrome 186
Glanzmann's thrombasthenia 428, 434, 435, 457, 458
    diagnosis of 435
Globin chain
    electrophoresis 147
    synthesis 13f
        measurement of 172
        studies 152, 172
    types of 153
Globin genes, structure of 11
Globulin 62, 116
Glossitis 86
Glucocerebrosidase gene 400, 401
Glucose-6-phosphate dehydrogenase 15, 80, 152
    deficiency 66, 194-197, 197b, 200
        clinical manifestations of 197b
        detection of 198
        effect of 196f
        prevalence of 194b
    enzyme, activity of 195
    quantitative assay of 199
    role of 196f
    variants of 195t
Glutathione 195
    peroxidase 195
    regeneration of reduced 15
    stability test 574
Glycerol lysis time test 171
Glycocalyx 41
Glycogen 20
Glycoprotein 94
    absence of 44
Glycosylphosphatidylinositol 221
Golgi region 19
Golgi zone 248
Graft rejection 117, 415, 416
Graft-versus-host disease 111, 117, 217, 270, 284, 416, 417, 541
    acute 416
    chronic 416
    prevention of 415
    transfusion associated 546
Gram's stain 544
Granules
    basophilic 282f
    primary 20
    secondary 20
    tertiary 20
    types of 22

Granulocyte 221, 299, 370, 532
 analysis of 225f
 concentrate 529, 532
  administration of 532
 disorders of 389
 function, loss of 525
 macrophage
  colony stimulating factor 555
  progenitor 6
 monocyte progenitor 22
Granulocytopenia, absolute 260
Granulopoiesis, stages of 18
Grape cell 570
Graves disease 32
Gray platelet syndrome 321, 450, 459
Guillain-Barré syndrome 405
Gum hypertrophy 272

H

H cell 569
H gene 499
Haemophilus influenzae 140, 184, 191, 193
Hair coloring agents 351
Hairy cell 335, 568
 leukemia 321, 325, 331, 335, 336, 336f, 338, 382
  clinical features 336
  complications of 339
  course and prognosis 339
  diagnosis of 337, 338b
  differential diagnosis of 337, 338t
  laboratory features 336
  treatment 339
  variant 325, 330, 335, 339
Half-ghost cells 197, 197f, 568
Ham's test 79, 115, 129, 224, 572
 principle of 224f
Hand foot syndrome 185
Hand mirror cell 568
Hand-Schuller-Christian disease 402
Hapten-protein carrier complex 209
Haptoglobin in blood, reduced 543
Hashimoto's thyroiditis 32, 104
Heat instability test 574
Heavy chain gene rearrangement 25
Heinz body 152, 152f, 195, 197f, 198, 569, 574
 hemolytic anemias, congenital 142
Helicobacter pylori 91, 378
HELLP syndrome 454
Helmet cells 485, 569
Hemagglutination 129
 assay, reverse passive 514
Hemangioblasts 3
Hemarthrosis 425
Hematocrit 63
Hematogones 266
Hematologic disorders 108, 230, 321, 392
Hematoma 425
 intramuscular 464
 large local 426

Hematopoiesis 315
 clonal 288
 extramedullary 4, 320
 hierarchy of 4
 ineffective 288
 normal 5f
 primitive 3
 principal steps in 6f
 regulates normal 273
 stages of 3f
Hematopoietic
 cell 3, 95, 287, 306, 328f
  normal 252
 growth factors 6, 554
 maturing cells 4
 microenvironment 8
 niche 288
 precursor cells 4, 6t
 progenitor cells 4, 237, 554
 stem cell 3, 4, 6, 111f, 221
  defective 111
  sources of 418
  transplantation 116, 180, 193, 270, 284, 350, 414, 417, 419
Hematuria 453, 484
Heme
 biosynthesis of 14
 iron 82
 oxidation of 195
Hemighost cell 567, 568
Hemochromatosis, primary 32
Hemodilution, acute normovolemic 552
Hemoglobin 11, 65, 80, 70, 78, 99, 142, 146, 147f, 523
 A 11
 abnormal 79, 184
 Bart's hydrops fetalis syndrome 167
 C disease 144, 188
 concentration 62, 317
  determination of 62
 D disease 66
 determination of 215
 disorders of 143, 144b
 E disease 66
 electrophoresis 79, 91, 144, 163, 166, 172, 188f
 estimation of 63t
 functions of 14
 H disease 167
 hereditary disorders of 140, 141b, 141t
 in urine 78
 inherited disorders of 140, 143f
 level
  falls 61
  maintain 551
 M 142
 normal 61
  levels of 61t
 reference ranges 557
 S 181
  combination of 181
  tests for 148

separation of 148f
solutions 555
structure of 14
unstable 142
variants of 11, 11b
Hemoglobinemia 78
Hemoglobinopathy 141
  nomenclature of 142
Hemoglobinuria 196, 223f, 543
  causes of 197b
Hemolysin, biphasic 208
Hemolysis 161, 200
  causes of 79
  chronic 186
  determine cause of 79
  evidence of 197, 538
  mechanism of 202f, 206f, 209f
  pathogenesis of 135f, 195
  presence of 76
  site of 78
  well-compensated 135
Hemolytic anemia 65, 71, 74, 76, 78b, 133t, 213b, 228
  cardiac 228
  causes of 79
  chronic intravascular 219
  diagnosis of 80f
  drug-induced 209f
    immune 204, 208
  evaluation of 79f
  hereditary 66b
  mechanical 65, 226
  mild to moderate 210
Hemolytic attack 200
Hemolytic crisis 136, 185
Hemolytic disease 210, 212f, 216f, 219f, 498, 537
Hemolytic episode
  acute 199
  severe 209
Hemolytic transfusion reaction 136, 500, 541, 542, 545
  causes of 536
  diagnosis of acute 543
  investigation of 543
  prevent 512
Hemolytic uremic syndrome 453, 454, 454t, 456
Hemophagocytosis syndrome 115, 115f
Hemophilia 463
  A 423, 462, 462f, 466, 466t
    clinical features 463
    coagulation profile 464
    diagnosis of 465
    differential diagnosis 465
    genetic defects in 468
    inheritance 462
    laboratory features 464
    management 467
    molecular genetics of 468
    severe 469f
    therapy of 466
  autosomal 476

B 423, 466, 466t, 478
  leiden 478
  classical 462
  diagnosis of 465b
  mild 486
  severity of 463t
Hemorrhage 76
  fetomaternal 212
  postpartum 186
Hemorrhagic disease 480, 480t
Hemorrhagic disorders 424t
Hemorrhagic telangiectasia 444
Hemosiderin 78
Hemosiderinuria 219, 223f
Hemostasis 40f, 43, 45, 47f, 433t
  cell based model of 51
  disorders of 421
  normal 39
  screening tests for 426t
  tests for 364
Hemostatic disorders 433
Hemostatic system 425
Hemothorax 75
HEMPAS antigen 130
Henoch-Schönlein purpura 442
Heparin 431, 480, 486
  in plasma, presence of 431
  therapy 489
Hepatitis 519, 541
  A virus 547
  B 162, 179
    surface antigen 524
    virus 191, 193, 514, 546, 547
  C virus 162, 179, 450, 514, 515, 546, 548
  transfusion of 549b
  viruses 547
Hepatobiliary system 186
Hepcidin 83
Hephaestin 83
Hereditary spherocytosis 66, 133, 134, 135f-137f
  clinical features 135
  diagnosis of 140, 140b
  differential diagnosis 140
  etiopathogenesis 134
  inheritance 135
  laboratory features 136
  treatment 140
Hereditary thrombocytopenia 450
Hermansky-Pudlak syndrome 459
Hess test 573
Heterocellular distribution 151
Heterophil antibody 406
  detection of 406
Heterophile agglutination test 574
Heterozygotes, detection of 199
High molecular weight kininogen 49, 50
Hinge region 34
Hip, fracture of 75
Histidine catabolism 97

Histiocytosis X 402
Hodgkin's disease 413
Hodgkin's lymphoma 236, 357, 369-371, 374t, 384, 401, 406
    classical 374
    classification of 370, 372
    clinical features 371
    course 376
    etiopathogenesis 370
    histopathology of 372
    lymphocyte
        depleted classical 375
        rich classical 375
    mixed cellularity classical 374
    nodular
        lymphocyte predominant 373
        sclerosis classical 374
    prognosis 376
    staging of 375
    treatment 376
    types of 373t
    WHO classification of 370b
Homocysteine 95, 102, 105
Horseshoe-shaped nucleus 38
Howell-Jolly bodies 67, 74, 98f, 99, 187, 569
Human activated protein C, recombinant 486
Human immunodeficiency virus 162, 413, 450, 514, 515, 547, 548
    infections 549b
Human leukocyte antigen 27, 414
    system 30
Human neutrophil antigen 33
Human red cells 555
Hunter's syndrome 397
Hurler's syndrome 397
Hyalomere 41
Hydrogen peroxide
    detoxification of 196f
    elutes 199
Hydroxycarbamide 193
Hydroxylase deficiency 32
Hydroxyurea 108, 193, 321, 323
Hypercalcemia 350, 351, 356
Hyperchromia 569
Hypereosinophilic syndrome 395
Hyperhemolytic crisis 185
Hyperhomocysteinemia 101
Hyperkalemia 550
Hyperleukocytosis 393
Hyperlipidemia 149
Hyperparathyroidism 321
Hyperplasia, granulocytic 321
Hyperreactive malarial splenomegaly syndrome 230
Hypersplenism 65, 114, 229, 315
Hypertonic cryohemolysis test 139, 574
Hypertransfusion program 179
Hyperventilation 523
Hypocalcemia 550
Hypocellular marrow 114
Hypocellular myelodysplastic syndrome 117
Hypochromia 75, 88, 165, 569
Hypoferremia 121
Hypofibrinogenemia 479
Hypogammaglobulinemia 329, 332, 355
Hypoglycemia 217
Hypokalemia, severe 108
Hypoplastic anemia, differentiation of 115
Hypoproteinemia 217
Hypothermia 550
Hypothyroidism 71
Hypoxia 217

I

Idiopathic thrombocytopenic purpura 446, 449f
    differential diagnosis of 450t
    pathogenesis of 447f
Imerslund-Gräsbeck syndrome 94
Immature cells 293
Immature plasma cell 354f
Immature precursors, abnormal localization of 293, 567
Immature reticulocyte fraction 70
Immune complex 209, 210
    formation 37
Immune dysregulation 288
    diseases of 409
Immune function 407
    laboratory tests for evaluation of 408t
Immune hemolytic anemias 65, 136, 200, 208, 209b
    classification 200, 200b
Immune system 33
Immune thrombocytopenia 445, 446, 456
    acute 448t, 451
    chronic 445, 451
    clinical features 447
    diagnosis of 449, 450
    differential diagnosis 449
    laboratory features 448
    management of 451f
    persistent 445
    primary 445
    secondary 445
    treatment of 451b
Immune thrombocytopenic purpura 446
Immunodeficiency disease 407
    classification of 408
    primary 408, 409
    severe combined 410, 412
Immunodeficiency disorder 407
    classification of primary 409t, 410f
Immunofixation 346, 347f, 350, 574
Immunoglobulin 535
    characteristics of 35t
    classes of 34
    gene 25
        rearrangement 25
        second 25
    molecule 34
        structure of 34f
    nonspecific 535

normal 535
secreting neoplasms 341
specific 535
structure of 33
Immunohistochemistry 254, 293
Immunological cell marker analysis 252
Immunophenotyping 262, 285, 574
Immunosuppressive therapy 116, 236
Indirect antiglobulin test 203, 512
Indirect serum bilirubin 78
Indolent lymphomas 381
Indomethacin 110
Infections 65, 117, 184, 265, 443
chronic 75, 120, 346
severe 482
Infectious diseases 230, 392, 519
risk of transmission of 517
Infectious mononucleosis 372, 404
clinical features 405
diagnosis 407
etiopathogenesis 404
laboratory features 405
treatment 407
Inflammation
acute 21f
anemia of 119
chronic 120
Inflammatory diseases 230
Influenza virus, seasonal 191
Inherited thrombocytopenia 448
causes of 450b
Inhibitor
nonspecific 486
tests 499
Innate immunity 409
Innocent bystander mechanism 209
Intensive consolidation therapy 284
Intensive therapy 270
International Myeloma Working Group 344
International Prognostic Index 386
International Prognostic Scoring System for Myelodysplastic Syndromes 296t
International Society of Blood Transfusion 497
International Union of Immunological Societies 408, 409t
Intracellular granules, deficiency of 459
Intracranial hemorrhage 464
risk of 452
Intracytoplasmic myeloperoxidase, detection of 561
Intravascular fibrin formation, pathogenesis of 484f
Intravascular hemolysis 77, 77f, 78t
diagnosis of 543
Intravenous fluids 541
Intrinsic immunity 409
Ionizing radiation 235
Iron 65
absorption 82, 83b
mechanism of 83f
amount of 93
binding capacity, total 87, 92, 578
chelation therapy 179

containing granules 123
deficiency anemia 65, 81, 86, 88f, 89, 89f, 91, 92, 122t, 127, 138, 165, 219, 444, 447
causes of 85, 85b
development of 87, 87b, 87f
diagnosis of 91b
differential diagnosis of 92t
high risk of 86b
treatment of 92
dietary sources of 82
incorporation of 85
metabolism
impairment of 121
normal 81, 81f
overload 161, 186, 550
pathogenesis of 162f
quantitation of 180
replacement therapy 93
requirements 82
daily 82b
storage of 85
studies, reference ranges 558
sucrose 93
therapy 122
transport of 84
Isopropanol precipitation test 574

J

Job's syndrome 398
Juvenile cell 569
Juvenile hemochromatosis 83
Juvenile myelomonocytic leukemia 310

K

Kaolin clotting time 574
Karyogram 306f
Kasabach-Merritt syndrome 483
K-dependent coagulation factors 478
Keratocyte 567, 569
Kidney
damage 556
loss of
endocrine function of 125
excretory function of 125
Kleihauer-Betke stain 574
Klinefelter's syndrome 19, 235
Koilonychias 86
Kostmann's syndrome 235, 394

L

L cell 569
Lactate dehydrogenase 102
Lacunar cell 569
Lambda light chain 328f
Laminin B receptor 396
Langerhans cell 402
histiocytosis 402
Latex agglutination test, principle of 439f
Laurell rocket immunoelectrophoresis method 476

Index

Lead poisoning 125
Leder stain 250
Leg ulcers, chronic 136
Leishman-Donovan body 569
Leishmania donovani 547
Lenalidomide 361
Leptocyte 569
Lesch-Nyhan syndrome 472
Letterer-Siwe disease 402
Leucapheresis 524
Leucocytosis, terms related to 393*b*
Leukemia 64, 139, 235*b*, 236, 254*f*, 381, 406, 448
    acute
        basophilic 279
        lymphoblastic 236, 240, 241, 243, 254, 281, 335, 560
        megakaryoblastic 248, 275, 279
        monoblastic 275, 279
        monocytic 275, 279
        myeloid 109, 118, 235, 236, 241, 242, 248*b*, 254, 265, 271, 274, 275, 279, 280*t*, 283*f*, 318, 396, 560
        myelomonocytic 279, 295
        promyelocytic 247, 253, 277
        undifferentiated 254
    associated immunophenotype 255
    B
        lymphoblastic 242, 260
        prolymphocytic 339
    categories of 381*b*
    chronic
        eosinophilic 299
        lymphoid 325, 325*t*, 330, 330*f*, 331*t*, 333
        myelogenous 282, 309*t*
        myelomonocytic 289, 310
        neutrophilic 299, 300, 310
    cutis 272
    development of 237, 237*f*
    risk of acute 235
    types of acute 237
Leukemic blasts 260
Leukemic cells 285
Leukemic lymphoblasts 261
Leukemogenesis 237
    mechanism of 301*f*
Leukemoid reaction 281, 309, 310*t*, 389, 392
    causes of 392*b*
    lymphoid type 569
    myeloid type 393, 569
Leukocyte 221, 398, 400, 530, 561
    adhesion deficiency 561
        congenital 398
    alkaline phosphatase score 574
    analysis 561
    count 20*f*
        reference ranges of differential 558
    depleted red cells 530
    disorders of 389
    poor red cells 529, 530
    qualitative disorders of 389
    quantitative disorders of 389, 389*b*
Leukocytosis 64, 149, 389, 392, 393

Leukoerythroblastic
    blood 128*f*
    reaction 320*f*, 389, 392, 393, 569
        causes of 392*b*
    smear 315
Leukoerythroblastosis 127
Leukopenia 98, 389
Lhermitte sign 105
Light chain gene rearrangement 25
Liley's graph 575
Liquid chromatography, high-performance 146, 147*f*, 164*f*, 189*f*, 574
Liver 319
    biopsy 180
    cells 95
    cirrhosis of 230, 481
    disease 71, 74, 77, 89, 138, 431, 481
        anemia of 127
        bleeding in 481
        chronic 431
    function tests 113
    in hemostasis, role of 481*t*
Loeffler's syndrome 394
Lumbar puncture 264
Lung injury, transfusion associated 541, 544
Lupus anticoagulant 487
    diagnosis of 488*b*
    identification of 488*f*
Lupus inhibitor 487
Lymph node
    biopsy 364, 384, 406
    enlargement of 404
Lymphoblast 245, 246*f*, 247, 264
    proportion of 260
Lymphoblastic leukemia 235
Lymphoblastic lymphoma 387
Lymphocyte 24, 341, 370
    atypical 405*f*, 567
    culture, mixed 576
    doubling time 333
    large 10*f*
    like lymphoblasts 260
    nucleus of small 88*f*
    reactive 567
    small 10*f*, 97*f*
    subsets, enumeration of 561
    types of 24
    typing
        primed 576
        test, primed 33
    vacuolated 572
Lymphocytic leukemia
    staging systems for chronic 332*t*
    types of chronic 326*f*
Lymphocytic lymphoma, small 27
Lymphocytosis 403
    acute infectious 403
    benign polyclonal 330
    causes of 403*b*
    reactive 265, 330
Lymphocytotoxicity test 575

Lymphohistiocytosis, hemophagocytic 115
Lymphoid
    antigens 254
    cells 301
    leukemoid reaction 392
    neoplasms 27*f*
        WHO classification of 379*b*
    progenitor, common 6
    proliferations 327
    tissues 369
Lymphoma 242, 243, 260, 321, 330, 359, 359*t*
    aggressive 381
    B lymphoblastic 242
    categories of 381*b*
    malignant 369
Lymphoplasmacytic lymphoma 339, 382
Lymphoproliferative disorder 445, 487
    X-linked 405
Lymphosarcoma cell leukemia 335
Lysosomal trafficking regulator gene 397
Lysosomes 23, 42
Lysozyme 23

M

M protein 344
Macrocytic anemia 71
    evaluation of 73, 73*f*
    severe 118
Macrocytosis 74, 291, 569
    oval 74*b*, 98
Macroglobulin 35
Macro-ovalocyte 570
Macrophages 8, 22, 25, 95, 134
    cell 7
Macropolycyte 570
Maintenance therapy 269
Malabsorption syndrome 480
Malaria 196, 514, 519
    parasite 516, 546, 547
Mannose-associated serine protease 36
Mannose-binding lectin 36
Mantle cell lymphoma 331, 378, 382
March hemoglobinuria 228
Marrow hypoplasia 108
Massive blood transfusion 550
Massive transfusion 455
Maternal blood group 211
Maturation 279
    arrest 570
Maurer's clefts 570
Maurer's dots 570
May-Hegglin anomaly 397, 450, 452, 452*f*
Mean cell
    hemoglobin 98
    volume 87, 92
Mean corpuscular
    hemoglobin 71, 575
        concentration 71, 184, 575
    volume 70, 575
Mean platelet volume 428, 575

Measles virus 443
Megakaryoblast 245, 247
Megakaryocyte 39*f*, 40, 305, 315, 324, 449*f*
    abnormal 323
    abnormalities in 293
    development of 38
    dysplastic 293
    erythroid progenitor 6
    fragments 291
    mature 39
Megakaryopoiesis 38
Megaloblastic anemia 65, 71, 77, 93, 97, 97*f*, 98*f*, 100, 101, 107, 108, 115, 127, 448
    causes of 100
    laboratory diagnosis of 103*f*
Megaloblastic crisis 136, 185
Megaloblastic madness 105
Megaloblasts 99
    hemolysis of 102
Megathrombocyte 449*f*
Memory cells 25
Meningitis 184
Menorrhagia 86, 91
Mental retardation syndromes 168
Mentzer index 575
Metabisulfite test 575
Metabolism, congenital defects of 108
Metamyelocyte 19
Metastatic carcinoma 321, 359
Metastatic tumors 265
Methemalbumin 78
Methemalbuminemia 78
Methemoglobin 62
    elution method 199, 575
    test 199, 575
Methionine, synthesis of 95
Methotrexate 65, 100
Methyldopa 65
Methylene blue 197, 199
Methylmalonic acid 102, 105
Meticulous anesthetic technique 554
Meticulous surgical technique 554
Mexican hat cell 572
Microangiopathic hemolytic anemia 227, 227*f*, 450, 453, 454
    causes of 227*b*
Microbiologic techniques 513
Microbiological agents 513
Microbiological techniques 504
Microcolumn chromatography 150
Microcytic anemia 71
Microcytic hypochromic
    anemia 87*f*, 123
        causes of 74
        evaluation of 74, 75*f*
        red cells 163*f*, 165*f*, 171*f*
Microcytosis 75, 88, 570
Micro-drepanocytic disease 165
Microhematocrit method 64

Micromegakaryocytes 293, 570
Microorganisms transmissible by transfusion 547*b*
Microspherocytes 197*f*
Minimal residual disease 270, 285
Mitogen-activated protein kinase 402
Molecular genetic
    analysis 321
        applications of 257*b*
    studies 257, 264
Molecular weight heparins, low 490
Monoblast 245, 247
Monoblastic leukemia 272
Monoclonal antibodies 253*t*
Monoclonal B-cell lymphocytosis 329, 331, 403
Monoclonal gammopathies, benign 366
Monoclonal gammopathy 341, 366
Monoclonal immunoglobulins 341, 343*b*
    quantitation of 347
Monoclonal protein 344
    demonstration of 343
    laboratory characterization of 344*b*
Monocyte 7, 10*f*, 22, 25, 221, 305
    and macrophages 413
        macrophage system 399
            hyperplasia of 136
Monocytopenia 336
Monocytosis 399
    causes of 400*b*
Monogenic diseases 472
Mononuclear cells 484*f*
Mononuclear phagocyte system 23*f*
Mononucleosis syndrome 403
Monospecific antisera 347*f*
Monospot test 576
Montreal platelet syndrome 450
Morphologic dysplasia 288
Morula cell 354, 570
Mott cell 354, 570
Motulsky dye reduction test 576
Mucosa-associated lymphoid tissue 27
Multilineage dysplasia 274, 310
Multilobated megakaryocytes 323*f*
Multimeric analysis 576
Multinucleated cells 354
Multiple myeloma 321, 350
Multiple plasma cell myeloma 360*t*
Multiple sclerosis 32
Multipotent progenitor cell 6
Muscle dystonia 222
Mushroom-shaped red cell 570
Mutation, direct detection of 191
Myasthenia gravis 104
Mycobacterial infections 117
Myeloblasts 9*f*, 18, 245, 246*f*, 247, 276
Myelocyte 19
    peak 311
Myelodysplasia 282, 448
    related changes 242, 243, 274, 277, 279
Myelodysplastic neoplasms 310

Myelodysplastic syndrome 8, 71, 100, 108, 168, 236, 240, 243, 271, 273-275, 281, 287, 290, 291, 292*f*, 294*b*, 295, 321, 396
    abnormal clones in 288
    cause of 288, 288*t*
    classification of 289
    clinical features 291
    diagnosis of 272
    differential diagnosis 295
    international prognostic scoring system for 296*t*
        revised 296*t*
    laboratory features 291
    pathogenesis of 287, 287*f*
    primary 288, 289*t*
    prognosis 295
    risk of 118
    treatment 297
Myelofibrosis 236, 248, 271, 275, 279, 315
    primary 299, 300, 318*f*, 319, 320*f*
Myeloid 221, 253, 254*f*, 272
    antigens, co-expression of 263
    cells, left-shifted 315
    leukemoid reaction 392
    metaplasia 319
    neoplasms 322
    precursors 9*f*
    progenitor, common 6
    proliferations 243, 275
    sarcoma 241-243, 275
    transcription factors 238, 240
    tumor, extramedullary 275
Myeloid : erythroid ratio 570
Myeloid leukemia
    lymphoid blast crisis of chronic 266
    molecular pathogenesis
        of acute 237
        of chronic 303*f*
    pathogenesis
        of acute 239*f*
        of chronic 303*f*
Myelokathexis 397, 570
Myeloma 345*f*, 352*f*, 357*f*
    asymptomatic 358, 362
    cells 351
    diagnosis of 357*f*
    signs of 348
    typical features of 357*f*
Myelomonocytic appearance 282*f*
Myeloperoxidase 23, 248, 249, 254, 399, 575
    deficiency of 293, 399
Myelophthisic anemia 127, 128*b*
    causes of 127
Myeloproliferative diseases 271, 300, 301, 310, 317
Myeloproliferative disorders 396
Myeloproliferative neoplasms 299, 300, 300*b*, 310, 311*t*, 314*f*, 321, 460
    diagnosis of 317, 318*f*
Myocardial infarction 318

N

Nalidixic acid 197
Napoleon hat cell 570
Naproxen 110
Natural killer cells 30, 221
Negakaryopoiesis 38f
Neisseria meningitides 191
Neonatal alloimmune thrombocytopenic purpura 43
Neonatal jaundice 197
Neonatal thrombocytopenia, causes of 452b
Neoplasia 487
Neoplasm 120, 341
    hematological 560
    types of 274
Neoplastic cells
    infiltration of 327
    morphology of 381
Neoplastic clone, part of 319
Neoplastic diseases 77
Neoplastic plasma cells 343t, 354
Neoplastic plasmacytosis 342
Neoplastic small lymphocytes 330
Nephrotic syndrome 186
Nestroft 576
Neural tube defects, development of 101
Neutropenia 8, 393
    absolute 98
    causes of 394b
    clinical features 394
    grading of 393t
Neutrophil 10f, 18, 20f, 568
    adhesion 21f
    alkaline phosphatase 316
        score 305, 576
    Botryoid nuclei of 567
    count, absolute 296
    Döhle body in 568
    doughnut nuclei of 571
    dysfunction 398b
    formation of mature 18f
    function 20, 408
        defect 399
        disorders of 397, 398f
        evaluation of 561
    granules 19, 20b
    hyposegmentation of 569
    kinetics 20f
    left in 391f
    morphological abnormalities of 396f
    ring of 571
    segmented 19
    series, shift to left in 391f
    specific antigens 33
    toxic granulation in 391f, 572
Neutrophilia 389, 390f
    causes of 390b
    dawn of 19
Neutrophilic leucocytosis 389, 390
    causes of 390b

New methylene blue 575
Nicotinamide adenine dinucleotide phosphate 399
Niemann-Pick cell 401f
    demonstration of 402
Niemann-Pick disease 392, 401, 402
    types of 402
Nile blue sulfate 199
    preferably 199
Nitroblue tetrazolium dye reduction test 576
Nitrocellulose membranes 175
Nitrofurantoin 197
Nitrous oxide 108
NK-cell neoplasms, mature 380
Nodular marginal zone lymphoma 382
Nonagglutinated cells 508
Non-hemolytic transfusion 542
    reactions, low-risk of 530
Non-Hodgkin's lymphoma 244, 330, 369, 369t, 377, 377b, 386, 386b
    acquired disorders 377
    aggressive 387
    classification of 379
    clinical features of 381
    congenital disorders 377
    diagnosis of 386b
    laboratory investigations 384
    leukemic phase of 265
    low-grade 387
    pathogenesis 377
    predisposing factors 377
    staging of 386
    treatment of 387
Noninvasive prenatal diagnosis 472
Nonmegaloblastic anemia 71
Nonmegaloblastic macrocytosis, causes of 109
Nonsecretory myeloma 349, 361
Nonsecretory plasma cell myeloma 362
Normoblast, basophilic 9
Normocytic anemia 71, 75, 79
    evaluation of 75, 76f
Nuclear budding 292
Nuclear cytoplasmic ratio, low 265
Nuclear hypersegmentation 291
Nucleated red cells 163f
Nucleic acid testing 515
Nucleophosmin 238, 239
Nucleotide sequence, normal 175f
Numerous target cells 144
Nurse cell 570
Nutritional deficiency 65

O

Obstructive jaundice 480
Oligoblastic leukemia 287
Oligonucleotide probe
    analysis 176, 177f, 470
    hybridization, sequence-specific 33
Oncogenesis, mechanism of 236
Opsonization 211

Index

Oral
　anticoagulant 490, 491
　　therapy 430, 491
　contraceptive pill 108, 192
　iron therapy 92
　vitamin B$_{12}$ 108
Organelle zone 42
Origin, cell of 325
Oropharyngeal mucositis 415
Orthostatic purpura 443
Osler-Weber-Rendu disease 444
Osmotic fragility 138
　test 137, 137f, 138, 138b, 576
　　limitations of 137
Osteoblasts 8
Osteoclast-activating factors 357
Osteolytic lesions 348
Osteomyelitis 184
Osteopetrosis 392
Osteoporosis 162
Oxidant stress 194
Oxygen
　affinity 15
　　low 142
　tension 184
Oxyhemoglobin 15, 62
　method 63

P

Packed cell volume 61, 61t, 64f
　determination of 63
　reference ranges 557
Packed red cell 527f, 529, 529b
　transfusion 192, 285, 536
Paget's disease of bone 321
Pagophagia 86
Pamaquine 197
Pancellular distribution 151
Pancytopenia 74, 114, 219, 339, 415
　causes of 114t
Panmyelosis, acute 248, 275, 279
Pappenheimer bodies 187, 570
Paracoagulation tests 438, 574, 576
Paranasal sinuses 272
Paraproteinemia 149, 341, 460, 492
Parasites 395
Parenteral fluid therapy, prolonged 101
Paroxysmal cold hemoglobinuria 197, 205, 207, 208t
Paroxysmal nocturnal hemoglobinuria 80, 111, 117, 130, 219, 221b, 226b, 562
　classification of 222t
Parvovirus B$_{19}$ 135
Paternal zygosity 214
Paternal zygosity testing 214
Patterson-Kelly syndrome 86
Paul-Bunnell test 265, 406, 576
Paul-Bunnell-Davidsohn test 406, 576
Pelger-Huet anomaly 396, 570
Pelvis 272

Pencil cell 88, 570
Penicillins 65
Pentagastrin test 576
Pentose phosphate shunt 15
Pentostatin 340
Percutaneous umbilical blood sampling 215
Perfluorocarbons 556
Periodic acid Schiff 249, 575
　reaction 248, 251
　stain 262f
Periodic neutropenia 394
Peripheral blood 20f, 97f, 98, 101, 128f, 129, 320, 331t, 333, 395f
　Examination of 88, 112, 136, 163, 186, 202, 223, 260, 276, 291, 341, 448
　lymphocytes, incubation of 118
　plasma cells in 404
　smear 88f, 123f, 292f, 353f, 458
　　examination of 66, 218
　stem cell mobilization and harvesting 418
Peripheral neuropathy 105
Perl's prussian blue 89, 249
Perls stain 575
Pernicious anemia 104, 104b
Peroxidase stain 575
Petechiae 425
pH chromosome, absence of 309
Phagocytic defects 409
Phagocytic leukocytes
　disorders of 396
　functional disorders of 397
Phagocytic system 401
Phenacetin 197
Phenotypic methods 470
Phenylbutazone 65, 110
Phenytoin 110
Pheresis 531b
Philadelphia chromosome 282, 306f
　formation of 301f
Phosphates 82
Phosphatidylcholine 41
Phosphatidylinositol 41, 221
Phospholipid 50
Phototherapy 217
Pincer cell 570
Piroxicam 110
Plasma
　column of 64f
　components 533, 537
　group 537
　haptoglobin 77, 78
　pink coloration of 543
　potassium level 525
　proteins 45
　transfusion of 537, 537t
　volume 62, 313f
Plasma cell 25, 341, 350, 354f, 370, 374, 404, 505
　abnormal 350
　differentiation 359, 359t

mature looking 353
morphological features of 354f
neoplasm 341, 357
Plasma cell dyscrasias 341, 341b, 342b, 346
salient features of 349t
Plasma cell myeloma 349, 350, 353f-355f, 358, 358b, 358t, 361, 362, 365, 365t, 367
   biochemical abnormalities 356
   bone marrow
      aspiration 353
      examination 353
   clinical features 351
   cytogenetic analysis 356
   diagnosis 357
   differential diagnosis 357
   etiology 351
   free light chain assay 355
   hemorrhagic tendencies 352
   hyperviscosity syndrome 352
   immunohistochemistry 356
   infections 352
   laboratory features 353
   pathogenesis of 350, 351f
   peripheral blood examination 353
   prognosis 360
   protein alterations 354
   radiological features 357
   renal failure 352
   skeletal system 351
   staging 360
      systems of 360
   treatment 360
   typical features of 357b
Plasmablastic lymphoma 382
Plasmablastic myeloma cells 354
Plasmacytoma
   extramedullary 363
   extraosseous 363
Plasmacytosis, reactive 358t
Plasmapheresis 523
Plasmin
   digests 52
   proteolytic action of 486
Plasminogen activators 54
Plasmodia, species of 228
Plasmodium
   falciparum 142, 399f
   ovale 571
   species 549
   vivax 571
Platelet 10f, 40, 99, 291, 299, 452, 486, 531, 531b
   abnormalities of 445
   activation 562
   aggregation of 40, 44f
      studies 433, 576
   aggregometry 434
   analysis 562
   and coagulation disorders 425t
   antibodies 449

antigens 43
concentrate 527f, 529-532
count 353, 427
   reference ranges 558
decreased production of 446
disorders of 445
distribution width 576
dysfunction 315, 445
fibrin thrombi 483
function
   acquired disorders of 460
   analyzer 427, 576
   defect 433
   defective 324
   disorders of 427, 435t, 457, 457t, 459f, 562
   inherited disorders of 457
   loss of 525
   tests 436
   tests for specific 433
   tests, salient features of 434t
granules 434
increased destruction of 446
lifespan of affected 460
membrane glycoproteins 42
normal-sized 450
on blood smear, normal distribution of 455f
organelles 42t
peripheral destruction of 452
phase 424
procoagulant activity 45, 45f
   tests for 435
reticulated 40, 428, 562
rich plasma 436, 531
role of 43
secretion, tests of 435
single large 449f
size abnormalities 570
small 450
transfusions 117
ultrastructure of 41, 41f
Plateletpheresis 523, 532
Pleomorphic mantle cell lymphoma 335
Plumbism 125
Plummer-Vinson syndrome 86
Pneumocystis
   carinii 413
   jiroveci 269
Pneumonia 196, 269, 412
POEMS syndrome 350, 357
Poikilocytosis 570
Polyacrylamide gel electrophoresis 17
Polyadenylation mutations 157, 157f
Polyagglutinable red cells 510
Polychromasia 163f, 571
Polychromatic cells 91, 136f, 197f, 202f, 216f, 485f
Polychromatic normoblast 9
Polychromatic red cells 67
Polychromatophilia 571
Polyclonal hypergammaglobulinemia 345f

Polyclonal immunoglobulins 341
Polycythemia 149, 313, 313f, 317t
    absolute 313
    apparent 313
    causes of 313t
    secondary 317, 317t
    types of 313f
Polycythemia vera 236, 271, 299, 300, 313, 315, 317t, 318f
    bone marrow examination 315
    clinical features 315
    course and prognosis 318
    diagnosis of 316b, 317
    differential diagnosis 317
    laboratory features 315
    pathogenesis of 314f
    peripheral blood examination 315
    treatment 319
Polycythemic blood samples 64f
Polyglutamates 96
Polymerase chain reaction 173, 174f, 271, 470, 472
    reverse transcriptase 256
Polymorphic mutations 194
Polymorphonuclear neutrophil 19
Polypeptide chain 49f
    elongation of 14
    pairs of 14
    primary 14
Popcorn cell 569, 571
Portal hypertension 481
    complications of 321
Postpolycythemic myelofibrosis 318, 319
Postremission therapy 284
Precursor cells, normal 266
Precursor lymphoid neoplasms 379
Predeposit autologous blood transfusion 551
Prednisolone 387
Predonation counseling 518
Preimplantation genetic diagnosis 191
Prekallikrein 49
Preleukemic syndrome 287
Proerythroblast 9
Prognostic scoring systems 295
Proliferative retinopathy 186
Prolonged thrombin time, evaluation of 439f
Prolymphocytic leukemia 265, 331-333, 334f
    clinical features 334
    course and prognosis 335
    differential diagnosis 334
    genetic analysis 334
    laboratory features 334
    treatment 335
Prolymphocytic transformation 335
Promyelocyte 9, 19, 245, 247, 273, 283f
    abnormal 252
Promyelocytic leukemia, treatment of acute 285
Protamine neutralization assay 576
Protamine sulfate test 576
Protease inhibitor 57
Protein
    abnormalities, investigation of 343
    C 57
        deficiency 491
        inhibitor 57
    coagulable 437
    major basic 22
    S 40
    synthesis of 481
    Z 57
        dependent protease inhibitor 57
Proteinuria 186, 453
Proteolytic enzyme papain 34
Prothrombin 47
    complex concentrate 478, 534
    time 576
Prothrombinase 47
    complex 51
Proton pump inhibitors 82
Prussian blue
    reaction 293
    stain 89f, 290, 575
Pseudo-Gaucher's cells 401, 571
Pseudogenes 12f
Pseudomonas 545, 547
Pseudoneutrophilia 393
Pseudo-Pelger-Huét
    anomaly 291, 293
    cell 292f, 396
Pseudothrombocytopenia 448, 455
Pseudovon Willebrand disease 475
Pteroylmonoglutamic acid 96
Pulmonary disorders 395
Punctate basophilia 67, 567
Pure red cell aplasia, acquired 119
Purines, synthesis of 97
Purpura 363, 425
    mechanical 443
    post-transfusion 453, 541, 546
    simplex 443
Pyknocyte 567, 571
Pyropoikilocytosis, hereditary 133

R

Radial immunodiffusion 347
Radioimmunoassay 515
Random donor platelets 531
Rapid slide tests 406
Rapoport-Luebering shunt 15
Raynaud's phenomenon 363
Reaction, release 435
Recipient blood group 537
Red blood cell 9, 206, 221, 291
    disorders of 59
    normal 322f
Red cell 62, 65, 98, 130, 134, 206, 299, 504, 504, 523, 529
    abnormalities 75
        early 72
        mild 72

agglutination 205
analysis 225*f*
antigen 210, 530, 545
    autoantibodies against 210
    loss of 510
    target 208
apheresis 523
aplasia, pure 119
artificially 514
autoagglutination of 207*f*, 567
coating of 510
column of 64*f*
components 529
concentrate 529*b*
count, reference ranges 557
destruction 18, 79, 134, 211, 219
    excessive 65, 133
detection of 562
dimorphic 67, 568
    population of 123*f*, 292*f*
distribution width 71, 92, 577
enumeration of 562
enzymes 15
    disorders of 194
extravascular destruction of 76
folate 74, 101
formation of mature 10*f*
hypochromic 91, 161
in additive solution 529, 530
in anemia 529
indices 70, 72, 88, 170
    reference ranges 557
irradiated 529, 531
layer 538
loss of viability of 524
mass 313, 313*f*, 315
    normal 313
mature 115*f*
membrane 16, 17*f*, 65, 209, 221*f*
    disorders of 133, 133*t*
    protein, types of 17
metabolic pathways in 16*b*, 16*f*
morphological abnormalities of 68*f*
production 69, 81, 121
    impaired 65
ranges of 70
stored 550
substitutes 555
survival 120
    shortening of 125
suspension 530
terminology 67*b*
transfusion, regular 178
types of 92
washed 529, 530
Redox dye 199
Reed-Sternberg cell 370, 406, 571
    classical 372
Refractory anemia 124, 289
Refractory cytopenia 290

Reiter syndrome 32
Relative proportions of hemoglobins,
    reference ranges 558
Remission induction 268, 284
Renal abnormalities 453
Renal diseases 492
Renal failure 454
    signs of chronic 126
    symptoms of chronic 126
Renal function tests 79
Renal insufficiency 350
Renal osteodystrophy 321
Renal papillary necrosis 194
Replacement blood donor 518
Replacement donors, types of 518
Replacement therapy, complications of 468
Respiratory
    burst 399
    distress 544
        syndrome 214, 550
    system 186
Responder cells 33
Restless leg syndrome 86
Restriction endonuclease analysis 470
Restriction enzymes 191
Restriction fragment length polymorphism 470
    analysis 176, 191
Reticulin fibers 319, 322
Reticulin fibrosis, abundant 248
Reticulin stain 575
Reticulocyte 69
    count 66, 67, 70, 75, 78, 121, 562
        absolute 67, 70
        corrected 67
        reference ranges 558
    enriched red cells 152
    hemoglobin 70, 88
    measures of 67
    production index 67, 70
    response 70
Reticulocytopenia 118
    causes of 69
Reticulocytosis 74, 215
    causes of 69
Reticuloendothelial cells 451
Reticuloendothelial system 121
    macrophages of 77*f*
Retinal damage 179
Reverse dot hybridization 174
Rh
    antibodies 502
    antigens 502
    hemolytic disease 211, 218, 500
        risk of 511
    immune globulin 217
    immunization, prevention of 217
    incompatible allograft 204
Rh negative 501, 511
    blood 537
    group 537

Rh positive 501
    blood 537
    fetus 211
Rh system 500
    antigens of 501
    genes of 501*f*
RhD groups 502*t*, 511
    method of 511
Rheumatoid arthritis 121, 32, 410
Ribosome-lamellar complexes 571
Richter's syndrome 332
Rickettsial organisms 443
Rieder cell 571
Ring sideroblasts 571
Ringer's lactate 539
Ristocetin cofactor assay 577
Ristocetin-induced platelet aggregation 476, 577
Romberg's sign 105
Rosette test 216
Rouleaux formation 353*f*, 509, 571
Rule of 3 63*b*
Rumpel-Leede test 573
Russell's bodies 571
Russell's viper venom time 577

S

Sahli's acid hematin method 63
Salmonella 184, 443
    osteomyelitis 186
Sarcoma, granulocytic 275
Saw-scaled viper 438
Schilling test 106, 577
    disadvantages of 106
    interpretation of 106*b*
Schistocyte 227*f*, 485, 568, 571
Schizocyte 571
Schuffner's dots 571
Schuffner's granules 571
Schumm's test 78, 577
Schwachman-Diamond syndrome 118
Scurvy 443
Sea-blue histiocytes 571
Sebastian syndrome 397, 450
Secretory vesicles 20
Semen sample 499
Senile purpura 443
Sepsis 184
    infection 482
Septicemia 217
Serological techniques 504
Serous atrophy 571
Serratia marcescens 399
Serum 344, 577
    alkaline phosphatase 356
    creatinine 356
    erythropoietin
        level 316
        subnormal 317

ferritin 89, 89*b*, 180
    concentration 87
folate 102
    estimation of 101
free light chain assay 348, 577
grouping 510, 536
haptoglobin 78, 577
holotranscobalamin 105
homocysteine 577
iron 89, 121
    low 121
lactate dehydrogenase 102
methylmalonic acid 577
protein 36
protein electrophoresis 344, 344*b*, 345*f*, 358
    densitometric scanning of 345*f*
vitamin B_{12} 101
    levels 102, 104
Sézary cell 571
Shwachman-Diamond syndrome 113
Sickle cell 188
    anemia 145, 145*f*, 146*f*, 165, 166, 181, 184-186,
        187*f*-189*f*, 191, 191*b*, 192, 193, 193*b*
        course of 193
        diagnosis of 176
        treatment of 191
    beta thalassemia 165, 181
    disease 138, 144, 160, 181, 185, 187, 192*b*
    disorder 66, 181, 182, 187, 188*t*
    gene 182
    solubility test 149*f*
    trait 146*f*, 181, 187, 181, 188, 188*f*, 189*f*, 193, 194*f*
Sickle hemoglobin 187
Sickled red cells, formation of 183*f*
Sickling syndrome 149
Sickling test 148, 148*f*
    limitations of 149
Sideroblast 571
Sideroblastic anemia 92, 122, 123*f*
    acquired 124
    causes of 123, 124*b*
    hereditary 124
    pathogenesis 124
    types 123
Sideroblasts 122, 123
    types of 123*f*
Siderocyte 572
Single donor platelets 532
Single tube osmotic fragility test 171*f*, 577
Single unit transfusions, avoidance of 554
Skeletal survey, normal 349
Skeletal system 186
Skin 186
    infiltration 272
Slide test 504
Small intestine, diseases of 104
Smoldering acute leukemia 287
Smoldering myeloma 358, 358*b*, 362
Smoldering plasma cell myeloma 341, 349

Smudge cell 567, 572
Snake venom 438
Snakebite 483
Sodium
    chloride 171f
    hydroxide 150
    sulfite 437
Soft tissues 272
Solitary eosinophilic granuloma 402
Solitary plasmacytoma 349
    of bone 362
Solubility test 149, 577
Soluble transferrin receptor 84, 90, 577
Somatic hypermutation 350
Southern blot analysis 175, 177f, 190f
    principle of 176f
Spherocyte 202f, 572
Sphingomyelin 41
Sphingomyelinase, assay of 402
Spin cross-match 512
Spleen 62, 161, 319
    enlargement of 315
    functions of 229
    normal structure of 229
Splenectomy 140, 180
    functional 184
Splenic lymphoma 331, 365
Splenic marginal zone lymphoma 331, 338, 365
Splenic sequestration crisis 185
Splenomegaly, common causes of 230b
Spliceosome complex 238
    genes 240
Sponge 41
Sporadic mutations 194
Spur cell 572
    anemia 127
Stab cell 572
Staghorn appearance 322
Staphylococci 547
Staphylococcus 545
    aureus 399
Starry sky appearance 572
Stem cell
    collection 524
    transplant 518
        autologous hematopoietic 418t
Sternum 272
Steroids, anabolic 118
Stimulator cells 32
Stomatocyte 572
Storage cells 401f
Storage disorders 392, 400
Storage pool deficiency 435, 457, 459
Stored blood 524
    massive transfusion of 492
Streptococcus pneumoniae 184, 191
Stress lymphocytosis 404
Stress-bearing joints 464
Stroke 185, 318
Stypven time 577

Sucrose hemolysis test 223, 577
Sugar water test 223
Sulfasalazine 100
Sulphamethoxazole 197
Superconducting quantum interference device 180
Superior vena cava syndrome 259
Supportive therapy 285
Supravital stain 69f
Surface membrane immunoglobulin 262
Symptomatic myeloma 361
Symptomatic thrombocytopenia, severe 452
Syncope 522
Syndromic immunodeficiencies 409
Syphilis 514, 516
Systemic lupus erythematosus 32, 117, 410
Systemic polyclonal immunoblastic proliferation 359

T

T cells 404, 413
    regulatory 28
T lymphoblastic leukemia 242, 260
T lymphocyte 24t, 27, 221
    functions of 28b, 408
T lymphoid 253
Tallqvist blotting paper method 63
Tannates 82
Target cell 167, 572
    presence of 91
Target joint 464
Tart cell 572
Tartrate-resistant acid phosphatase 575
Tay-Sachs disease 472
T-cell 333
    acute lymphoblastic leukemia 240
    development, stages of 29f
    helper-inducer 29
    lymphoma 342
    mature 29
    neoplasms, mature 265, 380, 383t
    ontogeny 29
    receptor 28
        complex 28f
Tear drop
    cells 67, 320f
    red cell 572
Telangiectasia 425
Telomere length assay 577
Tempi syndrome 350
Testicular biopsy 265
Tetanus vaccines 408
Tetracyclines 82
Tetrahydrofolate 96, 97
Tetrazolium linked cytochemical method 199, 577
Textarin: ecarin ratio 577
Thalassemia 71, 83, 138, 141-143, 152, 159b, 160, 168, 178, 180t, 183
    carrier state 171f
    classification of 153
    clinical feature of 160

dominant 158
intermedia 169
laboratory features of 160
minor 91, 165*f*
molecular basis of 153
nontransfusion-dependent 153
pathogenesis of 160
prenatal diagnosis of 178*f*
prevalence of 159
prevention of 169, 170
Thalidomide 361
Therapeutic agents 312
Therapeutic irradiation 236
Therapy-related myeloid neoplasms 242, 243, 274, 279
Thesaurocyte 572
Thrombin
generation of 484*f*
multiple actions of 47*f*
time 577
Thrombin-activated fibrinolytic inhibitor 53
Thrombocythemia, essential 299, 300, 318*f*, 322, 322*f*, 323*f*, 324*t*
Thrombocytopenia 99, 202, 260, 265, 291, 426, 428, 433, 445, 454, 485*f*
absent radii syndrome 452
artefactual 446
causes of 446*t*, 450, 456
chronic immune 448*t*
congenital amegakaryocytic 119
drug-induced 449
evaluation of 456*f*
isolated 450
mild-to-moderate 458
severe 546
Thrombocytosis 64, 322*f*, 428, 445, 457
causes of 457*t*
reactive 324*t*
Thromboelastography 440
Thrombolytic therapy 480
Thrombomodulin 40, 57
Thromboplastin 24, 47
generation test 436, 465, 578
interpretation of 437*t*
Thrombopoietin 7
receptor agonists 8
Thrombosis, risk of 319
Thrombotic microangiopathy 453
Thrombotic thrombocytopenic purpura 453, 454*t*, 456
Thromboxane synthesis 44*f*
defective 457, 460
Thromobocytopenia 277
Thymic hypoplasia 411
Ticlopidine 110
Tissue
factor 50
pathway inhibitor 56*f*, 57
thromboplastin inhibition test 578
T-lymphoid neoplasms, mature 561
Toluidine blue 575

Total leukocyte count 267, 389
reference ranges 558
Toxic granules 485*f*
Toxoplasma 413
gondii 547
Tranquilizers 110
Transcobalamin 94
Transcriptase-polymerase chain reaction 307
Transcription factor fusions 238, 239
Transferrin
receptor 87, 92
saturation 90, 578
transferrin receptor complex 84*f*
Transfusing blood 552
Transfusion 539
adverse effects of 541, 541*b*
monitored closely during 539
partial exchange 193
reactions 541
therapy
regular chronic 193
role of 192
Transgenic animals 555
Transient hypogammaglobulinemia 411
Transmembranous proteins 17
Transretinoid acid 285
Trauma, severe 482
Trephine biopsy 112
Treponema pallidum 516, 549
syphilis 546, 547
transmission of 549
Trimethoprim 65, 100
Tropical splenomegaly syndrome 230
Tropical sprue 101
Trypanosoma cruzi 547
Tuberculosis 104
Tumor
cells 255
lysis syndrome 269, 272, 285
necrosis factor-alpha 111*f*
suppressor genes 238, 239
Turk cell 567, 572
Turner's syndrome 463
Two-hit theory 237*f*
Typhoid fever 405
Tyrosine kinase 301
inhibitor 312

U

Umbilical cord 510
blood transplantation 419
Upshaw-Schulman syndrome 453
Urea clot solubility test 573
Uremia 460
Uric acid nephropathy, prevention of 269
Urinary system 484
Urine
examination 223

gross appearance of 223f
lysozyme 577
protein electrophoresis 346
test 344
Urticaria 363

V

Vascular disorder 425t, 427, 433
Vascular purpuras 442, 442t
    diagnosis of 442b
Vaso-occlusion, pathogenesis of 184
Vaso-occlusive
    crises 185
    episode, treatment of 191
Vasovagal attack 522
Venous thromboembolism 318
Verifynow test 435
Villous lymphocytes 331, 365, 572
Vinblastine 376
Vincristine 387
Viral capsid antigen 406
Viral hepatitis 113, 127
Viral infections 487
    transmission of 468
Viral vaccines, killed 520
Virus 236
Vitamin
    B_{12} 65, 93, 94, 97, 100, 102, 104, 105, 107, 107t, 108
        absorption of 94, 94f, 104, 106, 107
        diagnosis of 107
        functions of 95
        indicative of 103f
        metabolism, normal 93
        reference ranges 558
        role of 96f
        sources of 93
        transport of 95
    B_{12} deficiency 95, 99, 102-107
        causes of 103, 103b
        detection of 106
        treatment of 107
    C deficiency 443
    D deficiency 321
    K 480, 482, 490
        absence 490
        cycle 490f
        deficiency 430, 431, 480
        poor source of 480
        reductase 490f
        utilization of 481
    K dependent
        factors 45, 46, 482, 491
        glycoprotein 48
        proteins 481
    therapy 122
von Willebrand disease 423, 424, 433, 435, 463, 465, 466t, 472, 473, 576, 577
    acquired 477
    classification of 474, 474t
    clinical features 476
    laboratory
        features 476
        tests in 477t
    severe 427
    treatment 477
    types of 475f
von Willebrand factor 40, 43f, 467, 533
    functions of 473f
    role of 50
    structure of 473f
von Willebrand syndrome 316

W

Wafer cell 569
Waldenström's macroglobulinemia 342, 350, 359, 363, 365t
    clinical features 363
    differential diagnosis 365
    laboratory features 364
    prognosis 365
    treatment 365
Warfarin, side effects of 491
Waring Blender syndrome 228
Warm blood before transfusion 539
Watson-Schwartz test 578
Wharton's jelly 510
WHIM syndrome 397
Whipple's disease 104
White blood cells 18, 281, 291, 389
    disorders of 233
    mature 19f
White cell 98
    abnormalities 428
    antigens 30
Whole blood 526, 528, 528b, 536
    transfusion of 528
Window period 549
Wintrobe method 63
Wiskott-Aldrich syndrome 235, 412, 450, 452, 459, 570
World Health Organization Classification 242t, 260, 273, 289
    of myelodysplastic syndromes 290t
    of myeloproliferative neoplasms 299b
World Health Organization hemoglobin color scale 63
Worm infestation 92

X

X chromosome 463
    defective 469
X-linked disorder 423

Y

Yersinia enterocolitica 545

Z

Zidovudine 108
Zinc protoporphyrin 87
    formation of 90
Zygosity 212

www.ingramcontent.com/pod-product-compliance
Ingram Content Group UK Ltd.
Pitfield, Milton Keynes, MK11 3LW, UK
UKHW051106210325
456536UK00018B/11